Familial Adenomatous Polyposis

Familial Adenomatous Polyposis

Edited by

Lemuel Herrera

Cancer Research Surgeon
Roswell Park Memorial Institute
and
Assistant Professor of Surgery
State University of New York
Buffalo, New York

Alan R. Liss, Inc., New York

Address all Inquiries to the Publisher
Alan R. Liss, Inc., 41 East 11th Street, New York, NY 10003

Printed in United States of America

While the authors, editors, and publisher believe that drug selection and dosage and the specifications and usage of equipment and devices, as set forth in this book, are in accord with current recommendations and practice at the time of publication, they accept no legal responsibility for any errors or omissions, and make no warranty, express or implied, with respect to material contained herein. In view of ongoing research, equipment modifications, changes in governmental regulations and the constant flow of information relating to drug therapy, drug reactions and the use of equipment and devices, the reader is urged to review and evaluate the information provided in the package insert or instructions for each drug, piece of equipment or device for, among other things, any changes in the instructions or indications of dosage or usage and for added warnings and precautions.

Library of Congress Cataloging-in-Publication Data

Familial adenomatous polyposis / edited by Lemuel Herrera.
p. cm.
Includes index.
ISBN 0-471-56225-4
1. Intestinal polyps. I. Herrera, Lemuel.
RC280.I5F36 1989 89-7990
616.99'2347—dc20 CIP

To those who have shared with
us the gifts of life, love, knowledge,
and inquiry.

Contents

CLINICAL FEATURES

THE BASIS FOR TREATMENT MODALITIES

DIRECTIONS OF RESEARCH

Contributors

Joaquin S. Aldrete, Department of Surgery, University of Alabama at Birmingham, School of Medicine, University Station, Birmingham, AL 35294 [xix]

Concepcion Almoguera, Department of Biochemistry, State University of New York at Stony Brook, Stony Brook, NY 11794 [337]

Graham V.N. Appleton, Department of Surgery, Royal Postgraduate Medical School, Hammersmith Hospital, London W12 OHS, England [245]

Robert W. Beart Jr., Section of Colon and Rectal Surgery, Mayo Clinic and Mayo Foundation, Rochester MN 55905 [199]

Diana J. Beasley-Weigel, Information Systems, The Brown-Forman Corp., Louisville, KY 40201 [67]

Andrew M. Bell, Section of Colon and Rectal Surgery, Mayo Clinic and Mayo Foundation, Rochester, MN 55905 [185]

Theresa Berk, Division of General Surgery, Toronto General Hospital, and Department of Surgery, University of Toronto, Toronto, Ontario, Canada M5G 2C4 [91]

John S. Bertram, Basic Science Program, University of Hawaii of Manoa, Cancer Research Center of Hawaii, Honolulu, Hawaii 96813 [253]

C. Richard Boland, Department of Internal Medicine, University of Michigan Medical School, and Veterans Administration Medical Center, Ann Arbor, MI 48105 [305]

Bruce M. Boman, Creighton Cancer Center, Creighton University School of Medicine and the Hereditary Cancer Consultation Center, Omaha, NE 68178 [9]

Cor Breukel, Human Genetics Institute, University of Leiden, 2300 RA Leiden, The Netherlands [393]

Silke Brüderlein, Institut für Experimentelle Pathologie, Deutsches Krebsforschungszentrum, D-6900 Heidelberg, Federal Republic of Germany [351]

John J. Buchino, Departments of Pediatrics and Pathology, James Graham Brown Cancer Center, University of Louisville, Louisville, KY 40292 [67]

The number in brackets is the opening page number of the contributor's article

Steffen Bülow, Department of Surgical Gastroenterology, Hvidovre Hospital, University of Copenhagen, Copenhagen Denmark [109]

Randall W. Burt, Division of Gastroenterology, Department of Medicine, University of Utah, Salt Lake City, UT 84132 [17]

H.J.R. Bussey, The Polyposis Registry, St. Mark's Hospital, London EC1V 2PS, England [1]

Patricia M. Camuto, Department of Pathology, NYU School of Medicine, New York, NY [371]

Eira Cardenas-Gonzalez, Department of Physical Anthropology, National School of Anthropology and History, Public Education Secretariat, Mexico City, Mexico [121]

William Carl, Department of Dentistry and Maxillofacial Prosthetics, Roswell Park Memorial Institute, Buffalo, NY 14263 [115]

Aaron Carrel, School of Medicine, State University of New York at Buffalo, Buffalo, NY 14214 [133]

Ranajit Chakraborty, Center for Demographic and Population Genetics, University of Texas Graduate School of Biomedical Sciences, Houston, TX 77030 [77]

Chia-Cheng Chang, Department of Pediatrics/Human Development, Michigan State University, East Lansing, MI 48824 [279]

Zane Cohen, Division of General Surgery, Toronto General Hospital, and Department of Surgery, University of Toronto, Toronto, Ontario, Canada M5G 2C4 [91]

Freda C.A. den Hartog Jager, Netherlands Cancer Insitute, Amsterdam, The Netherlands [393]

Tusar K. Desai, Department of Medicine, Division of Gastroenterology, Wayne State University School of Medicine and Harper-Grace Hospitals, Detroit, MI 48201 [289]

Roger R. Dozois, Department of Surgery, Mayo Medical School, Section of Colon and Rectal Surgery, Mayo Clinic and Mayo Foundation, Rochester, MN 55905 [185]

Jordan Dunitz, Department of Biochemistry, State University of New York at Stony Brook, Stony Brook, NY 11794 [337]

Ghassan Farah, Department of Surgery, Jordan University Hospital, Amman, Jordan [215]

Andrew P. Feinberg, Howard Hughes Medical Center, Departments of Internal Medicine and Human Genetics, University of Michigan Medical School, Ann Arbor, MI 48109-0650 [371]

Kathleen Forrester, Department of Biochemistry, State University of New York at Stony Brook, Stony Brook, NY 11794-5215 [337]

Eileen A. Friedman, Gastroenterology Service and Laboratory of Gastrointestinal Cancer Research, Department of Medicine, Memorial Sloan-Kettering Cancer Center, New York, NY 10021 [227,275]

Francis M. Giardiello, Division of Gastroenterology, Department of Medicine, The Johns Hopkins University School of Medicine, Baltimore, MD 21205 [43]

Richard Alvin Greenberg, Department of Community Health, James Graham Brown Cancer Center, University of Louisville, Louisville, KY 40292 [67]

Gerrit Griffioen, Department of Gastroenterology, University Medical Center, Leiden, The Netherlands [393]

William E. Grizzle, Department of Pathology, University of Alabama at Birmingham and the Birmingham Veterans Administration Medical Center, Birmingham, AL 35294 **[337]**

José G. Guillem, Department of Surgery, Comprehensive Cancer Center, Columbia University, New York, NY 10032 **[325]**

Stanley R. Hamilton, Department of Pathology and Oncology Center, The Johns Hopkins University School of Medicine and Hospital, Baltimore, MD 21205 **[35]**

Kathleen M. Herold, Department of Human Genetics, Roswell Park Memorial Institute, Buffalo, NY; present address: Department of Macromolecular Sciences, Smith Kline and French Laboratories, King of Prussia, PA 19406 **[361]**

Lemuel Herrera, Familial Polyposis Registry, Cancer Research, Department of Surgical Oncology, Roswell Park Memorial Institute, and Department of Surgery, State University of New York at Buffalo, Buffalo, NY 14263 **[xvii, 115, 121, 133, 147, 155, 215, 333]**

Michael J. Hill, Public Health Laboratory Service Centre for Applied Metabolism and Research, Porton Down, Salisbury, England SP4 OJG **[263]**

Takeo Iwama, Second Department of Surgery, Tokyo Medical and Dental University, Tokyo, Japan **[101, 315, 383]**

David G. Jagelman, Department of Colorectal Surgery, The Cleveland Clinic Florida, Ft. Lauderdale, FL 33309 **[97]**

Heikki J. Järvinen, Second Department of Surgery, Helsinki University Central Hospital, 00290 Helsinki, Finland **[209]**

Noriyuki Kasahara, Graduate Program in Endocrinology, Department of Physiology, University of California, San Francisco, San Francisco, CA 94143-0444 **[315]**

Hidenori Kawanishi, Department of Pathology, VA Medical Center, Northport, NY 11768 **[337]**

P. Meera Khan, Human Genetics Institute, University of Leiden, 2300 RA Leiden, The Netherlands **[393]**

Levy Kopelovich, Departments of Pathology, and Cellular and Molecular Biology, University of South Florida College of Medicine, Tampa, and the Laboratory of Cancer Genetics and Cancer Prevention, VA Medical Center, Bay Pines, FL **[267]**

Anne J. Krush, Division of Medical Genetics, Department of Medicine, The Johns Hopkins University School of Medicine, Baltimore, MD 21205 **[43,151]**

T. Kuroki, Second Department of Surgery, Hyogo College of Medicine, Hyogo, Japan **[101]**

Concepcion Lama, Department of Biochemistry, State University of New York at Stony Brook, Stony Brook, NY 11794 **[337]**

Cock B.H.W. Lamers, Department of Gastroenterology, University of Medical Center, Leiden, The Netherlands **[393]**

Stephen J. Lanspa, Department of Medicine-Gastroenterology, Creighton University School of Medicine and the Hereditary Cancer Consultation Center, Omaha, NE 68178 **[9]**

Martin Lipkin, Gastroenterology Service and Laboratory of Gastrointestinal Cancer Research, Department of Medicine, and Memorial Sloan-Kettering Cancer Center, and Department of Medicine, Cornell University Medical College, Graduate School of Medical Sciences, New York, NY 10021 [227]

Gordon D. Luk, Division of Gastroenterology, Wayne State University School of Medicine and Harper-Grace Hospitals, Detroit, MI 48201 [289]

Henry T. Lynch, Department of Preventive Medicine/Public Health, Creighton University School of Medicine and the Hereditary Cancer Consultation Center, Omaha, NE 68178 [9]

Jane F. Lynch, Department of Preventive Medicine/Public Health, Creighton University School of Medicine and the Hereditary Cancer Consultation Center, Omaha, NE 68178 [9]

Irene H. Maumenee, The Wilmer Opthamologic Institute, The Johns Hopkins Hospitals, Baltimore, MD 21205 [125]

R.S. McLeod, Division of General Surgery, Toronto General Hospital, and Department of Surgery, University of Toronto, Toronto, Ontario, Canada M5G 2C4 [91]

Fabrizio Michelassi, Department of Surgery, University of Chicago Medical Center, Chicago, IL 60637 [347]

Y. Miki, Second Department of Surgery, Hyogo College of Medicine, Hyogo, Japan [101]

Michiko Miyaki, Department of Biochemistry, The Tokyo Metropolitan Institute of Medical Science, Honkomagome, Tokyo 113, Japan [383]

Tetsuichiro Muto, Department of Surgery 1, University of Tokyo, Tokyo, Japan 113 [299]

Kay Neale, The Polyposis Registry, St. Mark's Hospital, London, EC1V 2PS, England [61]

Harold Newmark, Gastroenterology Service and Laboratory of Gastrointestinal Cancer Research, Department of Medicine, Memorial Sloan-Kettering Cancer Center, New York, NY 10021 [227]

Mieko Okamoto, Department of Biochemistry, The Tokyo Metropolitan Institute of Medical Science, Honkomagome, Tokyo 113, Japan [383]

Masatoshi Ooya, Department of Surgery 1, University of Tokyo, Tokyo, Japan 113 [299]

Rafael Padilla-Longoria, Hospital de Oncologia, Centro Medico Nacional, Instituto Mexicano Seguro Social, Mexico City 06720, Mexico [121]

John H. Pemberton, Department of Surgery, Mayo Medical School, Section of Colon and Rectal Surgery, Mayo Clinic and Mayo Foundation, Rochester, MN 55905 [185]

Alberto Peña, Pediatric Surgery, Schneider Children's Hospital, Long Island Jewish Medical Center, Clinical Campus of State University of New York at Stony Brook, New Hyde Park, NY 11042 [169]

Ernestina Peña-Reyes, National School of Anthropology and History, Public Education Secretariat, Mexico City, Mexico [121]

Manuel Perucho, Department of Biochemistry, State University of New York at Stony Brook, NY 11794, and California Institute of Biological Research, La Jolla, CA 92037 [337]

Nicholas J. Petrelli, Department of Surgical Oncology, Roswell Park Memorial Institute, and Department of Surgery, State University of New York at Buffalo, Buffalo, NY 14263 [147,215,333]

Andrea Quaroni, Section of Physiology, Cornell University, Division of Biological Sciences, Ithaca, NY 14853 **[333]**

Raul Ramos, Department of Surgery, University of Texas Health Sciences Center at San Antonio, San Antonio, TX 78229 **[133]**

Sheila Ritchie, The Polyposis Registry, St. Mark's Hospital, London, EC1V 2PS, England **[61]**

Sergio Rodriguez-Cuevas, Hospital de Oncologia, Centro Medico Nacional, Instituto Mexicano Seguro Social, Mexico City 06720, Mexico **[121]**

Paul G. Rothberg, Department of Human Genetics, Roswell Park Memorial Institute, Buffalo, NY; present address: Department of Hematology/Oncology, The Children's Mercy Hospital, Kansas City, MO 64108 **[361]**

Victoriano Saenz, Department of Surgery Hospital Universitario, "Angel Leaño", Universidad Autonoma de Guadalajara, Guadalajara, Mexico **[147]**

Shinobu Sakamoto, Department of Endocrinology, Medical Research Institute and Dental University, Tokyo, 113 Japan **[315]**

Chieko Sato, Department of Biochemistry, The Tokyo Metropolitan Institute of Medical Science, Honkomagone, Tokyo 113, Japan **[383]**

Peter Schlag, Sektion Chirurgische Onkologie, Chirurgische Universitatsklinik, D-6900 Heidelberg, Federal Republic of Germany **[351]**

Manfred Schwab, Institut für Experimentelle Pathologie, Deutsches Krebsforschungszentrum, D-6900 Heidelberg, Federal Republic of Germany, **[351]**

Ahmed Shafik, Department of Surgery, Faculty of Medicine, Cairo University, Cairo, Egypt **[159]**

Ann L. Silverman, Division of Gastroenterology, Department of Medicine, Wayne State University School of Medicine and Harper-Grace Hospitals, Detroit, MI 48201 **[289]**

Tom Smyrk, Department of Pathology, Creighton University School of Medicine and the Hereditary Cancer Consultation Center, Omaha, NE 68178 **[9]**

Abdolkarim N. Sohrabi, Department of Surgery, University of Illinois, College of Medicine at Peoria, Peoria, IL 61603 **[23]**

John Stricklin Spratt, Department of Surgery, James Graham Brown Cancer Center, University of Louisville, Louisville, KY 40202 **[67]**

Kenichi Sugihara, Department of Surgery 1, University of Tokyo, Tokyo, Japan 113 **[299]**

Maureen A. Sullivan, Department of Dentistry and Maxillofacial Prosthetics, Roswell Park Memorial Institute, Buffalo, NY 14263 **[115]**

James P.S. Thomson, The Polyposis Registry, St. Mark's Hospital, London EC1V 2PS, England **[61]**

Carli M.J. Tops, Human Genetics Institute, University of Leiden, 2300 RA Leiden, The Netherlands **[393]**

Sergio Torres-Vargas, Hospital de Oncologia, Centro Medico Nacional, Instituto Mexicano Seguro Social, Mexico City, 06720 Mexico **[121]**

Elias I. Traboulsi, The Center for Sight, Georgetown University Medical Center, Washington, DC 20007 **[125]**

James E. Trosko, Department of Pediatrics/Human Development, Michigan State University, East Lansing, MI 48824 [279]

Joji Utsunomiya, Second Department of Surgery, Hyogo College of Medicine, Hyogo, 663, Japan [101]

Inge S.J. van Leeuwen-Cornelisse, Human Genetics Institute, University of Leiden, the Clinical Genetics Center, and National Familial Polyposis Registration Center, 2300 RA Leiden, The Netherlands, [393]

Kai van der Bosch, Institut für Experimentelle Pathologie, Deutsches Krebsforschungszentrum, D-6900 Heidelberg, Federal Republic of Germany [351]

Heleen M. van der Klift, Human Genetics Institute, University of Leiden, 2300 RA Leiden, The Netherlands [393]

Hans F.A. Vasen, National Familial Polyposis Registration Center, and Department of Gastroenterology, University Medical Center, Leiden, The Netherlands, [393]

Arnold Wald, Gastroenterology Unit, Department of Medicine, Montefiore Hospital, University of Pittsburgh School of Medicine, Pittsburgh, PA 15213 [175]

Alvin L. Watne, Department of Surgery, University of Illinois, College of Medicine at Peoria, Peoria, IL 61603 [23]

I. Bernard Weinstein, Institute of Cancer Research, Columbia University, New York, NY 10032 [325]

Milton M. Weiser, Division of Gastroenterology, Department of Medicine, State University of New York at Buffalo, Buffalo General Hospital, Buffalo, NY 14203 [223,333]

Kenneth M. Weiss, Department of Anthropology, and Graduate Program in Genetics, Penn State University, University Park, PA 16802 [77]

David R. Welling, Section of Gastroenterologic and General Surgery, Mayo Clinic and Mayo Foundation, Rochester, MN 55905 [199]

Juul Th. Wijnen, Human Genetics Institute, University of Leiden, 2300 RA Leiden, The Netherlands [393]

R.C.N. Williamson, Department of Surgery, Royal Postgraduate Medical School, University of London, Hammersmith Hospital, London W12 OHS, England [245]

Sidney J. Winawer, Gastroenterology Service and Laboratory of Gastrointestinal Cancer Research, Department of Medicine, Memorial Sloan-Kettering Cancer Center, and Department of Medicine, Cornell University Medical College, New York, NY 10021 [227]

Matthew Witten, Medical and Biological Supercomputing, ETA Systems, Inc., St. Paul, MN; present address: Computational Biology and Medicine, Control Data Corp., Minneapolis, MN 55440-4700 [67]

Sandra R. Wolman, Program in Cancer Genetics, Michigan Cancer Foundation, Detroit, MI 48226 [371]

Preface

The last ten years have seen a significant expansion in clinical and basic knowledge related to familial adenomatous polyposis (FAP), a premalignant entity precursor of colon cancer, also known as familial polyposis coli. A clearer understanding of pelvic anatomy and physiology has led to logical surgical interventions that have translated into substantial improvements in the patient's quality of life, while basic investigations have provided a glimpse into the mechanisms involved in the neoplastic transformation characteristic of both FAP and colon cancer.

This book is divided into two sections. The first and larger part is directed principally to clinicians; thus, it is highly focused. It provides practitioners with guidelines and answers relevant to the management of common and uncommon aspects of FAP, for which they are often consulted. The second part contains a series of articles that deal with future directions of research. We believe that advances may occur as a consequence to these research efforts; thus, clinicians must become familiar with them. Although part two is less focused than part one, it reflects well the heterogeneity of the multidisciplinary approaches to the study of FAP. The common denominator and catalyst in all research efforts centered around FAP is the desire for understanding of this basic biological model and the events that lead to uncontrolled cell proliferation and alterations in cell function, characteristics of both premalignant adenomatous polyps and colon cancer.

The possibility that laboratory research efforts may actually evolve into tests of clinical usefulness provides a bright outlook. This potential is best exemplified in this book by the results of the interaction between genetic investigations and FAP. Although the mutant gene responsible for the abnormal phenotype remains still unknown, linkage analysis using DNA polymorphic markers has revealed a relatively close relationship between selected DNA markers and FAP. Thus, for the first time, the possibility of carrier detection and prenatal diagnosis may be an option at hand for selected informative kindreds (families). With the knowledge of these two loci linked, one can follow the inheritance pattern of the DNA marker and predict the statistical likelihood that a relative at risk for FAP may have also inherited the disease locus. Even more exciting is the possibility of genetic-directed screening, using similar techniques, in populations with the so-called ''sporadic'' adenomatous polyps. The critical role of the endoscopist as the earliest surveyor and monitor of the phenotypical manifestations of FAP and his/her possible contribution towards the understanding of biomarkers of the disease emerges clearly from most chapters.

This publication constitutes a ''state-of-the-art'' assessment of a clinical syndrome that, although it is characterized by a mendelian dominant inheritance of more than 100 colonic adenomatous polyps, is often associated with protean, confusing, and misleading manifestations (i.e., up to 20% of the patients may be new mutants). The references cited in the articles will guide the reader to the major publications on the subject to date for an authoritative and comprehensive overview of FAP.

This book provides a nucleus of practical knowledge necessary for the understanding of current diagnostic and therapeutic approaches to FAP, a classic prototype for study of tumor biology. Specific clinical recommendations are carefully outlined, covering differential diagnosis, physical examinations, possible clinical markers, appropriate tests, therapeutic options and timing, pre- and post-surgical management, and follow-up strategies. This book also gives updated information on the recent biological advances necessary for sound and current clinical recommendations. It is hoped that it will broaden the perspective of the reader significantly, as it touches many different areas of clinical and basic knowledge not usually familiar to all practitioners. However, I must request the benevolence of the reader; because of the multinational, multiauthored chapters, differences in style and redundancy were inevitable. For this, I take full responsibility, but I feel that it was better to permit these occurrences than to try to rearrange the writings and risk out-of-context statements. After all, these chapters have been written by recognized experts.

If this book results in the better management of patients with FAP and of their relatives at risk, and if it provides the reader with a better understanding of the complex basic investigations related to this disorder, then the task of the authors and editor can be considered accomplished.

Lemuel Herrera

Introduction

Familial adenomatous polyposis (FAP) is the disease associated with the highest risk for the development of colorectal carcinoma; affected individuals are virtually certain to develop a carcinoma of their colorectum if colectomy is not performed. Furthermore, FAP is the best supportive model to test the hypothesis of the adenoma-carcinoma formation sequence. Because of its autosomal dominantly inherited characteristics, it has stimulated investigators to apply genetic and molecular biology approaches to elucidate the etiology of the disease. For these reasons, FAP has come into sharp focus for anyone interested in neoplastic disease of the intestines. Some of the noted investigational approaches have already produced important observations, such as the recently appreciated fact that the gene for FAP also causes polyps in the upper portion of the digestive tract. Several efforts have been made to identify the biological markers that would identify the presence of the FAP gene. Cytogenetic studies of adenomas in this syndrome have suggested that the patients affected with FAP may have non-random numerical chromosomal aberrations. A most important recent development has been the feasibility of mapping FAP to the long arm of chromosome 5 (5 q 21–22). At the present time, I am aware of three groups of investigators who have separately developed three closely related DNA probes that can be useful as genetic markers. In the very near future, these developments should result in the ability to accurately identify the members of families affected with FAP who have inherited the susceptibility for the disease. Hopefully, continuing investigations with now available molecular genetic techniques will eventually culminate in the specific identification of the gene responsible for FAP. The derivation of this new knowledge goes into the potential of fully understanding the subcellular mechanisms that determine the polyp-cancer pathogenesis with the tremendous implications of being able, through these mechanisms, to effectively treat or, even better, to prevent colorectal cancers.

Therefore, it is quite timely that Dr. Lemuel Herrera, Senior Surgical Clinician and Director of the Familial Polyposis Registry at the Roswell Park Memorial Institute, who has been one of the major forces in that Institution to form a Section of Surgical Developmental Oncology, has gathered many of the leading and respected experts in the field to be his co-authors and produce the most current and comprehensive textbook on FAP up-to-date. Dr. Herrera has orchestrated the contributions of his authoritative co-authors and has personally written some of the key chapters, resulting in a masterwork that covers the subject of FAP in a highly structured, sequential and logical manner. The co-authors are recognized investigators who, in recent years, have made and are still "making things happen" in the field of FAP.

The text begins with an engaging discussion of the historical development of FAP written by Dr. Bussey, one of the recognized pioneers in the field. The book covers the epidemiology, pathology, and data collection, the clinical aspects, the basis for the currently available operative treatment, and the pertinent current research directions; a separate introduction for this last part of the book has been written by Dr. Milton Weiser.

The first section of the book covers the inheritance character of FAP, followed by a lucid discussion of the histopathological considerations in the adenoma-carcinoma sequence. This first section is completed by a relevant discussion of the methods to screen the offsprings of patients with FAP, followed by several chapters that point out the need, advantages, and up-to-date methodology for having a genetics oriented registry for patients affected by this disease.

The eleven chapters of the second part of the book cover the clinical features of FAP by first ''getting down'' to the basics of how to evaluate patients with the disease. The chapter of phenotypic experiences of FAP is of particular interest because the Japanese authors discuss the similarities of the premalignant characteristics of this entity as observed in their country, in Great Britain, the USA, and Canada, thus adding an international dimension which is reinforced by several other chapters: one, describing the antropometrics of a Mexican kindred with FAP written by recognized Mexican authors in the field; another by Dr. S. Bulow from Denmark where he thoroughly describes and discusses the extracolonic manifestations of the disease, and several other chapters written by recognized authors from Canada, Egypt and Finland. The interrelations between desmoid tumors and FAP, and the pertinent therapeutic implications are nicely discussed, along with a chapter on how to counsel families and individuals with FAP. The editor and some of his associates round out this second section of clinical features with an innovative and specific approach to the decision-making process in kindreds with FAP, and a brief but highly pertinent chapter updating the information pertinent in the Leed's Castle polyposis group.

The third part of the book deals with the current modalities of therapy with emphasis on surgical treatment. It is initiated by a thorough but succinct discussion of the pertinent anatomical and physiological aspects of the anorectal region. The options for surgical treatment of FAP are discussed in a very comprehensible manner. The considerations relative to selecting the best timing to do the colectomy to prevent the development of carcinoma are also discussed. Other chapters describe in detail the new alternative for preserving anal continence by constructing an ileal pouch anastomosed to the preserved anal sphincter. One final chapter discusses the use of the Nd YAG laser to vaporize polyps. Each one of the above noted chapters has been written by a recognized worker and investigator in the management of patients with FAP.

In summary, this book fulfills the need to compile the most current available information pertaining to familial adenomatous polyposis. Because this goal has been accomplished, and because of the true expertise in FAP of the editor and his selected contributors, I would venture to predict that this book will become a landmark and a useful classical reference for physicians and non-physicians interested in the subject.

Joaquin S. Aldrete M.D.
Professor and Vice Chairman
Department of Surgery
University of Alabama Medical School
Birmingham, Alabama

1

Historical Developments in Familial Adenomatous Polyposis

H. J. R. Bussey

St. Mark's Hospital, London, England

INTRODUCTION

Conditions involving the presence of large numbers of polyps in the gastrointestinal tract had probably been observed long before 1721, when Menzelio recorded what is generally accepted as the first example in medical literature. It was certainly many decades after this that observation of such features as the number and anatomical distribution of the polyps, their histological nature, associated lesions, and possible familial incidence enabled the different types of polyposis syndromes to be grouped into the current classification. One of the first steps in this direction was the application of the new science of histopathology, initiated in the early 1860s, to intestinal polyps and the appearance of early subgrouping of the polyp types. In 1881, Woodward was dividing polyposis conditions into "primary" when there was no apparent antecedent disease and "secondary" when the polyps followed previous inflammation and ulceration of the colon.

The following year, 1882, W. Harrison Cripps reported polyposis coli in two members of the same family, a brother and sister. This was the first indication that the condition was familial and possibly of genetic origin, and it would be reasonable to suggest that this important observation dates the point at which the history of familial adenomatous polyposis started. A further report by Bickersteth [1890] of two affected members in two generations of a family, mother and son, strengthened the impression that polyposis was inherited. Increasing numbers of reports of familial cases soon confirmed the genetic origin of the condition as a definite fact, and a new parameter, useful in the separation and classification of gastrointestinal polyposis, was established. The mode of inheritance was subsequently accepted as being that of a Mendelian dominant characteristic by detailed analysis such as that of Veale [1965].

Thus, as the end of the 19th century approached, three of the four most prominent features of familial adenomatous polyposis had been recognized, the large number of polyps, that histologically the polyps were adenomas, and that the condition was inherited. The fourth feature, associated colorectal cancer, had begun to be noticed. Smith [1887] mentioned the presence of adenocarcinoma when reporting three members of a family with multiple polyps.

MALIGNANT POTENTIAL OF FAMILIAL ADENOMATOUS POLYPOSIS

With the growing interest in polyposis of the colon, more families became available for investigation in greater depth. It was not surprising that the high incidence of associated malignancy soon became apparent. Nor did it take long to realize that the average age of onset of colorectal cancer in polyposis patients was much lower than in the general population.

The records at St. Mark's Hospital for the early part of this century indicate that about two-thirds of the polyposis patients who presented because

Familial Adenomatous Polyposis, pages 1–7

of symptoms already had colorectal cancer. The usual reason for seeking medical advice was an increase in the severity of the usual symptoms of change of bowel habit and rectal bleeding from the development of cancer. Because of the high operative mortality following major abdominal surgery at that time, surgeons were reluctant to operate. As a result some of the patients diagnosed as having polyposis still at the benign stage subsequently developed cancer, raising the incidence above the 90% level. The probability was that few, if any, untreated patients living long enough would fail to develop large intestinal cancer.

The average age at diagnosis of cancer in patients first attending hospital because of symptoms was about 40 years, with most in the 25–50 years range. Cancer was uncommon in those under 20 years of age. In the general population, the average age is usually quoted as about 65 years, with the majority of cases falling into the 60–80 years range, i.e., about 25 years older than the polyposis group. The greater tendency for polyposis patients to develop intestinal malignancy is also reflected in the comparison of the number with synchronous large bowel malignancies, 50% vs. 4% of nonpolyposis patients treated at St. Mark's Hospital.

DEVELOPMENT OF A TREATMENT POLICY

A good deal of information about the more obvious features of polyposis coli had been collected by the beginning of the present century. However, before a policy of treatment could be formulated, more knowledge of the natural history was required. Little was known about the number and distribution of the adenomas, and, most important of all, the age range of their onset. The adenoma–carcinoma sequence [Hill et al. 1978; Morson et al. 1983] had by this time begun to be accepted. To prevent cancer developing in the polyposis patient by interrupting the sequence, it was necessary to know more about the earlier stages of the condition. The collection of this information really began after the end of World War I and was accelerated by the new technologies made available around this time. The sigmoidoscope, with its self-contained illumination, introduced at about the beginning of the century, afforded much more accurate assessment of lesions within the rectum. The increasing use of the barium enema examination and its subsequent improvement by the double-contrast technique gave a similar advantage with respect to the colon. Polypectomy via the sigmoidoscope and histological examination of the polyps became more frequent. Indirectly, this resulted in the setting up of the first register of polyposis families, which is discussed in more detail below. For the moment, it is necessary only to say that, to increase the number of patients available for investigation, Dr. Cuthbert Dukes, Consultant Pathologist at St Mark's Hospital, took advantage of the familial nature of the condition to look among the relatives for new cases. An affected person was interviewed about his family, and a pedigree was constructed. Family members, particularly siblings and children, were invited to attend for examination. If polyps were found in the rectum, one or more were usually removed for histological confirmation of the diagnosis.

THE CALL-UP POLICY

The procedure of making a family pedigree, recording the affected members, identifying other members who are at risk, and inviting the latter group to be checked not only identified new cases but also provided much needed information about the earlier stages of polyposis. More relatives were seen with adenomas but before cancer had developed. Younger members mostly were found to be asymptomatic even though polyps were present and sometimes free from polyps on first examination, although subsequent examinations might prove positive.

By the time World War II started, Dukes had decided that around puberty was the right time to commence regular annual sigmoidoscopic examination of the children of a polyposis patient. In the first place, he considered it important to have contact with the child who was still under parental control yet was old enough to understand the necessity of the periodic examinations and for their continuance into adulthood. Second, by the age of about 14 years, approximately half of the children destined to develop the condition were already showing evidence of polyps on examination. It was found that symptoms (usually occasional episodes of slight bleeding from the rectum, mucous discharge, or mild change of bowel habit) were infrequently present and cancer was rarely found before the age of 20 years. Malignancy increased in the 25–30 years of age period, reaching an incidence of about 50% in the fourth decade of life. Since most cases of polyposis could be diagnosed in the 15–25 year age range and the onset of cancer was mainly in the 30–35 year period, it was obvious that a considerable degree of cancer prevention could be obtained if affected family members were identified and treated by removal of the polyps before cancer appeared. The policy of constructing a family tree, identifying affected individuals, and "calling up" siblings and children was therefore put into practice.

There was, however, a major difficulty at this time in obtaining maximum benefit from the policy. To prevent cancer demanded removal of the adenomas and, because of the gross involvement of the whole colorectum, required some sort of surgical procedure approximating total colectomy. Before World War II, this could expose the patient to considerable risk, the mortality from such operations being on the order of 30–50%. The risk was likely to be even less acceptable with the increasing number of patients having polyposis diagnosed at ever younger ages.

Fortunately, by the end of World War II, the situation had been greatly improved by a number of factors. The need for correct blood electrolyte balance had been recognized, blood banks were available, antibiotics had been discovered, and improved anaesthetics reduced the mortality rate to about one-twentieth the prewar figure.

RESULTS OF THE CALL-UP POLICY

It has already been stated that, originally, two-thirds of polyposis patients presenting with symptoms at St. Mark's Hospital already had colorectal cancer, and, because of the inadequate treatment available at the time, the incidence of malignancy could rise to 90% or more. The first effect of the call-up policy was noticed in the gradual decline in the number of patients seen with carcinoma. Initially this was due to earlier examination of other family members, usually of the same generation as the propositus, whose siblings or cousins could be found to be affected even though they had no or only slight symptoms because cancer had not yet developed. This group was reinforced by the next generation of children called-up for examination at 14 years of age. The result has been that the former incidence of colorectal cancer on first examination of about 65%, has fallen to about 5%, a figure partly reflecting new mutation cases.

With the advent of safe surgical treatment, all patients found by earlier examination still to be in the benign stage of the condition could be prevented from developing colorectal cancer by total removal of the colon and rectum at this stage. Two schools of thought, however, emerged, the first advocating total proctocolectomy and ileostomy; the other school argued that an ileostomy was a severe handicap to inflict on an individual, particularly for a group who at the time were getting increasingly younger. The supporters of this school reasoned that the risk of rectal cancer following colectomy and ileorectal anastomosis would be minimal if six-monthly rectal examinations were carried out and any new adenomas destroyed. Moreover, should any cancers appear, these should be discovered at an early and curable stage. In general, the policy at St. Mark's Hospital has been to retain the rectum, the first ileorectal anastomosis being carried out in 1948. Now, 40 years later, just over 200 such operations have been carried out, with only one operative death (in 1953). Twelve patients subsequently developed rectal cancer, representing a cumulative risk of about 12% over a 25 year period. Four of these patients died from the rectal cancer, the cumulative risk of this event being about 6% over 25 years. These figures tend to decrease slightly as the numbers of cases under observation increase, an effect that may be due to reducing the amount of mucosal damage caused by excessive use of diathermy in attempting to destroy all polyps in the rectum however small.

In the last 2 decades, there has been increased

use of the ileal pelvic pouch to avoid the problem of an ileostomy. It will be some time, however, before the long-term disadvantages, if any, are known. One case of gross adenomatosis within the pouch has already been reported [Beart, 1982].

Until the middle of this century, familial adenomatous polyposis was thought to be a condition involving only the large intestine. The call-up policy for its treatment, started after World War II, soon showed that a considerable degree of cancer prevention could be achieved, giving the impression that the worst effects of the condition could be eliminated. However, further research on the increasing number of families being treated suggested that the condition was associated with other lesions and other organs. These extracolonic lesions fall mainly into three categories.

ASSOCIATED EXTRACOLONIC LESIONS

Gardner's Syndrome

Since chronic polyposis was first recognized, there have been reports of other lesions outside the colon, generally in isolated cases. Accounts of a more specific syndrome appeared in the early 1950s, when Gardner and his associates published a series of articles on a polyposis family among whom the affected members also exhibited multiple osteomas of the cranium and mandibles, multiple epidermoid cysts, and fibromas of the skin, the syndrome subsequently being called Gardner's syndrome [Gardner and Richards, 1953]. A later review of the family added dental abnormalities and desmoid tumors of the abdominal wall and abdomen, at the same time extending the site of osteomas to any part of the skeletal system [Gardner, 1969]. There has been a tendency to make a distinction between Gardner's syndrome and so-called "classic polyposis" coli, i.e., polyposis without extracolonic lesions. So far, it has not been easy to define precisely the boundary between the two groups; the extracolonic lesions may be found in variable numbers and in different permutations. Utsunomiya and Nakamura [1975] showed by X-rays of the mandibles that over 90% of all Japanese polyposis patients examined had occult osteomas in this area. This finding, confirmed later at other centers, has not helped in making classification easier, nor has the tendency to report any new associated lesion as a possible further facet of Gardner's syndrome.

More recently, another dimension has been introduced into the problem. Lewis et al. [1984] reported three families among whom features of Gardner's syndrome were accompanied by multiple bilateral patches of congenital hypertrophy of the retinal pigment epithelium. They suggested that this new feature might be used to identify at an early stage of life those members of a polyposis family who had inherited the condition. A further study by Traboulsi et al. [1987] also showed a high correlation between the presence of the extracolonic lesions of Gardner's syndrome and the retinal pigment abnormality. It is not clear from either of these reports if the pigmentation is a marker only for Gardner's syndrome. Polyposis patients without the extracolonic lesions of Gardner's syndrome do not appear to have been examined. Thus, there is a strong tendency to delete the eponym.

Adenomas of the Upper Gastrointestinal Tract

Occasional reports of polyps in the upper gastrointestinal tract found either at operation or, more commonly, at postmortem have appeared in the past, but, since in most cases the number and histological type were not mentioned, they excited little interest. During the 1960s, an increasing number of case reports of malignancy of the periampullary region and proximal duodenum appeared. These focussed attention on the upper gastrointestinal tract and resulted in a series of reports on gastroduodenoscopy of groups of polyposis patients, mainly from Japanese centers. The findings were startling. Most recorded that at least two-thirds of polyposis patients also had duodenal adenomas.

The examinations also revealed that about one-third of the patients also had gastric polyps [Bulow et al. 1985]. These polyps were mainly of two types, adenomas and the recently observed type, to which the term "gastric fundus polyp" has been applied. The figures given for the incidence of the two varieties vary greatly (12.5–55%

and 4–50% respectively) probably because of the small number of patients in the series investigated. In general, the higher incidence rates are from Japan, where gastric tumors tend to be more frequent in the general population.

Assessment of polyp frequency is less easy in the jejunal and ileal areas of the small bowel, but it appears that adenomas are fewer in number here than in the duodenum, although an example of adenomatosis in an ileal pouch has been already mentioned. Adenomas have also been found occasionally in the bile ducts and the gall bladder.

Malignancy of the Upper Gastrointestinal Tract

An obvious question is, "do the adenomas of the stomach and small bowel follow the adenoma-carcinoma sequence observed in the colorectum?" There is evidence suggesting that this is the case. An opportunity to examine an intussusception of the jejunum in a polyposis patient revealed the presence of all stages of adenoma formation from a few dysplastic crypts of Lieberkuhn to large pedunculated tumors exactly as found in the colorectum.

Malignancies of the upper gastrointestinal tract developed in several patients, the distribution of which around the tract roughly paralleled the distribution of adenomas. It has already been stated that colectomy and ileorectal anastomosis have been the major treatment for polyposis at St. Mark's Hospital, and this group of patients provides the best material for analysis. Starting in 1948, 191 patients have been followed. There have been six carcinomas of the duodenum and one each of stomach and jejunum. There have also been two malignancies each of the pancreas and the bile ducts. Three other patients died of carcinomatosis of unknown site, but which were highly suggestive of an upper gastrointestinal origin. These figures suggest that the cumulative risk of a patient developing a cancer of the upper gastrointestinal tract after colectomy and ileorectal anastomosis could be as high as 25% over a period of 30 years. Cancer prevention in this region will present the clinician with new problems.

Malignancies of Other Organs

The tendency to add to the Gardner's syndrome any new association of polyposis with other extragastrointestinal tract lesions has been mentioned. Until genetic studies have advanced further, it may be difficult to know if the association is merely coincidental. There are, however, some instances when the possibility of genetic linkage is less easily discarded. Plail et al. [1987] have suggested that papillary carcinoma of the thyroid is more common in polyposis patients than in the general population. Kingston et al. [1983] have found a similar increased incidence of hepatoblastoma in young children of polyposis parents, a few of whom survived long enough to develop adenomatous polyposis.

Desmoid tumors might also be included in this category. Although they have not been known to metastasize, they are generally regarded as locally invasive, aggressively so in some polyposis patients. Although often regarded as a manifestation of Gardner's syndrome, only half of the St. Mark's Hospital series patients had any of the syndrome lesions.

POLYPOSIS REGISTRIES

At present, increasing interest in gastrointestinal polyposis conditions is resulting in the establishment in many centers throughout the world of registers of polyposis families. There can be little doubt that this is a practical way of making sure that family members at risk of inheriting polyposis are made aware of that risk and of informing them when and where to obtain advice and, if they are found to be affected, treatment at the appropriate time.

The first register of polyposis patients arose out of a research project begun by two consultant members of the staff of St. Mark's Hospital. Founded in 1835 by a surgeon, Frederick Salmon, the Hospital has been concerned solely with colorectal conditions. Mr. J.P. Lockhart-Mummery, appointed Consultant Surgeon in 1903, was greatly interested in cancer and heredity, an interest probably fostered by the recently reported cases of polyposis coli. In 1922, Dr. Cuthbert Dukes was appointed Consultant Pathologist and soon started a research study of the histological structure of the various types of colorectal adenomas, a field to which polyposis had much to offer. At this time, Lockhart-Mummery had three polyposis families under his care as well as a few isolated patients, and it was from these patients that Dukes obtained histological material for his research. Because polyposis cases were rare, every effort was made to expand the family record and to increase the number of families. Fortunately what started as a mere list of research material was soon recognized as the means of maintaining permanent contact with the families and their future generations, and the register was established in 1925 with the three original families. Now, there are 510 families, 363 of whom show the adenomatous type; 1,238 members of these families have been considered to have had polyposis. Approximately one-third of these patients have been seen at St. Mark's Hospital. The other families recorded in the register include 37 with Peutz-Jeghers syndrome, 64 with juvenile polyposis, and 46 of miscellaneous type. In addition, there are about 150 cases for whom the information is insufficient to make a definite classification.

The advantage of having a central registry (preferably attached to a treatment center) is that duplication of family investigation can be avoided. Enquiry at the central registry about a new family may reveal that other branches of the family are already known and that their members are being treated. At the same time, the new contact with the family may be able to supply information about branches either unknown or, if known to exist, so far untraced.

Recently, there has been a tendency to establish local registers. For instance, in the United Kingdom, there is a register for Wales and another for Northeast England, with interest being shown in other areas. This move is to be welcomed in that it provides more centers with increased experience in the treatment of the condition. However, it is essential to maintain a feedback of information to the central registry.

INTERNATIONAL COOPERATION

Some degree of international cooperation has always existed. Over the years, many families have decided for various reasons to start a new life in another country. British families have gone to the United States and to the various Commonwealth countries and still do so. The St. Mark's Hospital Registry receives from time to time requests from abroad on the order of "We have a family originally from England; has the Registry any record of this?" There are also occasions when information is sought of family members who have emigrated to the United States or elsewhere. This type of information exchange is likely to increase as more registries are established.

Recently, however, another form of international cooperation has begun. In 1985, some 1,300 doctors concerned with gastroenterology assembled in London from many parts of the world to commemorate the 150th Anniversary of the founding of St. Mark's Hospital. Mr. Ian Todd, then Senior Surgical Consultant at the Hospital, took the opportunity to arrange a meeting of a small group of those known to be especially interested in familial adenomatous polyposis to consider the possibility of pooling information to accelerate research into the new problems of treatment for the upper gastrointestinal malignancies as well as old ones, such as the aggressive abdominal desmoid tumours. The suggestion was received with enthusiasm, and the subsequent activities of the group, now known as the Leeds Castle Polyposis Group, are described elsewhere in this volume.

CHROMOSOME 5

Reliable markers for the identification of familial adenomatous polyposis before the intestinal polyps appear have been eagerly sought in the past. If found, one-half of the children of affected parents could be eliminated from screening. Earlier hopes were based on physical signs, such as the skin cysts and osteomas of Gardner's syndrome, which are not, however, sufficiently specific. More recently, congenital hypertrophy of retinal pigment epithelium appears to be more consistent, although false-positive results may occur, and results from larger series of cases have yet to be collected. With the advances in genetic analysis it was only a matter of time before a chromosomal solution would be found.

Herrera et al. [1986] investigated a patient who had a number of developmental abnormalities as well as familial adenomatous polyposis and an interstitial deletion of chromosome 5. Working with a DNA probe with a close linkage with polyposis and which localized in the same region described by Herrera et al., Bodmer et al. [1987] were able to provide overwhelming evidence that the familial adenomatous polyposis gene was sited on chromosome 5. The exact position has not yet been determined, but, with the modern techniques available, the identity of the gene and its functions should soon be known. A more detailed account of the assigning of the gene to chromosome 5 is to be found in a subsequent chapter.

Familial adenomatous polyposis has already provided much of the evidence for the adenoma–carcinoma sequence. There are several genetic conditions in which adenomas and adenocarcinomas of the gastrointestinal tract occur in varying degree as a common factor. Familial adenomatous polyposis is the outstanding example; others are colorectal cancer, Cowden's disease, Muir-Torre syndrome, Turcot's syndrome, and the Peutz-Jeghers syndrome. Solomon et al. [1987] have also shown that more than 20% of sporadic colorectal carcinomas became homo- or hemizygous for chromosome 5 alleles. It would not be surprizing if analysis of chromosome 5 eventually provides clues to the small changes in genetic patterns that must exist between those conditions, and it may pinpoint the genetic defect causing cells to overgrow and produce the abnormal structures of the adenoma–carcinoma sequence.

References

Beart RW Jr, Fleming R, Banks PM: Tubulovillous adenomas in a continent ileostomy after proctocolectomy for familial polyposis. Digest Dis Sci 27:533–556, 1982.

Bickersteth RA: Multiple polypi of the rectum occurring in a mother and child. St Bartholomew's Hosp Rep 26:299–301, 1890.

Bodmer WF, Bailey CJ, Bodmer J, Bussey HJR, Ellis A, Gorman P, Lucibello FC, Murday VA, Rider SH, Scambler P, Sheer D, Solomon D, Solomon E, Spurr NK: Localization of the gene for familial adenomatous polyposis on chromosome 5. Nature 328:614–616, 1987.

Bulow S, Lauritsen KB, Johansen A, Svendsen LB, Sondergaard JO: Gastroduodenal polyps in familial polyposis. Dis Colon Rectum 28:90–93, 1985.

Cripps WH: Two cases of disseminated polyps of the rectum. Trans Pathol Soc London 33:165–168, 1882.

Gardner EJ: Gardner's syndrome re-evaluated after twenty years. Proc Utah Acad 46:1–11, 1969.

Gardner EJ, Richards RC: Multiple cutaneous and subcutaneous lesions occurring simultaneously with hereditary polyposis and osteomatosis. Am J Hum Genet 5:139–147, 1953.

Herrera L, Kakati S, Gibas L, Pietrzak E, Sandberg AA: Brief clinical report: Gardner's syndrome in a man with an interstitial deletion of 5q. Am J Med Genet 25:473–476, 1986.

Hill MJ, Morson BC, Bussey HJR: Aetiology of adenoma–carcinoma sequence in large bowel. Lancet 1:245–247, 1978.

Kingston JE, Herbert A, Draper GJ, Mann JR: Association between hepatoblastoma and polyposis coli. Arch Dis Child 58:959–962, 1983.

Lewis RA, Crowder WE, Eierman LA: The Gardner syndrome. Significance of ocular features. Ophthalmology 91:916–925, 1984.

Menzelio D: De excrescentals verrucosa cristosis in intestinis crassis dysenteriam passi observatis. Ast Med Berolinensium 4(7):68–71, 1721.

Morson BC, Bussey HJR, Day DW, Hill MJ: Adenomas of large bowel. Cancer Surv 2:451–477, 1983.

Plail RO, Bussey HJR, Glazer G, Thomson JPS: Adenomatous polyposis: An association with carcinoma of the thyroid. Br J Surg 74:377–380, 1987.

Smith T: Three cases of multiple polypi of the lower bowel occurring in one family. St Bartholomew's Hosp Rep 23:225–229, 1887.

Solomon E, Voss R, Hall Z, Bodmer W, Jass JR, Jeffreys AJ, Lucibello FC, Patel I, Rider SH: Chromosome 5 allele loss in human colorectal carcinomas. Nature 328:616–619, 1987.

Traboulsi EI, Krush AJ, Gardner EJ, Booker SV, Offerhaus GJA, Yardley JH, Hamilton SR, Luk GD, Giardiello FM, Welsh SB, Hughes JP, Maumenee IH: Prevalence and importance of pigmented ocular fundus lesions in Gardner's syndrome. N Engl J Med 316:661–667, 1987.

Utsunomiya J, Nakamura T: The occult osteomatous changes in the mandible in patients with familial polyposis coli. Br J Surg 62:45–51, 1975.

Veale AMO: Intestinal Polyposis. Eugenics Laboratory Memoirs Series 40. New York: Cambridge University Press, 1965.

Woodward JJ: Pseudo-polypi of the colon: An anomalous result of follicular ulceration. Am J Med Sci 81:142–155, 1881.

2

Heritage of Colonic Polyps

Henry T. Lynch, Bruce M. Boman, Stephen J. Lanspa, Tom Smyrk, and Jane F. Lynch

Department of Preventive Medicine/Public Health (H.T.L., J.F.L.), Creighton Cancer Center (B.M.B.), Department of Medicine—Gastroenterology (S.J.L.), and Department of Pathology (T.S.), Creighton University School of Medicine and the Hereditary Cancer Consultation Center, Omaha, Nebraska

HISTORY OF FAMILIAL ADENOMATOUS POLYPOSIS (FAP)

Bulow [1987] has traced the history of FAP to a report in 1861 by Luschka that "may have been FAP." However, the first definite example of a patient with multiple colonic polyposis was published in 1881 by Sklifasowski [1881]. The first "familial" example was that of a brother and sister with FAP reported by Cripps in 1882. Examples of colorectal carcinoma occurring in patients with FAP were reported by Smith in 1887. Discussion of the histologic findings of the changes from adenoma to adenocarcinoma was first described by Handford [1890]. Finally, Lockhart-Mummery [1925] was the first to express the concern that the hereditary factor was not for cancer per se in this disease but, rather, for the presence of multiple adenomas because of their tendency to undergo malignant transformation. This report was in context with findings in the histories from three families and has formed the basis for the now-renowned St. Mark's Hospital Polyposis Registry (London, England). As will be evident in this chapter, much has been learned about FAP since these early historical accounts.

FAP: A MULTIFACETED PHENOTYPE

Understanding the heritage of colonic polyps requires an appreciation of the fact that genes show variable expressivity, a characteristic particularly of autosomal dominantly inherited disorders. In the case of FAP, this matter has been inadequately investigated. These phenomenon not only pertain to the polyp phenotype but moreover may involve extracolonic sites and a wide spectrum of cancer. This is particularly important in the face of Jagelman's statement [1987] that FAP is primarily a problem involving an inherited predisposition to aberrant growth disorganization.

The phenotype of FAP has become more complex in direct proportion to the number and scope of investigations of FAP patients and their at-risk relatives. FAP's phenotype is characterized by an array of colonic polyps, cancer (multiple sites), and extracolonic manifestations (osteomas, cutaneous signs, congenital hypertrophy of the retinal pigment epithelium [CHRPE], and others). The full spectrum of tumors integrally associated with FAP remains to be determined. The polyp is only one, albeit the cardinal, component of the FAP story.

VARIABLE PHENOTYPIC EXPRESSION OF POLYPS

Individual patients from FAP kindreds may or may not express the textbook picture of florid carpeting of the colon with hundreds or even thousands of polyps. It is imperative that this fact be seriously considered when assessing patients who are potentially at risk for FAP. These facts are seen in high relief in our pedigree (Fig. 1). Note that the proband (IV-2) had isolated polyps and that her father (III-2), also with isolated polyps, manifested colon cancer at age 46 years. His sis-

Familial Adenomatous Polyposis, pages 9–15

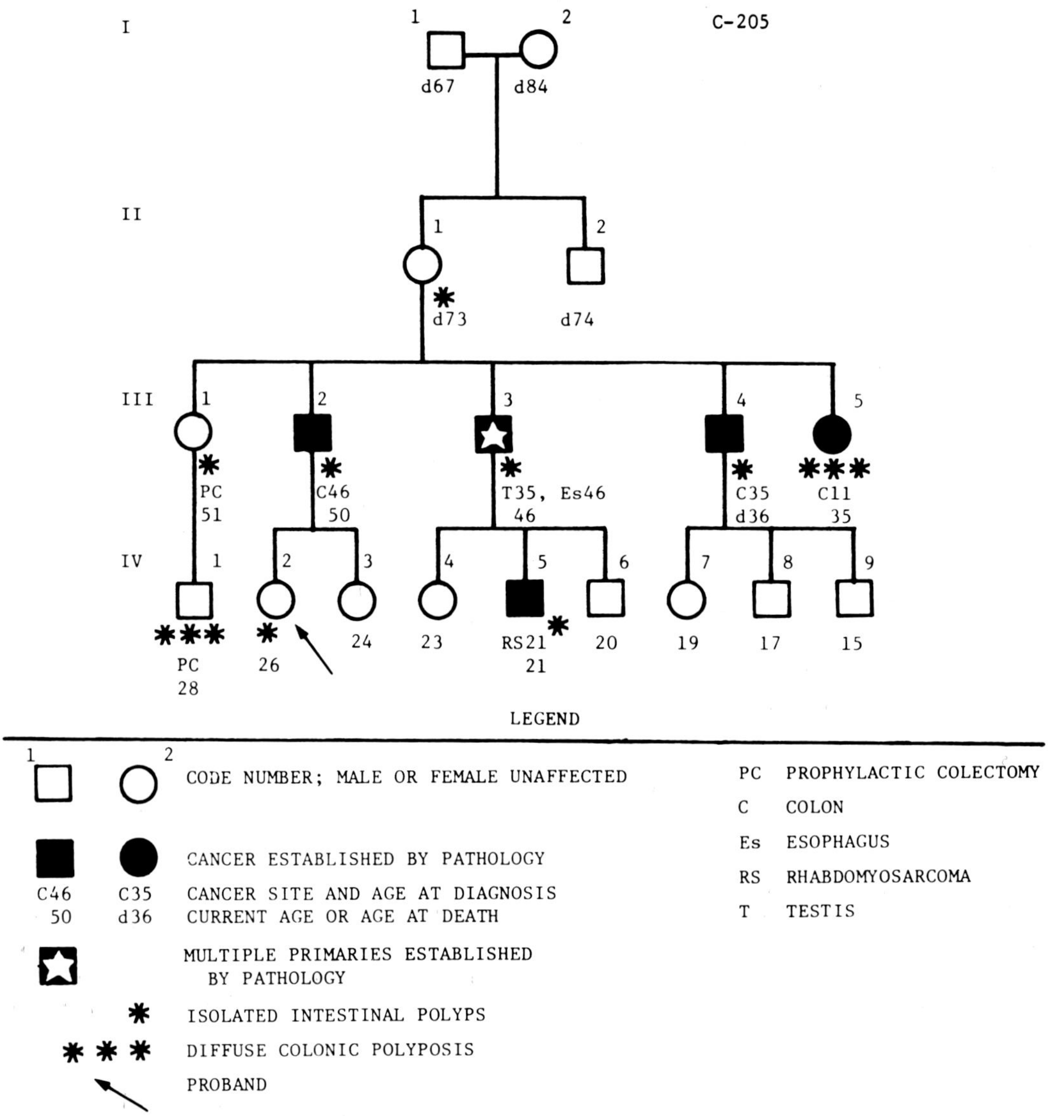

Fig. 1. Pedigree of family, depicting marked variation in the adenomatous polyposis phenotype and variable cancer expression. (Reproduced from Lynch et al., 1982; with permission of Lippincott/Harper & Row.)

ter (III-5) had myriad colonic polyps and manifested colonic cancer at age 11 years. Critical to our thesis is the finding of *isolated* polyps in the proband's maternal aunt (III-1) and the fact that her son (IV-1), the proband's first cousin, had *myriad* colonic polyposis and underwent a prophylactic colectomy at age 28 years. Note also that the proband's maternal uncle (III-3), also with isolated colonic polyps, manifested seminoma of the testis at age 35 years and esophageal cancer at age 46 years. His son (IV-5), also with isolated polyps, manifested rhabdomyosarcoma. Thus cancer of variable anatomic sites was observed.

This pedigree clearly depicts the phenomenon of variable phenotypic expression of the polyposis phenotype, ranging from isolated to diffuse colonic polyposis, in a given family. We have observed similar clinical findings in other kindreds [Lynch and Lynch, 1985]. However, the accuracy of this type of polyp phenotype assessment requires careful attention to examination of the *entire* colonic mucosa, with reporting of all variations in polyp expression observed during colonoscopy, double air contrast barium enema, or pathologic description of the resected colon. Such description of the polyposis phenotype must be made in context with as many at-risk members of the FAP pedigree as possible. Thus the heterogeneity observed in adenomatous colorectal polyps (and polyps at extracolonic sites) as well as cancer (all sites) in FAP necessitates reassessment of our traditional understanding of the polyp phenotype in FAP [Lynch et al., 1982].

The description of families with variable polyp expression has been hampered by the reluctance or inability of many investigators to focus on the problem of heterogeneity per se. This has been due in part to 1) inadequate or nonexistent surgical pathological description of the quantity, distribution, and histological classification of colonic polyps, particularly in patients who were affected before the advent of modern diagnostic and surgical techniques and 2) uncritical acceptance by geneticists and clinicians of inadequately documented cases in whom diffuse colonic polyposis was inferred, with its genetic implications then ascribed within pedigrees. For example, Asman and Pierce [1970] reported a large kindred that included eight patients categorized as having "deduced polyposis," those who died of colon cancer and had a child with polyposis, notwithstanding the fact that records of the patients with "deduced polyposis" showed no documented evidence of this trait. The authors also described a class of "polyposis carriers," those having no clinical evidence of a gastrointestinal tract disorder but who had children with polyposis.

Age of onset of symptoms, diagnosis, and onset of cancer have shown extreme variation in FAP [Veale, 1985]. It is clear that the frequency and variable expression of colonic polyps, including variation in age of onset, both within and between families, require further systematic investigation.

The problem of variable colon polyp expression with FAP brings serious concerns for patient management. Options would include prophylactic colectomy in the presence of isolated colonic polyps, notwithstanding the uncertainty regarding the patient's genotypic status (are the polyps associated or unassociated with the FAP gene?); should surveillance be an acceptable option as opposed to prophylactic surgery, then we would recommend annual colonoscopy and/or barium enema with air contrast and biannual evaluation of fecal occult blood in the stool, and, should colonic polyps show a progressive increase in number and/or size, then prophylactic colectomy should be performed, given the greater confidence that the patient is expressing the deleterious effects of the FAP genotype. These diagnostic and surveillance/management dilemmas may be effectively resolved through biomolecular/genetic strategies, with the goal of establishing the presence or absence of the deleterious FAP gene.

FAP AND OVERLAP OF PHENOTYPIC FEATURES

A vexing problem is the classification of FAP. Noteworthy is whether there is a "pure" form of the syndrome characterized by a predominance of adenomatous colonic polyps in the absence of extracolonic phenotypic characteristics vs. a more complex version of the syndrome as seen classically in so-called Gardner's syndrome showing an array of extracolonic manifestations, including osteomas, cutaneous signs, CHRPE, periampullary carcinoma, an excess frequency of desmoid tumors, sarcomas, adrenocortical carcinoma, thyroid carcinoma, and brain tumors as well as other forms of cancer. Are FAP and Gardner's syndrome distinct clinical entities (see addendum) or is FAP primarily a problem involving an inherited predisposition to aberrant growth disorganization involving a diverse number of organs and systems in addition to the colon, as proposed by Jagelman [1987]? Evidence [Lynch and Lynch, 1985; Utsunomiya and Iwama, 1980] suggests that, when meticulous studies of all facets of the phenotype are evaluated in FAP, overlap appears to be the rule so far as benign as well as malignant neoplastic phenotype is concerned. For example, Bulow [1987] and others have clearly identified osteomas as occurring in patients with the relatively pure form of FAP, in Gardner's syndrome, and, indeed, in the cancer family syndrome (CFS; Lynch's syndromes I and II) the recent finding of Sondergaard et al. [1986] of mandibular osteomas in the CFS serves, in the absence of other malignancies, as an accessible physical marker for phenotypic expression of the syndrome. CHRPE was originally described in Gardner's syndrome [Lewis et al., 1984; Lyons et al., 1988; Traboulsi et al., 1987]; however, Lynch et al. [1987] found clear evidence of CHRPE in patients from two FAP families in whom there was a total absence of other features consonant with Gardner's syndrome.

GENETIC IMPLICATIONS: A NOSOLOGIC DILEMMA

The traditional concept of the heritage of colonic polyps has been almost exclusively that diffuse carpeting of the entire colonic mucosa with adenomatous polyps is ncessary for diagnostic purposes. This concept ignored voluminous evidence showing variation in expression of the polyposis phenotype within and between patients/families. Thus, clinically, one finds a spectrum of colonic polyp expression ranging from discrete polyps to variable occurrence of polyps throughout the colon as well as in extracolonic sites of the small bowel and stomach. Histologically, one also may find polyps with adenomatous, juvenile, and hamartomous as well as mixed features. Extracolonic signs must be considered to discern the role of primary genetic factors in FAP's etiology. We must consider the sum total of these phenotypic findings, since they provide compelling evidence for a reappraisal of the etiologic significance of colorectal polyps with respect to the genetics, classification, and expression of cancer in FAP.

Burt et al. [1985] described the occurrence of an autosomal dominant inheritance pattern for discrete colorectal polyps and colorectal cancer in a large Utah pedigree. This kindred lacked those natural history characteristics of the "typical" FAP presentation; namely, early age of onset of multiple colonic polyps, an excess of synchronous and metachronous colonic cancer, cancer of extracolonic sites, and variable extracolonic phenotypic stigmata. Indeed, the findings of colonic cancer in association with discrete polyps in the colorectum were more in accord with expectations from the general population. A reasonable question is whether the heritage of colorectal polyps in families with discrete colorectal polyps represents one end of the colonic mucosal polyp expression with respect to a host factor susceptibility to colorectal cancer.

The hereditary non-polyposis colorectal cancer (HNPCC) syndromes have heretofore been considered to be unassociated with an excess of colonic polyps. However, this problem may be much more complex than was previously imagined, as will be seen in the following discussion of flat adenomas.

FLAT ADENOMAS

An even more subtle phenomenon appears to relate to the finding of Muto et al. [1985] of flat adenomas occurring apparently sporadically (family history not reported) as a putative link in the polyp-to-cancer sequence. Further description of flat adenomas has been provided by Adachi et al. [1988], who found flat adenomas in two patients with proximal colonic cancer, but, again, they failed to discuss the family history. More recently, flat adenomas of colonic mucosa (Fig. 2) were described by Lynch et al. [1988] in a family with findings consonant with Lynch's syndrome II. One therefore wonders whether the flat adenoma might represent some of the most minimal phenotypic expression of genetic susceptibility to colorectal cancer. Is this a heterogeneous variant of FAP, and, if so, are the Lynch's syndromes an extreme end of the spectrum of FAP, with discrete polyps in association with colorectal cancer [as described by Burt et al., 1985] another heterogeneous form of FAP but with a more intermediate polyp phenotype? Again, this provides fodder to the lumpers and splitters in the nosology of colonic polyps and cancer.

In summary, it is clear that the traditional clas-

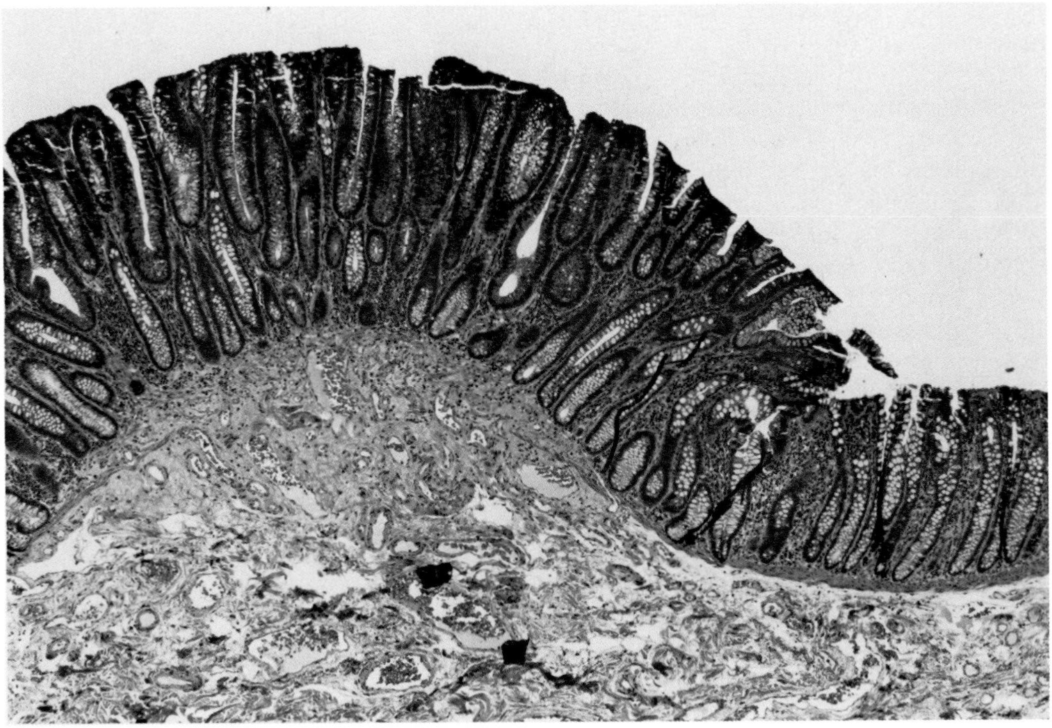

Fig. 2. Section through the center of a 0.3 cm sessile, tubular adenoma with features typical of flat adenomas; the lesion is less than twice as thick as adjacent mucosa, and adenomatous tubules are concentrated near the lumenal surface. Occasional nonneoplastic crypts are interspersed between the adenomatous tubules ×66.

sification of hereditary colon cancer requires more reflection in light of problems in heterogeneity of phenotype. One must raise the question of whether all so-called variants of hereditary colon cancer represent a spectrum in the heritage of colonic polyps, since there is significant variability in the expression of colonic polyps within each of the so-called discrete hereditary colon cancer-prone syndromes; namely, FAP, hereditary discrete colonic polyps, and HNPCC.

MOLECULAR GENETICS

Despite the variable expressivity of the FAP gene, this remains an excellent model system to study the molecular genetics of colonic polyp heritage, because the gene shows essentially 100% penetrance [Boman and Levin, 1986]. The FAP trait has recently been mapped to chromosome 5 through molecular linkage studies [Bodmer et al., 1987; Leppert et al., 1987; Meera Khan et al., in press]. This single mutant allele, which is transmitted through the germline, appears to be the primary genetic event associated with the predisposition to develop multiple adenomatous polyps of the colon in FAP.

The molecular genetics of the HNPCC syndromes have been diffficult to characterize because of the lack of a premonitory biomolecular marker or phenotypic manifestation for this disease [Boman et al. 1987]. Based on positive linkage of the CFS (Lynch's syndrome II) to the JK blood group, an HNPCC gene has tentatively been assigned to chromosome 18 [Boman et al., in press; Lynch et al., 1985]. The recent observation of flat mucosal adenomas in an HNPCC family suggests that the germline mutation in this syndrome is another genetic event associated with the predisposition to develop adenomatous polyps [Lynch et al., 1988].

Future molecular biological studies will be important in defining the genetic mutations associated with the predisposition to develop adenomatous polyps. For example, it should be possible to determine using linked genetic markers whether Gardner's syndrome and FAP are due to mutations of the same gene on chromosome 5. Genetic markers for the hereditary colon cancer syndromes will be useful in classification of genetic disorders and in cancer prevention through identification of individuals who are at risk.

CONCLUSIONS

Central to the elucidation of the heritage of colonic polyps is the need for extended and thoroughly documented pedigree studies of individuals with colonic polyps (all histologic varieties—adenomatous, hamartomatous, juvenile, mixed) in context with a full description of all known potential phenotypic signs involving the colon, other portions of the gastrointestinal tract, extragastrointestinal tract, and cancer (all sites). There have been many reviews purporting to depict the role of primary genetic factors in the etiology of both colonic polyps and colonic cancer. However, the bulk of these studies suffer from a dearth of detailed, comprehensive family investigations, with documentation of phenotype in all available at-risk relatives. Needed, therefore, are more uniform reporting methods describing in sufficient detail the histopathology of polyps, and their precise location and number in the colon as well as in the remainder of the gastrointestinal tract. Comparable consideration must be given to cancer (all anatomic sites) and those noncancer but potentially significant phenotypic stigmata that might aid in FAP syndrome identification. More interdisciplinary studies are needed, with attention to the integration of basic biomolecular genetic research with the clinical programs, so that through this knowledge we will be in a better position to understand hereditary colon cancer's classification and the genetics of the heritage of colonic polyps.

ADDENDUM

While this paper was in press, two important papers have been published on the heritage of colonic polyps. Nakamura et al. [1988] studied six pedigrees, three having the FAP phenotype and three having Gardner's syndrome, by linkage analysis and found no evidence of genetic heterogeneity between the two phenotypes. Although the possibility that two different defective genes located close together on chromosome 5 cannot be eliminated, the simplest interpretation is that separate mutations within the same gene are generating the difference between the phenotypes. Cannon-Albright et al. [1988] studied 34 kindreds with discrete colorectal adenomas and carcinomas by likelihood analysis that provided evidence for a dominantly inherited susceptibility to adenomatous polyps and subsequent carcinoma which is present in a sizable segment of the general population.

ACKNOWLEDGMENTS

Support for this effort was provided by NIH grants 1 RO1 CA42705 and 5 RO1 CA41371.

References

Adachi M, Muto T, Morioka Y, Ikenaga T, Hara M: Flat adenoma and flat mucosal carcinoma (IIb type)—A new precursor of colorectal carcinoma? Dis Colon Rectum 31:236–243, 1988.

Asman HB, Pierce ER: Familial multiple polyposis: a statistical study of a large Kentucky kindred. Cancer 25:972–981, 1970.

Bodmer WF, Bailey CJ, Bodmer J, Bussey HJR, Ellis A, Gorman P, Lucibello FC, Murday VA, Rider SH, Scambler P, Sheer D, Solomon E, Spurr NK: Localization of the gene for familial adenomatous polyposis on chromosome 5. Nature 328:614–616, 1987.

Boman BM, Levin B: Familial polyposis. Hosp Pract 21:155–170, 1986.

Boman BM, Lynch HT, Kimberling WJ, Wildrick DM: Reassignment of a cancer family syndrome gene to chromosome 18. Cancer Genet Cytogenet (in press).

Boman BM, Polyzos A, Levin B: Problems in the identification of a cancer family: Clinical case reports. Am J Clin Oncol 10:531–534, 1987.

Bulow S: Familial polyposis coli. Danish Med Bull 34:1–15, 1987.

Burt RW, Bishop DT, Cannon LA, Dowdle MA, Lee RE, Skolnick MH: Dominant inheritance of adenomatous colonic polyps and colorectal cancer. N Engl J Med 312:1540–1544, 1985.

Cannon-Albright LA, Skolnick MH, Bishop T, Lee RG, Burt, RW: Common inheritance of susceptibility to colonic adenomatous polyps and associated colorectal cancer. N Engl J Med 319:533–537, 1988.

Cripps WH: Two cases of disseminatec polyps of the rectum. Trans Pathol Soc London 33:165– 168, 1882.

Glass RE, Fazio VW, Jagelman DG, L ivery IC, Weakley SL, Forsythe SR: The results of surgic il treatment of cancer of the colon at the Cleveland Clir ic from 1965–1975: Classification of the spread of coloı cancer and long-term survival. Int J Colorect Dis 1:33- 39, 1986.
cation of a cancer family: Clinical case reports. Am J Clin Oncol 10:531–534, 1987.

Handford H: Disseminated polypi of the large intestine becoming malignant: strictures (malignant adenoma) of the rectum and of the splenic flexure of the colon; secondary growths in the liver. Trans Pathol Soc London 41:133–137, 1890.

Jagelman DG: Extracolonic manifestations of familial polyposis coli. Cancer Genet Cytogenet 27:319–325, 1987.

Leppert M, Dobbs M, Scambler P, O'Connel P, Nakamura Y, Stauffer D, Woodward S, Burt R, Hughes J, Garder E, Lathrop M, Wasmuth J, Lalouel JM, White R: The gene for familial polyposis coli maps to the long arm of chromosome 5. Science 238:1411–1413, 1987.

Lewis RA, Crowder WE, Eierman LA, Nussbaum RL, Ferrell RE: The Gardner syndrome: significance of ocular features. Ophthalmology 91:916–925, 1984.

Lockhart-Mummery P: Cancer and heredity. Lancet i:427–429, 1925.

Luschka H: Ueber polypöse Vegetationen der gesammten Dickdarmschleimhaut. Arch Pathol Anat Phys Klin Med 20:133–142, 1861.

Lynch HT, Kimberling WJ, Albano WA, Scnelke GS, Lynch JF, Biscone KA, Lipkin ML, Deschner EE, Mikol YB, Sandberg AA, Elston RC, Bailey-Wilson JE, Danes BS: Hereditary nonpolyposis colorectal cancer (Lynch syndromes I and II), parts I and II. Cancer 56:934–951, 1985.

Lynch HT, Priluck I, Fitzsimmons ML: Congenital hypertrophy of the retinal pigment epithelium (CHRPE) in non-Gardner's polyposis kindreds. Letter to the editor. Lancet ii:333, 1987.

Lynch HT, Ruma TA, Albano WA, Lynch JF, Lynch PM: Phenotypic variation in hereditary adenomatosis: unusual tumor spectrum. Dis Colon Rectum 25:235–238, 1982.

Lynch HT, Smyrk T, Lanspa SJ, Marcus JN, Kriegler M, Lynch JF, Appelman HD: Flat adenomas in a colon cancer-prone kindred. JNCI 80:278–282, 1988.

Lynch PM, Lynch HT: "Colon Cancer Genetics." New York; Van Nostrand Reinhold Co, 1985.

Lyons LA, Lewis RA, Strong LC, Zuckerbrod S, Ferrell RE: A genetic study of Gardner syndrome and congenital hypertrophy of the retinal pigment epithelium. Am J Hum Genet 42:290–296, 1988.

Meera Khan P, Tops CMJ, Broek MVD, Breukel C, Wijnen JT, Oldenburg M, Bos J, Van Leeuwen-Cornelisse ISJ, Vassen HFA, Griffioen G, Verspaget HM, den Hartog Jager FCA, Lamers C: Close linkage of a highly polymorphic marker (D5S37) to familial adenomatous polyposis (FAP) and confirmation of FAP localization on chromosome 5q21–q22. Hum Genet 79:183–185.

Muto T, Kamiya J, Sawada T, Konishi F, Sugihara K, Kubota Y, Adachi M, Agawa S, Saito Y, Morioka Y, Tanprayoon T: Small "flat adenoma" of the large bowel with special reference to its clinical pathologic features. Dis Colon Rectum 28:847–851, 1985.

Sklifasowski NW: Polyadenoma tractus intestinalis. Vrac 4:55–57, 1881.

Nakamura Y, Lathrop M, Leppert M, Dobbs M, Wasmuth J, Wolff E, Carlson M, Fujimoto E, Krapcho K, Sears T, Woodward S, Hughes J, Burt R, Gardner E, Lalouel JM, White R: Localization of the genetic defect in familial adenomatous polyposis within a small region of chromosome 5. Am J Hum Genet 43:638–644, 1988.

Smith T: Three cases of multiple polypi of the lower bowel occurring in one family. St Bartholomew's Hosp Rep 23:225–229, 1887.

Sondergaard J, Svendsen L, Witt I, Bulow S, Lauritsen KB, Tetens G: "Mandibular Osteomas in the Cancer Family Syndrome." Br J Cancer 52:941, 1986.

Traboulsi EI, Krush AJ, Gardner EJ, Booker SV, Offerhaus G, Yardley JH, Hamilton SR, Luk GD, Giardiello FM, Welsh SB, Hughes JP, Maumenee IH: Prevalence and importance of pigmented ocular fundus lesions in Gardner's syndrome. N Engl J Med 316:661–667, 1987.

Utsunomiya J, Iwama T: Adenomatosis coli in Japan: In Winawer S, Schottenfeld D, Sherlock P (eds); "Colorectal Cancer: Prevention, Epidemiology, and Screening." New York; Raven Press, 1980.

Veale AMO: Investigation of a genetic model. In Lynch PM, Lynch HT (eds); "Colon Cancer Genetics." New York; Van Nostrand Reinhold Co, 1985, pp 17–29.

3

Mode of Inheritance of "Sporadic" Adenomatous Polyps

Randall W. Burt

Division of Gastroenterology, Department of Medicine, University of Utah, Salt Lake City, Utah

INTRODUCTION

The hypothesis that inherited factors play a role in the development of both "sporadic" adenomatous polyps and "common" colorectal cancers derives from the observation that colorectal cancers and adenomatous polyps frequently exhibit an increased familial occurrence. Epidemiological studies consistently have demonstrated that, in addition to the well-characterized inherited syndromes of familial polyposis coli, Gardner's syndrome, and nonpolyposis inherited colorectal cancer, colorectal cancers occur in families in excess of that expected by chance [1–7]. Even when the rare syndromes are excluded, first-degree relatives of those with large bowel cancer or adenomatous polyps have a twofold to threefold increased risk of colonic cancer. Since monogenetic segregation patterns seldom have been apparent in these studies, investigators have suggested other mechanisms to account for the familial excess of cases [4,8]. These have included multifactorial or polygenic inheritance, environmental factors common to family members, or partially penetrant Mendelian factors.

To clarify which of these mechanisms is responsible for the common familial clustering of cases, the occurrence of adenomatous polyps, the precursor to colorectal cancer, has been examined in pedigrees [9]. Because adenomatous polyps are more common than colon cancer, and because only a fraction of them become malignant, it is likely that they are a more penetrant expression of underlying genetic or environmental susceptibilities to colon cancer than colorectal cancer itself. Examining the pedigree occurrence of adenomatous polyps together with available pedigree analysis techniques has proved very helpful in defining the mechanisms of familial clustering.

The epidemiologic studies examining the familiality of common colorectal cancer first will be reviewed because of their pertinence to polyp inheritance. More recent studies that have included polyps then are summarized in addition to a genealogic data base study of colon cancer. Studies of polyp occurrence in pedigrees are then reviewed.

FAMILIAL STUDIES OF COLORECTAL CANCER

The first familial studies examined the frequency of large bowel cancer among first-degree relatives of individuals with this malignancy. This frequency was then compared either to an appropriate control group or to an expected population frequency. The first such study was performed in the late 1950s [1]. Death certificates in Utah from 1931 to 1951 were examined. First-degree relatives of all those who had died of colorectal cancer were identified through the Utah Genealogical Society. Death certificates of these first-degree relatives were then located, together with an equal number of controls matched for age, sex, and county of birth. Colorectal cancer had occurred in 26 or 763 first-degree rela-

Familial Adenomatous Polyposis, pages 17–22

tives but in only 8 of 763 controls, a statistically significant difference. Cases of polyposis coli were excluded. An equivalent number of "other cancers" occurred among relatives and controls (81 and 83, respectively).

A similar study was published in 1960 [2]. The frequency of large bowel cancer cases among relatives of individuals with colorectal cancer in Ohio was compared to the expected frequency based on death rates for the state. Thirty-one of 392 first-degree relatives were affected, whereas only 9.7 were expected. Excess colorectal cancer occurred in parents as well as siblings. Second-degree relatives also exhibited excessive numbers of large bowel cancers. Tumors of other sites occurred with the expected frequency. Polyposis coli cases were excluded. There was no evidence of single-gene inheritance in the families studied.

An investigation undertaken in the mid-1970s, in London, determined the occurrence of colorectal cancer among first-degree relatives of patients with that tumor admitted to the St. Mark's Hospital over a four year period [3,4]. Individuals with polyposis coli, as well as all those who had been referred because of a family history of large bowel cancer, were excluded. Forty-one of 352 relatives had died of colorectal cancer, whereas only 11.7 were expected from U.K. mortality rates. An equivalent excess was noted among fathers, mothers, brothers, and sisters. The likelihood of cancer in a relative was increased if the proband exhibited multiple benign or malignant neoplasms, a previous history of large bowel cancer, or early age of onset of colorectal cancer. The investigator could not identify evidence of single-gene inheritance among the families studied.

Medical records of first-degree relatives of 50 consecutive large bowel cancer patients admitted to the Aberdeen Hospitals in Scotland were examined recently for the presence of colorectal cancer [5]. Controls were the first-degree relatives of 50 randomly selected age- and sex-matched hospital patients. Eight of the 50 colorectal cancer patients, but only one of the 50 controls, had affected relatives.

FAMILIAL STUDIES INCLUDING POLYPS

Recent studies from several countries have consistently verified the familial clustering of colorectal cancer. Many of these studies have included colorectal adenomatous polyps.

A study in Paris in 1984 demonstrated that a patient with colorectal cancer was 6.3 times more likely to have an affected first-degree relative than a control patient [6]. A patient with a colonic adenomatous polyp was 4.7 times more likely than a control to have a first-degree relative affected with colorectal cancer. Patients with polyposis coli and cancer family syndrome (CFS) were excluded.

An investigation from a tumor registry in Italy involving more than 2,000 first-degree relatives in both the study and control group revealed a 4.5-fold excess of colorectal cancer among relatives of individuals with colonic neoplasms (polyps or cancer) [7]. The excess was seen in parents, siblings, and other relatives of probands with either adenomatous polyps or cancer.

GENEALOGIC DATA BASE STUDY

A different approach to discerning familial clustering in colorectal cancer was recently reported. It involved assessing the relatedness of all individuals with colorectal cancer in the Utah population database [10–13]. This database combines genealogic, cancer, and death record information on over 1.5 million individuals who are living or have lived in Utah. There were 1,520 cases of colorectal cancer in the database. The relatedness of these persons with colorectal cancer was significantly greater than the relatedness of a group of age-, sex-, and birthplace-matched controls. The relatedness among those with colorectal cancer was also greater than for most other cancers. Excess relatedness was also apparent among very distant relatives, suggesting a genetic cause for the familial clustering. It is noteworthy that equivalent excess relatedness was observed among individuals with proximal colonic cancers and those with distal colonic cancers when these groups were considered separately. This approach is important for assessing familial clustering in common diseases, because ascertainment is complete and the genetic relationship between all individuals is known.

PEDIGREE STUDIES

An investigation was recently undertaken at our institution to determine which of the suggested mechanisms of familial clustering (polygenic inheritance, shared environmental factors, or decreased penetrance of mendelian factors) might account for the familial clustering of colon cancer. The possibility of inheritance of adenomatous polyps, the clinical precursor of colorectal cancer, was examined specifically [9].

The study began with the examination of a large pedigree selected on the basis of colorectal cancer in a brother, a sister, and their nephew. Extensive pedigree evaluation revealed moderate clustering of colorectal cancer but no Mendelian inheritance patterns when cancer alone was analyzed. Cancers in the pedigree were typical of common large bowel cancer in terms of age of onset and colonic distribution. Asymptomatic members of four branches of the pedigree were then studied by 60 cm flexible proctosigmoidoscopy to determine the prevalence of colorectal polyps. Spouses served as controls to ensure demographic similarity in the control group. On examination, one or more adenomatous polyps were found in 41 of 191 family members (21%) but in only 12 of 132 controls (9%) ($P < 0.005$). Hyperplastic polyps were found in equivalent numbers of family members and controls, 46 of 191 (24%) and 38 of 132 (29%), respectively.

Pedigree analysis was then performed considering both colorectal cancer and adenomatous polyps as the positive phenotype. The analysis used likelihood methods to determine whether random clustering, autosomal recessive inheritance, or autosomal dominant inheritance best explained the excess of adenomatous polyps and colonic cancer in the pedigree. The $\log_{10}$ of the probability of the dominant model over the random model was 16.16, and that of the dominant model over the recessive model was 6.43. Autosomal dominant inheritance was therefore many orders of magnitude more likely to explain the distribution of adenomas and cancer in the pedigree than autosomal recessive inheritance or random clustering. Random clustering would have been expected if shared environmental factors were the basis of familial excess.

To determine the population frequency of a gene or genes that confer susceptibility to adenomatous polyps, and to determine what fraction of "common" colonic adenomas arise from this purported gene, 33 additional pedigrees were examined for evidence of polyp inheritance [14]. The pedigrees were systematically selected from three different sources. The first group of pedigrees was selected on the basis of a sibling pair with colorectal cancer. This group was studied to verify the initial observation of polyp inheritance in a pedigree with a cluster of cases of colorectal cancer. Four pedigrees in addition to the original large pedigree were studied and analyzed from this group. The second set of pedigrees consisted of 19 families of probands who were selected from pathology files for the presence of an adenomatous polyp or polyps. This set represented a random sequential series of adenomas identified clinically. The third set of pedigrees consisted of the families of spouses who were found to have an adenomatous polyp during the investigation. Spouses were used as controls throughout the study to assure similarity of demographics and lifestyle characteristics. Whenever a spouse was found to have an adenoma, that individual then also became a proband for a new pedigree to be studied. This set of 10 pedigrees represented a random sampling of adenomas in the population. This group of pedigrees was chosen to provide an estimate of the fraction of adenomas in the general population that arise on the basis of an inherited susceptibility.

Neoplasms in all pedigrees studied appeared to represent "common" colonic adenomatous polyps and colorectal cancers, that is, polyps and cancers not associated with known syndromes. Inheritance was not apparent in any set of pedigrees when cancer patients alone were considered.

Flexible proctosigmoidoscopy was used to

identify polyps, and likelihood methods were applied to compare single-locus autosomal genetic models to random occurrence. Of the 670 subjects from the three pedigree groups analyzed (including the initial large pedigree described above), 407 were relatives and 263 were spouse controls. The prevalence of adenomatous polyps among relatives was 19.2% (78 of 407) and among spouse controls was 12.2% (32 of 263; $P < 0.02$).

Analysis of the observations was first performed considering all pedigree groups and the initial large pedigree together. This pedigree analysis again employed likelihood methods and compared the probability of autosomal dominant, autosomal recessive, and random models. Because multiple pedigrees were involved, the analysis also was able to provide a reasonable estimate of gene frequency. The results strongly favor dominant inheritance of susceptibility to adenomatous polyps, with a gene frequency of 19%. The 95% confidence interval for this frequency was 14–28%. The penetrance (the presence of an adenomatous polyp or colon cancer) in individuals with the susceptible genotype was estimated to be 63% by age 80 years. The proportion of nongenetic cases was estimated by the model to be zero. Computations indicated that, for individuals who had adenomatous polyps, the 95% confidence interval for the proportion of these who carried the susceptibility allele extended from 53% to 100%. These results suggest that most polyps that were apparent by proctosigmoidoscopy arose, at least in part, because of an inherited susceptibility.

Each of the groups of pedigrees was then analyzed separately, considering the original large pedigree separately from the other three groups. The results were consistent, in each case, with the model obtained when all the pedigrees were analyzed jointly.

These results suggest the presence of an underlying genetic susceptibility for the majority of common colonic adenomatous polyps and colorectal cancers. They also suggest that a majority of individuals with endoscopically identifiable adenomatous polyps or colorectal cancer are affected because of a common, dominantly inherited susceptibility.

The preliminary nature of this specific genetic model, however, must be noted. The results are based on only 34 pedigrees, consisting of observations on 670 individuals. Complete understanding of the genetics will require a much larger data set. The underlying genetic mechanisms may, in fact, be much more complex than indicated by the present model. There may be multiple disease loci with several different penetrance levels. Polygenic inheritance may also be involved, since the analysis focused on utilizing a major gene hypothesis to eliminate the nongenetic hypothesis and to provide evidence for a strong genetic component yet to be fully described. The interaction of environmental and genetic factors also needs to be investigated. It is likely that inherited susceptibilities to adenomatous polyps are not expressed without certain environmental exposures. It is anticipated that inherited susceptibility loci can soon be mapped to DNA linkage markers. When gene markers are available, it can be determined which environmental factors completely suppress expression of the purported susceptibility gene or genes, which lead to expression of an adenomatous polyp, and which environmental exposures are needed to cause large polyps and finally cancer.

MOLECULAR STUDIES

Several of the recent molecular genetic studies addressing colorectal cancer bear some relationship to the inherited susceptibilities discussed in this chapter. Loss of DNA sequences from the same chromosomal location identified for familial adenomatous polyposis (5q21–q22) [15,16] was found in the cancer tissue of 20% of random colon cancers [17]. In a different laboratory, loss of DNA sequences from an area of the short arm of chromosome 17 was found in cancer tissue from 76% of random colon cancers tested [18]. Loss of heterozygosity has also been noted in a small percentage of polyps and cancers from familial adenomatous polyposis patients on chromosomes 5, 6, 12, 15, and 22 [19]. Similar findings were noted from random colorectal cancers [19]. In two separate studies, expression of the Ki-ras oncogene was observed in 40% of random colorectal cancers and in some premalignant villous adenomas [20,21].

Despite the importance of these studies, the DNA abnormalities observed are not germline mutations but instead mutations that occur late in the process of benign to malignant change. Nevertheless, the findings suggest candidate chromosomal locations for genes that might confer inherited susceptibility to colorectal adenomas and cancer. Whether the susceptibility genes for adenomatous polyps suggested by the pedigree studies presented are at or allelic to genes at any of these locations is presently under investigation.

SUMMARY

Although the exact etiology of "common" or "sporadic" colonic adenomatous polyps is unknown, familial aggregation of these polyps and common colorectal cancer is a consistent observation. The pedigree studies presented suggest that underlying inherited susceptibility to colonic adenomatous polyps is the most likely explanation for this familial occurrence. These studies also imply that the gene or genes that confer susceptibility are common and are present in most of the clinically identified colonic adenomas. Investigations to determine the chromosomal location and molecular basis of this purported susceptibility are underway. Once genotype markers are available, studies of environmental (specifically dietary) factors can be performed to determine how environmental factors interact with susceptibility genes to determine which individuals develop polyps and which finally develop colon cancer.

ACKNOWLEDGMENTS

This study was supported by NIH research grants CA-40641 and CA-28854 and PHS grant RR-64.

References

1. Woolf CM: A genetic study of carcinoma of the large intestine. Am J Hum Genet 10:42–47, 1958.
2. Macklin MT: Inheritance of cancer of the stomach and large intestine in man. J Natl Cancer Inst 24:551–571, 1960.
3. Lovett E: Familial factors in the etiology of carcinoma of the large bowel. Proc R Soc Med 67:21–22, 1974.
4. Lovett E: Family studies in cancer of the colon and rectum. Br J Surg 63:13–18, 1976.
5. Duncan JL, Kyle J: Family incidence of carcinoma of the colon and rectum in north-east Scotland. Gut 23:169–171, 1982.
6. Maire P, Morichau-Beauchant M, Drucker J, Barboteau M-A, Barbier J, Matuchansky C: Prevalence familiale due cancer du colon et du rectum: Resultats d'une enquete "cas-temoins" de 3 ans. Gastroenterol Clin Biol 8:22–27, 1984.
7. Ponz de Leon M, Ascari A, Antonioli A, Manenti F, Melotti G, Pezcoller C, Piccagli I, Grisendi A, Mazzeo D, Miselli A: Frequency of colorectal cancer among the first-degree relatives of patients with cancer or polyps of the large bowel. Gut 26:A1153, 1985.
8. Lynch HT, Lynch PM, Keathley J: Epidemiology of colon cancer. In Lynch PM, Lynch HT (eds): "Colon Cancer Genetics." New York: Van Nostrand Reinhold Company, 1985, pp 1–16.
9. Burt RW, Bishop DT, Cannon LA, Dowdell MA, Lee RG, Skolnick MH: Dominant inheritance of adenomatous colonic polyps and colorectal cancer. N Engl J Med 312:1540–1544, 1985.
10. Skolnick M: The Utah genealogical data base: a resource for genetic epidemiology. In Cairns J, Lyon JL, Skolnick M (eds): Banbury Report 4: Cancer Incidence in Defined Populations. Cold Spring Harbor, NY: Cold Spring Harbor Laboratory, 1980, pp 285–297.
11. Bishop DT, Skolnick MH: Genetic epidemiology of cancer in Utah genealogies: A prelude to the molecular genetics of common cancers. J Cell Physiol Suppl, Vol 3:63–77, 1984.
12. Cannon L, Bishop DT, Skolnick M, Hunt S, Lyon JL, Smart CR: Genetic epidemiology of prostate cancer in the Utah Mormon genealogy. Cancer Surv 1:47–69, 1982.
13. Cairns J: A survey of cancer sites by kinship in the Utah Mormon population. In Cairns J, Lyon JL, Skolnick M (eds): Banbury Report 4: Cancer Incidence in Defined Populations. Cold Spring Harbor, NY: Cold Spring Harbor Laboratory, 1980, pp 299–318.
14. Cannon-Albright, Skolnick MH, Bishop DT, Lee RG, Burt RW: Common inheritance of susceptibility to colonic adenomatous polyps and associated colorectal cancers. N Engl J Med 319:533–537, 1988.
15. Leppert M, Dobbs M, Scambler P, O'Connell P, Nakamura Y, Stauffer D, Woodward S, Burt R, Hughes J, Gardner E, Lathrop M, Wasmuth J, Lalouel J-M, White R: The Gene for familial polyposis coli maps to the long arm of chromosome 5. Science 28:1411–1413, 1987.
16. Bodmer WF, Bailey CJ, Bodmer J, Bussey HJR, Ellis A, Gorman P, Lucibello FC, Murday VA, Rider SH, Scambler P, Sherr D, Solomon E, Spurr NK: Localization of the gene for familial adenomatous polyposis on chromosome 5. Nature 328:614–616, 1987.
17. Solomon E, Voss R, Hall V, Bodmer WF, Jass JR, Jeffreys AJ, Lucibello FC, Patel I, Rider SH: Chromosome

5 allele loss in human colorectal carcinomas. Nature 328:616–619, 1987.

18. Fearon ER, Hamilton SR, Vogelstein B: Clonal analysis of human colorectal tumors. Science 238:193–197, 1987.

19. Okamoto M, Sasaki M, Sugio K, Sato C, Iwama T, Ikeuchi T, Tonomura A, Sasazuki T, Miyaki M: Loss of constitutional heterozygosity in colon carcinoma from patients with familial polyposis coli. Nature 331:273–277, 1988.

20. Bos JL, Fearon ER, Hamilton SR, Verlaan-deVries M, vanBoom JH, vanderEB AJ, Vogelstein B: Prevalence of ras gene mutation in human colorectal cancers. Nature 327:293–297, 1987.

21. Forrester K, Almoguera C, Han K, Grizzle WE, Perucho M: Detection of high incidence K-ras oncogenes during human colon tumorigenesis. Nature 327:298–301, 1987.

4

Criteria for Diagnosis of Inherited Colonic Polyposis Syndromes

Alvin L. Watne and Abdolkarim Sohrabi

Department of Surgery, University of Illinois, College of Medicine at Peoria, Peoria, Illinois

Observation of any polypoid lesion of the colon or rectum should alert the clinician to the potential possibility of the patient having one of the genetically inherited syndromes for developing the colon polyp cancer sequence. The differential diagnosis of the lesion and its possible familial tendency are among the intellectual exercises that make the practice of medicine the finest profession. Diagnosis at the present time is absolutely dependent on the histological identification of the type of growth under observation. The sophisticated aspects of this histologic diagnosis are beautifully described in the report by Fenoglio-Preiser and Hutter [1]. Assuming that the patient will undergo a physical examination, endoscopy, and/or barium enema evaluation and eventual biopsy and histologic confirmation of the polypoid lesion, let us first consider the noninherited polyposis syndromes.

Table 1 lists the noninherited gastrointestinal polyposis syndromes. First and foremost among these are the hyperplastic polyps. Although they were first described in 1927 [2], it was not until 1959 that it was recognized that the hyperplastic polyps have a cellular proliferation different from that of the adenomatous polyp [3]. Subsequent studies showed that 75% of autopsy patients older than 40 years of age had hyperplastic polyps present in the colon [4]. Whereas recent reports have indicated that hyperplastic polyps can be associated with adenomatous polyps, it is not clear that hyperplastic polyps in any way proceed or develop into invasive neoplasms. To the endoscopist, the polypoid lesions all appear similar, as shown in Figure 1. The histologic features of differentiated and mature cells lining the epithelial crypts with thickened collagen fibers and some increased density of pericryptic collagen under the mucosal surface of the epithelium near the opening of the crypt, and the picture of a reduced rate of extrusion of the cells from the surface of the crypt, rather than cellular crowding and hyperchromatism, identify the hyperplastic polyp, and place the patient among those with the noninherited syndrome. Figure 2 illustrates the histology of the hyperplastic polyp.

TABLE 1.
Gastrointestinal Polyposis: Nonhereditary Polyposis

Hyperplastic
Inflammatory
Benign lymphoid
Cronkhite-Canada syndrome
Juvenile polyps
Neoplastic polyps

Inflammatory polyposis is exemplified by the lymphoid polyps and pseudopolyps of ulcerative colitis shown in Figure 3. The pseudopolyps of ulcerative colitis should not be mistaken for polyposis coli. On biopsy, they show inflammatory round cells and regenerating mucosal epithelium. Ulcerative colitis is recognized as a premalignant condition, which with time will show a high incidence of malignant degenera-

Familial Adenomatous Polyposis, pages 23–34

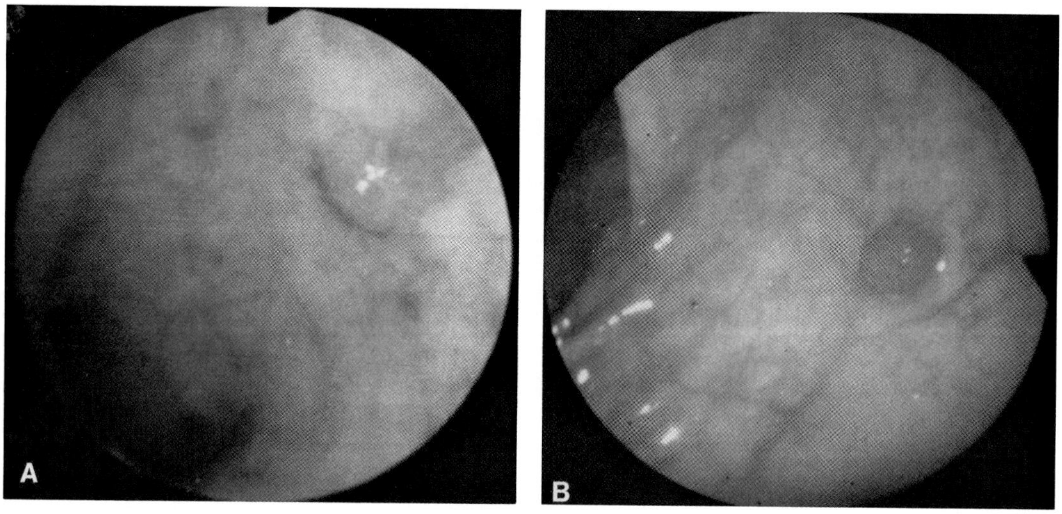

Fig. 1. Endoscopic view of Hyperplastic polyp **(A)** and Adenomatous polyp **(B)**.

tion, and the pseudopolyps make the differential diagnosis more difficult. There is no familial or inherited characteristic of this disease.

Gastrointestinal tract lymphoid hyperplasia was reviewed by Ranchod et al. in 1978 [5]. Lymphoid hyperplasia of the colon was considered a specific entity and was differentiated from lymphoid polyps by the smaller size of the lesions, the more diffuse distribution, and the larger number of lesions. The polypoid lesions are typically sessile but may be pedunculated and arise predominantly in the rectum. The patients classically have no family history; however, familial occurrence has been reported [6]. Lymphoid hyperplasia polyps have a rich submucosal lymphoid aggregate, and, although there may be a familial incidence for this problem, it is probably not genetic in origin. Figure 4 shows benign lymphoid hyperplasia. The polyps tend to disappear spontaneously with maturity, and there is no indication that they are premalignant. It is imperative for the endoscopist to biopsy and recognize the polyps for what they are. A colectomy must not be carried out for benign lymphoid hyperplasia polyposis.

Schistosomiasis occurs in large areas of the world, and bilharzial polyposis is endemic where this acquired parasitic disease occurs. With long-standing bilharzial infection, colon cancer may develop. There is of course no inheritance pattern with this disease.

The Cronkhite-Canada syndrome is a fascinating entity with abnormal pigmentation of the skin, alopecia, and atrophy of the fingernails and toenails along with polyposis of the entire gastrointestinal tract as shown in Figure 5. Originally, the polyps were thought to be adenomas; however, it is now clear that the polyps are a hamartoma of the juvenile or retention type [7]. There have been reports of adenomatous change of the colonic polyps in Cronkhite-Canada syndrome associated with the development of rectal cancer; however, this is a very rare occurrence. The syndrome is nonhereditary, and, with its response to antiinflammatory drugs, we are gaining further insight into the general problem of gastrointestinal tract polyposis [8].

Juvenile polyps of the large intestine were initially described by Verse [9]. The polyps are frequently pedunculated, vary in size from under 1 cm to more than 5 cm in diameter, and are difficult to distinguish grossly from periadenomatous polyp (Fig. 6). Their characteristic pattern shows cystically dilated glands and stroma, which led to the hypothesis that they arise from mucosal inflammation, causing blockade of the glands and

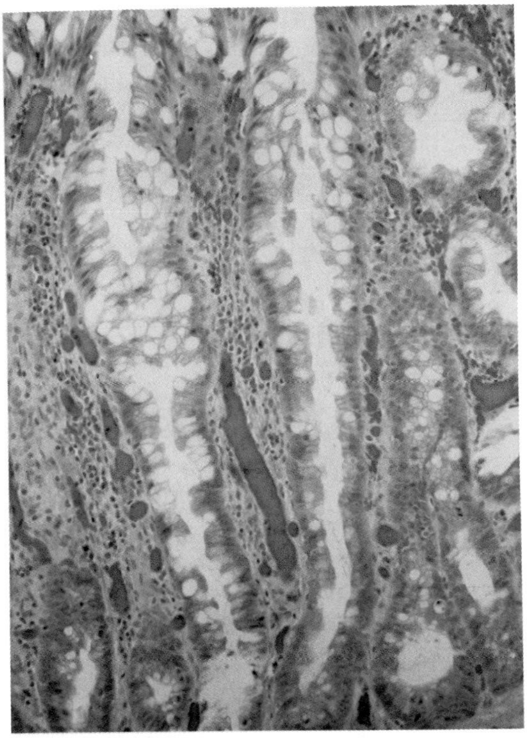

Fig. 2. Hyperplastic polyp. Note lengthening of the tubules and serrated appearance of the epithelium because of patchy flattening of the columnar cells, with a decrease in the number of goblet cells and variable hyperplasia of the cells in the depth of the crypts. Hematoxylin-eosin. ×40. (Courtesy of W. Chang, MD.) (Reproduced with permission from Watne [66] courtesy of Year Book Medical Publishers.)

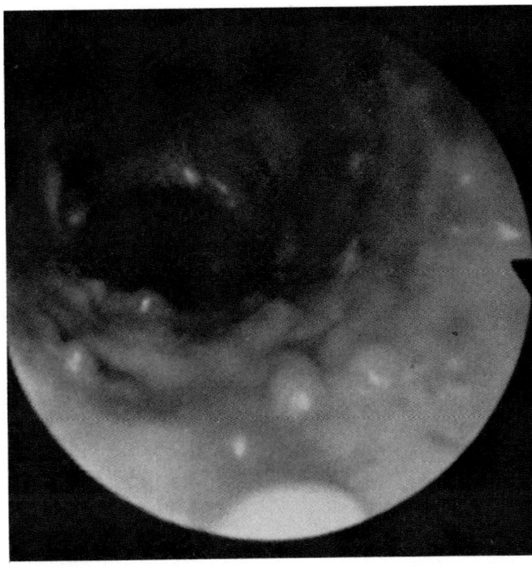

Fig. 3. Endoscopic appearance of pseudopolyps in ulcerative colitis.

formation of cystic spaces. The polyps frequently do not have a muscularis mucosa in the attached pedicle, and this allows autoamputation to occur. Figure 6 shows the histology of a juvenile polyp. Sporadic juvenile polyps arise most frequently in the pediatric patient but may be seen in the adult. They are classically single; however, multiple polyps can occur in 10–25% of patients.

Table 2 lists the hereditary polyposis syndromes of the nonneoplastic variety. Although they are classified this way, as the discussion develops it will become obvious that there is an intermixing of these syndromes so that what appears to be uniquely partitioned into respective disease complexes becomes more vague and overlapping.

The hamartomas do follow a familial pattern, and the classic is the Peutz-Jeghers syndrome, originally described by Peutz [10] and subsequently clarified by Jeghers et al. in 1949 [11]. The Peutz-Jeghers syndrome has a Mendelian dominant inheritance pattern. The pigmented spots around the mouth, hands, and feet are associated with intestinal polyposis. Figure 7 shows pigmented lesions of Peutz-Jeghers syndrome. These polyps are hamartomas and show involvement of the muscularis mucosa layer. The tumors are most commonly found in the small intestine but may occur throughout the gastrointestinal tract. There are reports of colonic carcinoma associated with Peutz-Jeghers syndrome, but these patients also had adenomas of the colon [12,13]. In addition, about 5% of female patients with Peutz-Jeghers syndrome develop ovarian tumors [14]. These frequently are sex cord tumors, and a high percentage of these tumors are hormonally active. Non-gastrointestinal tumors account for about half of the malignancies, among them ovarian, fallopian tube, thyroid, lung, basal cell cancer, and unknown primaries. Juvenile polyps can have a familial tendency. Among fifty patients

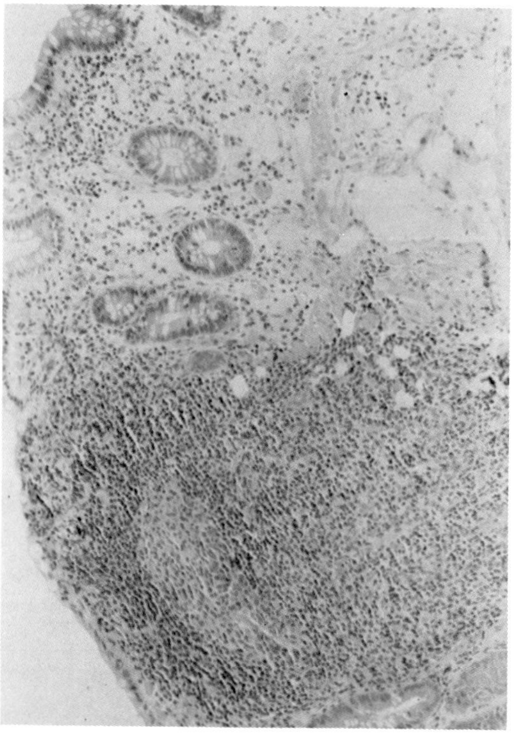

Fig. 4. Nodular lymphoid hyperplasia removed from the rectum of a 14-year-old girl. Hypertrophy of the normal lymphoid tissue causes mucosal protuberances resembling polyps. These rare lesions are seen most frequently in children. Hematoxylin-eosin. ×10. (Reproduced with permission from Watne [66] courtesy of Year Book Medical Publishers.)

with juvenile polyposis listed in the St. Mark's Polyposis Registry, one-fourth of the families with two to five members had polyps, suggesting a genetic origin for the polyps. Veale et al. [15] put forward the hypothesis that if the patient received the gene for polyposis coli (P) and the gene for juvenile polyps (j), the resultant genotype would be a (Pj), and juvenile polyposis would develop. Sachatello and Griffin [16] found that patients with juvenile polyps showed one of three syndromes: 1) juvenile polyposis of infancy, 2) juvenile polyposis coli, and 3) generalized juvenile and gastrointestinal polyposis. The risk of carcinoma in these patients was not increased, and there were no extracolonic manifestations. Sachatello et al. [17] did report on generalized juvenile gastrointestinal polyposis in three members of a kindred and believed that generalized gastrointestinal polyposis was a hereditary syndrome distinct from juvenile polyposis coli. Originally, it was thought that these polyps were not associated with an increase in cancer development; however, it became apparent that some patients had both juvenile and adenomatous polyps [18–20] and that dysplasia could be identified in the crypts of the juvenile polyps, which can progress to frank cancer [21]. Currently, it is believed that the relative risk of gastrointestinal cancer is 13 (confidence intervals 2.7–38.1) and the relative risk for all malignancies is 9 (confidence intervals 4.2–17.3). These authors also pointed out that the relatives of patients with juvenile polyps are at increased risk for development of gastrointestinal cancers [18–21]. The problem was further compounded by the description in 1963 by Lloyd and Dennis [22] of Cowden's disease, an autosomal dominant, general dermatosis with numerous systemic manifestations, including hamartomatous polyps of the gastrointestinal tract. In addition to the hamartomatous polyps, lipomatous polyps, fibromatous polyps, and lymphoid polyps of the colon have been described in other reports. It is important to recognize this syndrome because of the high frequency of associated malignancies, which appear to be particularly high in women. Malignant tumors observed in patients with Cowden's disease include breast cancer, thyroid carcinoma, ovarian carcinoma, uterine carcinoma, bladder carcinoma, lung carcinoma, liposarcoma, colon carcinoma, malignant melanoma, and squamous cell carcinoma of the skin [23]. Cowden's disease falls into the group of inherited conditions in which the patients develop multiple systemic tumors, and these are associated with cutaneous markers. Indeed breast carcinoma in middle-aged women affected with this syndrome is so common that it has recently been recommended that these patients have a prophylactic total mastectomy [24].

It has been recognized that ganglioneurofibromatosis is inherited as a Mendelian dominant characteristic [25] and gives rise to polypoid ganglioneurofibromatosis of the intestinal tract, including the colon. Recently, Mendelshon and Diamond [26] reported both a sporadic patient with polypoid ganglioneurofibromatosis involv-

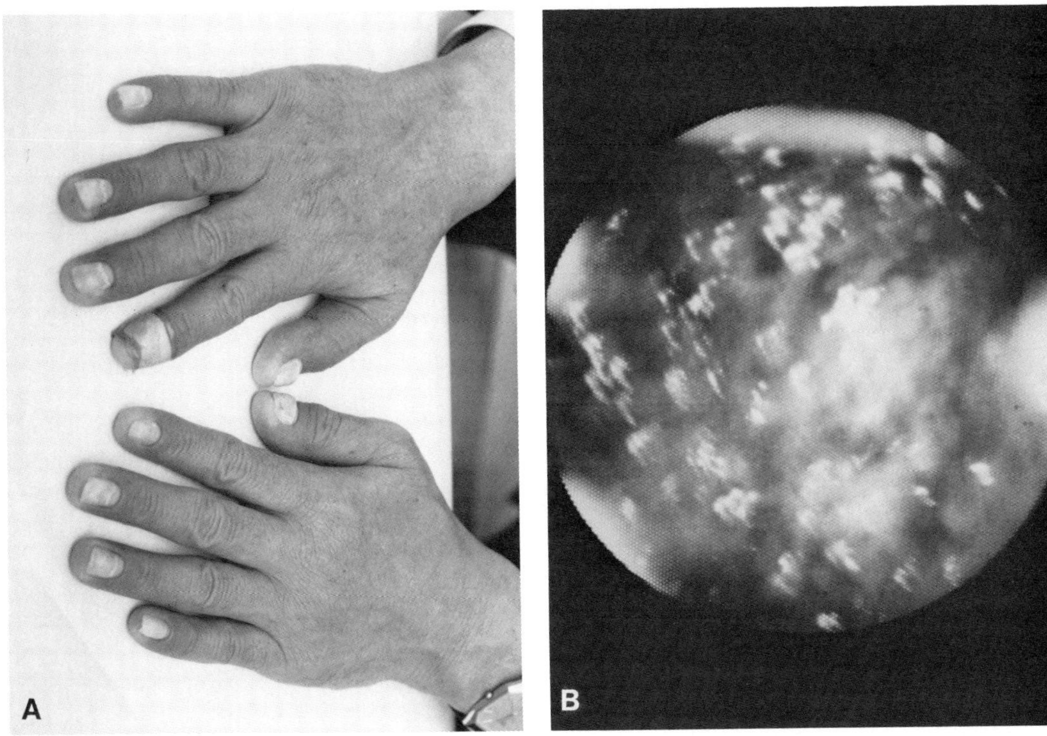

Fig. 5. **A:** Nail atrophy in a 57-year-old man with Cronkhite-Canada syndrome. The patient had been under treatment for 1 year. **B:** Endoscopic view of hamartomatous polyps of the ileum in a 57-year-old man with Cronkhite-Canada syndrome. The patient had undergone a total colectomy 1 year earlier for hamartomatous polyps and adenocarcinoma. He had been taking steroids and antiinflammatory drugs since that time. The polyps show both cystic changes and inflammatory reaction. (A and B courtesy of A. Goto, MD, Gifu University, Japan.) (Reproduced with permission from Watne [66] courtesy of Year Book Medical Publishers.)

ing the large bowel in a child and a 38-year-old man and his three children, all of whom had juvenile polyps and ganglioneuromatous polyps of the colon. None of these patients exhibited any other manifestations of neurofibromatosis. One patient has been reported by Snover et al. [27] with diffuse mucosal ganglioneuromatosis and adenocarcinoma of the colon. Familial ganglioneuromatosis of the alimentary tract including the colon has been seen in the multiple endocrine neoplasia (MEN) syndrome type 2B. MEN-2B differs from the common MEN-2A in that hyperparathyroidism is rarely seen and in that the polypoid ganglioneuromata of the gastrointestinal tract occur. Patients with both syndromes have medullary thyroid cancer and pheochromocytomas. This rare disorder, MEN-2B, may occur sporadically or as an autosomal dominant characteristic [28]. A recent report has described a young man with MEN-2B with adenomatous polyposis coli. The patient demonstrated a metastatic medullary carcinoma of the thyroid, a pheochromocytoma, and peripheral nerve abnormalities, including ganglioneuromatosis of the colonic mucosa and neuromas of the laryngeal mucosa. The patient also had tubular and villous adenomas of the colon and an adenoma of the duodenum. The authors proposed the two-hit mutational theory of carcinogenesis described by Knudson [29] as applying to this particular patient and these

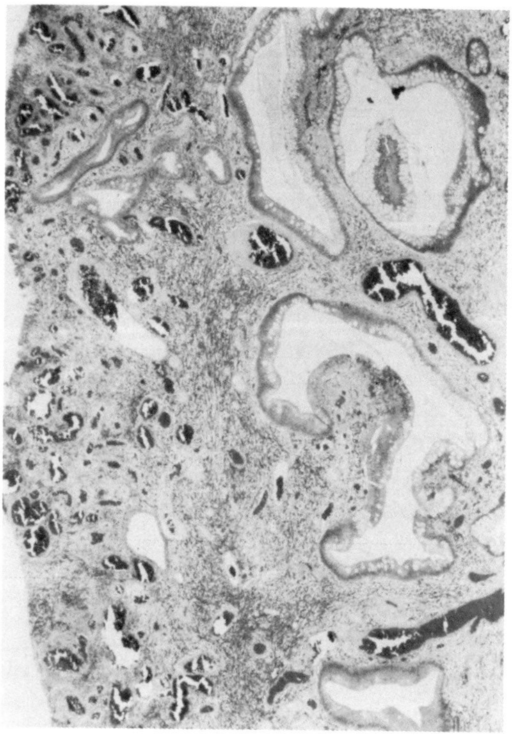

Fig. 6. Juvenile polyp, also called retention polyps. The cut section shows numerous cysts of various size, with mucus-secreting epithelium surrounded by a great deal of mesenchymal-appearing connective tissue. Hematolysin-eosin. ×40. (Courtesy of W. Chang, MD.) (Reproduced with permission from Watne [66] courtesy of Year Book Medical Publishers.)

TABLE 2.
Gastrointestinal Polyposis: Hereditary Polyposis

Hamartomatous
Juvenile polyposis
Peutz-Jeghers syndrome
Cowden's syndrome
Ganglioneuromatosis
MEN-2B

particular syndromes [30]. The first hit is the genetically transmittable "germinal mutation," and the second is a "somatic mutation" in the target tissue, with the result of multiple tumors at a younger age.

Table 3 lists the hereditary gastrointestinal polyposis of the neoplastic type. In 1985, Burt et al. [31] published a classic article describing a large Utah pedigree with multiple cases of common colorectal cancer, which, when analyzed for the association of adenomatous polyps, showed an inherited autosomal dominant gene for susceptibility to discrete adenomatous polyps and/or the colorectal cancers. It is believed that this may account for more than 10% of the colorectal cancer patients treated each year. Lynch et al. [31] have published extensively on the cancer family syndrome (CFS). This syndrome of carcinoma arising in the right colon, ovary, and breast shows a Mendelian dominant inheritance pattern. Whereas the CFS is not associated with adenomatous polyposis of the colon, the picture was further complicated by the description in 1967 by Torre [33] of a patient with numerous sebaceous adenoma, sebaceous carcinoma, basal cell carcinoma, and a history of carcinoma of the ampulla of Vater and primary carcinoma of the colon. Almost simultaneously Muir, Bell, and Barlow [34] published a report of a patient with multiple primary carcinoma of the colon, duodenum, and larynx associated with keratoacanthomas of the face. This syndrome, with the family history of internal carcinomas, has been reported with concomitant colonic polyposis and cutaneous markers of the visceral carcinomas. The syndromes were related even further by the subsequent observation of a cutaneous phenotypic linkage of Torre's syndrome with the CFS [35]. The coexistence of the rare sebaceous neoplasia and visceral cancer associated with four families showing the CFS made the authors think that some cases of Muir-Torre's syndrome represent a full phenotypic expression of the gene responsible for the CFS.

Over a century ago, in 1882, W. Harrison Cripps [36] presented a paper before the Pathological Society of London establishing familial polyposis of the colon as a clinical entity and noting the familial nature of the disease and its malig-

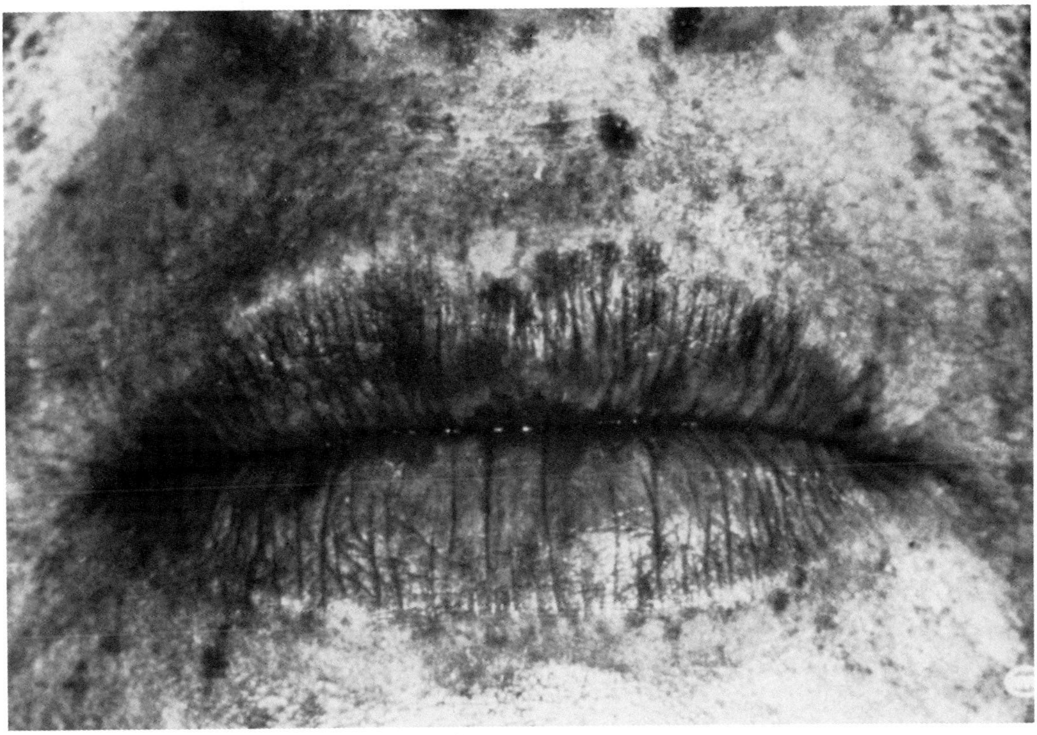

Fig. 7. Pigmented lesions Peutz-Jeghers syndrome.

TABLE 3.
Gastrointestinal Polyposis: Hereditary Polyposis and Neoplastic Polyposis

Discrete polyps and cancer
Torre's syndrome
Familal adenomatous polyposis
Gardner's syndrome
Turcot's syndrome

nant potential. Smith [37] and Handford [38] stressed the familial pattern of the disease and the early malignant degeneration of the polyps. It was not until 1927 that Cockayne [39] recognized that multiple polyposis was inherited as a Mendelian dominant trait. Then, in 1930, Dukes [40] published his classic paper on review of polyposis intestini or multiple adenomas and the role of heredity. He and Lockhart-Mummery [41] subsequently clearly established the autosomal dominant inheritance pattern for the disease, reporting on the occurrence of the disease in 10 families over three or four successive generations. In the same year, McKenney described 21 patients in three families all in their third generation of a Mendelian dominant inherited disease pattern [42]. In 1943, Freidell and Wakefield [43] described 49 members of a family descended to the third generation from a brother and a sister with polyposis coli. Among these 49 family members, 19 had either polyposis coli or colorectal carcinoma. Guptill [44] collected 347 reported cases of polyposis coli from the world literature by 1947. He added five cases, four of whom had malignant degeneration and two of whom had multiple colon cancers. Among these collected case reports was the sporadic patient with polyposis coli who had associated extracolonic findings. The first such report is credited to Devic and Bussey [45], who, in 1912, described a woman with osteoma of the mandible, sebaceous cyst of the scalp. subcutaneous lipomas, and multiple polyposis coli. Cabot [46] described a 36-year-old man with multiple polyposis of the duodenum, jejunum, ileum, and large bowel; multiple bony exostosis; a history of fibrosarcoma removed from three ribs; multiple sebaceous cysts; and carcinoma of the ampulla of Vater. In 1937, Miller and Sweet [47] described a 21-year-old woman with polyposis coli who had a desmoid tumor of the abdominal scar. A few years later, Fitzgerald [48] described a 36-year-old woman with recurring desmoid tumors of the abdominal wall, bony exostosis, multiple compound odontomas, torus palatinus, and multiple polyps of the bowel. This led to the series of papers beginning in 1950 by Eldon J. Gardner [49–53] describing the syndrome that bears his name. Gardner's syndrome includes soft tissue tumors, sebaceous cysts and fibromas, bony tumors, osteomas, and adenomatous polyps of the colon. The latter had the same growth pattern and malignant potential as the polyps seen in the patients with familial polyposis. The development of periampullary carcinoma as part of the syndrome was emphasized by McDonald et al. [54] when in 1967 they were able to review 118 patients reported in the literature with this manifestation.

In 1959, Turcot et al. [55] described two young siblings with documented familial polyposis of the colon and central nervous system tumors, a 15-year old boy who developed a medulloblastoma invading the medulla spinalis and a 13-year girl who died at age 21 years with a left frontal glioblastoma and a small chromophobe adenoma. Most recently, Hamilton et al. have suggested that "Turcot syndrome" is a manifestation of pleiotropy in Familial Adenomatous Polyposis, rather than a distinct inherited condition [80]. In our own study of 280 patients from 11 families, we concluded that Gardner's syndrome represents a complete expression of a number of extracolonic manifestations that may be present in any patient with polyposis coli [56].

These extracolonic manifestations may be used to signal the need for additional clinical care in at-risk propositi. Table 4 lists many of these. Gardner [57] has established the importance of subcutaneous cysts and fibrous tumors as a marker for these patients from birth through later life. These skin growths, common in adults, appear during childhood, generally manifest on face or scalp, and may appear as isolated lesions [58]. Osteomas of the skull and jaw have been seen in children 5–10 years before the appearance of colon polyps [59]. Orthopantomography has demonstrated the presence of multiple small mandibular osteomas [60], and this relatively simple noninvasive examination has been suggested for screening of first-degree relatives [61]; however, age dependence and the occurrence of mandibulary osteomas have not been determined. Associated dental abnormalities, including impacted teeth, supernumerary teeth, congenitally missing teeth, and fused roots of first and second molars, occur in 80% of patients with familial polyposis coli and may also be used to recognize the relative at risk for polyposis coli [62].

Recently, benign ocular patches, identified as congenital hypertrophy of the retinal pigment epithelium (CHRPE) has been postulated as an ophthalmologic marker for polyposis coli [63]. In a study of four kindreds of patients Lewis et al. [64] found the CHRPE lesions to be familial, congenital, and multiple in nature as compared to the isolated fundus lesion seen in the general population. They found each child positive for CHRPE to have an involved parent. Negative testing for CHRPE did not mean the patient did not have or would not develop colonic polyps. The recent report by Berk et al. [65] revealed

TABLE 4.
Extracolonic Manifestations of Gardner's Syndrome

Soft tissue tumors
Osteomas
Dental abnormalities
CHRPE

CHRPE lesions in 87.5% of patients with polyposis coli regardless of other extracolonic manifestations. The authors are also following 11 offspring, eight of whom have CHRPE lesions, and one of whom has been diagnosed with polyposis coli. Additional follow-up will document the role of CHRPE as a phenotypic marker.

The inheritance pattern for all these manifestations is Mendelian dominant, not sex-linked, and they may be inherited from either sex, by either sex, in equal ratio. Each offspring of a FAP patient has a 50/50 chance of inheriting the disease, and, when the disease is present, the development of colon cancer is at a much earlier age than the usual sixth or seventh decade for sporadic colon cancer. Dukes [40] reported colon cancer arising at age 40 years for his patients, and cancer arose at an average age of 41 years in our series of patients [66]. Many reports have presented single cases of polyposis coli in which the patient had no apparently affected relatives. Freidell and Wakefield [43] saw a positive family history in only 50% of their patients. Dukes [67] found only one isolated person with polyposis coli among 11 of his 33 families. Reed and Neel [68] detected a solitary patient among their families with polyposis coli in 35.5% of their propositi. Utsunomiya and Iwama [69] reported that 46% of their families from the Japanese Polyposis Center had no affected patient other than the propositus; however, the proportion of these sporadic cases decreased as the survey progressed. In his classic monograph on the subject, Bussey [70] reported that 98 of 200 families in the St. Mark's Registry represented possible new mutations. He thought that this number, almost one-half, was abnormally high and that perhaps one-third of the new patients would be from mutations. He did find that mutations occurred in males more frequently than in females (at a ratio of 3:2). The Japanese Polyposis Registry reported a sex ratio of the proband of 1.7, with females less frequently affected with no significant difference in the patients other than the probands [69]. Our own experience has been different. With vigorous family data collection, including traveling about the country to interview relatives, we have only one propositus who presented as an isolated case. Thus one of 18 families with 1,155 patients at risk for the disease could be attributed to a mutation [71]. Supporting the possibility of increased mutations was a report of Veale [72] showing that birth rank was increased for the polyposis patients, as was paternal age. Both these factors contributed to the association of fresh mutations.

The question of whether familial polyposis coli and Gardner's syndrome are controlled at the same or at different DNA sequences has been studied [73]. Smith [74], in a careful evaluation, agreed that Gardner's syndrome, familial polyposis coli, and Turcot's syndrome were a "molecular disease" and were the expression of one genetic entity. Bussey [70] thought that all the polyposis coli syndromes were different degrees of manifestations of the Gardner's syndrome, which represented the full expression of the inherited disease. In 1983, Gardner [57] called the disease a "systemic overgrowth" problem with familial polyposis coli and Gardner's syndrome being different manifestations of the same underlying disease.

A great deal of work has gone into chromosome studies to identify and diagnose the patient with one of the inherited polyposis coli syndromes. Opinions have varied on the value of such studies [75]. In favor of a useful diagnostic criterion for the polyposis coli syndromes are the reports of chromosomal instability, i.e., presence of numeral and structural aberrations both in vivo in solid tumor and in vitro in cultured lymphocytes and fibroblasts. Increased tetraploidy is a feature of polyposis coli cells. However, similar observations led to the conclusion that chromosomal studies are not useful as a diagnostic test for familial polyposis coli [76]. Sandberg [75] in his review brought up the problem of "to what extent changes observed in vitro reflect cyto-genetic events in vivo remains an unknown entity."

In 1986, Herrera et al. [77] reported a 42-year-old man with mental retardation, colon polyps and carcinoma, horseshoe kidney, absence of left lobe of liver, agenesis of the gallbladder, and development of a fatal abdominal desmoid tumor after colectomy. Cultured peripheral blood cells showed a marker chromosome from deletion (5) (q13–q15) or cell (5) (q15–q22). A subsequent report by Bodmer et al. [78] showed that the familial adenomatous polyposis gene is on chromosome 5, most probably near band 5q21–q22. In December of 1987 Leppert et al. [79] presented work supporting the localization of the polyposis coli gene to the long arm of chromosome 5, probably in the region of 5q22. Needless to say, these exciting developments of an accurate gene marker for the polyposis coli syndromes would provide an invaluable diagnostic test to select the patient at risk for vigorous clinical screening to detect and prevent subsequent cancer development.

References

1. Fenoglio-Preiser CM, Hutter RV: Colorectal polyps: Pathologic diagnosis and clinical significance. Cancer 35:322–344, 1985.
2. Schmieden V, Westhues H: Zur Klinik und Pathologie der Dickdarm polypen und deren klinische und pathologish—anatomischen Beziehungen zum Dickdarmkarzinom. Deutsch Z Chir 202:1–124, 1927.
3. Wattenberg LW: A histochemical study of succinic dehydrogenase and cytochrome oxidase in proliferative lesions of the large intestine. Cancer Res 19:1118–1123, 1959.
4. Arthur JF: Structure and significance of metaplastic nodules in the rectal mucosa. J Clin Pathol 21:735–743, 1968.
5. Ronchod M, Lewin KJ, Dorfman RF: Lymphoid hyperplasia of the gastrointestinal tract: A study of 26 cases and review of the literature. Am J Surg Pathol 2:383–400, 1978.
6. Louw JH: Polypoid lesions of the large bowel in children with particular reference to benign lymphoid polyposis. J Pediatric Surg 3:195–209, 1968.
7. Daniel ES, Ludwig SL, Lewin KJ, Ruprecht RM, Rajacich GM, Schwabe AD: The Cronkhite-Canada syndrome and analysis of clinical and pathologic features and therapy in 55 patients. Medicine 61:293–309, 1982.
8. Katayama Y, Kimura M, Konn M: Cronkhite-Canada syndrome associated with a rectal cancer and adenomatous changes in colonic polyps. Am J Surg Pathol 9:65–71, 1985.
9. Verse M: Ueber die Hestogenes der Schleim hart carcinome. Vech Deutsch Ges Pathol 12:95, 1908.
10. Peutz JLA: Over een zeer merkwaardige gecombineerde familiare polyposis van de slijmvliezen van den tractus intestinalis met die van de neuskeelholte en gepaard met eigenaardige pigmentaties van huid-en slijmvliezen. Nederlandsh Maandschr Geneesckunde 10:134–146, 1921.
11. Jeghers H, McKusick VA, Kathy KH: Generalized intestinal polyposis and melasia spots of the oral mucosa, lips, and digits. N Engl J Med 241:993–1005, 1949.
12. Shrbata HR, Phillips MJ: Peutz-Jeghers syndrome with jejunal and colonic adenocarcinomas. Can Med Assoc J 103:285–287, 1970.
13. Dodd WJ, Schulte WJ, Hensley GT, et al.: Peutz-Jeghers syndrome and gastrointestinal malignancy. Am J Roentgenol Radium Ther Nuclear Med 115:374–377, 1972.
14. Scully RE: Sex-cord tumor with annular lubules: A distinctive ovarian tumor of the Peutz-Jeghers syndrome. Cancer 25:1107–1121, 1970.
15. Veale AMO, McColl I, Bussey HJR, Morson BC: Juvenile polyposis coli. J Med Genet 3:5–16, 1966.
16. Sachatello CR, Griffin WO: Hereditary polyposis disease of the gastrointestinal tract. Am J Surg 129:198–203, 1975.
17. Sachatello CR, Pechren JW, Grace JT: Generalized juvenile gastrointestinal polyposis. Gastroenterology 58:699–708, 1970.
18. Smilow PC, Pryor CA Jr, Svinton NW: Juvenile polyposis coli: A report of three patients in three generations in one family. Dis Colon Rectum 9:248–254, 1966.
19. Kaschula ROC: Mixed juvenile adenomatous and intermediate polyposis coli. Report of a case. Dis Colon Rectum 14:368–374, 1971.
20. Goodman IO, Yardley JH, Milligan FD: Pathogenesis of colonic polyps in multiple juvenile polyposis. Report of a case associated with gastric polyps and carcinoma of the rectum. Cancer 43:1906–1913, 1979.
21. Friedman CJ, Fehner RE: A solitary juvenile polyp with hyperplastic and adenomatous glands. Digest Dis Sci 27:946–948, 1982.
22. Lloyd KM, Dennis M: Cowden's disease. A possible new symptom complex with multiple system involvement. Ann Intern Med 58:136–142, 1963.
23. Ortonne JP, Lambert R, Daudet J, Berthet P, Gianadda E: Involvement of the digestive tract in Cowden's disease. Int J Dermatol 19:570–576, 1980.
24. Walton BJ, Morain WD, Baughman RD, Jordan A, Crichlow RW: Cowden's disease: A further indication for prophylactic mastectomy. Surgery 99:82–86, 1986.
25. Donnelly WH, Seeber WK, Yunis EJ: Polypoid ganglioneurofibromatosis of the large bowel. Arch Pathol 87:537–541, 1969.
26. Mendelshon G, Diamond MP: Familial ganglioneuromatous polyposis of the large bowel. Am J Surg Pathol 8:515–520, 1984.
27. Snover DC, Weigent CE, Sumner HW: Diffuse/Mucosal ganglioneuromatosis of the colon associated with adenocarcinoma. Am J Clin Pathol 75:225–229, 1981.
28. Carney JA, Go VL, Sizemore GW, Hayles AB: Alimentary tract ganglioneuromatosis. A major component of the syndrome of multiple endocrine neoplasia type 2B. N Engl J Med 295:1287–1291, 1976.
29. Knudson AG: Mutation and cancer: Statistical study of retinoblastoma. Proc Natl Acad Sci USA 68:820–823, 1971.
30. Perkins JT, Blackstone MO, Riddell RH: Adenomatous polyposis coli and multiple endocrine neoplasia type 2B. Cancer 55:375–381, 1985.

31. Burt RW, Bishop T, Cannon LA, Dowdle MA, Lee AG, Sholneds MH: Dominant inheritance of adenomatous colonic polyps and colorectal cancer. N Engl J Med 312:1540–1544, 1985.

32. Lynch HT, Harris RE, Organ CH, et al.: The surgeon, genetics, and cancer control: The cancer family syndrome. Ann Surg 16:434–440, 1977.

33. Torre O: Multiple sebaceous tumors. Arch Dermatol 98:549–551, 1968.

34. Muir EG, Bell AJY, Barlow KA: Multiple primary carcinomata of the colon, duodenum, and larynx associated with kerato-acanthomata of the face. Br J Surg 54:191–195, 1967.

35. Lynch HT, Lynch PM, Pester J, Fusaro RM: The cancer family syndrome: Rare cutaneous phenotypic linkage of Torre's syndrome. Arch Intern Med 141:607–611, 1981.

36. Cripps WH: Two cases of disseminated polyps of the rectum. Trans Pathol Soc London 33:165–168, 1882.

37. Smith T: Three cases of disseminated polyps of the lower bowel occurring in one family. St Bartholonew's Hosp Reg 23:225–229, 1882.

38. Handford H: Disseminated polypi of the large intestines becoming malignant with stricture (malignant adenoma) of the rectum and of the splenic flexure of the colon: Secondary growths in the liver. Trans Pathol Soc London 41:133–137, 1890.

39. Cokayne EA: Heredity in relation to cancer. Cancer Rev 2:337–347, 1927.

40. Dukes C: The hereditary factor in polyposis intestini or multiple adenomata. Cancer Rev 5:241–256, 1930.

41. Lockhart-Mummery JP, Dukes CE: Familial adenomatosis of the colon and rectum: Its relationship to cancer. Lancet 2:586–589, 1939.

42. McKenney DC: Multiple polyposis: Congenital heredofamilial malignant. Am J Surg 46:204–216, 1939.

43. Friedell MT, Wakefield EG: Familial Polyposis of the Colon. J. AMA 1943; 121:830.

44. Guptill P: Familial polyposis of the colon: Two families, five cases. Surgery 22:286–304, 1947.

45. Devic A, Bussey HR: Un cas de polypose adenomateuse generalisee a tout de L'intestin. Arch Mal App Digest 6:278–289, 1912.

46. Cabot RC: Case records of the Massachusetts General Hospital: Case no. 21061. N Engl J Med 212:263–267, 1935.

47. Miller RH, Sweet RH: Multiple polyposis of colon: Familial disease. Ann Surg 105:511–515, 1937.

48. Fitzgerald GM: Multiple composite odontomes coincidental with other tumorous conditions: Report of a case. J Am Dent Assoc 30:1408–1417, 1943.

49. Gardner EJ, Stephens FE: Cancer of the lower digestive tract in one family group. Am J Hum Genet 2:41–48, 1950.

50. Gardner EJ: A genetic and clinical study of intestinal polyposis, a predisposing factor for carcinoma of the colon and rectum. Am J Hum Genet 3:167–176, 1951.

51. Gardner EJ, Plenk HP: Hereditary pattern for multiple osteomas in a family group. Am J Hum Genet 4:31–36, 1952.

52. Gardner EJ, Richards RC: Multiple cutaneous and subcutaneous lesions occurring simultaneously with hereditary polyposis and osteomatosis. Am J Hum Genet 5:137–147, 1953.

53. Plenk HP, Gardner EJ: Osteomatosis (leontiosis ossea): Herditary disease of membranous bone formation association in one family with polyposis of the colon. Radiology 62:830–840, 1954.

54. MacDonald JM, Davis WC, Crago HR, Turcot J, Despres JP, St Piere F: Gardner's syndrome and periamullary malignancy. Am J Surg 113:425–430, 1967.

55. Turcot J, Despres JP, St. Pierre F: Malignant tumors of the central nervous system associated with familial polyposis of the colon: A report of two cases. Dis Colon Rectum 2:465–468, 1959.

56. Watne AL, Core S, Carrier JM: Gardner's syndrome. Surg Gynecol Obstet 141:53–56, 1975.

57. Gardner EJ: Familial polyposis coli and Gardner's syndrome. Is there a difference? In Ingall JRF, Mastromarino AJ (eds): "Prevention of Hereditary Large Bowel Cancer." New York: Alan R. Liss, Inc., 1983, pp 39–60.

58. Cohen SB, Pauledes GP, Krush AJ, Levin LS: Familial polyposis coli. Maryland State Med J 27(7):64–67, 1978.

59. Watne AL, Lai HY, Carrier J, Coppala W: The diagnosis and surgical treatment of patients with Gardner's syndrome. Surgery 82:327–333, 1977.

60. Utsunomiya J, Nakamura T: The occult osteomatous changes in the mandible in patients with familial polyposis coli. Br J Surg 62:45–51, 1975.

61. Bulow S, Holm NV, Sondergaard JO, Witt IN, Tetens G: Manidibular osteomas in unaffected sibs and children of patients with familial polyposis coli. Scand J Gastroenterol 21:744–748, 1986.

62. Carl W, Herrera L: Dental and bone abnormalities in patients with familial polyposis coli. Semin Surg Oncol 3:77–83, 1987.

63. Blair NP, Trempe CL: Hypertrophy of the retinal pigment epithelium associated with Gardner's syndrome. Am J Ophthalmol 90:661–667, 1980.

64. Lewis RA, Crowder WE, Eierman LA, Nussbaum RL, Ferrell RE: The Gardner syndrome. Significance of ocular features. Ophthalmology 91:916–925, 1984.

65. Berk T, Cohen Z, McLeod RS, Parker JA: Congenital hypertrophy off the retinal pigment epithelium, as a marker for familial adenomatous polyposis. Dis Colon Rectum 31:253–257, 1988.

66. Watne AL: Syndromes of intestinal polyposis. Curr Prob Surg 24:271–340, 1987.

67. Dukes CE: Familial intestinal polyposis. Ann Eugen 17:1–29, 1952.

68. Reed TE, Neel JA: A genetic study of multiple polyposis of the colon (with an appendix deriving a method of estimating relative fitness). Am J Hum Genet 7:236–263, 1955.

69. Utsunomiya J, Iwama T: Adenomatosis coli in Japan. In Winawer SJ, Schottenfield D, Sherlock P (eds): "Colorectal Cancer: Prevention, Epidemiology, and Screening." New York: Raven Press, 1980, pp 83–95.

70. Bussey HJR: "Familial Polyposis Coli." Baltimore: Johns Hopkins University Press, 1975.

71. Watne AL: Patterns of inheritance of colonic polyps. Semin Surg Oncol 3:71–76, 1987.

72. Veale AMO: "Intestinal Polyposis." Cambridge: Cambridge University Press, 1965.

73. Kussin SZ, Lipkin M, Winawer SJ: Inherited colon cancer: Clinical implications. Am J Gastroenterol 72:448–457, 1979.

74. Smith WG: Familial multiple polyposis: Research tool for investigating the etiology of carcinoma of the colon. Dis Colon Rectum 11:17–31, 1968.

75. Sandberg AA: Chromosomal abnormalities in patients with familial polyposis and colorectal cancer. Semin Surg Oncol 3:133–136, 1987.

76. Nielsen KB, Balow S, Tommerrey N: Chromosomal studies in familial polyposis coli. Cancer Genet Cytogenet 17:355–357, 1985.

77. Herrera L, Kakati S, Gebas L, Pietzak E, Sandberg AA: Brief clinical report: Gardner syndrome in man with an interstital delection of 5q. Am J Med Genet 25:473–476, 1986.

78. Bodmer WF, Bailey CJ, Bodmer J, Bussey HJR, Ellis A, Gorman P, Lucibella FC, Murday VA, Rider SA, Scambler P, Sheer D, Soloman E, Spurr NK: Localization of the gene for familial adenomatosus polyposis on chromosome 5. Nature 328:614–619, 1987.

79. Leppert M, Dobbs M, Scrambler P, O'Connell P, Naksamara Y, Stauffer I, Woodward S, Burt R, Hughes J, Gardner E, Lathrop M, Wasmuth J, Talouel JM, White R: The gene for familial polyposis coli maps to the long arm of chromosome 5. Science 238:1411–1413, 1987.

80. Hamilton SR, Krush AJ, Taqui F, Giardello FM, Bookr SV: The third meeting of the Leed's Castle Polyposis Group. Proceedings, June 1989.

5

Histopathologic Considerations in the Adenoma–Carcinoma Sequence

Stanley R. Hamilton

Department of Pathology and Oncology Center, The Johns Hopkins University School of Medicine and Hospital, Baltimore, Maryland

INTRODUCTION

The phenotypic hallmark of adenomatous polyposis syndrome is the occurrence of hundreds to thousands of adenomas in the large bowel, usually during childhood or adolescence. The natural history of the syndrome is characterized by the eventual development of colorectal adenocarcinoma in virtually all untreated, affected patients, i.e., an adenoma–carcinoma sequence. Adenomas also appear to be the usual precursor to adenocarcinoma in hereditary nonpolyposis colorectal cancer syndrome (Lynch's syndrome) and in ordinary "sporadic" colorectal carcinoma (recent reports suggest that heredity also plays an important role in seemingly sporadic cases). Histopathologic considerations in the adenoma–carcinoma sequence include three aspects: 1) occurrence of adenomas as a marker for risk of colorectal carcinoma, 2) characteristics of adenomas as markers for synchronous and metachronous colorectal neoplasms, and 3) management of patients with adenocarcinoma found in a colonoscopic polypectomy specimen.

OCCURRENCE OF ADENOMAS AS A MARKER FOR RISK OF COLORECTAL CARCINOMA

The occurrence of numerous adenomas is well known to be a definitive phenotypic marker for affected patients among persons at risk for adenomatous polyposis syndrome [1]. In any patient with a polyp (generic term for a localized structure protruding above the mucosal surface), the first consideration in clinical management is histopathologic classification. Adenomas show characteristic dysplastic epithelium, representing unequivocal neoplastic epithelial proliferation, and are usually recognized easily by pathologists. However, the differential diagnosis of polyps, and of polyposis if multiple polyps are present, must be considered in each patient (Table 1).

In the past, colorectal adenocarcinoma in patients with hereditary nonpolyposis colorectal cancer syndrome was said to arise "de novo," i.e., in the absence of a precursor adenoma. Some patients with the syndrome have adenomas synchronous with colorectal carcinoma (S.R. Hamilton, unpublished observations), and recently a prospective study of at-risk persons showed that affected patients do, in fact, develop adenomas. These adenomas have been reported to have a propensity to grow in plaque-like fashion, making their endoscopic detection difficult, and have been termed "flat adenomas" [2]. As a result, it appears that the occurrence of an adenoma in an at-risk member of a pedigree with hereditary nonpolyposis colorectal cancer syndrome provides a phenotypic marker for an affected patient who probably requires prophylactic colectomy. The clinical situation is thus analogous to the patient with multiple adenomas in a pedigree with adenomatous polyposis syndrome.

The occurrence of an adenoma is also well known to be a risk factor for colorectal carci-

Familial Adenomatous Polyposis, pages 35–41

TABLE 1.
Histopathologic Classification of Polyposis

Inflammatory polyps
Multiple inflammatory (pseudo) polyps in chronic idiopathic inflammatory bowel disease and schistosomiasis
Nodular lymphoid hyperplasia with combined variable immunodeficiency
Juvenile polyposis(?)
Cronkhite-Canada syndrome(?)
Hamartomatous polyps
Peutz-Jeghers syndrome
Juvenile polyposis(?)
Cronkhite-Canada syndrome(?)
Neurofibromatosis/ganglioneuromatosis
Hyperplastic (metaplastic) polyps
Neoplastic polyps
Adenomatous polyposis syndrome (>100 colorectal adenomas)
Lymphoma/leukemia
Kaposi's sarcoma
Carcinoid tumors

noma and adenoma in persons with no apparent family history. Recent studies have suggested that these seemingly ordinary, sporadic cases may often have a familial basis, possibly autosomal dominant inheritance [3]. Thus adenomas may be clinical markers in individual patients and in pedigrees.

CHARACTERISTICS OF ADENOMAS AS MARKERS FOR SYNCHRONOUS AND METACHRONOUS COLORECTAL NEOPLASMS

Larger size, greater proportion of villous architecture, and greater severity of dysplasia have been known for many years to be associated with higher prevalence of adenocarcinoma in an adenoma [4]. In addition, these characteristics may be related to the risk of synchronous (simultaneous) and metachronous (subsequent) colorectal neoplasms. For example, in one study of colectomy specimens containing carcinoma and synchronous adenoma, patients who developed metachronous carcinoma showed higher grades of dysplasia in the initial synchronous adenoma than those patients who did not develop carcinoma subsequently [5]. Another study showed that "carcinoma in situ" was almost seven times more frequent in adenomas in resection specimens containing adenocarcinoma than in adenomas excised as solitary lesions [6]. In another study, patients with adenoma showing "carcinoma in situ" had a higher rate of synchronous colorectal carcinomas than those with less severe dysplasia [7]. Thus the presence of high-grade dysplasia (so-called "carcinoma in situ") in an adenoma may mark a patient population at higher risk for synchronous and metachronous colorectal neoplasms than patients whose adenomas show lesser grades of dysplasia. Retrospective studies have suggested that the occurrence of both synchronous and metachronous carcinoma also increases with the number of adenomas [4,8]. A large prospective study, the National Polyp Study, will probably provide more definitive answers about the utility of adenoma characteristics as clinical markers in individual patients.

MANAGEMENT OF PATIENTS WITH ADENOCARCINOMA FOUND IN A COLONOSCOPIC POLYPECTOMY SPECIMEN

The pathology of colonoscopic polypectomy specimens is an important determinant of clinical management, and interaction between clinicians and pathologists is essential. The pathologist's role in the process (Table 2) begins with appropriate specimen processing. Procedures are described in various textbooks of surgical pathology and gastrointestinal pathology. Microscopic assessment of the resulting histopathologic sections includes consideration of pseudocarcinomatous epithelial entrapment [9,10], which may be difficult to distinguish from carcinoma (Table 3). Reporting of findings is as important as the microscopic assessment of the specimen, because clinical decision-making is based in part on the surgical pathology report. An important consideration in this regard is use of the term "carcinoma." In the large bowel, the occurrence of metastases is extremely rare unless the tumor has breeched the muscularis mucosae (Fig. 1) and involved the submucosa [11,12]. In contrast to gastric adenocarcinoma, colorectal carcinoma does not seem to have access to the lymphatics in the lamina propria and muscularis mucosae. As a result, morphologic carcinoma confined to the epithelium (''carcinoma in situ'') or invading only the lamina propria (''intramucosal carcinoma'') does not behave clinically as malignant tumor. As a result, the term ''carcinoma'' is best

TABLE 2.
Pathologist's Role in Assessment of Colonoscopic Polypectomy Specimens

Appropriate specimen processing
Describe size and configuration
Fix and section to show stalk
Embed in entirety
Cut multiple sections from each block
Microscopic assessment
Evaluate characteristics of adenoma and carcinoma if present
Consider pseudocarcinomatous epithelial entrapment
Reporting of findings
Carcinoma (invasion through muscularis mucosae—don't use the "c" word unless you really mean it)
Grade of differentiation
Depth of invasion
Angiolymphatic involvement
Transection of, or proximity to, margin of excision
Adenoma
Architecture
High-grade dysplasia
Completeness of excision
Discussion with endoscopist/surgeon

TABLE 3.
Criteria Favoring Pseudocarcinomatous Epithelial Entrapment

Lamina propria-type connective tissue and muscularis mucosae, rather than desmoplastic fibrous tissue, surrounding the worrisome glands
Comparable severity of dysplasia between the worrisome glands and those in the remainder of the adenoma
Prominent hemosiderin deposition
Cystic dilatation of the worrisome glands

restricted to those tumors that involve the submucosa because of the emotive clinical implications of ''carcinoma'' despite virtual absence of metastasis with ''carcinoma in situ'' or ''intramucosal carcinoma'' alone [12].

Approximately 3% of polypectomy specimens will be found to contain a carcinoma [13] (also, S.R. Hamilton, unpublished data). In such cases, questions will be raised about the need for the patient to undergo further therapy, usually surgical resection. As a result, pathologic reporting of appropriate criteria is needed. The rationale for the clinical decisions is based on the mechanisms of spread of large bowel cancer. These tumors extend by direct invasion or gain access to lymphatic vessels and/or veins that are portal vein tributaries to produce lymph node and hepatic metastases, respectively. Thus a patient who has undergone polypectomy, with the specimen containing a carcinoma, may have residual disease at the polypectomy site, local metastases in the wall or in the regional lymph nodes, or distant metastases. Surgical resection has the potential to remove all residual tumor and local or regional metastases, thereby prolonging the patient's life. On the other hand, morbidity and mortality are associated with general anesthesia and colonic resection, and disseminated disease from distant metastases may already be present. As a result, the potential benefit to the patient must be weighed against the operative risk.

A large number of studies have evaluated criteria that may predict the presence of residual or locally metastatic tumor whose resection would be beneficial to the patient [reviewed in 14, 15]. Unfortunately, these studies use variable criteria and sometimes reach conflicting conclusions. Furthermore, a large number of factors enter into the decision-making process, as illustrated in Table 4.

No hard and fast criteria are yet available, and many of the reported criteria represent interrelated features (e.g., poorly differentiated carcinomas often show angiolymphatic involvement, as illustrated in Fig. 1). In addition, there is disagreement about some criteria [12,16,17]. For example, in a study from St. Mark's Hospital,

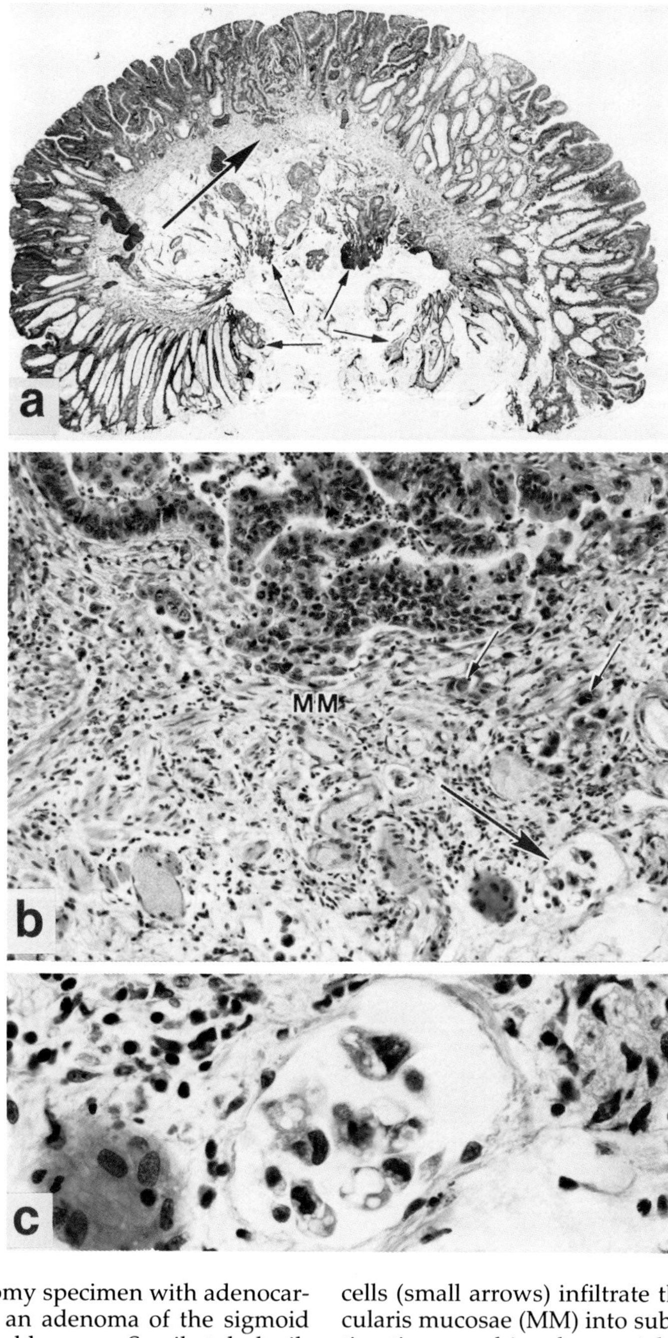

Fig. 1. Polypectomy specimen with adenocarcinoma arising in an adenoma of the sigmoid colon in a 64-year-old man. **a:** Sessile tubulovillous adenoma contains a focus of adenocarcinoma in the area indicated by the large arrow (see b). The margin of excision is indicated by small arrows and shows cautery artifact on nonadenomatous epithelium and submucosal connective tissue. Hematoxylin-eosin. ×15. **b:** Area indicated by large arrow in a. Poorly differentiated adenocarcinoma is present in the lamina propria and submucosa. Individual tumor cells (small arrows) infiltrate through the muscularis mucosae (MM) into submucosal connective tissue and involve angiolymphatic spaces, as indicated by large arrow (see c). Hematoxylin-eosin. ×155. **c:** Angiolymphatic space indicated by large arrow in b. Individual mucin-containing tumor cells are present in this lymphatic space. Hematoxylin-eosin. ×350. This patient underwent segmental resection; no residual or metastatic colorectal carcinoma was found at laparotomy or in the resection specimen.

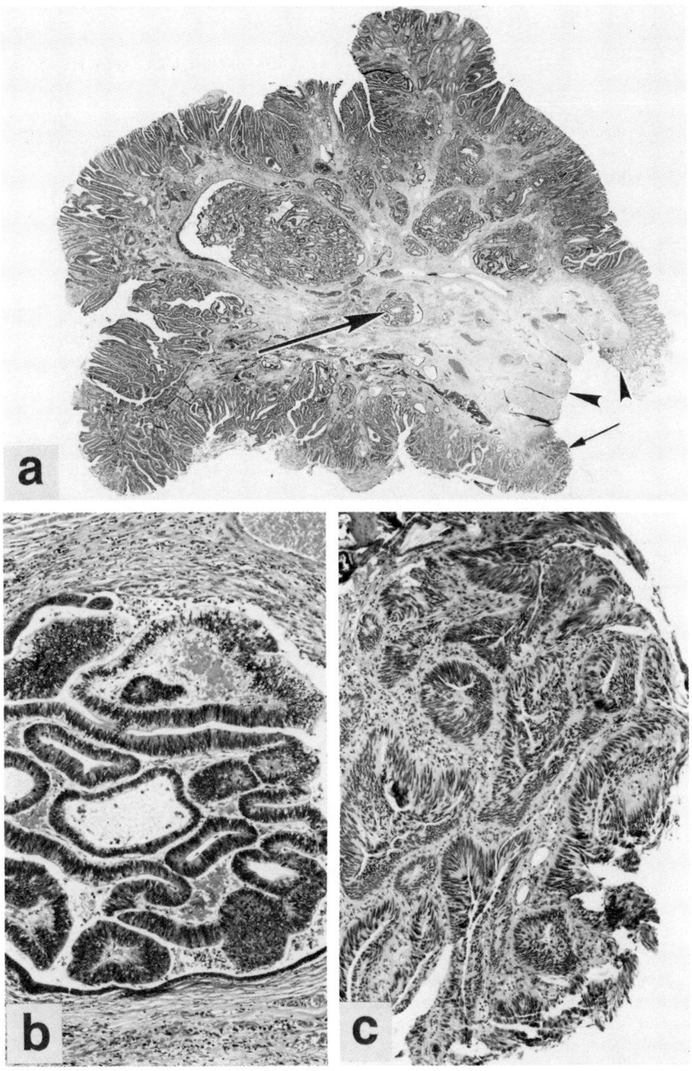

Fig. 2. Polypectomy specimen with adenocarcinoma arising in an adenoma of the sigmoid colon in a 59-year-old man. **a:** Pedunculated villous adenoma contains gland-forming adenocarcinoma, which invades the submucosa of the head of the polyp. The greatest depth of extension is indicated by the large arrow (see b). The margin of excision is indicated by cautery artifact on adenomatous epithelium in the area indicated by the small arrow (see c) and on submucosal connective tissue and nonadenomatous mucosa in the area indicated by arrowheads. Hematoxylin-eosin. ×7. **b:** Moderately differentiated gland-forming adenocarcinoma in the submucosa in area indicated by large arrow in a. Hematoxylin-eosin. ×75. **c:** Margin of excision with adenomatous epithelium in area indicated by small arrow in b. The adenomatous epithelium shows cautery artifact and high-grade dysplasia morphologically equivalent to "carcinoma in situ." Hematoxylin-eosin. ×75. Follow-up sigmoidoscopy showed no residual tumor. (Follow-up examination courtesy of Dr. Hon-Chiu Yu.)

patients with apparently transected, incompletely excised carcinoma had no evidence of unsatisfactory outcome in a follow-up study [16]. In part, this result may be due to the effects of electrocautery (Fig. 2). The specimen that the pathologist examines is not entirely representative of what is removed from the patient. Because of tissue necrosis associated with cautery, additional tissue that will not be examined pathologically is ''excised'' from the patient by sloughing into the lumen of the large bowel. Thus, despite the histopathologic appearance of incomplete excision, it is not uncommon to find no evidence of residual carcinoma or adenoma on reexamination and biopsy. As another consideration, level of invasion relative to the bowel wall is often difficult to define histopathologically [12], as is the configuration of the adenoma. Finally, most of the studies are retrospective and include patients assessed for outcome on the basis of findings at colectomy as well as follow-up alone after polypectomy. Thus the validity of the criteria remains to be established. Table 5 represents our current criteria favoring resection.

TABLE 4.
Factors in Decision-Making for Surgical Resection After Colonoscopic Polypectomy With the Specimen Showing Carcinoma

Probability of residual disease and local metastases in the absence of distant metastases
Operative efficacy in "curing" residual and locally metastatic disease (few data available)
Operative mortality
Operative morbidity
Medical economics
Life expectancy of patient
Patient preference

The clinician responsible for management of the patient is in the uncomfortable position of having to take the histopathologic information provided by the pathologist and then factor in the patient characteristics in a ''risk-benefit'' type of analysis regarding surgical resection. The reported criteria favoring resection have high

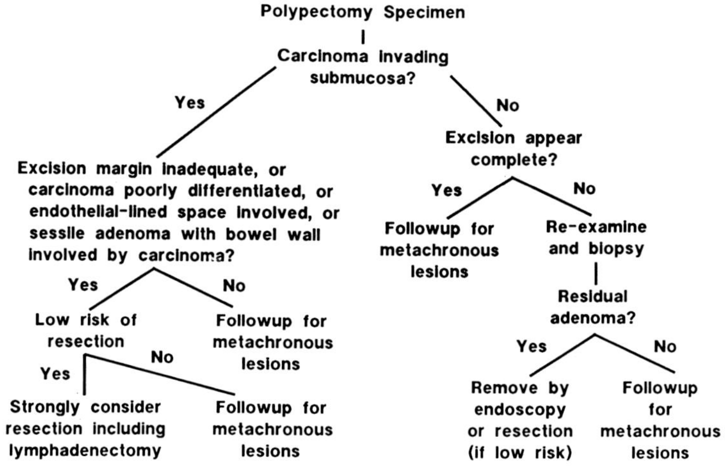

Fig. 3. An approach to management of a patient with adenocarcinoma found in a colonoscopic polypectomy specimen.

TABLE 5.
Histopathologic Criteria Favoring Surgical Resection After Colonoscopic Polypectomy With the Specimen Showing Carcinoma

Incomplete excision:	Carcinoma at or adjoining excision margin as evidenced by cautery artifact
Poor differentiation:	"Grade III" poorly differentiated, signet-ring cell, or mucinous carcinoma
Angiolymphatic involvement:	Carcinoma in endothelial-lined space representing lymphatic or blood vessel
Sessile configuration:	Involvement of wall likely from shape of tumor

sensitivity and high predictive value of a negative result; i.e., if all patients showing these criteria undergo resection, very few will have poor outcome as defined by subsequent recurrent carcinoma. Furthermore, one study based on theoretical mathematical modeling suggested that all patients at low risk of operative mortality should undergo resection [18]. On the other hand, the criteria show low specificity and predictive value of a positive result, indicating that they identify patients with poor prognosis at the expense of "unneeded" surgery in a relatively high proportion of cases. Careful explanation of these circumstances to the patient and family is necessary. Malpractice suits have resulted from "unnecessary" surgery when no residual tumor or locally or regionally metastatic carcinoma was found (S.R. Hamilton, unpublished observations). The results of further studies should help to clarify this difficult management problem. Our current approach to management is summarized in Figure 3; the importance of pathologic reporting in decision-making is evident.

References

1. Bussey HJR: "Familial Polyposis Coli. Family Studies, Histopathology, Differential Diagnosis, and Results of Treatment." Baltimore; The Johns Hopkins University Press, 1975.
2. Lynch HT, Smyrk T, Lanspa SJ, Marcus JN, Kriegler M, Lynch JF, Appelman HD: Flat adenomas in a colon cancer-prone kindred. JNCI 80:278–282, 1988.
3. Cannon-Albright LA, Skolnick MH, Bishop T, Lee RG, Burt RW: Common inheritance of susceptibility to colorectal cancers. N Engl J Med 319:533–537, 1988.
4. Muto T, Bussey HJR, Morson BC: The evolution of cancer of the colon and rectum. Cancer 36:2251–2270, 1975.
5. Morson BC, Konishi F: Contribution of the pathologist to the radiology and management of colorectal polyps. Gastrointest Radiol 7:275–281, 1982.
6. Kalus M: Carcinoma and adenomatous polyps of the rectum and biopsy and organ tissue culture. Cancer 30:972–981, 1972.
7. Rittenhouse MC, Copeland EM: Carcinoma in situ of the distal part of the colon and of the rectum. Surg Gynecol Obstet 146:225–229, 1978.
8. Shinya H, Wolff WI: Morphology, anatomic distribution, and cancer potential of colonic polyps. Ann Surg 190:679–683, 1979.
9. Greene FL: Epithelial misplacement in adenomatous polyps of the colon and rectum. Cancer 33:206–217, 1974.
10. Muto T, Bussey HJR, Morson BC: Pseudo-carcinomatous invasion in adenomatous polyps of the colon and rectum. J Clin Pathol 26:25–31, 1976.
11. Fenoglio CM, Kay GI, Lane N: Distribution of human colonic lymphatics in normal, hyperplastic and adenomatous tissue. Its relationship to metastasis from small carcinomas in pedunculated adenomas, with two case reports. Gastroenterology 46:51–66, 1973.
12. Haggitt RC, Glotzbach RE, Soffer EE, Wruble LD: Prognostic factors in colorectal carcinomas arising in adenomas: Implications for lesions removed by endoscopic polypectomy. Gastroenterology 89:328–336, 1985.
13. Gillespie PE, Chambers TJ, Chan KW, Doronzo F, Morson BC, Williams CB: Colonic adenomas—A colonoscopic survey. Gut 20:240–245, 1979.
14. Marcial MA: Colorectal adenomas: Identification and management. Bol Asoc Med Puerto Rico 78:287–292, 1986.
15. Listrom MB, Fenoglio-Preiser CM: The malignant polyp. An analysis of the procedures for handling polyps. Endosc Rev September-October, 1985, pp 21–37.
16. Morson BC, Whiteway JE, Jones EA, Macrae FA, Williams CB: Histopathology and prognosis of malignant colorectal polyps treated by endoscopic polypectomy. Gut 25:437–444, 1984.
17. Cranley JP, Petras RE, Carey WD, Paradis K, Sivak MV: When is endoscopic polypectomy adequate therapy for colonic polyps containing invasive carcinoma? Gastroenterology 91:419–427, 1986.
18. Wilcox GM, Beck JR: Early invasive cancer in adenomatous colonic polyps ("malignant polyps"). Evaluation of the therapeutic options by decision analysis. Gastroenterology 92:1159–1168, 1987.

6

Development of a Genetics Registry: Hereditary Intestinal Polyposis and Hereditary Colon Cancer Registry at the Johns Hopkins Hospital, 1973–1988

Anne J. Krush and Francis M. Giardiello

Divisions of Medical Genetics (A.J.K.) and Gastroenterology (F.M.G.), Department of Medicine, The Johns Hopkins University School of Medicine, Baltimore, Maryland

CREATION OF THE REGISTRY

In the summer of 1972, the National Large Bowel Cancer Project was organized by the National Cancer Institute of the National Cancer Institute of the National Institutes of Health, with the objective to support both basic and clinical research leading to the prevention and control of large bowel cancer. Dr. Murray N. Copeland at the M.D. Anderson Hospital and Tumor Institute, Houston, was appointed Program Director, and Dr. Rulon W. Rawson was appointed Associate Director and Chairman of the Working Cadre [Copeland, 1975].

Research concerning large bowel cancer was encouraged through grants; an application for one, entitled Families at High Risk of Colorectal Cancer, was submitted by the Johns Hopkins Hospital, and funding was awarded for a 3 year period. The Johns Hopkins Familial Polyposis and Hereditary Colon Cancer Registry was then established in 1973.

AIMS AND OBJECTIVES OF THE STUDY

The initial and continuing aims of the Polyposis and Hereditary Colon Cancer Project are the following.

1. To study the natural history and genetics of precancerous and cancerous lesions of the large bowel, particularly familial adenomatous polyposis coli (FAP)
2. To establish a regional registry of families to detect those with the disorders and to follow the at-risk family members
3. To investigate the sensitivity and specificity of clinical, radiological, cytologic, endoscopic, and immunological methods of detecting malignant change
4. To study the premalignant characteristics of colonic epithelium in persons carrying the mutant gene(s) and to explore the mechanism by which they lead to cancer

HISTORICAL ASPECTS OF THE DEVELOPMENT OF POLYPOSIS REGISTRIES

When the Johns Hopkins Registry was begun in 1973, it was not called a registry; it was called simply The Polyposis Study. As early as 1975, however, groups working with polyposis patients in other cities of the United States and Canada conferred with and visited us to learn how we managed the information concerning the polyposis families in our "registry."

In 1982, a conference was arranged by Dr. John R.F. Ingall of the Comprehensive Cancer Center in Detroit and Dr. Anthony Mastromarino

Familial Adenomatous Polyposis, pages 43–59

of the National Large Bowel Cancer Project in Houston to consider The Prevention of Hereditary Large Bowel Cancer and the possibility of establishing a National Registry. It was decided to call our registries, collectively, a "National Pedigree and Linkage Data Bank to Facilitate Prevention of Hereditary Large Bowel Cancer" and to seek funding for this project at a future date [Cohen, 1983]. In the meantime, each registry was to try to standardize the computerization of its medical and demographic information.

In 1983, a meeting of registry coordinators was held at Memorial Sloan-Kettering Cancer Center in New York City to discuss standardization and pooling of information from polyposis registries (or data banks). Consensus among the conference participants included 1) the need for a one-page computerized data sheet for each person in the registry. Included on this page would be research interests and studies in progress at the institution. 2) Requests for biological specimens from another institution for research purposes should be addressed directly to the polyposis registry coordinator to preserve the relationships with family members. In no case should the requesting group contact such individuals without the permission and cooperation of the second institution. 3) Surveillance or follow-up of affected and at-risk family members should be computerized. 4) Other pages of information would include all results of examinations, placed only in the institution's registry, *not* in the pooled registry. Although the question of confidentiality of a regional or national registry was raised, the consensus was that it could be adequately safeguarded.

IDENTIFICATION OF PATIENTS AND FAMILIES

Families to be identified were those with members at high risk for hereditary colon cancer. They included the hereditary polyposes and hereditary colon cancer occurring before age 40 years, in the nearby six-state area (Maryland, Delaware, Virginia, West Virginia, New Jersey, Pennsylvania, and the District of Columbia).

All first- and second-degree relatives at risk for polyps and/or colon cancer were to be urged to have a complete physical examination, including examination of the colon. The at-risk family members were to be placed on follow-up for longitudinal estimation of the cumulative risk for malignancy. Specific entities within these categories of families (such as those with desmoids or tumors of specific sites) were to be identified and the genetics of each studied.

Channels of access of patients within the Johns Hopkins Hospital included 1) patients who had received treatment at this institution for one of the hereditary intestinal polyposes from 1963 to 1973, 2) families recorded in the medical genetic register of the Moore Genetics Clinic, and 3) referrals of hospitalized and clinic FAP and hereditary colon cancer patients by staff physicians. Channels of access outside the institution included 1) referrals from physicians in the six-state area who were aware of the ongoing polyposis study at our institution and 2) letters of inquiry sent to area physicians asking for names of patients in their practice with one of the hereditary kinds of polyposis (Appendix A). Physicians who were polled included general practitioners, family practice physicians, gastroenterologists, internists, surgeons, pathologists, dermatologists, and dentists. With 7,000 letters sent, 642 responses were received; 214 physicians identified such patients in their practice. Since this was only 9% of the total number, it was assumed that many of the 6,300 physicians who did not respond had not treated patients with FAP. 3) Because we were confident that not all the physicians in the area who were treating patients with polyposis had received the original letter of request, letters of inquiry were sent to medical records departments and the administrators of 378 accredited hospitals in the area asking for a list of all their patients who had received treatment for one of the hereditary polyposes during a specified period of time (Appendix B). (However, the 1979 International Classification of Diseases, 9th Revision, Clinical Modification [ICDA.9.CM] does not code specific diagnoses such as familial polyposis coli or Gardner syndrome but lists only benign and malignant neoplasms of specific sites in the intestinal tract.) The hereditary intestinal polyposes can usually be found in the categories 211.3,

211.4, and 211.9. Our conclusion, from visits to seven of the 72 hospitals that had granted us permission to abstract records, was that, unless specific hereditary polyposis diagnoses (excluding the hereditary single or scattered discrete polyp diagnoses) can be located in medical records departments, it is not efficient use of time to abstract records at outside hospitals (Table 1).

In December, 1978, following an interview with one of the principal investigators of the polyposis project at our institution, the Associated Press erroneously released the following item to newspapers throughout the United States.

> Researchers at the genetics center at Johns Hopkins Hospital are looking for people who suffer from hereditary colon cancer. They hope to learn enough to design a diagnostic test for early identification of the disease, which is now undetectable before cancerous growths appear.
>
> A son or daughter has a 50-50 chance of inheriting the disease from a parent who has it. The growths do not appear until adulthood and often people who have the disease bear children before they know they have it.

That article, followed by a radio announcement by Paul Harvey, resulted in our receiving more than 100 letters and phone calls from individuals from all parts of the United States. From them, we added 11 new FAP families to our registry and about 100 families with hereditary colon cancer. If one is asked to publicize his registry, we suggest that he make sure that the information is correctly interpreted, because, at the time of this release, the mechanism of inheritance of colon cancer was not certain.

INCOMPLETE ASCERTAINMENT

Even after 15 years, we do not have complete ascertainment of all families in the area with FAP or hereditary colon cancer. Physicians are being made aware of our registry through articles prepared for state medical journals [Cohen et al. 1978], research articles in medical journals, publications from the registry in a newsletter entitled "Newsletter: G.I. Polyposis & Related Conditions," and booklets concerning polyposis and colon cancer that we send to patients as well as their physicians.

OBTAINING MEDICAL INFORMATION: CONFIDENTIALITY

The matter of confidentiality of records should be considered carefully when obtaining medical

TABLE 1.
Patients With Hereditary Polyposis Ascertained by Abstracting Medical Records*

Location	Number of records abstracted	Patients with single discrete polyps	Patients with hereditary polyposis	Percent of total with hereditary polyposis	Number of days to complete study
Falls Church	390	381	9	2	4.5
Reading	40	35	5	13	1
Annapolis	31	29	2	6	1
Newport News	264	253	11	4	0[a]
Richmond 1	20	18	2	10	0[a]
Richmond 2	60	59	1	2	½
Richmond 3	181	160	21	12	3
Total	986	935	51	5	10 days

*Reproduced from Krush AJ, 1976, with permission of the *Journal of the American Medical Record Association*.
[a]Records were abstracted by medical records librarian.

information. When a record reveals hereditary polyposis, a letter is written to the patient's physician, explaining the polyposis study and registry, asking permission for the patient to be sent a medical and genealogical questionnaire. The physician usually discusses the matter with the patient and the patient's family.

When the physician's approval for a family study is received, or a request is made for a study by a family member or other professional person working with the family, a personal letter and a medical and genealogical questionnaire are sent to the patient. If the patient is deceased, the letter is sent to the closest living relative. The letter explains the study and asks permission to include the family in the registry. A five-page questionnaire requests demographic, medical, and genealogical information and includes an authorization form for the investigators to send for past medical history (Appendix C).

After the completed questionnaire is received, a "working" pedigree (not for publication) is drawn. Then all members of the family over the age of 10 years at risk for polyps are urged to begin a medical surveillance program if they are not already being followed medically. If family members wish to have medical care at our institution, results of those examinations are later sent to the family physician.

At all times, patients under our care, and those whose medical records and pathology slides are received from other hospitals, are assured that the information is confidential and is shared only with physicians and other individuals they designate to receive it. When family members participate in research projects, personal identity is protected. It is explained that patients' names will not be used in subsequent publications.

DISSEMINATION OF INFORMATION TO FAMILIES

Family members participating in a research study frequently ask to receive the results of the study. This information is sometimes provided by discussions or by letter from the principal investigator; also, the research team may place a written report in a newsletter that is received by most of the registry families. Sometimes it is necessary to explain that the results of the study will not apply to a single person or family but will be a group result that may not be available until a large number of individuals have been tested. Relationships with family members, some of their psychosocial problems that are encountered, and a support organization, IMPACC (or Intestinal Multiple Polyposis And Colorectal Cancer) are discussed in the chapter on counseling.

TEAM PERSONNEL

The number of persons on the team varies as clinical and research functions change. However, it is important, initally, that roles be delineated, although as the study progresses roles may need to be changed. Three essential roles that should be assumed are: team leader, or medical director, who is responsible for the design and execution of the study; coordinator, who is responsible for the clinical and research aspects of the study, including record keeping and research logistics (carrying out the study in the most efficient manner); and family investigator, who develops a relationship with families and encourages their participation in the clinical follow-up and research studies; this person usually manages the registry. Qualifications for this team member are that he or she should enjoy working with people; a medical social work background, courses and on-the-job training in medical genetics, and some additional knowledge of medicine are advantageous.

When studies are requested either by members of the team or by collaborators from outside institutions, the family investigator makes contact with family members, encourages their participation, and accompanies the investigators on home visits or field trips when biological specimens are collected [Krush and Evans, 1984] (Fig. 1). We have found that very few members of our registry families have refused to cooperate with investigators once they understand the reason for the study.

THE COMPUTER AND THE REGISTRY

Computerization of a polyposis registry is a useful but often difficult endeavor. Unfortunately, standardization of data entry has not yet been

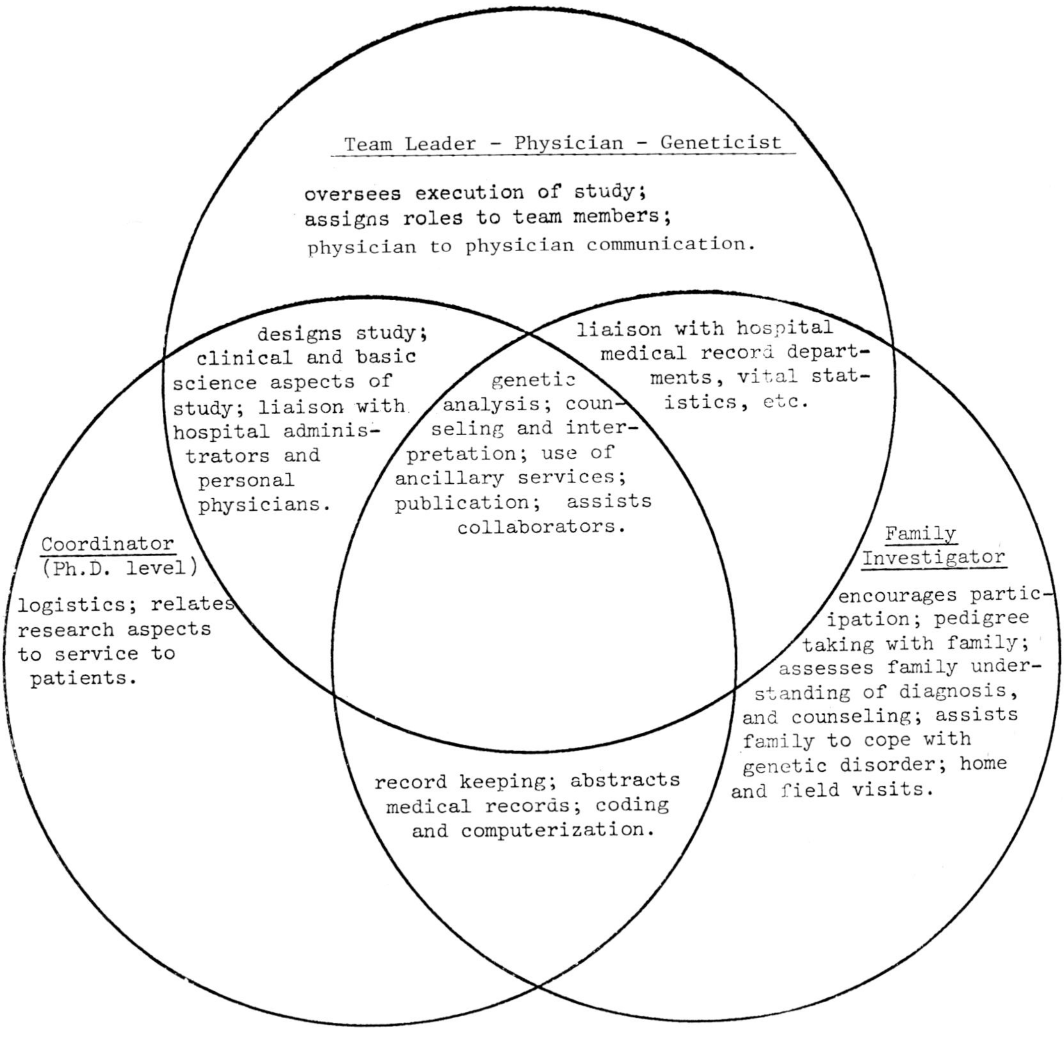

Fig. 1. Diagram for team personnel. (Reproduced from Krush and Evans, *Family Studies in Genetic Disorders*, 1984. Courtesy of Charles C. Thomas, Publisher, Springfield, Illinois.)

achieved among the several different registries in the United States and Canada.

Very early in our polyposis study we decided that the information for each individual and family should be placed on the computer. However, changes in personnel who were knowledgeable about computers, changes in the kinds of computers used in the Genetics Division at Johns Hopkins Hospital, and increasing knowledge about the various polyposis conditions frequently led to changes in data entry. In the meantime, investigators continually asked for detailed patient information, necessitating review of large numbers of records many times to satisfy the inquiries. Although tables and forms were filled out, it was almost impossible to keep the information up to date as additional families were enrolled in the registry and new patient information was accumulated.

In 1984, a clinical form was devised to be used for each individual in the registry. A pathology form was also devised and was to be merged with the clinical form. It was soon learned, however, that the clinical form was quite incomplete. Following an international meeting of members of polyposis registries held in England in 1985 (Leeds Castle Group), certain information concerning our patients was requested but could not be obtained from the clinical forms, and, again, all family records had to be reviewed.

In 1987, after the second meeting of the international group in Washington DC, computerization at our institution was expanded to include six different modules (Appendix D). A registration module gives the patient's demographic data. A history module gives family history and the patient's past medical history. A treatment module records surgical treatment of the patient. Encounter and procedure modules record clinic visits and results of all examinations (Appendix E). A research module categorizes the studies in which the patient is involved.

In addition to the above modules, an "overview" form was devised for each family in the registry (Appendix F). It identifies families with a specific polyposis or hereditary colon cancer diagnosis who may be recruited for research studies. It serves also to determine the total number of individuals in the registry, both deceased and living. In addition, computer programs for the identification of patients needing follow-up and letter-writing programs have been developed.

REGISTRY FUNCTIONS

Registries are valuable for a number of reasons.

1. Estimation of the prevalence of a condition in a specific geographical area
2. Ascertainment of all members of a family at risk to develop the condition
3. Assessment of risks and development of surveillance and follow-up plans for affected family members and those at risk for polyps and/or colon cancer (Appendix G)
4. Detection of the condition in other family members at earlier and more treatable ages or stages of the condition because of accrued pedigree information
5. Observation and recording of the natural history and course of a disorder
6. Long-term patient follow-up; as the patient's care changes between medical and surgical physicians, often the follow-up care in the family is disrupted; the registry functions to tie the entire family to follow-up care; so the registry encourages a working relationship among the surgeon, the gastroenterologist or other physician who has responsibility for ongoing patient care, and the registry coordinator; if all medical, surgical, and pathology reports are routed to the registry, as well as the patient's medical record, follow-up can be systematized
7. Linking families in different areas of a country as well as in other countries for more complete ascertainment and surveillance
8. Permitting research studies of large numbers of families with a relatively rare disorder, such as epidemiological, etiological, pathogenetic, clinical, medical management, etc.
9. Creation of permanent records; information may be coded and placed on the computer for easy retrieval
10. Retrieval of data for statistical and mathematical analysis; a computerized registry is essential for research projects, and it is our hope that soon we will be able to standardize information input so that national and international registries will have comparable data
11. Initiation of collaborative studies with investigators in different countries and different areas of one country [Krush and Evans, 1984]

In summary, a registry serves the affected patient and his family by providing access to clinical information and the identification and screening of patients. It also serves patient care by fostering research.

PATIENTS' CONCERNS ABOUT REGISTRIES

We have found that most patients and their families want to be included in a registry of a large institution. Altruistically, they hope that information learned about their condition will benefit others and that they, themselves, might benefit from new kinds of treatment emanating from research.

There are others, however, who have reservations about registries. Those with a diagnosis of cancer may fear that they will be stigmatized. They are also concerned that inclusion in a registry might be inadvertently disclosed to life or health insurance personnel or employers. Some persons affected with FAP or hereditary colon cancer may be willing to have their own names listed in a registry but be unwilling to have other family members included. When this happens, it is reasonable to explain how confidentiality is secured through the use of codes and passwords so that access to computerized registry information by outsiders is virtually impossible. Some family members may object to the use of the word registry or register, although these terms are now almost universally accepted [Krush and Evans, 1984].

INTERACTION AMONG REGISTRIES

As more polyposis registries are started, it is obvious that there will be overlap among them. For example, we have been following several families in eastern Pennsylvania whose medical needs are being managed by physicians in Philadelphia and elsewhere. Recently, two registries have begun operation in the Philadelphia area and undoubtedly some of "our" families will also be registered there. We approve of this because we can pool the Baltimore registry information with that in Philadelphia, where additional family members may be ascertained, producing more complete family pedigrees.

We have had a similar experience with a large kindred with members living in Minneapolis and Seattle as well as in the Baltimore area. So long as all agree that we are not "usurping" other patients and families, there should be no problem with overlapping in registries. Noteworthy is the fact that two physicians in two different states are planning statewide registries and hope to apply for funds, one from his state legislature, and the other from his state cancer council. The first physician plans to incorporate IMPACC into his grant request for a state registry.

SUMMARY

The Johns Hopkins Polyposis Registry, begun in 1973, can also be considered a longitudinal study of families in the nearby six-state area with diagnoses of one of the hereditary kinds of intestinal polyposis and colon cancer. Placing family medical and genealogical information on the computer is a continuous process and is proving to be helpful in planning research studies as well as in follow-up of patients. As new registries are organized in different parts of the United States and Canada, it will be important to standardize computerized information. Meetings to consider this matter have taken place and are being planned for the future both nationally and internationally.

ACKNOWLEDGMENT

We thank Mrs. Susan Booker, coordinator of the Johns Hopkins Hospital Polyposis Clinic and programmer for the Polyposis and Hereditary Colon Cancer Registry, for her revisions of the clinical modules and programming of the overview, follow-up, and patient letter forms. The Polyposis and Hereditary Colon Cancer Registry is supported in part by the Clayton Fund, the Johns Hopkins University School of Medicine.

References

Cohen SB, Pavlides GP, Krush AJ, Levin LS: Familial polyposis coli. Maryland State Med J 27:64–67, 1978.

Cohen Z: What is the potential for a national pedigree and linkage data bank to facilitate prevention of hereditary large bowel cancer? In Ingall JRF, Mastromarino AJ (eds): "Prevention of Hereditary Large Bowel Cancer." New York: Alan R. Liss, Inc. 1983, pp 177–180.

Copeland MM: The national large bowel cancer project: Its goals and objectives. Cancer 36:2308–2313, 1975.

Krush AJ: Hereditary intestinal polyps: Finding families in a six-state area. Med Rec News 47:13, 1976.

Krush AJ, Evans KA: "Family Studies in Genetic Disorders." Springfield, IL: Charles C. Thomas, Inc, 1984, pp 36–39.

APPENDIX A. LETTER OF INQUIRY TO PHYSICIAN IN SIX-STATE AREA, ASKING IF HE OR SHE HAS PATIENTS WITH POLYPOSIS

THE JOHNS HOPKINS HOSPITAL
BALTIMORE, MARYLAND 21205

DEPARTMENT OF MEDICINE
JOHNS HOPKINS UNIVERSITY SCHOOL OF MEDICINE

DIVISION OF MEDICAL GENETICS
TEL: (301) 955-3875

Dear Doctor:

I am writing to ask your assistance in a clinical and genetic study of intestinal polyposis disorders which Dr. Victor A. McKusick and I are planning. We are particularly interested in those having a familial component and risk of malignancy.

The initial phase of our work involves the ascertainment of all cases of polyposis in Delaware, District of Columbia, Maryland, New Jersey, Pennsylvania, Virginia, and West Virginia. The objective is to determine if enough cases can be obtained to justify the establishment of a regional polyposis center where members of these families may be quickly studied to determine who, if any, are actually at risk for these tumors and malignancy.

Should the ascertainment survey indicate that such a center is feasible, reports of the diagnostic and predictive tests, genetic counseling, and other services we provide will be sent to you and augment, rather than in any way interfere with your primary care of these patients.

If you have patients with polyposis you would like to have included in our ascertainment survey, please indicate so on the enclosed form and return it to us in the addressed stamped envelope.

Thank you in advance for your kindnesses and considerations.

Sincerely yours,

Edward R. Pierce, Ph.D., M.P.H.
Assistant in Medicine

ERP:aa

THE JOHNS HOPKINS HOSPITAL
BALTIMORE, MARYLAND 21205

DEPARTMENT OF MEDICINE
JOHNS HOPKINS UNIVERSITY SCHOOL OF MEDICINE

DIVISION OF MEDICAL GENETICS
TEL: (301) 955-3875

INTESTINAL POLYPOSIS SURVEY

PATIENT: ______________________________

ADDRESS: ______________________________

____

PATIENT: ______________________________

ADDRESS: ______________________________

____

PATIENT: ______________________________

ADDRESS: ______________________________

____

COMMENTS:

SIGNATURE: ____________________

PHYSICIAN: ____________________

ADDRESS: ____________________

____

APPENDIX B. LETTER TO MEDICAL RECORDS DEPARTMENT AND ADMINISTRATOR OF HOSPITAL ASKING FOR LIST OF PATIENTS WITH POLYPOSIS DURING A FIVE-YEAR PERIOD

THE JOHNS HOPKINS HOSPITAL
BALTIMORE, MARYLAND 21205

DEPARTMENT OF MEDICINE
JOHNS HOPKINS UNIVERSITY SCHOOL OF MEDICINE

DIVISION OF MEDICAL GENETICS
TEL: (301) 955-3875

Dear Colleague:

With the assistance of a National Institutes of Health Large Bowel Cancer Project grant, our medical group is engaged in the study of families (in Maryland and the surrounding states of Delaware, Virginia, West Virginia, Pennsylvania, New Jersey, and the District of Columbia) at least one member of which has received a diagnosis of intestinal polyposis. We are conducting medical genetic studies of all of those families in which the polyposis appears to be an hereditary type. Each available family member over the age of ten is offered colonoscopy, barium enema, complete physical examination, including a dental examination, and a number of blood studies for chromosome, linkage, CEA, PHA, and AHH analyses. These findings are then shared with the family's physicians.

We hope, eventually, to establish a Polyposis Center in this area for longitudinal family studies. All family members who are found to have polyposis will be referred to their own physicians and hospitals for treatment and follow up care.

The diagnoses in which we are interested include: familial polyposis coli, Peutz-Jeghers syndrome, Gardner syndrome, juvenile polyposis coli, multiple polyposis coli, and Turcot syndrome/ These are ICDA numbers 211.0, 211.1, 211.2, 211.3, 211.4, and 211.9.

I am writing now to ask if you will kindly enumerate for us on the enclosed sheet the hospital numbers of the patients who have been treated in your hospital for any of the above conditions in the past five years. May we also have your permission to abstract the records of those patients and to communicate with the attending or referring physician in order to secure his permission to begin a medical and family study?

We shall appreciate any information you may share with us and wish to assure you that it will be held in strict medical confidence. An addressed envelope is enclosed for your reply.

Sincerely,

Edmond A. Murphy, M.D.
Principal Investigator
Medical Genetics Division

EAM:dv
enc.

HOSPITAL NUMBERS OF PATIENTS WITH:

FAMILIAL POLYPOSIS COLI (FPC OR FAPC)

PEUTZ-JEGHERS SYNDROME

GARDNER SYNDROME (GS OR FAPC)

JUVENILE POLYPOSIS COLI

MULTIPLE POLYPOSIS COLI (OR SCATTERED DISCRETE POLYPS)

TURCOT SYNDROME

OR ICDA #

211.0

211.1

211.2

211.3

211.4

211.9

APPENDIX C. POLYPOSIS QUESTIONNAIRE

POLYPOSIS
QUESTIONNAIRE

NAME______________________________________ DATE______________________

ADDRESS____ ZIP__________
(Street, City, Stste)

BIRTHDATE______________ BIRTH PLACE__________________ SOC. SECURITY #__________

OCCUPATION__________

HOSPITAL NUMBER____________ PEDIGREE NUMBER 9780:________ TELEPHONE # Home__________
Work__________

I. 1. Have you ever been examined for polyps in the intestine? YES____ NO____
If so, a) sigmoidoscopy YES____ NO____ DATE__________ WHERE__________

b) Colonoscopy YES____ NO____ DATE__________ WHERE__________

c) Barium enema YES____ NO____ DATE__________ WHERE__________

Were polyps detected? YES____ NO____

2. Have you had surgery for intestinal polyps? YES____ NO____ If so, please write hospital & address

____

____

____

DATES:______________

3. Have you had cysts (lumps) on the skin? YES____ NO____

Location of cysts______________________

Age when first cyst found______________________

Surgery for cysts? YES____ NO____ WHERE? HOSPITAL______________________
ADDRESS______________________

4. Have you had growths on bony areas? YES____ NO____

Location of "lumps" or "bumps"______________________

Age when first noted______________________

Surgery for bone growths? YES____ NO____ HOSPITAL______________________

ADDRESS______________________

____

DATE______________________

5. Please describe any other unusual features of your skin: ______________________

____

6. Have you ever been told by a physician that you have cancer or a tumor? YES____ NO____

SURGERY? YES____ NO____ HOSPITAL______________________

ADDRESS______________________

DATE______________________

LOCATION OR KIND OF CANCER OR TUMOR______________________

7. If you know it, please give your blood type ______________

II. Information concerning your immediate family:

NAME	ADDRESS	BIRTHDATE	DATE OF DEATH	CAUSE (if known)	PLACE OF DEATH

My Mother ______________________________
(maiden name also)

My Father ______________________________

My Children ______________________________

____

____

____
(Names of additional children may be added on page 4)

My wife ______________________________
(maiden name also)

My husband ______________________________
(PLEASE USE BACK OF SHEET TO DESCRIBE ANY ILLNESSES IN ABOVE FAMILY MEMBERS).

My Brothers & Sisters ______________________________

____

____

____

(maternal)
My Grandmother ______________________________
(maiden name also)
My Grandfather ______________________________
(paternal)
My Grandmother ______________________________
(maiden name also)
My Grandfather ______________________________

(PLEASE USE BACK OF SHEET TO DESCRIBE ANY ILLNESSES IN YOUR GRANDPARENTS)

OTHER RELATIVES WHO HAVE HAD DIAGNOSES OF TUMOR AND/OR CANCER:

NAME	ADDRESS	HOW RELATED TO YOU	DIAGNOSIS	HOSPITAL OR PHYSICIAN	DATE & PLACE OF DIAGNOSIS

I know of NO family members with tumors or cancer ____________

Comments:

AUTHORIZATION TO OBTAIN MEDICAL INFORMATION

Patient's Name______________________________ Date__________

Family Number________________ Date of Birth________

I hereby give my permission to the Polyposis and Colon Cancer Registry of the Johns Hopkins Hospital to obtain medical information from physicians and hospitals where I or my ______________________received treatment.
(relationship)

Hospital______________________Address_____________________Dates_________

Hospital______________________Address_____________________Dates_________

Hospital______________________Address_____________________Dates_________

Doctor________________________Address_____________________Dates_________

Doctor________________________Address_____________________Dates_________

Witness_______________________Signed__________________________________
(Person giving permission)

Medical Genetics
Johns Hopkins Hospital
600 North Wolfe Street
Baltimore, MD 21205

APPENDIX D. SIX MODULES FOR COMPUTERIZING THE POLYPOSIS REGISTRY

REGISTRY COMPUTER MODULES

REGISTRATION MODULE

1 History #
2 Prefix to name
3 First name
4 Middle name
5 Last name
6 Suffix to name
7 Former name
8 Send mail c/o - name
9 Street address
10 City name
11 State name
12 Zip code
13 Home area code
14 Home phone #
15 Work area code
16 Work phone #
17 Pedigree #
18 Diagnosis
19 Diagnosis confirmed
20 Risk status
21 Type and location of follow up
22 Follow up interval
23 Date of birth
24 Sex
25 Race
26 Spouse
27 Mother
28 Father
29 Referring physician
30 Date of death
31 Cause of death
32 Death related to registry dx
33 Death information confirmed
34 Source of death information
35 Date initial registry review
36 Most recent update

HISTORY MODULE

1 History #
2 Related family names
3 Family hx of polyps
4 Family hx of colon ca
5 Family hx of fibroma/cyst
6 Family hx of other neoplasms
7 Family comment
8 Prior symptoms
9 Hx of extra-colonic lesions
10 History comment
11 Cancer present
12 Type/location cancer
13 Stage/extent of cancer
14 Cancer confirmed
15 Clinic visit date
16 Date of diagnosis
17 Age at diagnosis in years
18 Pathology comment
19 Pathology reference number

TREATMENT MODULE

1 History #
2 Date of surgery
3 Type of surgery
4 Location of surgery
5 Confirmation
6 Treatment comment

ENCOUNTER MODULE

1 History #
2 Date of encounter
3 Type of encounter
4 Symptoms - bleeding
5 Symptoms - diarrhea
6 Symptoms - pain
7 Symptoms - other
8 Extra-colonic lesions
9 Abstract of note
10 Physician reporting encounter

PROCEDURE MODULE

1 History #
2 Procedure type
3 Procedure date
4 Location procedure
5 # polyps/rect
6 # polyps/sig
7 # polyps/dc
8 # polyps/tc
9 # polyps/ac
10 # polyps/sb
11 # polyps/duod
12 # polyps/stom
13 Pathology reference
14 Clinical review/flat mucosa
15 Clinical review/polyp type
16 Clinical review/polyp size
17 Clinical review/hx of cancer

RESEARCH MODULE

1 History #
2 Jaw lesions / describe
3 Number of jaw lesions
4 Date jaw x-ray
5 Jaw lesion size
6 Jaw lesion location
7 Odontomas
8 Location odontoma
9 Other jaw lesions
10 Jaw comment
11 Eye lesions
12 Date eye exam
13 # eye lesions - right eye
14 # eye lesions - left eye
15 Blood studies

APPENDIX E. ENCOUNTER FORM

ENCOUNTER FORM

Date ____/____/____
Type ____________

Name ______________________ Hx # ______________

Dx ____ DOB ________ Pedigree ______ Phone ______________

Location ____________ Time ______ Physician ______________

Referred by ______________ Billing ______________

Prior consent ____

Note ____

____

____

==

PROCEDURE	Planned	Completed		Planned	Completed
Sigmoidoscopy	____	____	Upper Endoscopy	____	____
Colonoscopy	____	____	Barium swallow	____	____
Barium enema	____	____	Surgery - type	____________	
					____

RESULTS

Rect ____ Sig ____ DC ____ TC ____ AC ____ SB ____ Duod ____ Stom ____

Tissue collected: Y N Case # ______

____

BLOOD STUDIES

Chromosome	____	____	grn	Bank	____	____	red
DNA ________	____	____	yel		____	____	lav
EBV trans	____	____	yel		____	____	grn
CEA	____	____	lav				

____

Eye exam ____ ____ Panorex ____ ____

Consent ____ ____ # ________

==

Symptoms: Bleeding ____ Diarrhea(#bm/day) ____ Pain ____ Other ______

Extra-colonic findings ______________________

Note ____

____

____

____

Risk code ____ FU code ____ FU interval ____(yrs) Billing code ____

==

Next visit ________ Procedures planned ______________

APPENDIX F. "OVERVIEW" FORM

Date________________________________

A. Pedigree #_______________________

B. Propositus/a___________________________________

C. Family diagnosis_______________________________

D. Diagnosis confirmed? YES______ NO___________

E. Number members_____________

F. Number affected (may be estimated)___________

G. Number members with clinical review___________

H. Number generations________

I. Availability for study (geographic or otherwise)

J. Individual studies in which family members were included:

K. Publications in which family was included:

BT = brain tumor study	G6PD = G6PD study
CEA = CEA study	HPB = hepatoblastoma study
DER = dermatoglyphics study	JL = jaw lesions study
DES = desmoid study	JP = juvenile polyposis study
DNA = DNA chromosome study	PJS = PJS study
EL = CHRPE study	PL = ploidy study_

APPENDIX G. FOLLOW-UP EXAMINATION GUIDELINES

FOLLOW UP EXAMINATION GUIDELINES

PERSONS AT RISK FOR FAPC

AGE	EXAMINATION
10-24	Flexible sigmoidoscopy yearly
25-34	Flexible sigmoidoscopy every 2 years
35-44	Flexible sigmoidoscopy every 3 years
>44	Flexible sigmoidoscopy every 3-5 years and follow ACS guidelines

IF POLYPS ARE DETECTED, SURGERY WILL BE RECOMMENDED

PERSONS WITH FAPC - FOLLOW UP AFTER SURGERY

1. Flexible sigmoidoscopy every 6 months to 3 years (depending on type of surgery.
2. Upper endoscopy every 4 years
3. Complete physical examination every 1-2 years
4. Follow ACS guidelines for cancer surveillance

7

Screening of Offspring of Patients With Familial Adenomatous Polyposis: The St. Mark's Hospital Polyposis Register Experience

Kay Neale, Sheila Ritchie, and James P. S. Thomson

St. Mark's Hospital, London, England

INTRODUCTION

The registration of families of St. Mark's Hospital patients with polyposis of the colon began in 1925. As this special interest in polyposis became known, physicians, surgeons, and pathologists from other hospitals sent details of their patients to the registry. At the end of 1987, 351 families with familial adenomatous polyposis (FAP) had been entered in the register. Another 37 with Peutz-Jeghers syndrome and 61 with juvenile polyposis were also registered. Families are admitted to the register only when histological evidence has been obtained on at least one family member.

A substantial number of families is awaiting registration when the diagnosis is not established beyond doubt. These families are some of those reported to the registry from other centers without supporting histology. Each family, as it is identified as having FAP, is given a number and a family tree is constructed (Fig. 1). From this, each member is given an individual number corresponding to his generation and position within that generation. Thus, in a hypothetical family 997, grandfather would be 997.I.1, his two sons 997.II.1 and 997.II.2, and their children 997.III.1, etc.

Persons at risk of having inherited the disease are entered into the screening program at St. Mark's or are advised to attend for screening nearer their homes if they prefer. The initial contact is usually made through a member of the family known to the registry. This informal type of approach has the advantage of involving the family in discussion of the need for screening and certainly adds to their understanding of the mode of inheritance. When it is apparent that for one reason or another there is little contact existing or wanted by members of a family, the registry will make a direct approach to the person at risk or will contact his general practitioner. Because each family has its own peculiarities, it is difficult to generalize about the best way to achieve total family screening.

Occasionally it transpires that children have been adopted out of the family and their whereabouts are unknown. The registry has successfully traced a number of such cases and arranged for the adoptive parents to be advised of the risk. The strictest confidence is always maintained to avoid any possible cause of embarrassment or annoyance to either party.

WHAT AGE TO START SCREENING?

The practice has long been established here of examining the children of polyposis patients at or about the age of 14 years to determine whether they have inherited the condition. The best age

Familial Adenomatous Polyposis, pages 61–66

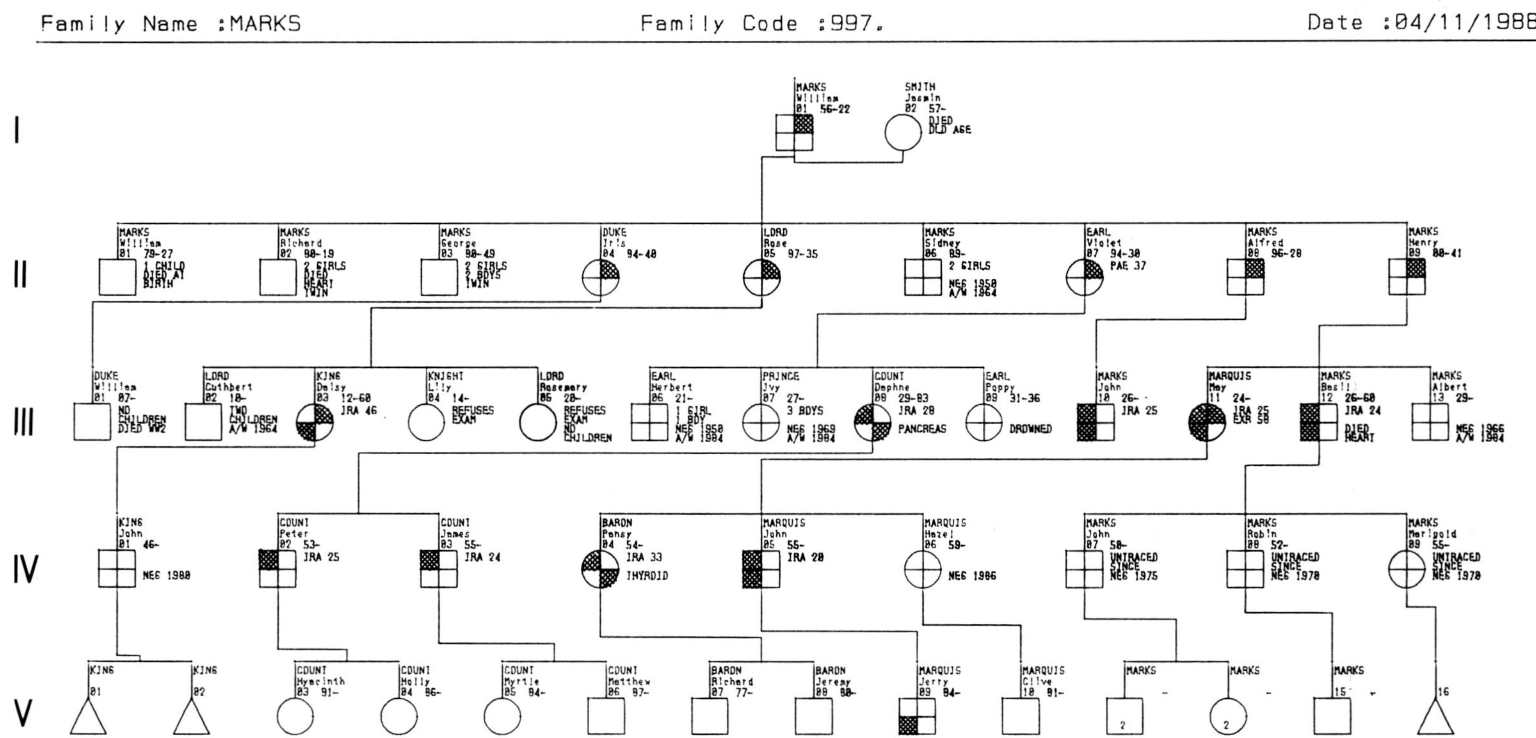

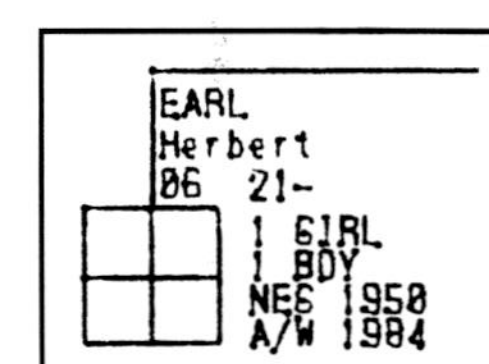

Fig. 1. Above: 80% reduced, B&W reproduction of a family tree generated by the Epson Hi-80 plotter. **Right:** Enlarged section of the tree.

to initiate regular screening of those at risk has been the subject of much international debate. There is general agreement among the surgeons at St. Mark's that, in *most* cases when polyps are present in 14-year-old children, surgery is not needed for several years. It follows that earlier diagnosis at St. Mark's Hospital would not lead to earlier treatment and that examination of children under about 14 years of age is not necessary. Indeed, it could prove sufficiently traumatic to alienate the child and make further surveillance difficult. There are instances in which parental concern necessitates an earlier examination being made, and, of course, younger children may present with bowel symptoms that warrant investigation. It might be argued that examination need not start until later, when surgical treatment is most likely to be undertaken. However, if screening is delayed, there is a risk that the young adult will refuse to attend for examination and, too, it is necessary to be alert to the occasional case requiring early treatment. Cases of colorectal cancer in people under 20 years of age have been known.

Nonetheless, there are times when offspring are older when called to hospital for their first visit. For example, a patient newly diagnosed as having FAP may have children already well over 14 years of age. It is also possible that the new patient will be found to have siblings or other adult relatives, possibly parents, at risk. Parents of an apparently new case of polyposis are never considered too old to be at risk and are, whenever possible, examined. There is, therefore, a wider range than might be expected in those being screened for the first time.

SCREENING CLINICS

Members of polyposis families are normally seen by a surgeon in clinics set aside every 3 months. This facilitates the monitoring of their attendances and enables a rapport to be developed with the staff of the polyposis registry. Many of the young patients regularly bring their children to these clinics before they are of an age to be screened. They are therefore quite familiar with the hospital, the clinicians, the nurses, and the registry staff when the time comes for them to be examined. It is usual for one of the six surgeons at St. Mark's to be responsible for a whole family. It has been found that, in both those at risk and those affected with the disease, compliance is improved when several members of a family are seen at the same time. If, however, there are reasons why members of a family prefer not to see each other, arrangements can be made for them to attend different clinics and so avoid chance encounters. Since the registry was established, a record has been kept of every attendance at the hospital by any family member whether affected by the disease or not.

SCREENING METHODS

For people at risk, examination is by rigid sigmoidoscopy. No bowel preparation is given unless it is impossible to get a good view of the

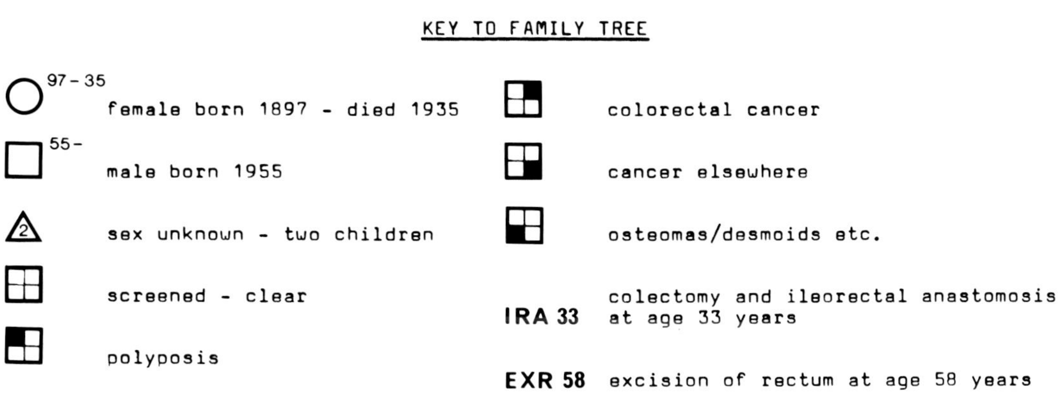

Fig. 2. Key to family tree on facing page.

mucosa. It is very important to minimize disturbance to the patient that might deter him from making further visits.

If polyps are seen in the rectum, a biopsy must be obtained to confirm the presence of adenomas before telling the patient that he has inherited the condition. Lymphoid follicles are not an unusual finding in the rectum of a young person. If no polyps are seen in the rectum, the person is advised to return for a similar examination the following year.

Barium enema or colonoscopy examination is requested by a surgeon if he wishes to 1) satisfy himself that the colon is polyp-free in an older patient before reducing the number of screening visits or 2) confirm a positive diagnosis.

AT WHAT AGE SHOULD SCREENING STOP?

Some surgeons say "never." In practice, it depends on several factors. It is well known that the risk of developing polyps after adequate negative examinations diminishes with age. Family members are aware of this, and some may decide that they no longer wish to attend regularly. In these cases it is made clear that, should the patient at any time be worried or have any bowel symptoms, he or she would be well advised to return to St. Mark's. There would appear to be a tendency for the members of a particular family to produce adenomas at more or less the same age, so it would be unwise to assess the diminution of risk with increasing age in a particular patient without reference to the trend in that family. Certainly there are families for whom the age of onset of polyps is greater than that found in the more "classical" case of polyposis.

In the 36 years to the end of 1987, 357 offspring of polyposis patients had been screened for polyps by rigid sigmoidoscopy. The age at first examination ranged from 5 to 40+ years. One hundred twenty four (34.7%) were found to have adenomas in the rectum at first screening. Thirty one of the remaining 233 have, so far, had polyps seen on second or subsequent examination. This makes a total of 155 (43.4%) of the original 357 screened having inherited the condition. (It should be remembered that propositus cases are omitted from screening figures, and this has an effect on the overall percentage found to be positive. For example, a young person presenting with symptoms and found to have polyposis and evidence that a parent had polyposis will not be included, but the brothers and sisters who are then called for screening will be included.)

In theory, one could deduce the age of appearance of polyps in the rectum by taking a mean of the last negative and first positive sighting. However, in some cases, the interval is far too great to be of value. Also, it is not usual for any bowel preparation before a routine screening examination. It is perhaps wiser only to make general observations as a result of studying the figures, bearing in mind that they have been collected over 62 years.

1. Twenty percent of patients were not diagnosed at first examination.
2. Approximately two thirds of those not diagnosed at first examination were diagnosed by 20 years of age (put another way, roughly one third were not.)
3. Although in most cases there is a tendency for members of a sibship to develop polyps at about the same age, there have been exceptions.
4. It appears that there may be families in whom the onset of polyps is much much later. Unless we maintain a screening program that allows for this possibility, we are likely to make mistakes and lose the chance of learning more about the variable nature of FAP.

Thus during a 62 year period only 31 people who have been seen and found negative have subsequently developed rectal polyps. In one case, after four negative examinations at ages 13, 16, 19, and 22 years, one polyp was seen at 26 years, which was not thought to be an adenoma. There were three subsequent negative examinations at ages 28, 29, and 33 years before a positive diagnosis was made at age 34 years. These observations highlight the difficulty of knowing when to stop screening.

COMPUTERS AND POLYPOSIS

The register of polyposis patients has been maintained at St. Mark's for more than 60 years, and in that time Dr. Bussey has developed a system of documenting information about polyposis that made retrieval of that information an easy matter. His system and beautifully produced family trees had served so well that it was with some reluctance, and with great caution, that computerization was implemented in 1985.

In recent years, the registry has been equipped with an 80386 MHz microprocessor, with a 60 megabyte hard disc, two mega-bytes of memory, and an integral tape back-up unit. This computer runs two operating systems, C DOS 386 and MS DOS 3.3. The C DOS 386 enables the computer to be used by up to five users at any time.

When the computer was introduced, it was realized that much effort and time would be needed just to enter the vast accumulation of data. To avoid any disruption to the work of the registry, it was clear that it would be necessary to maintain the existing system while developing the new. Although this has meant a great deal of duplication of work, it has been a considerable advantage to be able to reconcile figures obtained from the computer with those in the Bussey system.

To provide an accurate database for both retrospective and prospective studies, much thought was given to the categorization of the patients. It would be naive to believe that every person diagnosed as having polyposis and admitted to the register could be entered into every study. For example, there are those patients who, having been screened at St. Mark's and had their surgery here, are still being seen twice each year some 30–40 years later. This group will have complete documentation. However, others, having been screened and treated surgically here, choose to have their follow-up examinations nearer to their homes. Others have surgery elsewhere and then attend St. Mark's for follow-up, and some people are registered when diagnosis and follow-up events are reported to us by a family member or doctor working elsewhere. Since we are careful to include in our studies only those people on whom we have adequate—and more often than not first-hand—information, it is essential that the computer can distinguish easily these and many other groups.

Consequently, the program has been designed to answer the various and variable needs of the registry. It is a flexible program, which is subject to constant review and modification.

In addition to providing a database for statistics, the computer is used to produce family trees. These are drawn by an Epson Hi-80 plotter using single sheets of A4 paper and four-colored pens (Fig. 1). The facility for giving personal information about each family member allows plotting of the person's name, year of birth and death, and four lines, each of eight characters, free text beside each symbol. These lines usually are used to indicate the type of operation, with the age of the person at the time of surgery, the site of carcinoma, the cause of death, or the date of the last negative examination; however, in some cases they are used for other information that is of importance or interest.

The family trees are working documents, and it is essential they they are clear and easy to use and to interpret. There is a limit of 15 symbols (people) to any one line (generation) on each sheet of paper, and it is the registry staff who decide, when dealing with a large family, how the tree should be constructed. In some cases, family members who are not at risk can be omitted with a note of their existence in the free text of their unaffected parent. In some cases, the facility for grouping family members will be used; the appropriate symbol then bears the number of people it represents plotted within it. In the case of a family where more than 15 family members in one generation need to be included in detail, it is up to the staff of the registry to decide the breaking point(s). The aim is to construct the tree so that the family members under the care of St. Mark's are on one sheet while allowing the make-up of the whole family to be examined if the sheets are laid end to end. A well constructed tree allows a clinician to see at a glance not only the way in which family members under his care relate to each other but also the state of health of every individual.

As far as is possible, the clinicians see the patients at the polyposis clinics held by each consultant every 3 months in the outpatient department. Clinic appointments can be made up to 1 year in advance, which means that most people leave the hospital with a confirmed appointment for their next visit. However, if patients are asked to return after a longer period, the due date can be entered into the polyposis registry computer. Similarly, babies at risk of having inherited the disease can have their first screening visit date 14 years ahead entered onto their computer record. Thus the registry list can be compared with the outpatient clinic list every 3 months and appointments arranged as necessary. Computerization also allows the registry staff to keep track of people booked for X-ray examination, endoscopy, or admission to hospital more efficiently.

8

Use of Computers in the Management of Registries for Familial Adenomatous Polyposis

John Stricklin Spratt, Richard Alvin Greenberg, John J. Buchino, Matthew Witten, and Diana J. Beasley-Weigel

Departments of Surgery (J.S.S.), Community Health (R.A.G.), and Pediatrics and Pathology (J.J.B.), James Graham Brown Cancer Center, University of Louisville, Louisville, Kentucky; Medical and Biological Supercomputing, ETA Systems, Inc., St. Paul, Minnesota (M.W.), and Information Systems, The Brown-Forman Corporation, Louisville, Kentucky (D.J.B.-W.)

INTRODUCTION

The purposes of a genetic registry may be to monitor genetic penetrance of a known disorder, to assess risk and to counsel those at risk, to research unknown multifactorial aspects of the expression of a disorder with genetic associations, and to engage in epidemiological studies—clinical, reference, monitoring, research, and prevention [1]. Registries can be extremely expensive to operate and often there are problems in justifying necessary funding. The highest cost in registry development and maintenance is attributable to manpower. These manpower costs roughly divide into two areas: 1) the costs of initial planning and ultimate use by accredited scientific authorities and 2) the ongoing costs of actually acquiring, accessing, managing, analyzing, and reporting quality-controlled data. In this second area, the computer comes into its own as a tireless workhorse, unbiased critic for quality-control checks, database manager, and iterative calculator and analyzer. To use the computer effectively requires concise planning.

The problem, which the registry is expected to address, must be defined. Then, each portion of the problem must be stated as a succinct objective. Objectives, characteristically, have measurable end points. An inventory of resources potentially available for use by the registry must be compiled—demographic characteristics of the study population, estimated prevalence and incidence of problems to be studied, state of knowledge, manpower, software, and computers.

With problem identified, objectives stated, and resources identified, the approaches possible to obtain the objectives must now be enumerated. As the final step, in the process, the tasks required by each approach must be listed and outlined graphically. Tasks require people, time, resources, and money. Tasks have to be phased in an appropriate time sequence. Budgets are justified only by defined and justified tasks. The planning process, if properly and objectively carried out, should define the most economical way to attain the objectives of the registry.

Obviously, a chapter such as this cannot lay out the perfect registry, for all users, because of variations in objectives and resources. However, we can review progress made toward computerized genetic registries as applied to the monitoring of familial adenomatous polyposis.

Tracing the impact of any genetically transmitted disease, through an ever-arborizing population, presents a complex problem in data management as well as statistical analysis, one that requires melding the needs of the registry

Familial Adenomatous Polyposis, pages 67–75

design with the capabilities of the computer. This, the effort, must ensure that a useful genetic disease registry results.

DEFINITION OF FAMILIAL ADENOMATOUS POLYPOSIS (FAP)

By definition, FAP is a Mendelian dominant disorder associated with the early appearance in life of adenomatous polyps of the colon and rectum, succeeded by the appearance of adenocarcinoma. There are a variety of associated anomalies that may be related to the inherited genetic defect.

Since the term ''polyp'' can be used to describe any intraluminal projection caused by a mass, one must be careful to differentiate FAP from other multiple polyposis conditions. Grossly, there must be at least 100 colorectal polyps present in the generally accepted criteria set forth by Bussey [2]. These polyps of polyposis are identical to sporadically occurring adenomatous polyps. These lesions have a somewhat characteristic gross appearance, usually being slightly less than 1 cm in diameter but varying from 0.1 to 3.0 cm. They typically have an irregular, darker, somewhat redder surface than the surrounding mucosa and are attached by a short stalk. However, they can easily be confused with several other epithelial lesions on endoscopy or gross pathological examination. Therefore, definitive diagnosis rests on histologic confirmation of the lesion.

Histologically, as the name implies, adenomatous polyps are glandular. These glands differ from those of the normal colonic mucosa in several ways. First, goblet cells are few. Second, the columnar epithelial cells present lack the usual basal orientation of nuclei. Rather, there is stratification of nuclei. Third, nuclei may show mild pleomorphism and are frequently elongated. Finally, mitotic figures are not uncommon. These glands are usually supported by a loose fibrovascular stroma, with a mild mononuclear inflammatory infiltrate similar to the normal lamina propria [3,4].

REVIEW OF EXTANT REGISTRIES

In the case of FAP, we are dealing with a disease with which a considerable effort has already been put forth [1,5–12]. The primary purpose of this review is to provide the reader with an overview of the progress to date.

A genetic registry may be for service and/or research. In the area of service, the objective is to monitor families or populations at risk—for the purpose of genetic counselling [13–16] and for the recommendation of preventive therapy to specific members of the family, applying known genetic information. A registry may be utilized as a means to survey data or as a metholological schema for clinical management review of the characteristics of a specific family or population. Such a registry would be expected to access and display data in a clinically useful manner. The concept of a registry for research is far more complex.

The research registry, whose purpose is to test specific hypotheses, may well require controls and will clearly necessitate detailed statistical planning to ensure that the appropriate statistical tests can be performed, thereby allowing for the rejection of null hypotheses with sufficient power to be clinically and biologically meaningful. Since the various hypotheses will be unique to the research purposes of the specific investigator, an extensive review of potential research objectives is beyond the scope of this chapter. The necessary chromosomal parameters can certainly be coded as part of genetics registry research program when data and design indicate.

In the United States today, there are several well tested, on-line systems that we have selected to review as good registry models. Notable examples are located in the Department of Medical Genetics, The University of Indiana (Helios Software Works, Indianapolis, IN) [17]; The Cleveland Clinic [18,19]; Roswell Park Memorial Institute [20,21]; and Louisiana State University at New Orleans [10] as well as that of The Leeds Castle Group [22].

The Cleveland Clinic Foundation developed a familial polyposis registry, in 1979, for families with a 100% genetically determined risk for developing colorectal cancer [19]. The registry is intended to codify the pedigree of individuals who have actually developed FAP for the express purpose of informing relatives of their risk for colon cancer.

FAP is autosomal dominant, associated with a 50% risk of developing FAP in offspring. The only present measure for preventing cancer of the colon in the presence of established FAP is total proctocolectomy. A protocol exists, with this registry, that permits follow-up and management of the noncolonic manifestations of the syndrome, desmoids, polyps elsewhere in the gastrointestinal tract, medulloblastomas, pancreatic cancers, thyroid tumors, adrenal tumors, and other tumors.

The registry is designed to operate on a VAX computer with VMS operating system, a BASIC compiler, Mass-11, and FMS. The programs consist of several software packages, all written in BASIC. Further information about this program can be obtained from Thomas K. Schroeder, M.D., Research Coordinator, Department of Colorectal Surgery, Cleveland Clinic Foundation [19].

The Department of Biometry and Genetics at Louisiana State University Medical Center has available, for marketing, a package of computer programs entitled The Statistical Analysis for Genetic Epidemiology (S.A.G.E.). The programs in this package are written in ANSI Standard FORTRAN 77 for operation on any computer with the appropriate compiler and enough memory and disk space [10]. The following programs are presently available in the current release of S.A.G.E.

1. Family Structure Program (FSP)—a program that checks pedigree data for 20 common structural errors, such as married individuals having the same sex code, an individual who is his own ancestor, or two or more individuals having the same identification number. It also identifies consanguineous matings and loops in the pedigree and sends an error message if the pedigree structure is too complex to be analyzed by the programs in the current package. S.A.G.E. generates a linked list pointer scheme with pointers to father, mother, sibling, mate, and offspring and multiple secondary records for each individual record. This flexible pointer scheme is then used to generate the appropriate pointer structure for the other programs in the package. It can also be used to generate all possible pedigree plots using the commercially available MEGADATS PROGRAM.

2. Segregation Analysis Programs—a set of six programs, all of which assume that any major gene inheritance is through a single two-allele autosomal locus. An option to allow for single ascertainment (simplex or multiplex) is available in all the programs.

A. Segregation Analysis of a Continuous Trait Under a Regressive Model (REGC)—pedigree analysis under class A regressive model is included as a special case. Covariates may be included in the analysis.

B. Segregation Analysis of a Discrete Trait Under a Regressive Logistic Model (REGD)—segregation analysis of a discrete trait coded as either a dichotomy of or a trichotomy of the trait under a regressive logistic class A model. Covariates may be included in the analysis.

C. Segregation Analysis of a Truncated (Censored) Trait With Logistic probability density function (p.d.f.)—model 1 (REGTL1)—Segregation analysis of a disease trait under a regressive class A model allowing for variable age of onset. The genotype of an individual is presumed to influence age of onset through location and scale parameters but not to affect susceptibility (defined as the probability of being affected at age "infinity"). Susceptibility may be different for up to two affections classes. Covariates may be included in the analysis.

D. Segregation Analysis of a Truncated (Censored) Trait With Logistic p.d.f.—model 2 (REGTL2)—segregation analysis of a disease trait under class A regressive model allowing for variable age of onset. Genotype is presumed to influence susceptibility to the affected state but not to affect age of onset. Covariates may be included in the analysis.

E. Segregation Analysis of a Truncated (Censored) Trait With Normal p.d.f.—model 1 (REGTN2)—segregation analysis of a disease trait under a transmission probability model allowing for variable age of onset. Genotype is presumed to influence age of onset (which is normally distributed) through location and scale parameters but not susceptibility. Susceptibility may be different for up to two affection classes.

F. Segregation of a Truncated (Censored) Trait With a Normal p.d.f.—model 2 (REGTN2)—segregation analysis of a disease trait under a transmission probability model allowing for variable age of onset. Genotype is presumed to influence susceptibility to the affected state, but not age of onset (which is normally distributed).

3. Familial Correlations Program (FCOR)—this program first generates all possible relevant pairs of relatives and classifies them into the following ten main types (and 88 subtypes defined by the sexes of the individuals involved).

1) Marital (spouses)
2) Parental (four subtypes, e.g., father-daughter)
3) Siblings (three subtypes)
4) Half siblings (six subtypes)
5) Grandparental (eight subtypes)
6) Avuncular (eight subtypes)
7) Cousins (ten subtypes)
8) Great-grandparental (16 subtypes)
9) Great-avuncular (16 subtypes)
10) Half-avuncular (16 subtypes)

Then unvariate and/or multivariate familial correlations for up to five traits are computed for the main and/or subtypes of relatives. Several different weightings can be used in the analysis: equal weights to pairs of individuals, equal weights to nuclear families, or equal weights to pedigrees. The user also has the option to assume the mean in age, sex, or user-specified class.

4. Sib-Pair Linkage Analysis Program (SIBPAL)—this is a general program to screen for genetic linkage on the basis of the sib-pair relationship. It can be used for ordering marker loci and for robust linkage analysis between putative genes and a set of marker loci. It does not assume a specific genetic model. This program can also be used to estimate, for each sib pair and each marker locus, the proportion of genes shared identical by descent. The purchase price is $110.00 [10].

The applicability of S.A.G.E is discussed in a review article by George et al. [17]. The statistical method reviewed is logistic regression. This method can be used to identify familial aggregations and can be adapted to incorporate information on age of disease onset. The flexibility can accommodate "a wide range of skewness and kurtosis" and will allow the incorporation of covariates into the model. This method may even be extended to permit "segregation of major genes."

A cancer preventive registry for familial adenomatous polyposis is also operated at Toronto General Hospital [5]. A previous issue of *Seminars in Surgical Oncology* (Vol. 3, No. 2, 1987) contains a collection of reviews on various aspects of FAP as a genetic syndrome, including registry surveillance, associated manifestations, counselling, and treatment. These references and others contain a great wealth of information that should be reviewed as background for registry planning and management [6,13,18,20–27]. The review and planning considerations should include the diversity of disorders associated with the genetic expression of the polyposis [25].

The Department of Medical Genetics at the University of Indiana has been a sustained contributor to the development of computer software essential for the operation of a registry for genetic diseases. The major system there is called MEGADATS (Helios Software Works).

MEGADATS can store on disks many pedigrees and can retrieve any single pedigree or set of pedigrees from the archived file. Therefore, the MEGADATS storage mechanism for data is an excellent starting point for data analysis. The relational database and query language allow for easy selection of and easy reformatting of data on individuals for use with standard statistical packages.

More important, the MEGADATS system can make use of the pedigree structure to prepare automatic input for programs such as PEDIG and LIPED. Separate pedigree and marker data files can be combined and the output formatted for direct input to the analysis program. The conversion process is saved as a MEGADATS playback file and can be activated by entering the name of the file, so data collection, storage, and display features can be used as a "front end" for an analysis effort.

MEGADATS offers useful plot options. The standard printer plot is 8.5″ × 11″ across the page (for Epson/IBM or equivalent dot matrix printers with graphics capabilities). A new option of 11″ × 8.5″ down the page has been added. This new option connects the lines across page perforations to produce a continuous strip plot. A CRT graphics display, for previewing files, is now a part of the MEGADATS plot system (for PC systems with graphics cards).

The user can select the information to be displayed in the plot text block and the relative sizes of the lettering and symbols. The plot now includes letters centered in the symbols for carrier markings or off page correction as well as shading by quarters within the symbols.

MINI/PLOT is a subset of MEGADATS. MINI/PLOT is a software system designed specifically for pedigree drawing. One part of the system, MINIdats, is the MEGADATS pedigree inputs from the MEGADATS-3 system. The other part, PLOT, is the PC plot process from the MEGADATS-3 system.

Very minimal computer hardware is required to use the MINI/PLOT system on an IBM/PC/XT/AT or compatible system:

Memory—256K bytes
Disk—one 5.25″ disk drive (360K bytes)
Printer—Epson, IBM, or compatible parallel printer with the graphics option
Optional—second 5.25″ disk (convenience), graphic card (pedigree screen plot), hard drive (speed, and storage capacity)

The price of the MINI/PLOT system is $995 for the two-diskette set that includes the MINIdats and PLOT programs as well as system files to start the system.

When specific chromosomal defects are associated with inherited disorders, it is desirable to register these defects. In dominant familial cases, susceptibility seems inherited through a germline mutation. Cancer may develop after a somatic change in the homologous allele. In the case of FAP and colonic cancer, chromosomes 5q has been implicated [28]. Other biological and genetic markers should be carefully considered for inclusion during registry planning [26,27].

In summary, there is a rich and accessible experience base for anyone wishing to set up a computerized registry for FAP. The neophyte does not need to reinvent the wheel. He does need to define registry objectives concisely and adapt any of the existing systems to the fulfillment of his registry objectives. He needs to have access to the required data base management systems, hardware, and software and have the well trained personnel necessary to run the system. In some situations, a remote entry station to an existing registry may serve the purpose. Careful initial planning remains the key to ultimate success of any registry.

PLANNING THE REGISTRY

The disease to be registered has been defined. The second step is to define the purpose of the registry. Following this, we must specify the data to be recorded; doing so in an unambiguous way to meet the purposes of the registry. The final step, before going to the computer, is to determine what data elements are to be acquired and the relationship of these data elements to each other and to the entire structure of the database system. From this analysis a determination can be made on the maximum amount of data that will be stored within the system. Other important factors concerned in collecting large amounts of data are to establish and maintain a mechanism to check for accuracy and completeness. After this initial design and analysis, one must determine and develop an interface to the system in order to enter this information to the computer, examine for data integrity and quality within the computer system, and process for useful output (i.e., specification for design of useful reports and audit systems). Having performed the aforementioned sequence of predesigned decisions and steps, programming the appropriate computer to do the essential, vital, and iterative work is much easier. Paralleling all the above steps is a running design and development cost. In the last analysis, the utility value of the registry has to justify that cost. Cost is no minor problem in the management of any registry and overly expensive registries have a history of floundering when money is short. The surest way to contain costs is to engage in careful initial planning to avoid the costly acquisition of unnecessary/unusable data. This planning effort should not "reinvent the wheel," but rather it should begin with an analytical look at the state of the art in registry design.

The fundamentals of clinical research design, data collection, and basic statistical testing have been reviewed elsewhere, and the reader is referred to this discussion [29]. There are basic principles for the design of data collection. After the specific objects of the investigation have been detailed, the method of analysis to be used must be known. Finally, the volume of detailed information actually required must be identified. In designing the data–acquisition system, important rules of thumb are that 1) paper is cheaper than time; 2) exact data should be coded as is rather than using a coding scheme; 3) simple codes should be used; 4) all questions must be stated clearly, constructing a parallel glossary of explicit definitions to eliminate ambiguity; 5) all protocols must be identified and outlined; 6) all possible answers with codes should be specified; "unknown" and "none" can often be coded similarly; 7) codes for combinations of answers should be avoided; 8) the use of "zeroes" in answers, except where part of exact data, should be avoided; only number codes should be used; and 9) the acquisition/input of all answers should be in the order in which they will be encountered for coding. Once the code sheets have been designed, they should be "debugged" by a trial run on a sample of the data sources. Errors or incumbrances should be corrected, and "debugging" should be repeated until the data collection forms and codes are well tested. The above steps are necessary even if direct data entry into a computer terminal will be used. Quite obviously, the computer system administrator, system programmers, and database managers have to participate in the entire planning process. The computer must always be regarded as the labor-saving device that it is. It will faithfully carry out the work needed to complete the well planned project.

CONCEPTS IN COMPUTERIZED REGISTRY DESIGN

When one contemplates the design/implementation of a genetic registry, there are two levels of discussion involved: hardware and software needs. Concomitant with these needs are the important factors of available finances and whether this registry is to be a single- or a multiple-user system. The planner must decide whether it is more costly to purchase a prepackaged system and pay to have it tailored to individual needs or to design a system from the ground up. Should the system start small and grow as demand increases? Should a larger system be implemented, in anticipation of increasing need? These are but a small fraction of the important questions that one should ask before jumping into the computer registry domain. All these questions lead to what is often called "systems design requirements."

Think of a genetic registry as a collection of modules in the same sense as a high-quality component audio system. Each module of the registry is a specialized piece of software performing an important task. Some software modules may be more generally used and more important. If the tape deck fails, you cannot play a tape. If the amplifier fails, the system is unusable. In the same sense, the design of a computerized registry hinges on two software factors; the various component software programs and a program that allows the user to communicate with those programs, "the user interface." The actual software packages (modules) and how to use them are unimportant to the user. This is handled by the interface program.

The interface program, itself, is actually a very sophisticated set of programs. Usually, the interface programs contain an entry/security routine protecting the system from unauthorized users and limiting users from various other program sections. The master interface menu allows the user to choose from a variety of registry options. Options, for example, to review patient records, to perform statistical analyses, to create a pedigree, to output various information, to print a letter, or to execute other options.

Let us examine, first, some of the more important general software features of a genetic registry. Clearly, the ideal registry will 1) contain a "statistics module" capable of performing relevent statistical analyses; 2) contain an "output module," which can a) output relevent graphics, such as pedigrees, graphs, and charts; and b) output letters and reports, preferably in low- and high-quality resolution; 3) contain an "input module," which allows for the input of a) patient data, b) familial data, c) other data, such as histological photos; 4) contain an "editor," which allows for the editing/correction of records in the computer and checking for completeness and accuracy; 5) contain a "report generator," which allows for generation of standardized reports including recall and follow-up schedules; 6) contain a "report form generator," which allows for the creation of customized reports; 7) contain a "pedigree generator"; and 8) contain a "basic graphics module," which allows the user to generate certain standardized graphs, such as histograms, line plots, and pie charts. If a system is going to be used by remote users and if we wish to access remote systems, we will need 9) a "communications module," which defines correct remote tie-in to the registry.

System software routines all work from data records, either patient data or familial data. When a user must deal with large amounts of data, he often stores those data in an organized manner, for example, in a file system (filing cabinets). The same is true for computerized records. Any registry must have a way of organizing and managing the stored data. Such a program or system is an integral part of the software and is called a database management system (DBMS).

Having the data stored in an organized form is important. A database provides a mechanism for centralized control of all data associated within the system, thus facilitating easier access and retrieval of quality data. One general question that should be examined by the general user is the ease of user access to and interface with the data. Database systems today offer various mechanisms to interface with the data. Relational database systems, the new vogue in database technology, offer a standard query language (SQL) that allows novice computer users a standard access mechanism to retrieve and report on necessary data elements. Whether one uses hierarchial, relational, or any other of the numerous database structures, an easy mechanism should be present that allows nonprofessional computer users to retrieve, report, and update the necessary data elements of the system in an easy and timely fashion. As demands on databases become more and more sophisticated, and the questions become more demanding, software designers are integrating artificial intelligence (AI) concepts into the DBMS systems. AI shell packages, an artificial intelligence development package, allowing the user to build his or her own expert system and interface to and from data elements within a defined database system, are now available from Texas Instruments, Inc. (Austin, TX), and Information Builders, Inc. (New York, NY).

To this point, we have discussed a generic software structure requirement for a computerized genetic registry. We have been purposefully general to allow the potential user/designer to tailor his or her system as necessary for his or her particular needs. Let us now examine generic hardware requirements for our registry.

Hardware is much more difficult to specify. Rather than worry about the financial constraints, and worry about the restrictions that often exist because of such constraints, consider a generic computer system.

We begin with the input devices. The standard input device is the familiar computer keyboard. However, depending on user requirements and software design, there are a variety of other devices that are also suitable as input devices: 1) a light pen, 2) a mouse, 3) an optical scanner, 4) a bar code scanner, 5) a digitizing tablet, 6) magnetic tape, and 7) information directly communicated from other computers.

At the other end of the computer, we have the output devices. These can range from simple paper printers, to laser jets, to full-blown laser printers with the ability to print publishable-quality text and to generate high-resolution graphics. Additionally, for higher-quality graphics, liquid ink pen plotters can be added to the system, as can tape drives and floppy disk communication devices. Every computer system requires a power supply. Even in the best of environments, occasional voltage changes, surges, and the more dangerous lightening spikes, can damage and/or destroy the delicate microchips (the most sensitive and important part of the computer). Therefore, particularly in an environment in which the system is continuously operating, it is essential that a voltage/line surge protection device be purchased. The reader is cautioned to be wary of the cheap, discount store protectors. Rarely are these as good as the box states. With the cost of a computer on the line, a high-quality surge device is more than worth the investment. A back-up system on a remote computer or stored files of data is an additional safeguard. Most computer centers routinely back up their files on a weekly and/or monthly basis.

Multiple-user systems and remote-user systems place further hardware demands on the genetic registry. Remote users must have a modem to access the registry via a phone line that will accept transmissions without interruption. The registry computer must have the necessary equipment to recognize a dial-in call. Furthermore, the calls can come in at different communication speeds (BAUD rates). Standard rates are 300, 600, 1,200, 4,800, and 9,600 BAUD, although higher speeds are also available. Fixing the BAUD rate at a specific value is cheaper, but it restricts the remote users to a particular communication rate. Allowing any communication rate (AUTOBAUD) facilitates the general user but is more expensive.

Multiple users, in the same building, for example, might also wish to communicate with the registry. One way to do this is to dial into the system through the dial-in lines. However, this ties up the lines for remote users. One solution to this problem is to install some sort of local area network (LAN). Another consideration in database design for multiple users is to allow for synchronization of data use (i.e., multiple users may go against the same data record or data element, but a mechanism must be in place to allow for lock out of that element or record during the process of update or deletion; this mechanism ensures data integrity and quality; there are many ways to do this, and it is beyond the scope of this chapter to discuss them).

Before we close with a discussion of the central computer itself, it is important to note that software, programming languages, and database systems all require memory. This memory can be resident in the machine itself or, as is more often the case, an additional peripheral storage device can be used. This is particularly true when the memory capacity is limited by structural requirements. For example, in a microcomputer, there are a limited number of "expansion" slots into which one can slide additional memory boards. Hence a "hard-disk" peripheral device becomes crucial. External memory is also important in a scenario in which one might start with a small database of patients and expect it to grow.

The central piece of registry hardware is the computer itself. This is, perhaps, the most difficult of all the hardware to specify. To a great extent, the choice depends on which of the previously described demands will be placed on the machine. The more complex the demands, the more carefully one must choose the computer. Computers range from the desktop microcomputer, to the desktop minicomputer, to the workstation, on to the mainframe machine, and finally reaching the supercomputer.

The preceding excursion through the complexities of genetic registry construction is meant to stress the importance of careful, comprehensive planning. It also serves as an introduction to the various aspects of systems design. Genetic registries are important clinical tools, tools that should be of great value when designed carefully. Although the computing power of computers is increasing, the increase will be explosive with the next generation of supercomputer.

In conclusion, evolving knowledge, software, and computer technology foreshadow the day when supercomputers will handle thousands of requests with no delay, when exhaustive statistical analyses can be performed on vast datasets in nanoseconds. Instead of analyzing 10 or 20 variables from 100 individuals, we will be able to analyze 10–20,000 variables from 100,000 or more patients. Clearly, the frontier for the genetic registry is exciting.

References

1. Emery AEH: "A Computerized "At Risk" for Genetic Disease." New York: Associated Scientific Publishers, 1976.
2. Bussey HS: "Familial Polyposis Coli: Familial Studies, Histopathology, Differential Diagnosis, and Results of Treatment." Baltimore: John Hopkins University Press, 1975.
3. Spjut HS, Estrada RG: The significance of epithelial polyps of the large bowel. Pathol Annu 12:147–170, 1977.
4. Spjut HS: Pathology of neoplasms. In Spratt JS (ed): "Neoplasms of the Colon, Rectum and Anus." Philadelphia; WB Saunders Co., 1984, pp 168–170.
5. Berk T, Cohen Z, Cullen JB: Familial polyposis and the role of the preventive registry. Can Med J 124:1427–1428, 1981.
6. Berk T, Cohen Z, McLeod RS, Cullen JB: Surveillance in relatives of patients with adenomatous polyposis. Semin Surg Oncol 3:105–108, 1987.
7. Robertson PE: Genetic registers. In Emery AEH, Rimoin DL (eds): "Principles and Practice of Medical Genetics." Vol 2. New York; Churchill Livingstone, 1983, pp 1481–1487.
8. Conneally PM, Heuch I: Letter to the editor: A computer program to determine genetic risks: a simplified version of PEDIG. Am J Hum Genet 26:773–775, 1974.
9. Smith C: Computers in medicine: Computer programme to estimate recurrence risks for multifactorial familial disease. Br Med J 1:495–497, 1972.
10. Elston RC: For the study of familial cancer. Personal communication, 1988.
11. Stevenson AC: The load of hereditary defects in human populations. Radiat Res Suppl 1:306–325, 1959.
12. Emery AEH, Brough C, Crawfurd M, Harper P, Harris R, Oakshott G: A report on genetic registers, based on the report of the Clinical Genetics Society Working Party. J Med Genet 15:435–442, 1978.
13. Krush AJ: Counseling families with hereditary gastrointestinal polyposis syndromes. Semin Surg Oncol 3:137–139, 1987.
14. Emery AEH, Elliott D, Moores M, Smith C: A genetic register system (RAPID). J Med Genet 11:145–151, 1974.
15. Tips RL, Lynch HT: The impact of genetic counseling upon the family milieu. J Am Med Assoc 184:117–120, 1970.
16. Emery AEH, Smith C: Ascertainment and prevention of genetic disease. Br Med J 3:636–637, 1970.
17. George VT, Elston RC, Lynch HT, Hirayama T: Biostatistical methods for the familial study of cancer. Lynch HT, Hirayama T (eds). Boca Raton, FL: CRC Press, in press.
18. Jagelman DG: Extracolonic manifestations of familial polyposis coli. Semin Surg Oncol 3:88–91, 1987.
19. Schroeder TK: Personal communications, 1988.
20. Herrera-Ornelas L, Elsiah S, Petrelli N, Mittelman A: Causes of death in patients with familial polyposis coli (FPC). Semin Surg Oncol 3:109–117, 1987.
21. Carl W, Herrera L: Dental and bone abnormalities in patients with familial polyposis coli. Semin Surg Oncol 3:77–83, 1987.
22. Northover JMA: Activities of the Leeds Castle polyposis group. Semin Surg Oncol 3:118–119, 1987.
23. Sandberg AA: Chromosomal abnormalities in patients with familial polyposis and colorectal cancer. Semin Surg Oncol 3:133–136, 1987.
24. Watne AL: Patterns of inheritance of colonic polyps. Semin Surg Oncol 3:71–76, 1987.
25. Bulow S: Incidence of associated diseases in familial polyposis coli. Semin Surg Oncol 3:84–87, 1987.
26. Luk GD, Silverman AL, Giardeillo FM: Biochemical markers in patients with familial colonic neoplasia. Semin Surg Oncol 3:126–132, 1987.
27. Wolman SR: Genetic markers of colonic neoplasia. Semin Surg Oncol 3:120–125, 1987.
28. Solomon E, Voss R, Hall V, Bodmer WF, Jass JR, Jeffreys AJ, Lucibellow FC, Pafel I, Rider SH: Chromosome 5 allele loss in human colorectal carcinomas. Nature 328:616–619, 1987.
29. Watson FR, Greenberg RA, Spratt JS: Statistical methods in cancer research. In Donegan WL, Spratt JS (eds): "Cancer of the Breast." Philadelphia: 1988, pp 739–767, WB Saunders Co.

9

Multistage Models and the Age Patterns of Cancer: Does the Statistical Analogy Imply Genetic Homology?

Kenneth M. Weiss and Ranajit Chakraborty

Department of Anthropology, and Graduate Program in Genetics, Penn State University, University Park, Pennsylvania (K.M.W.); Center for Demographic and Population Genetics, University of Texas Graduate School of Biomedical Sciences, Houston, Texas (R.C.)

INTRODUCTION

One of the most insightful hypotheses ever suggested in regard to cancer is Knudson's [1971] somatic mutation hypothesis, which was first offered to explain retinoblastoma (RB) and other embryonal tumors. This has been strikingly borne out by molecular genetic studies of cancer. In response to the discovery of somatic mutation in RB, numerous investigators have searched for and found that similar mechanisms are also involved in many other tumors. This now includes colorectal cancer, including cancer in familial adenomatous polyps (FAP).

Such processes at the cellular level should be reflected at the level of the whole organism in terms of age-specific incidence or mortality rates. This has been one rationale for the widespread application of multistage risk models in cancer epidemiology. Several years ago, we discussed the use of multistage models to fit the age patterns of onset of cancers [Weiss and Chakraborty, 1984]. Many such models have been suggested, including multihit-single cell, multihit-multicell, and initiation-promotion models [reviewed by Whittemore and Keller, 1978].

Although formulated in many different ways, these models shared the feature that they were based on exponential waiting-time distributions, in which the number of events and their rates of occurrence were parameters of the model. By introducing a first-order power series approximation for exponential terms, the age-specific risk, or hazard function, at age x would take the form

$$h(x) \approx ax^b, \tag{1}$$

where the model hypothesizes b events to be required for transformation. The parameter a is a composite parameter whose interpretation is not important to the current discussion.

The number of hits, i.e., value of the parameter b, estimated from a variety of human cancers using these models was about four to six [Cook et al., 1969]. A small number of stages seemed reasonable, based on what was known from experimental carcinogenesis (even before the molecular documentation of the somatic loss of heterozygosity), and on the well established concept of cancer resulting from initiation and promotion events. The fact that cancer was genetic at the cellular level, since most carcinogens were shown to be mutagens, and that mammals are diploid, also made a small number of events seem reasonable. From the fit of these models to cancer epidemiological data, it was assumed by many investigators that the number and nature of the events being modeled at the cellular level were, more or less, correctly understood at the epidemiologic level.

Familial Adenomatous Polyposis, pages 77–89

We looked at the nature of the approximation that led from models derived from first principles to the approximation in Equation 1 and found that, when we fitted a variety of multistages models to data without using the numerical approximation, the number of stages estimated was much greater than four to six (the fit also improved slightly). To us, this meant that although Equation 1 was empirically close, it was not an accurate way to estimate the parameters of the original model, a point also noted by Moolgavkar [1978]. More importantly, the number of stages estimated without using the approximation, on the order of ten or so, was too great to be consistent with contemporary concepts of carcinogenesis [Weiss and Chakraborty, 1984].

We also noted some other disturbing facts [Weiss and Chakraborty, 1984]. For example, if the model was to be believed, different racial groups, or even different sexes, seemed to require different numbers of "hits" to produce the same type of cancer. This makes little biological sense, and casts doubt on the epidemiological value of multistage models of cancer.

One of the epidemiologically clearest forms of cancer is FAP and its association with colorectal cancer. This disease is inherited as a mendelian dominant disorder. Because the probablity of polyps, and of subsequent colorectal cancer, is nearly 100% without prophylactical treatment, and because this risk is similar in Japan, the United States and Europe, where baseline colorectal cancer rates are very different, cancer in an FAP gene carrier does not seem to depend on exogenous environmental risk factors. Given the plausibility of mechanisms such as those suggested by Knudson [1971, 1977], it seemed likely that a different, presumably lower, number of "hits" would be required to transform cells in the FAP patient than in the population at large, a result that various investigators had suggested from the data using the approximation of Equation 1 [Weiss and Chakraborty, 1984].

In fitting FAP data, however, we found quite a different pattern. The number of stages estimated from applying multistage models to the FAP data was greater—much greater—not less, than that in the general population. When the approximate model was used (Equation 1), the number was about ten, but when the original models were tested, the estimated number of stages was much larger and depending on the method is as high as 95 ×.

These observations raise doubts about the use of multistage models to make inferences about the underlying cellular processes, for example, whether different racial groups require the same number of stages for a given cancer, or to make

TABLE 1.
Cumulative Incidence (%) for Second Tumors* in Retinoblastoma Patients

Source		Time since treatment (≈ age) 10	20	30
Tucker et al., 1987		3	14	Unavailable
Abramson et al., 1984	In radiation field	20	50	90
	Not in field	10	30	68
Draper et al., 1987	In field	3	7	Unavailable
	Not in field	2	3	Unavailable
	Orbit, sporadic RB	0	0	Unavailable
Francois et al., 1980	In field			>>7.7[a]
	Not in field			>>13[a]
Population risk at 20 years	All osteosarcomas =		0.0001	
	Orbital osteosarcomas =		≈0.0	

*Majority are osteosarcomas.
[a]These are percent of cases with tumors, observed for variable times 4–30 years, but not computing risk by actuarial methods.

inferences concerning human exposures to carcinogens, such as chemicals and radiation, for purposes such as determining whether the carcinogen does its damage by affecting early, or late, stages in the process [Whittemore, 1977; Day and Brown, 1980; Brown, 1987; Brown and Chu, 1987].

Rather than estimating the number of stages in carcinogenesis, Moolgavkar, Knudson, and colleagues developed an explicit two-stage model that fits many aspects of cancer epidemiology, including Knudson's somatic mutation hypothesis [see, e.g., Moolgavkar and Venzon, 1978; Moolgavkar and Knudson, 1981]. In this model, the first stage is a mutational stage that occurs with a specified rate in an age-specific number of at-risk stem cells. After a cell has suffered the first mutation, it will produce a clone of daughter cells by mitosis whose size can be quantified by a stochastic birth-death process. At any subsequent time, the second carcinogenic event may take place in one of these cells.

This model can fit population data for many tumors, including hormonal cancer, as well as the effects of environmental risk factors, including a discrimination, at least qualitatively, between the consequences of chronic and single exposures to risk factors that affect different parts of the carcinogenic process [Moolgavkar and Knudson, 1981; Moolgavkar, 1983]. However, because it assumes two stages, a goodness of fit does not provide support for the assertion that two stages are in fact involved in carcinogenesis but only that, however many stages are actually involved at the cellular level, this two-stage model fits the epidemiological data well.

Because of the molecular genetic support for it, there is now obvious enthusiasm to pursue Knudson's idea, and that idea is clearly being incorporated into the working model of cancer molecular epidemiology. This chapter looks at age patterns of colorectal and other cancers to determine if a new set of cautions might be in order.

FAP AND COLORECTAL CANCER

Several studies have now shown an association between the FAP phenotype and polymorphic DNA markers on the long arm of chromosome 5 [Bodmer et al., 1987; Leppert et al., 1987; Khan et al., 1988]. Somatic loss of heterozygosity in the FAP region has been found in colorectal carcinoma in FAP patients as well as in sporadic colorectal carcinomas [Okamoto et al., 1988; Solomon et al., 1987], which strongly suggests that this region contains an allele, which we can denote FAP+ (using the + to represent the affected allele, regardless of its physiological function), generally involved in colorectal cancer. Molecular genetic studies have shown that malignant transformation within a polyp occurs after somatic loss of heterozygosity at this FAP locus but that this is not required for the formation of the polyps themselves [Bodmer et al., 1987; Okamoto et al., 1988]. However, segregation analysis in families with the FAP gene has used polyps, rather than cancer, as the defining phenotype, and this shows that the FAP locus acts as a nearly fully penetrant dominant; therefore, the FAP locus must be involved in the adenomas as well as cancer. Bodmer et al. [1987] speculate that cellular heterozygosity for FAP+/− can lead to polyp growth through a dose of effect, with final transformation involving the somatic loss of the remaining normal FAP− locus allele (conversion to FAP+/+). This fits with Knudson's model for embryonal tumors, if not his early speculations on FAP [Knudson, 1977].

It is still an open question whether there is a second locus involved in the FAP syndrome. Because untreated FAP+ carriers are at nearly 100% risk of both polyps and colorectal cancer [Lipkin et al., 1980], if any other loci are required for the final transformation to colorectal cancer, the probability of a mutation occurring at those loci, in at least some colorectal stem cells, must also be nearly 100%. There is evidence for systematic changes in heterozygosity at other chromosome locations in colorectal cancer. Okamoto et al. [1988] found frequent cellular loss of heterozygosity at chromosome 22 in colorectal cancer, and Fearon et al. [1987] found similar loss in chromosome 17 (these authors also find other chromosome segments involved with lower frequency). Something similar may be occurring in multiple endocrine neoplasia type 2 (MEN-2), in which the main susceptibility gene is on chromosome 10 but loss of heterozygosity is on chromosome 1 [Mathew et al., 1987a, b; Simpson et al., 1987]. If such a multilocus mechanism is involved in colorectal cancer, one may wonder why there is no evidence for a comparable familial colorectal cancer syndrome involving the other loci themselves. Is it that, without the FAP+ allele present, the penetrance of the second locus as colorectal cancer is too small to appear to be mendelian?

Either view is in principle plausible: 1) FAP is a single-locus system, with the observed homozygosity at other loci merely coincidental or unrelated to the etiology of the cancer; 2) FAP is part of a genuine two-locus system. However, in practice these two mechanisms should produce different age-onset patterns. In the first model, FAP +/− individuals would only need to await the occurrence of somatic homozygosity (FAP +/+), a one-stage process, but, in the second instance, they would also need to await cellular homozygosity at another locus; this process might require three steps, somatic FAP +/+ conversion, loss of first allele aat second locus, and somatic loss of heterozygosity at the second locus in the same cell.

None of these scenarios fits the hazard function of equation 1, for reasons discussed above, and only the single-locus version should fit Moolgavkar's two-stage model (this appears not to have been tried). In the following, we examine the age-onset pattern of cancers in which the number of steps in the process may be known. We also study the effects on the age of onset distribution of exposure to environmental agents that appear to alter the rate at which those steps occur.

ONE-STAGE TUMORS?

The tumor for which we have the best data on the age of onset data in a known single-gene process to compare with FAP is retinoblastoma (RB), which involves a locus, denoted RB or RB1, on chromosome 13; this is the first tumor for which the somatic mutation model was suggested [Knudson, 1971]. At present, there is little or no evidence that a second locus is involved in RB. By birth, heritable RB is frequently bilateral and/or multifocal, whereas sporadic RB, in which both events must occur during gestation, is almost always unilateral and unifocal. Both heritable and sporadic RB appear to be cytologically RB +/+. Unlike FAP vs. other colorectal cancer, the age of onset is very similar in both sporadic and heritable RB; this appears to be due to the histological dynamics of the retina. Retinoblasts are essentially all differentiated before birth, with little or no further mitotic activity and hence little postnatal opportunity for cell transformation. Thus both sporadic and familial tumor transformation have essentially occurred by the time of birth, and the clinical occurrence of the subsequent tumors is due essentially to variation in tumor growth itself.

However, there are many more cell divisions, and many more stem cells, in the neonatal large intestine than in the retina, and these cells are actively dividing throughout life. If nothing other than somatic loss of heterozygosity was required in FAP, one would expect FAP+ individuals to be affected at or soon after birth. This supports the idea that the formation of polyps is not a sufficient, even if it is perhaps a necessarily prior, step in the process.

Individuals who have inherited the RB gene are also at elevated risk for osteosarcomas, but, like colon cancer in FAP, these are not manifest at birth. They arise in childhood in tissue sites and at ages at which sporadic osteosarcomas arise. Presumably this age pattern is related to the tissue dynamics of bone growth and development. There is now molecular evidence to suggest that somatic RB homozygosity is involved in the production of osteosarcomas (even in sporadic cases) [Dryja et al., 1986; Hansen et al., 1985]. In osteosarcomas, a precursor lesion analogous to adenomatous polyps is not known, so it is somewhat surprizing that the osteosarcomas occur over such a dispersed time period whereas the much smaller bed of retinoblasts generates tumors—often many tumors—in a brief perinatal period. This again suggests the presence of other factors, perhaps other gene loci, in osteosarcomas, but some tests have failed to show evidence of any locus other than the RB locus on chromosome 13 [Hansen et al., 1985].

A ZERO-STAGE PROCESS?

Even more remarkable is the age of onset pattern of second sarcomas occurring in the field of therapeutic irradiation in heritable RB patients. In these individuals, the bone and connective tissue of the orbit are exposed to a point-source risk factor. Although the doses involved may sterilize many of the recipient nonocular orbital cells, one would expect that a sizeable fraction would experience the secondary events needed to produce tumors if these are solely mutational in nature. Irradiated RB patients would then experience a zero-stage processes in the irradiated field, just as they appear to do for RB itself. Indeed, the risk of sarcoma is much increased, but the age of onset pattern does not suggest that cells are fully transformed at the time of irradiation. In fact, the excess risk appears to persist for 20 or even 30 years after exposure and occurs past the age at which normal childhood osteosarcoma risk has disappeared.

There have been three sizeable studies of the risk of subsequent osteosarcomas in RB patients, including tumors in, as well as outside, the field of irradiation [Abramson et al., 1984; Draper et al., 1986; Tucker et al., 1987]. In these studies, we may compare the risk of second tumors in individuals not irradiated and/or of tumors in nonirradiated tissues. A summary of these data is given in Table 1.

There is wide disagreement on the absolute risk values in these studies, for reasons not yet clear, probably involving variation in dosage and treatment method, ascertainment, and method of computation of risk. Even the lowest estimate (7% after 20 years) represents a large relative risk for any childhood cancer, yet nonocular orbital osteosarcomas are not found in irradiated sporadic-RB patients (i.e., in those who do not carry a susceptibility gene), so that radiation alone may not be sufficient to generate these tumors. The long latency period for these tumors in heritable-RB patients also suggests that, whatever the absolute risk, irradiation does not produce the final event required to transform exposed cells, and that those events occur over a period probably in relation to the dynamics of mitosis in those cells. It is also interesting that this latency period for in-field second tumors is very similar in time, but different in scale, to not-in-field second tumors, again suggesting that radiation is only increasing the number of partially transformed cells rather than completing the transformation process. As with FAP, but unlike with ocular RB, might there be a second locus? There are similar relationships between radiation and second tumors in other heritable childhood tumors [UNSCEAR, 1988].

EXPOSURE TO ENVIRONMENTAL RISKS AND THE AGE PATTERN OF COLORECTAL CANCER

Somatic homozygosity has now been demonstrated in at least some instances in colon, breast, and lung cancer as well as in a variety of childhood tumors, suggesting that this mechanism is common, perhaps even general, in carcinogenesis. Current data suggest that a small number of gene loci are responsible for these changes in a wide variety of tumors [Okamoto et al., 1988]. Cancers of different organs thus might be analogous, or even evolutionarily *homologous,* diseases. The different age patterns of cancers in different organs may reflect the same mechanisms, scaled to tissue-specific details: intensity of exposure to environmental mutagens, tissue size, turnover rate of at-risk cells, and the like. The observation that many cancer risks increase as the fourth to sixth power of age is the kind of evidence we would expect.

To look at this, we have elsewhere obtained multistage parameter estimates for the age- and sex-specific mortality patterns of a wide variety of tumors, using international mortality data for 1970 from the World Health Organization [Weiss et al., 1988]. The particular model used specifies that b events are required to transform a cell lineage, and that each of these events occurs at rate a per unit time. As was mentioned above, we do not think such estimates can represent the underlying process accurately, so the fitting must be viewed as *only* empirical. In this model, the probability that disease occurs by age t is P(t), where

$$P(t) = [1 - \exp(-at)]^b. \quad (2)$$

from which h(t), the age-specific mortality rate, is

$$h(t) = [dP(t)/dt]/[1 - P(t)]. \quad (3)$$

Maximum likelihood estimates of the parameters a and b of the model were determined by fitting Equation 3 to the population count and number of deaths in each 5-year age/sex group in each tested population, from age 35 to age 75 years, assuming h(t) to be the parameter in a binomial process. Thus, for each population, and separately for males and females within each, we determined the best fitting values of a and b. The results of this parameter estimation for colon cancer are given in Table 2. From a statistical point of view, the model fit most age-specific mortality patterns quite well.

It is generally assumed that interpopulation differences in cancer risks are largely the result of differences in exposure to environmental mutagens [see, e.g., Doll and Peto, 1981]. Differences in exposure should change the *rate* of occurrence of cancer but not the *shape* of the age-onset curve, which presumably is determined by histology and genetics. We found a regular pattern consistent with this. There is a correlation of over 0.9 between the estimates of a and b across the populations tested. That is, we were able to fit a regression line, a = (0.0014)b − 0.0013, to the (a,b) points fitted to the set of populations. Higher-risk populations are generally to the right along this line. Figure 1 provides a

TABLE 2.
Fitting of 1970 Colon Cancer Mortality Data*

Country	Sex	Pop. $\times 10^6$	a	b	$\hat{a}$	ASCR	χ^2	Signif?
Switzerland	M	3.0	.01835	14.90	.01927	184	7.48	1
Austria	M	3.5	.01874	14.56	.01894	223	22.16	1
France	M	24.8	.01793	14.35	.01851	191	18.79	1
Canada	M	10.7	.01846	14.21	.01832	237	6.90	1
Hungary	M	5.0	.01685	13.74	.01767	142	20.78	1
Singapore	M	1.1	.01596	13.70	.01762	63	10.93	1
Scotland	F	2.7	.01775	13.54	.01739	237	2.98	1
U.S.	M	99.6	.01782	13.54	.01739	218	33.20	0
Belgium	F	4.9	.01749	13.52	.01737	216	7.36	1
Denmark	M	2.4	.01685	13.13	.01682	192	6.26	1
West Germany	M	28.9	.01690	12.87	.01647	196	89.81	1
Argentina	M	11.5	.01665	12.70	.01624	202	17.83	1
Belgium	M	4.7	.01655	12.59	.01608	214	12.22	1
Switzerland	F	3.2	.01555	12.58	.01607	139	23.46	1
Puerto Rico	M	1.3	.01429	12.53	.01601	56	14.20	1
Israel	F	1.3	.01550	12.48	.01593	115	13.15	1
Norway	M	1.9	.01534	12.39	.01581	145	4.40	1
Uruguay	M	1.4	.01680	12.28	.01566	231	8.39	1
Peru	M	6.8	.01272	12.17	.01551	25	11.97	0
France	F	26.0	.01529	12.15	.01548	151	15.27	1
Uruguay	F	1.4	.01622	11.85	.01506	264	9.77	1
Italy	M	26.2	.01530	11.77	.01495	155	26.01	1
Hungary	F	5.3	.01477	11.62	.01475	140	6.96	1
Denmark	F	2.5	.01568	11.62	.01475	205	8.35	1
U.K.	M	23.7	.01557	11.61	.01473	193	37.08	1
N. Ireland	M	0.7	.01595	11.46	.01453	213	3.5	1
U.S.	F	104.6	.01562	11.45	.01451	197	10.19	0
West Germany	F	31.8	.01504	11.35	.01437	175	62.40	1
Holland	M	6.5	.01493	11.28	.01428	183	8.46	1

(continued)

TABLE 2.
Fitting of 1970 Colon Cancer Mortality Data* (continued)

Country	Sex	Pop. $\times 10^6$	a	b	â	ASCR	χ^2	Signif?
Australia	M	6.3	.01544	11.25	.01424	205	19.22	1
Argentina	F	11.7	.01494	11.20	.01417	178	11.36	1
Austria	F	3.9	.01464	11.19	.01415	163	4.81	1
Sweden	M	4.0	.01456	11.15	.01410	175	4.35	1
Venezuela	M	5.2	.01207	11.12	.01406	59	29.65	1
Canada	F	10.6	.01561	11.05	.01396	235	2.51	0
Holland	F	6.5	.01469	10.91	.01377	193	1.37	1
Italy	F	27.4	.01374	10.76	.01356	125	10.83	1
Spain	F	17.3	.01309	10.58	.01331	104	23.38	1
Mexico	F	25.4	.01102	10.47	.01316	34	2.88	0
Ecuador	F	3.0	.01120	10.47	.01316	37	59.13	1
Czechoslovakia	M	7.0	.01381	10.44	.01312	129	9.59	1
U.K.	F	25.1	.01418	10.36	.01301	181	5.53	0
Spain	M	16.5	.01265	10.33	.01297	89	25.42	1
Finland	F	2.4	.01229	10.25	.01286	93	11.50	1
Peru	F	6.7	.01067	10.14	.01271	25	14.03	1
Israel	M	1.3	.01318	10.04	.01257	124	2.93	1
Czechoslovakia	F	7.4	.01268	10.03	.01255	103	8.09	1
Poland	F	16.7	.01170	9.96	.01246	60	27.60	1
Finland	M	2.2	.01239	9.93	.01242	114	8.49	1
Singapore	F	1.0	.01260	9.79	.01222	76	1.45	1
N. Ireland	F	0.8	.01394	9.71	.01212	228	2.92	1
Chile	M	4.5	.01128	9.54	.01188	63	3.29	1
Chile	F	4.7	.01151	9.44	.01174	83	7.31	1
Paraguay	F	0.6	.01169	9.35	.01161	128	5.29	1
Greece	F	4.5	.01126	9.34	.01159	73	6.19	1
Sweden	F	4.0	.01230	9.21	.01142	152	9.74	1
Australia	F	6.2	.01311	9.02	.01116	218	4.94	1
Norway	F	1.9	.01165	8.87	.01095	129	7.55	1
Bulgaria	M	4.2	.01026	8.81	.01087	50	4.62	1
Yugoslavia	F	10.4	.00972	8.64	.01063	45	6.66	1
Bulgaria	F	4.2	.00999	8.57	.01054	48	6.85	1
New Zealand	M	1.4	.01298	8.51	.01046	260	5.10	1
Romania	M	9.9	.00962	8.36	.01025	51	9.34	1
Romania	F	10.3	.00939	8.26	.01011	45	14.08	1
Poland	M	15.8	.00997	8.14	.00994	69	17.17	1
Mexico	M	25.3	.00826	8.04	.00980	25	16.22	1
Yugoslavia	M	10.0	.00908	7.90	.00962	51	3.61	1
Japan	M	50.6	.00927	7.82	.00951	58	20.91	1
Puerto Rico	F	1.4	.00952	7.81	.00949	59	26.06	1
New Zealand	F	1.4	.01113	7.40	.00893	218	5.32	1
Greece	M	4.3	.00874	7.27	.00874	71	7.99	1
Paraguay	M	0.6	.00996	7.21	.00867	164	9.88	1
Hong Kong	M	2.0	.00954	7.17	.00860	132	8.94	1
Ecuador	M	3.0	.00668	7.07	.00047	19	25.33	1
Hong Kong	F	2.0	.00775	6.47	.00764	69	2.47	1
Thailand	M	18.2	.00614	6.23	.00731	20	6.65	1
Thailand	F	18.1	.00409	5.23	.00593	10	4.55	1

*Data from WHO (1970). a and b are estimated from the data using Equation 3. â is the nearest point on the a-b line to the point (a,b). χ^2 values have 6 d.f. for goodness of fit of mortality rates to those predicted by Equation 3 with parameters â and $\hat{b}$. 'Signif?' equals 0 when the point (a,b) is beyond the ± 2 SE ellipse around the point (â,$\hat{b}$), and 1 if it is within the ellipse.

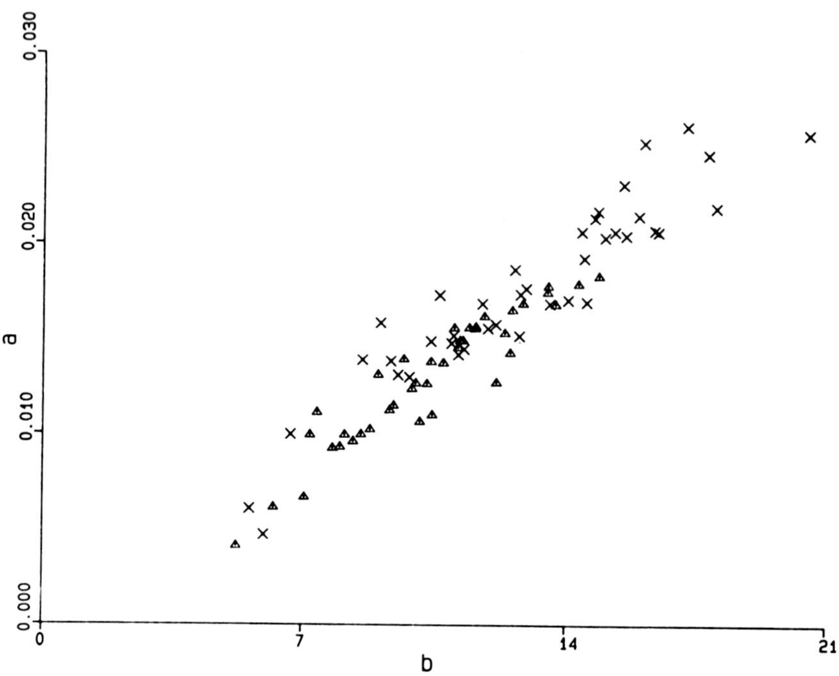

Fig. 1. Scatter plot of (a,b) values fitted to a multistage risk model for males, and separately to females, from 40 countries based on 1970 World Health Organization mortality data for colon cancer (△) and for stomach cancer (×).

scatter plot of the (a,b) values for the data shown in Table 2. We also fitted a variety of other multistage models with similar results.

The reality of this finding receives interesting confirmation from the FAP data. For comparable ages, the parameters (a,b) estimated for FAP cancer onset lie essentially on the regression line determined from "normal" populations (Fig. 1), even though the parameter values are nearly a full order of magnitude higher than in any of the populations from which the line was derived. This is true, with basically the same parameter estimates, for Japanese, English, and U.S. FAP data. FAP appears to speed up risk in the same way that other risk factors do, except much more so. (There is some indication that the distribution of onset age in FAP is a composite one, with a small subset having even younger onset than the majority [Utsonomiya et al., 1980]).

We repeated this analysis for many other cancers, including hematopoietic cancers, with results shown in Table 3. We found a similar relationship among the parameters. More interesting is the fact that, as is shown in Figures 1 and 2, we obtain a very similar regression line for *different* tumor sites. This finding is comparable to the observation by Cook et al. [1969] that cancer hazard functions for different tumor sites were approximate multiples of each other.

Real populations are undoubtedly mixtures of risk groups, and, in at least some instances, this has been shown in detail within populations. We found this for intrapopulational sex differences, and for FAP, and a similar result was obtained by Lustbader et al. [1988], who showed that a subset of childhood sarcoma families appear to be at genetically elevated risk. We found by numerical simulation that the pattern in Table 3

TABLE 3.
Summary of Fitted Data for Various Cancer Sites

Site	Min. a	Max. a	Min. b	Max. b	a–b Line parameters Slope	a–b Line parameters Intercept	a–b Correlation[b]
Esophagus	.0023	.0238	3.94	28.67	0.00084	0.00251	0.82
Stomach	.0044	.0263	5.04	20.53	0.00136	-0.00021	0.96
Colon	.0041	.0187	5.23	14.90	0.00128	-0.00138	0.94
Lung	.0039	.0311	5.09	24.32	0.00148	-0.00141	0.98
Bone	.0003	.0092	2.18	9.98	0.00117	-0.00210	0.90
Skin	.0007	.0092	1.91	11.20	0.00111	-0.00150	0.96
Breast[a]	.0035	.0237	4.48	14.22	0.00194	-0.00282	0.96
Cervix[a]	.0032	.0169	3.38	11.35	0.00161	-0.00130	0.90
Uterus[a]	.0050	.0230	4.92	18.16	0.00121	-0.00112	0.94
Prostate	.0151	.0331	15.43	49.14	0.00049	-0.01024	0.97
Leukemia	.0003	.0104	1.73	8.88	0.00158	-0.00269	0.99
Lymphoma	.0004	.0129	1.70	11.06	0.00150	-0.00209	0.96

[a]Site fitted for ages 25–44 years only; others fitted for 35–74 years. "Uterus" refers to endometrium.
[b]Correlation between values of a and b for the populations fitted for the specified site.

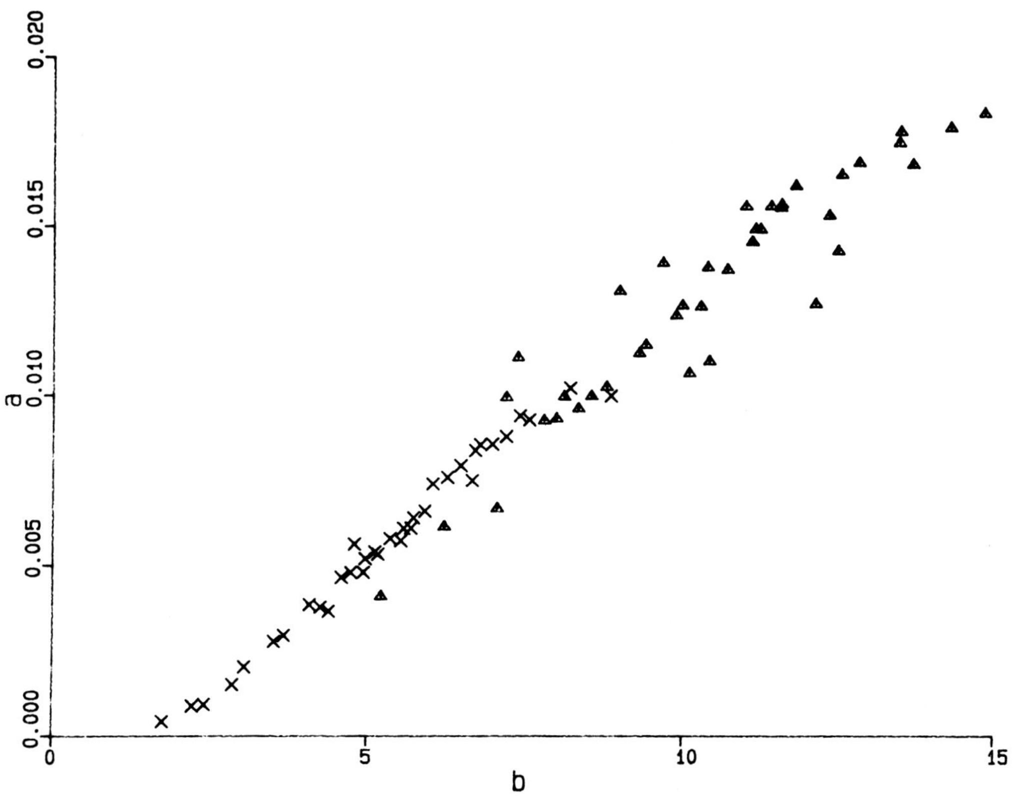

Fig. 2. Scatter plot of (a,b) values fitted to a multistage risk model for males, and separately to females, from 40 countries based on 1970 World Health Organization mortality data for colon cancer (△) and for leukemia (×).

holds, to a close approximation, if we consider a population to be a mixture of distributions (the whole-population [a,b] values are approximately equal the average of the values of $[a,b]_i$ for the subpopulations, weighted by their mixing proportions.

These results show that, to a reasonable degree, the effect of exposure to environmental agents on cancer age-onset patterns is in some sense approximately linear. This supports the idea that cancers of different organs are cytologically analogous and/or genetically *homologous,* the latter because the molecular genetic evidence shows that the same few loci may be involved in a variety of tumors and because some of the known oncogenes are evolutionarily homologous genes.

Let us return briefly to the subject of radiation carcinogenesis. The most recent and reliable reports of colon cancer in adults subject to irradiation of the colon are from survivors of the atomic bombings in Hiroshima and Nagasaki [Shimizu et al., 1987, 1988; Preston et al., 1986; UNSCEAR, 1988]. The best fitting model of the effect of a single exposure to a modest level of ionizing radiation is that, for a given sex and age at irradiation, and after a 10 year latency period, the subsequent risks of colorectal cancer are a roughly constant multiple of the baseline risks for 30 years or more (there is some evidence of a slight decline after 30 years). Most of the excess cancers occur in the ages at which that cancer would normally occur. There are no published reports of chromosome 5 typing in Japanese atomic bomb survivors. Qualitatively similar patterns are found for most adult-onset solid carcinomas. Because there is a 10+ years latency time, it appears unlikely that radiation is inducing the second (or last) stage in adult carcinogenesis. The exposure, as in RB therapy, is a point-source exposure. It appears to increase the fraction of singly or partially hit cells, which then await the occurrence of a later event(s) to become transformed.

DISCUSSION

We believe that molecular data have corroborated our concern about literal interpretations of multistage model parameters applied to human cancer data. This does not mean that multistage models are of no use, but it does mean they must be interpreted with caution. Molecular data show that cancer is clonal and involves a small number of events (two to four perhaps). That at least some of these events can be induced by mutations seems clear, and these are probably the prior events, because subsequent changes apparently often involve somatic recombination rather than point mutation.

From epidemiological data as well, it appears to be possible that, properly parameterized, environmental risk factors have relatively simple effects on the incidence function, suggesting that they may affect only one, probably an early, stage required to transform cells (a point made from a different perspective by Whittemore [1977], Day and Brown [1980], Day [1984], Brown and Chu [1987]).

We never pursued our work showing a linear-like effect of environmental risk factors (reported in Weiss et al. [1988], but completed in 1984), because it did not appear possible that carcinogenesis could be a one-step process, and we were unable to reformulate the model we were using (Equation 2) to address the problem adequately. However, it may be productive to speculate about its possible meaning.

Not enough attention may have been given to the fact that the genesis of loss of somatic heterozygosity, presumably a late stage in carcinogenesis, may not represent the classical mutational process [Hansen et al., 1985]. Somatic recombinations may occur at mitosis, when other mutations also become manifest, and in that sense the two may share time-related characteristics. However, somatic recombinations may not share response patterns identical to those of environmental mutagens; the RB and FAP data suggest that environmental mutations are not needed to induce the transforming somatic recombinations. Perhaps the major environmental mutational effects affect only the first stage(s) of the process, the later stages being histologically, but not environmentally, determined (except, perhaps, when these involve tissue growth promotors). For example, radiation may not be effective in inducing in vivo somatic recombination of the observed type or may do so only rarely. If somatic recombination is relatively independent of environmental effects, we might find a one- or two-hit relationship to the environment. This should have consequences for comparing risk schedules among different exposure categories.

FAP+ individuals have a course of cancer onset that reflects the fact that they begin life with *all* their cells affected by this stage. Their waiting time may reflect a pure b − 1 stage process. In the general population, the same first stage will be caused by exposure to a carcinogens (e.g., in the diet) but only in a limited number of cells. This difference in the number and age of occurrence of partially transformed cells is enough to raise FAP cancer risks by orders of magnitude. However, the number of colorectal stem cells is very large, and their turnover rapid, so, if environmental mutations were all that were required, everyone should experience colorectal cancer in the normal lifetime.

It is interesting to recall Peto's speculation on the importance of the fact that a human has many orders of magnitude, more cells and longer exposure time relative to a mouse, yet both species have about the same lifetime probabilities of cancer [Peto et al., 1975]. Might this also be explained by the tissue-dynamic dependence of somatic recombinational events in the two species?

If FAP+ individuals reflect a cell population wholly affected by one mutational event, we might view the general population as a mixture of individuals with dose-dependent fractions of their cells mutationally affected (i.e., made FAP+/-). The dose-response pattern should be reflected in the difference between the whole-population and FAP age-onset patterns. General environmental exposures could be regarded as a stand-in for dose measurements.

In light of the molecular data, the relative absence of single-gene, dominantly expressed tumors seems surprising. Given the great similarity in genetic mechanisms among many tumors, why do we not have clearly mendelian families like FAP for many other sites? Knudson's model may be generally accurate in regard to many human cancers. However, we have tried to note some cautions about complexities or subtleties that might be overlooked. Just as multistage models must be used with great circumspection, we suggest proceeding with care before adopting two-stage models too enthusiastically.

SUMMARY

Carcinogenesis is a multistage process at the cellular level, which yields characteristic age-specific risk patterns at the population level. These fit closely to a variety of related stochastic multistage models, which hypothesize a small number of stages required to transform a cell lineage. In an earlier paper, we showed that a commonly used but inaccurate mathematical approximation has led to erroneous interpretations of such models in regard to the number of stages in the carcinogenic process. We showed that this problem applied to the case of FAP. Recently, the nature of some of the causal stages in colorectal carcinogenesis has been discovered. In this paper, we explore how that new knowledge and data on the effects of environmental risk factors relate to the interpretation of the age pattern of colorectal and other cancers. The common structure of cancer risks between populations for the same site, and between sites, suggests a common underlying biological process, with a simple, perhaps nearly linear relationship to levels of environmental risk factors. This is interpreted in light of molecular data to reflect the possibility that only one or two stages in carcinogenesis are due to environmental mutations, the others being due to mitotic recombinational events that may be relatively unrelated to environmental exposures.

References

Abramson DH, Ellsworth RM, Kitchin FD, et al.: Second nonocular tumors in retinoblastoma survivors. Ophthalmology 91:1351–1355,1984.

Bodmer WF, Bailey CJ, Bodmer J, Bussey HJR, Ellis A, Gorman P, Lucibello FC, Murday VA, Rider SH, Scambler P, Sheer D, Solomon E, Spurr NK: Localization of the gene for familial adenomatous polyps on chromosome 5. Nature 328:614–616, 1987.

Brown CC, Chu KC: Use of multistage models to infer

stage affected by carcinogenic exposure: Example of lung cancer. J Chronic Dis 40 [Suppl 2]:171S–179S, 1987.

Chu KC: A nonmathematical view of mathematical models for cancer. J Chronic Dis 40 [Suppl 2]:163S–170S, 1987.

Cook P, Doll R, Fellingham S: A mathematical model for the age distribution of cancer in man. Int J Cancer 4:93–112, 1969.

Darby SC, Nakashima E, Kato H: A parallel analysis of cancer mortality among atomic bomb survivors and patients with ankylosing spondylitis given x-ray therapy. Radiation Effects Research Foundation, Technical Report No. TR 4-84, 1984.

Day N: Radiation and multistage carcinogenesis. In Boice JD, Fraumeni JF (eds): "Radiation Carcinogenesis: Epidemiology and Biological Significance," New York: Raven Press, 1984, pp 437–443.

Day N, Brown C: Multistage models and primary prevention of cancer. J Natl Cancer Inst 64:977–989, 1980.

Doll R, Peto R: The causes of cancer: Quantitative assessment of avoidable risks of cancer in the United States today. J Natl Cancer Inst 66:1192–1308, 1981.

Draper G, Sanders BM, Kingston JC: Second primary neoplasms in patients with retinoblastoma. Br J Cancer 53:661–671, 1986.

Dryja TP, Rapaport JM, Epstein J, et al.: Chromosome 13 homozygosity in osteosarcoma without retinoblastoma. Am J. Hum Genet 38:59–66, 1986.

Fearon ER, Hamilton SR, Vogelstein B: Clonal analysis of human colorectal tumors. Science 238:193–197, 1987.

Francois J, De Sutter E., Coppieters R, De Bie S: Late extraocular tumours in retinoblastoma survivors. Ophthalmalogica 181:93, 1980.

Hansen MF, Koufos A, Gallie BL, Phillips RA, Fodstad Ø, Brogger A, Gedde-Dahl T, Cavenee WK: Osteosarcoma and retinoblastoma: A shared chromosomal mechanism revealing recessive predisposition. Proc Natl Acad Sci USA 82:6216–6220, 1985.

Khan PM, Tops CMJ, Bruekel C, et al.: Close linkage of a highly polymorphic marker (D5S37) to familial adenomatous polyposis (FAP) and confirmation of FAP localization on chromosome 5q21–q22. Hum Genet 79:183–185.

Knudson AG: Mutation and cancer: Statistical study of retinoblastoma. Proc Natl Acad Sci USA 68:820–823, 1971.

Knudson AG: Genetic and environmental interactions in the origin of human cancer. In Mulvihill JJ, Miller RW, Fraumeni JF (eds): "Genetics of Human Cancer," New York: Raven Press, 1977, pp 39–97.

Leppert M, Dobbs M, Scambler P, O'Connell P, Nakamura Y, Stauffer D, Woodward S, Burt R, Hughes J, Gardner E, Lathrap M, Wasmuth J, Lalouel J-M, White R: The gene for familial polyposis coli maps to the long arm of chromosome 5. Science 238:1411–1413, 1987.

Lipkin M, Scherf S, Schechter L, et al.: Memorial Hospital registry of population groups at high risk for cancer of the large intestine: age of onset of neoplasms. Prevent Med 9:335–345, 1980.

Lustbader ED, Williams WR, Strong LC: Analysis of cohort data with uncertainty in stratification. Biometrics (in press).

Mathew CGP, Chin KS, Easton DF, Thorpe K, Carter C, Liou GI, Fong S-L, Bridges CDB, Haak H, Kruseman ACN, Schifter S, Hansen HH, Telenius H, Telenius-Berg M, Ponder BAJ: A linked genetic marker for multiple endocrine neoplasia type 2A on chromosome 10. Nature 238:527–528, 1987a.

Mathew CGP, Smith BA, Thorpe K, Wong Z, Royle NJ, Jeffreys AJ, Ponder BAJ: Deletion of genes on chromosome 1 in endocrine neoplasia. Nature 238:524–526, 1987.

Moolgavkar SH: The multistage theory of carcinogenesis and the age distribution of cancer in man. J Natl Cancer Inst 61:49–52, 1978b.

Moolgavkar SH: Model for human carcinogenesis: Action of environmental agents. Environ Health Perspect 50:285–291, 1983.

Moolgavkar SH, Knudson A: Mutation and cancer: A model for human carcinogenesis. J Natl Cancer Inst 66:1037–1052, 1981.

Moolgavkar SH, Venzon DJ: Two-event models for carcinogenesis: Incidence curves for childhood and adult tumors. Math Biosci 47:55–77, 1979.

Okamoto M, Sasaki M, Sugio K, Sato C, Iwama T, Ikeuchi T, Tonomura A, Sasazuki T, Miyaki M: Loss of constitutional heterozygosity in colon carcinoma from patients with familial polyposis coli. Nature 331:273–277, 1988.

Peto R, Gore FJC, Lee PN, Levy L, Clack J: Cancer and ageing in mice and men. Br J Cancer 32:411–425, 1975.

Preston DL, Kato H, Kopecky KJ, Fujita S: Life span study report No. 10. Part 1. Cancer mortality among A-bomb survivors in Hiroshima and Nagasaki, 1950–82. Radiation Effects Research Foundation Technical Report, No. TR 1-86, 1986.

Shimizu Y, Kato H, Schull WJ: Life span study report 11. Part II. Cancer mortality in the years 1950–85 based on the recently revised doses (DS86). Hiroshima: Radiation Effects Research Foundation, Technical Report No. TR5-88, 1988.

Shimizu Y, Kato H, Schull WJ, Peston DL, Fujita S, Pierce DA: Life span study report 11. Part 1. Comparison of risk coefficients for site-specific cancer mortality based on the DS86 and T65DR shielded Kerma and organ doses. Hiroshima: Radiation Effects Research Foundation, Technical Report No. TR 12-87, 1987.

Simpson NE, Kidd KK, Goodfellow PH, et al.: Assignment of multiple endocrine neoplasia type 2A to chromosome 10 by linkage. Nature 328:528–530, 1987.

Solomon E, Voss R, Hall V, Bodmer WF, Jass JR, Jeffreys AJ, Lucibello FC, Patel I, Rider SH: Chromosome 5 allele loss in human colorectal carcinomas. Nature 328:616–619, 1987.

Tucker MA, D'Angio GJ, Boice JD, et al.: Bone sarcomas linked to radiotherapy and chemotherapy in children. N Engl J Med 317:588–593, 1987.

United Nations Scientific Committee on the Effects of Atomic Radiation (UNSCEAR): "Radiation Carcinogenesis in Man." Vienna: United Nations, 1988.

Utsonomiya J, Murata M, Tanimura M: An analysis of the age distribution of colon cancer in adenomatosis coli. Cancer 45:198–205, 1980.

Weiss KM, Chakraborty R: Multistage models and the age patterns in familial polyposis coli. Cancer Invest 2:443–448, 1984.

Weiss KM, Chakraborty R, Ward RH, Yucel MK: Estimating the parameters that define age-specific risks for cancer. Sankhya (in press).

Weiss KM, Schull WJ: Identifying groups at high risk of colorectal cancer. In Ingall JRF, Mastromarino AJ (eds); "Prevention of Hereditary Large Bowel Cancer." New York, Alan R. Liss, Inc, 1983, pp 81–104.

Whittemore A: The age distribution of human cancer for carcinogenic exposures of varying intensity. Am J Epidemiol 106:418–432, 1977.

Whittemore A, Keller JB: Quantitative theories of carcinogenesis. SIAM Rev 20:1–30, 1978.

10

A Clinician's-Office Approach to Patients With Familial Adenomatous Polyposis and Their First-Degree Relatives

Z. Cohen, T. Berk, and R.S. McLeod

Division of General Surgery, Toronto General Hospital, and Department of Surgery, University of Toronto, Toronto, Ontario, Canada

INTRODUCTION

Early diagnosis and surgical intervention have decreased the mortality associated with familial adenomatous polyposis (FAP). However, clinicians should consider the chronic multifocal nature of this gastrointestinal disorder. New guidelines are required for long-term screening of affected kindreds, focussing on the preventive rather than only the surgical aspects of FAP. Awareness of known risk factors associated with FAP should be incorporated into the management of the pre- and postoperative patient. Similarly, identification of common psychosocial concerns may improve compliance with surveillance by first-degree relatives (offspring and siblings) at risk for FAP.

INITIAL DIAGNOSIS

Patients referred to the familial polyposis registry at The Toronto General Hospital are assessed for any clinical and family history of bowel disease or early death. Presenting symptoms may include rectal bleeding, diarrhea, or cramp-like abdominal pain, although the complete absence of symptoms is not uncommon. In a survey of 97 at-risk offspring and siblings, 70 (72.2%) were asymptomatic at the time of diagnosis [1]. Since the age of onset of FAP is variable, from puberty onward, external features related to this disease may be overlooked. A physician may remove one or more epidermoid cysts from the scalp or face of an at-risk child without attempting to correlate cysts with possible colonic pathology. The rarity of these lesions in children, not adults, should indicate close follow-up of the colon at an appropriate age [2]. In addition, an oral surgeon may excise a benign mandibular osteoma or a full set of tiny supernumerary teeth, unaware that dental anomalies may antedate the development of colonic adenomas [3]. Our registry provides a written guide for the family practice and dentistry units of regional hospitals, highlighting the potential significance of these extracolonic manifestations (ECM) and their possible association with FAP.

CLINICAL INVESTIGATION

Colorectum

Flexible sigmoidoscopy is our procedure of choice for screening and is performed on all patients along with biopsy of any lesions identified. All histopathology is verified by one pathologist with a particular interest in FAP, and the sections are retained for further review if necessary. Histopathology reports are filed separately from clinical data and are updated accordingly to establish an ongoing record of the natural history of FAP in each patient. Only when adenomas are confirmed on biopsy would assessment of the rest of the colon be carried out, prefera-

Familial Adenomatous Polyposis, pages 91–95

bly with colonoscopy. These guidelines have been advocated by other centers that also emphasize the need to confirm histopathology prior to colonic surgery [4–6]. The importance of histologic documentation was demonstrated to us in 11 of 17 surgically treated patients referred to our registry with an apparent diagnosis of FAP and reclassified by our pathologist as nonpolyposis patients. These patients were diagnosed and treated on clinical grounds rather than on more accurate histologic evidence. Screening of family members for a misperceived chronic disease was a further unwarranted sequela [7].

Upper Gastrointestinal Tract

Our patients undergo esophagogastroduodenoscopy, repeated annually for duodenal adenomas or every 3 years for nonneoplastic polyps in the stomach. The side-viewing instrument is used to visualize the ampulla when duodenal adenomas are observed. Recent reports from familial polyposis registries on upper gastrointestinal tract lesions cite a predominance of duodenal adenomas in patients with and without other ECM: 33 of 100 (33%) [8], 25 of 50 (50%) [9], 12 of 26 (46.1%) [10], and 10 of 41 (24.4%) [11]. The association between gastric adenomas and gastric carcinoma is uncertain outside Japan, and few cases have been reported in North America [12–14]. However, a potential adenoma–carcinoma sequence in the duodenum may be expected to resemble that in the colon. The approximated 12% incidence of periampullary carcinoma may be an underestimate because of lack of uniform investigation and reporting [15]. Sporadic accounts of an intrafamilial correlation for gastroduodenal lesions have not been confirmed as a predisposing factor [8]. Six of our 414 cases (1.4%) have died of periampullary carcinoma up to 22 years postcolectomy. Synchronous duodenal adenomas were present in only three of these patients.

Histologically discrete adenomas identified in duodenal mucosa that appears endoscopically normal have prompted suggestions for biopsies even when no overt lesions are noted [8,10]. The multiple sessile nature of duodenal adenomas has sparked controversy about management, its effect on the natural history of the disease, and the long-term prognosis. The need for controlled trials over a prolonged period was described from a preliminary sample of patients with duodenal lesions [16]. Different forms of endoscopic removal are being compared with surgery or observation and biopsy alone in an effort to determine their efficacy.

In some centers, patients may undergo esophagogastroduodenoscopy from age 20 years as part of their diagnostic evaluation, whereas others initiate upper endoscopy at age 30 years [4,11]. A review of 1,255 cases from ten polyposis registries participating in an international study group indicated that only 42% of the patients had undergone endoscopy, including 14% of 57 patients with duodenal cancer [17]. Questions about treatment modalities and screening intervals require assessment of cancer risk in the upper gastrointestinal tract, which will, in turn, improve cancer control.

OUTPATIENT FOLLOW-UP

Rigid sigmoidoscopy is our procedure of choice for all patients who have undergone colectomy and ileorectal anastomosis. Patients are followed initially every 3–6 months until the rectum is clear, and then they may be seen yearly depending on their individual status. Similar to the St. Mark's Hospital protocol, fulguration is performed on small adenomas [18]. Patients are admitted for day surgery if confluent rectal adenomas require removal. Adenocarcinoma has resulted in proctectomy and ileostomy in two patients, aged 26 and 63 years, both of whom had malignancy (Dukes' A for the former and Dukes' C for the latter).

Ileal adenomas have been documented in eight patients in our Registry; five of these were recorded at the time of colectomy. Recurrent tubular adenomas, as well as lymphoid polyps, have appeared around the ileostomy stoma in one patient. A single lesion was documented in three patients after colectomy and ileorectal anastomosis (age range 16–28 years). The ileal mucosa must continue to be scrutinized since adenomas are being identified in conventional ileostomies, continent ileostomies, and pelvic pouches [19,20].

Patients with FAP and the pelvic pouch should have periodic inspection and biopsy of the pouch.

EXTRACOLONIC MANIFESTATIONS

Desmoid Tumors

Forty-three of our patients (25 female, 18 male) have been diagnosed with desmoid tumors. These are benign but diffusely infiltrating lesions, which are particularly difficult to treat when located within the mesentery [21]. Surgery may be extremely dangerous and may be contraindicated because of the high incidence of recurrence. Surgery must at all times be weighed against impending obstruction or compromise of the small bowel. In our series, desmoid tumors occurred an average of 3.5 years (range 1–19 years) postoperatively. Pregnancy may also be a desmoid growth promoter, and five of eight patients in our series were postpartum. Eight of fourteen patients who died with surgically unresectable mesenteric desmoids were female. The 19 patients with mesenteric lesions remaining for follow-up are monitored with computerized axial tomography (CAT) scanning. Some of our desmoid tumor patients have been entered into a trial using a combination of tamoxifen and Clinoril. The results of this treatment await further patient entry and analysis. A family history of a desmoid tumor exists in six of 168 kindreds in our registry. This tendency may represent the variable expression of the FAP gene or a predilection for fibrous proliferation, which has been suggested from two other registries [20,22]. The appearance of a desmoid tumor may not always be associated with FAP; desmoids can occur in otherwise-healthy postpartum patients. However, the significance of rectal investigation in such patients is illustrated by one of our outside cases, an apparent mutation, aged 31 years, documented with Dukes' C adenocarcinoma of the rectum was diagnosed 2 years after excision of a postpartum desmoid in the abdominal wall. At present, unfortunately, there is no consistently effective treatment for these tumors.

Retinal Lesions

The appearance of a congenital ocular abnormality has been identified in 51 of 61 patients (84%) and 12 of 22 offspring (55%) in our registry. Characterized by pigmented patches, some are surrounded by a halo and others completely depigmented. These lesions appear to be heterogeneous within and between kindreds. Twenty-six of sixty-one patients (42.6%) are positive for retinal lesions but have no other ECM. This observation has been confirmed in another study of two FAP kindreds [23]. We did not find any retinal pigment changes in a small sample of eight nonpolyposis colon cancer patients [24]. All consenting patients in our registry are examined by one ophthalmologist using indirect ophthalmoscopy, which involves diligent scanning of the retina. This is important because lesions as small as 1/10 mm may be otherwise hidden in the periphery. The specificity of this test cannot be assessed because of the young age (range 7 months to 27 years) and short follow-up time of the offspring at risk for FAP. Histopathologic studies will determine whether the altered pigment epithelium is hypertrophic or hyperplastic. Chromosomal studies may further define the reason for the inconsistent heterogeneity of FAP when this manifestation of the primary defect is explored.

Mandibular Osteomas

Orthopantomography has demonstrated benign bony jaw lesions in 76–90% of FAP patients, older individuals showing more lesions [10]. Mandibular osteomas were reported in three of 34 at-risk offspring and siblings (age range 12–47 years) in the Danish Polyposis Registry [25]. However, radiopaque densities have also been noted in 4% of the normal population. Perhaps a more precise radiologic definition is necessary for another potential clinical marker, especially in children [20]. Currently, a baseline panorex film may be an adjunctive noninvasive test for patients diagnosed with FAP.

Associated Lesions

Despite the presence of papillary thyroid adenocarcinoma in five patients, medulloblastoma in four patients and hepatoblastoma in two patients, we do not advocate additional screening for our patients or at-risk first-degree relatives. The term cancerophobia aptly describes the reaction to ongoing tests and may negatively influence compliance with follow-up or screening sigmoidoscopy and esophagogastroduodenoscopy [26]. The high cost of medical insurance and refusal by some third-party carriers to cover repeated examinations should also be considered.

FAMILY HISTORY

A working pedigree is developed by the registry coordinator so that an overview is available for the clinician at the time of examination. This can be extremely helpful in ascertaining the other potentially susceptible family members who require examination. The presentation of a seemingly isolated case (mutation) should not preclude surveillance of parents and siblings since delayed age of onset, illegitimacy, or early parental death may mask their actual risk factors. Thirty-eight percent of our cases represent apparent mutations, but their first-degree relatives continue to be followed at regular intervals. Two apparent mutations each had a parent diagnosed with FAP at ages 57 and 43 years. No evidence of adenocarcinoma was present in the former asymptomatic patient, but the latter had metastases at the time of colectomy.

SCREENING OF OFFSPRING AND SIBLINGS

From the age of 12 years, flexible sigmoidoscopy is recommended for all at-risk offspring and siblings. Complete rectal sparing has not been observed in any of our patients who have FAP. Biopsy of apparently normal mucosa in the rectum has been suggested to adequately assess unaffected family members [15]. The soft tip and less rigid nature of the flexible sigmoidoscope result in less discomfort than the standard instrument while allowing visualization of up to 60cm of the colon and rectum. Careful dietary instruction and preparation of the bowel are required for each examination, although some prefer to administer a cleansing agent after the patient arrives. A printed examination reminder sheet is sent to patients and is reinforced by a telephone call prior to the test. Screening intervals depend on the age and circumstances of the patient.

Compliance with regular testing is a fundamental concern; consequently, at-risk offspring and siblings are not subjected to colonoscopy or air-contrast barium enema unless warranted. The first deterrent to follow-up mentioned by unaffected relatives is excess screening. Other barriers include denial of risk, cost, and misconceptions about the variable age of onset [27]. The young age and frequent lack of symptoms in this at-risk population require alternatives for teaching cancer prevention. Patient education is integral to surveillance, since patient anxiety may result in incomplete understanding of any information about FAP. A patient guide and lay library have been developed by our registry because of our observation that coping is improved when affected kindreds are better prepared. To achieve prolonged survival, patients must learn to understand the chronic nature of the disease. Patient attitudes toward screening may be determined by a perceived rather than an actual interpretation. Care should be taken to reinforce current ideas about this generalized disorder before and after colonic surgery. Those individuals who receive counselling when they first enter the health-care system may be more accepting of clinical intervention. In the future, it is our hope that a preclinical marker testing program will be developed. This will require built-in support systems and counselling to minimize any negative effects in all FAP gene carriers.

ACKNOWLEDGMENTS

This work was supported by a grant from the Stavro Polyposis Registry.

References

1. Bussey HJR: "Familial Polyposis Coli." Baltimore; The Johns Hopkins University Press, 1975, pp 67–70.
2. Leppard B: Epidermoid cysts and polyposis coli. Proc R Soc Med 67:1036–1037, 1974.
3. Sondergaard JO, Bulow S, Jarvinen H, Wolf J, Witt IN, Tetens G: Dental anomalies in familial adenomatous polyposis coli. Acta Odontol Scand 45:61–63, 1987.
4. Herrera-Ornelas L, Elsiah S, Petrelli N, Mittelman A: Causes of death in patients with familial polyposis coli. Semin Surg Oncol 3:109–117, 1987.
5. Gebert HF, Jagelman DG, McGannon E: Familial polyposis coli. Am Fam Physician 33:127–137, 1986.
6. Boman BM, Levin B: Familial polyposis. Hosp Practice 21:155–170, 1986.

7. Berk T, Cohen Z, McLeod RS, Cullen JB: Surgery based on misdiagnosis of adenomatous polyposis. The Canadian polyposis registry experience. Dis Colon Rectum 30:588–590, 1987.

8. Sarre RG, Frost AG, Jagleman DG, Petras RE, Sivak MV, McGannon E: Gastric and duodenal polyps in familial adenomatous polyposis: A prospective study of the nature and prevalence of upper gastrointestinal polyps. Gut 28:306–314, 1987.

9. Jarvinen HG, Sipponen P: Gastroduodenal polyps in familial adenomatous and juvenile polyposis. Endoscopy 18:230–234, 1986.

10. Bulow S: Familial polyposis coli. Danish Med Bull 34:1–15, 1987.

11. Kurtz RC, Sternberg SS, Miller HH, DeCosse JJ: Upper gastrointestinal neoplasia in familial polyposis. Digest Dis Sci 32:459–465, 1987.

12. Iida M, Yao T, Itoh H, Watanabe H, Matsui T, Iwashita A, Fijishima M: Natural history of gastric adenomas in patients with familial adenomatosis coli/Gardner's syndrome. Cancer 61:605–611, 1988.

13. Design G, Wang M, Dunn GD, Halter S, Vaughan S: Intramucosal gastric carcinoma in a patient with familial polyposis coli. Am J Gastroenterol 81:19–22, 1986.

14. Jagelman DG, Bussey HJR, DeCosse JJ: Upper gastrointestinal cancer in familial adenomatous polyposis. Lancet 2:1149–1151, 1988.

15. Haggitt RC, Reid BJ: Hereditary gastrointestinal polyposis syndromes. Am J Surg Pathol 10:871–887, 1986.

16. van Stolk R, Sivak MV Jr, Petrini JL, Petras R, Ferguson DR, Jagelman D: Endoscopic management of upper gastrointestinal polyps and periampullary lesions in familial adenomatous polyposis and Gardner's syndrome. Endoscopy 19:19–22, 1987.

17. Leeds Castle Polyposis Group Meeting, Washington, May 1987.

18. Bussey HJR, Eyers AA, Ritchie SM, Thomson JPS: The rectum in adenomatous polyposis: The St. Mark's policy. Br J Surg 72[Suppl]:S29–S35, 1985.

19. Nakahara S, Itoh H, Iida M, Iwashita A, Ohsato K: Ileal adenomas in familial polyposis coli. Differences before and after colectomy. Dis Colon Rectum 28:875–877, 1985.

20. Jagelman DG: Extracolonic manifestations of familial polyposis coli. Semin Surg Oncol 3:88–91, 1987.

21. Suehiro S, Inai K: Mesenteric fibromatosis in familial polyposis. A case report and a review of Japanese cases. Acta Pathol Jpn 37:1837–1843, 1987.

22. Klemmer S, Pascoe L, DeCosse J: Occurrence of desmoids in patients with familial adenomatous polyposis of the colon. Am J Med Genet 38:385–392, 1987.

23. Lynch HT, Priluck I, Fitzsimmons ML: Congenital hypertrophy of retinal pigment epithelium in non-Gardner's polyposis kindreds. Lancet 2:333, 1987.

24. Berk T, Cohen Z, McLeod RS, Parker JA: Congenital hypertrophy of the retinal pigment epithelium as a marker for familial adenomatous polyposis. Dis Colon Rectum 31:253–257, 1988.

25. Bulow S, Holm NV, Sondergaard JO, Witt IN, Tetens G: Mandibular osteomas in unaffected sibs and children of patients with familial polyposis coli. Scand J Gastroenterol 21:744–748, 1986.

26. Bulow S, Holm NV, Mellemgaard A: Papillary thyroid carcinoma in Dutch patients with familial adenomatous polyposis. Int J Colorectal Dis 3:29–31, 1988.

27. Berk T, Cohen Z, McLeod RS, Cullen JB: Surveillance in relatives of patients with adenomatous polyposis. Semin Surg Oncol 3:105–108, 1987.

11

Evaluation of the Gastrointestinal Tract in Patients with Familial Adenomatous Polyposis

David G. Jagelman

The Cleveland Clinic Florida, Clearwater, Florida

INTRODUCTION

Familial adenomatous polyposis (FAP) is the term currently used to describe a genetically determined disease that leads to the development of multiple intestinal polyps that inevitably degenerate to carcinoma of the large intestine. The disease was previously termed familial polyposis coli (FPC), hereditary adenomatosis (HA), or Gardner's syndrome (GS). There is much more to the disease than gastrointestinal polyposis alone; there are a number of associated benign and malignant extracolonic manifestations that confirm that the disease is a genetically determined generalized growth disorder and not just a colonic or gastrointestinal disease. The gastrointestinal polyposis feature is, however, significant; death from colorectal cancer is invitable if left untreated. This chapter reviews the gastrointestinal pathology of FAP and overviews the methods of evaluation and recommendations for management of the gastrointestinal tract in terms of both detection of the disease and long-term surveillance.

COLORECTAL PATHOLOGY

FAP is a genetically determined condition in which adenomas arise in the large intestine. They are predominately tubular adenomas, but tubulovillous and villous adenomas may also arise. They arise in small numbers and increase in size and number with time, with inevitable progression to malignant degeneration. The cancers may be multicentric. Bussey [1], in his monograph, evaluated a number of colon specimens and found that they all contained at least 100 adenomas and often many more. The range was from 104 to over 5,000 adenomas, the average being 988 adenomas. These polyps are sometimes discrete lesions, but on occasion the adenomatous change is confluent, making counting of these lesions difficult. This study led to the belief that it was necessary to have 100 polyps to make a conclusive diagnosis of FAP. With today's greater knowledge of the disease, we realize that adenoma formation is a progressive phenomenon, with polyps being absent at birth and arising at varying intervals later in life and then progressing gradually in sheer numbers. The colonic specimens examined by Bussey were diagnosed late in the patients' lives, mostly from symptomatic patients old enough to have developed more than 100 polyps. By beginning intestinal surveillance at puberty in at-risk children, the diagnosis can often be made with five to twenty adenomas. It is just a question of the point of diagnosis in the natural history of the disease. The adenomas are usually scattered throughout the large intestine, even the appendix, but there may be a preponderance of polyps on the left side of the colon.

Malignant degeneration appears to be 100%, although some patients obviously have prophylactic colectomy by being diagnosed early, often in a presymptomatic stage. Bussey [1] also noted

Familial Adenomatous Polyposis, pages 97–100

that 194 (66%) of the 293 patients seen initially with symptoms of FAP had already developed a cancer. It is obvious, therefore, that the detection of this disease should not be reliant on the development of symptoms and that early diagnosis should be the aim. The average age of diagnosis in Bussey's study was 39.2 years. It should not be forgotten that cancer can arise in these patients in the teenage years and is common in the 20–30 year age group.

Bulow [2] found that the median age at the time of development of adenomas was 16 years (range 5–38) and the development of colorectal cancer was 36 years (range 17–67). This information regarding the age of first adenoma formation was obtained from the Danish Polyposis Registry, for which at-risk patients were examined by proctosigmoidoscopy from a negative examination to the development of adenomas at subsequent examinations. Adenomas may initially develop from early childhood or even later in life, even up to the age of 40 years, although this has has not truly been confirmed. Similar findings have been reported by Alm and Licznerski [3] and Cohen [4].

SCREENING OF THE LARGE INTESTINE

Based on our knowledge of the natural history of the disease regarding the early development of adenomas and the later development of cancer, certain guidelines can be recommended for early detection. The questions are what tests should be used, when should they be started, when can they be safely stopped, and how frequently should they be performed.

Clinically, for the past 25 years, simple proctosigmoidoscopy has been the only method used for at-risk individuals at our institution. We have yet to see a patient with a conclusive diagnosis of FAP who did not have at least one visible rectal adenoma. Bulow [2] found that all 247 Danish patients with FAP had rectal adenomas. Alm and Licznerski [3] and Bussey [1] also found rectal adenomas in all cases. No patient in our study population or that of the Danish, Swedish, or English reports developed a colon cancer while proctosigmoidoscopy was negative. Simple proctosigmoidoscopy alone would therefore appear to be not only adequate but also safe as a screening examination for the disease. The detection of a rectal adenoma confirmed on biopsy would demand a colonoscopic examination to assess the number and extent of colonic polyps and of course to exclude cancer. Biopsies should be taken to confirm adenoma and to be certain that hyperplastic and juvenile polyposis is excluded. A confirmed diagnosis would seem to be an indication for prophylactic colectomy. Repeated colonoscopy or attempts at multiple polypectomy have no place in the long-term management of FAP even with early diagnosis. There seems no point in delaying surgical intervention. Why wait for the inevitable cancer that will occur? Barium contrast studies have little place in surveillance. The polyps are often small and not easily seen, and, if they are profuse, they may appear to suggest that the preparation of the colon was poor. Simple proctosigmoidoscopy with biopsy followed by a single colonscopy is all that is required.

When to start the examinations and how often to perform them is debatable. Cancer arose in a single patient of age 16 years in the Danish Registry [2] and at 17 years in the St. Mark's Registry [1]. We have seen an 18-year-old with cancer among our patient population. We have elected as a routine to recommend commencing examination at age 10 years not because we are unduly concerned about cancer at that age but we wish to make an early diagnosis and have the child become familiar with the examination and the registry personnel. Ten-year-old children tend to follow the advice of their parents to have the examination, whereas teenagers are more independent, and we have found it very difficult to persuade them to have the examination in later years. Starting at a younger age seems to improve compliance with a follow-up program in later life. We have recommended yearly proctosigmoidoscopy examination to maintain compliance and to keep in touch with the patients rather than suggesting biannual or four-yearly examinations.

When to stop the examinations is a most difficult question. Polyps have been seen to develop for the first time as late as age 37 years in some series, so it seems reasonable to continue up to age 40 years. General guidelines would support continuing follow-up past this point if there is a family history of colon cancer. At present, there is no evidence to suggest that nonaffected members of FAP kindreds have a higher risk of subsequent nonpolyposis colon cancer, but long-term follow-up in this group has never truly been performed. In reviewing the kindreds within our registry, this certainly does not appear to be the case. With longer follow-up, this point should be clarified. In time, maybe a blood test to detect the genetic defect will be available and will supersede simple proctosigmoidoscopy as the screening test of choice of FAP.

GASTRODUODENAL PATHOLOGY

Periampullary malignancy has been reported with some frequency in association with FAP over the years [5]. It is only recently that detailed observations of premalignant lesions of the stomach and duodenum have been defined with the use of gastroduodenoscopy. It has been determined that a large number of patients with FAP have polypoid lesions in the stomach or duodenum. Most of the gastric lesions have been shown to be fundic gland polyps and are not adenomas. However, a few adenomas in the antrum of the stomach have been noted. All the polypoid lesions in the duodenum seem to be adenomatous, mostly tubular adenomas but also tubulovillous adenomas and villous adenomas. They are concentrated in the second and on occasion in the third part of the duodenum and are frequently closely related to the papilla of Vater. The adenomatous change frequently extends into the papilla and may extend up into the common bile duct. In a prospective study of 100 patients with FAP undergoing gastroduodenoscopy in our institution [6], 46 patients had polypoid lesions in the stomach and duodenum. Among them, 35 had adenomas (33 in the duodenum and two in the gastric antrum), 26 patients had fundic gland polyps, and some patients had both types of polyps. Adenomas of the duodenum were present in 33% of patients overall, and that percentage increased with age. The nature of upper gastrointestinal polyps in FAP has been clarified. In the stomach, there may be a variable number of hemispheric polyps. These may be profuse and are usually located in the fundus. Histologically, they have been termed fundic gland polyps. True adenomas in the stomach seem to be rare, most cases having been reported in the Japanese patients of Utsunomiya et al. [7]. Duodenal polyps tend to be concentrated around the papilla of Vater and the second portion of the duodenum and are frequently multiple. Histologically, they are adenomas and are generally thought to be premalignant. The prevalence of these lesions does not seem to be related to the presence of other extracolonic manifestations of FAP. Periampullary carcinoma has been well documented in association with FAP [1,5], the malignancy being associated with adjacent villous adenomas in many cases. A disturbing feature, noted by us and by others [8–10] is the presence of histological villous changes in flat, apparently normal-appearing mucosa in and around the site of the papilla of Vater.

UPPER GASTROINTESTINAL SCREENING

Present knowledge confirms that gastroduodenal polyps in patients with FAP are more common than was previously thought. The true incidence of periampullary cancer is still unknown, although when it does occur it seems to be associated with adenomatous change in the duodenum. The detection of the duodenal adenomas in particular would demand at least long-term surveillance because of the risk of malignancy. The use of both an end and side view gastroduodenoscope, with biopsies of macroscopic lesions, together with random biopsies of apparently normal mucosa in the region of the papilla, is supported. Gastric polyps also should be biopsied, but most will be fundic gland polyps, and these do not seem to carry an premalignant potential. We have decided on a purely empirical basis that the presence of histologically proved adenoma in the duodenum demands annual upper endoscopic evaluation with biopsy. Attempts to ablate the lesions endoscopically, if they numerous, with bipolar electrocautery (Bicap) have been made. Large lesions or villous adenomas with dysplasia are recommended for surgical resection by a modified Whipple technique. We are starting a prospective clinical study, randomizing duodenal adenoma patients to one of two arms of the study, one group to have annual endoscopy, with biopsy, with surgical intervention for large adenomas and those with villous changes and dysplasia, the second group to be treated with extensive electrocautery destruction of all adenomatous tissue, which may involve two or three treatments followed by annual surveillance. This group may also require sphincterotomy, stenting of the papilla, and snare excision of adenomas, especially those extending into the bile duct. It is hoped that this clinical study will eventually define the true incidence of periampullary carcinoma in patients with FAP and also whether this can be influenced positively by electrocautery destruction.

SMALL BOWEL POLYPS

The information on the prevalence of small bowel adenomas is limited because of the difficulty in accurate examination with radiological contrast studies and endoscopy. Small bowel carcinoma has been reported in FAP patients, but with much less frequency than duodenal carcinoma [11]. However, we have seen adenomas on ileostomy in a continent ileostomy, in the ileum above an ileorectal anastomosis, and more recently in an ileoanal pouch. Ohsato et al. [12] reported small adenomas in patients undergoing intraoperative fiberoptic endoscopy of the small intestine. Hamilton et al. [13] reported ileal adenomas in nine patients following colectomy. More recently, Stryker et al. [14] described ileal adenomas arising in a patient with a continent ileostomy. Jejunal or ileal cancer in FAP seems to be rare. Adenomas, however, are well documented in the ileum, but it is probably not necessary to institute routine small bowel surveillance following colectomy, but ileoscopy would be indicated in patients with FAP who develop gastrointestinal symptoms following surgery whether that surgery was ileostomy, ileorectal anastomosis, ileoanal pouch, or continent ileostomy, because an adenoma or carcinoma may have developed.

References

1. Bussey HJR: "Familial polyposis coli: Family Studies, Histopathology, Differential Diagnosis, and Results of Treatment." Baltimore; The Johns Hopkins University Press, 1975, pp 65–66.
2. Bulow S: "Familial Polyposis Coli: A Clinical and Epidemiological Study." Laegeforeningens Forlag, 1986, p 18.
3. Alm T, Licznerski G: The intestinal polyposes. Clin Gastroenterol 2:577–602, 1973.
4. Cohen S: Familial polyposis coli and its extracolonic manifestations. Med Genet 19:193–203, 1982.
5. Sugihara K, Muto T, Kamiya J, Konishi F, Sawada T, Morioka Y: Gardner's Syndrome associated with periampullary carcinoma, duodenal and gastric adenomatosis. Dis Colon Rectum 25:766–771, 1982.
6. Sarre RG, Frost AG, Jagelman DG, Petras RE, Sivak MV, McGannon E: Gastric and duodenal polyps in familial polyposis: A prospective study of the nature and prevalence of upper gastrointestinal polyps. Gut 28:306–314, 1987.
7. Utsunomiya J, Maki T, Iwama T, Matsunaga Y, Ichikawa T, Shimomura T, Hamaguchi E, Aoki N: Gastric lesions of familial polyposis coli. Cancer 34: 745–754, 1974.
8. Yao T, Iida M, Ohsato K, Watanabe H, Omae T: Duodenal lesions in familial polyposis of the colon. Gastroenterology 73:1086–92, 1977.
9. Burt RW, Berenson MM, Lee RG, Tolman KG, Freston JW, Gardner EJ: Upper gastrointestinal polyps in Gardner's syndrome. Gastroenterology 86:295–301, 1984.
10. Bulow S, Lauitsen KB, Johansen A, Svendsen LB, Sondergaard JO: Gastroduodenal polyps in familial polyposis coli. Dis Colon Rectum 28:90–93, 1985.
11. Ross JE, Mara JE: Small bowel polyps and carcinoma in multiple intestinal polyposis. Arch Surg 108:736–738, 1974.
12. Ohsato K, Yao T, Watanabe H, Iida M, Itoh H: Small-intestinal involvement in familial polyposis diagnosed by operative intestinal fiberscopy. Dis Colon Rectum 20:414–420, 1977.
13. Hamilton SR, Bussey HJR, Mendelsohn G, Diamond MP, Pavlides G, Hutcheon D, Harbison M, Shermeta D, Morson BC, Yardley JH: Ileal adenomas after colectomy in nine patients with adenomatous polyposis coli/Gardner's Syndrome. Gastroenterology 77:1252–1257, 1979.
14. Stryker SJ, Carney JA, Dozois RR: Multiple adenomatous polyps arising in a continent reservoir ileostomy. Int J Colorectal Dis 2:43–45, 1987.

12

Phenotypic Expressions of Japanese Patients With Familial Adenomatous Polyposis

J. Utsunomiya, Y. Miki, T. Kuroki, and T. Iwama

Second Department of Surgery, Hyogo College of Medicine, Hyogo, Japan (J.U., Y.M., T.K.); Polyposis Center, Tokyo Medical and Dental University, Tokyo, Japan (T.I.)

INTRODUCTION

Familial adenomatous polyposis (FAP) or adenomatosis coli is the condition in which adenomas are distributed throughout the large bowel, principally in numbers of 100 or more. Its subtypes include simple FAP, Gardner's syndrome, and other rare specific condition such as Turcot's syndrome and Zanca's syndrome.

The first well studied case of FAP in the Japanese literature was reported by Matsubara in 1923: this was followed with many clinical presentations. Systematic genetic study, however, was not made until 1961, when the first nationwide survey was carried out by Komatsu [1]. With his collaboration, one of the authors (J.U.) extended the study to establish the Polyposis Center (JPC) at the Tokyo Medical and Dental University in 1976, which documented the status of FAP in Japan [2–7]. By 1987, 793 cases (555 families) of FAP (including Turcot's syndrome), 163 cases (155 families) of Peutz-Jeghers syndrome, and cases with other polyposes has been registered. The family survey has now been completed on 528 FAP families and has revealed the presence of 1,564 patients, including 590 deduced cases [8]. This chapter reviews our studies using these materials as well as other Japanese literature comparing that with data from representative Western literature.

Familial Adenomatous Polyposis, pages 101–107

PATHOLOGICAL ASPECTS

Lesions in the Large Bowel

Polyps. It may be reasonable to define FAP as described above and as Bussey also commented [9]. FAP is further divided into two types—the profuse type and the sparse type—by the number of polyps (Fig. 1) [4,5]. The criteria for delineating these clusters were a total count of 5,000 polyps or a unit count of $10/cm^2$ by macroscopic observation and two adenomatous foci detected in 1 cm of a histological section, or adenomatous foci estimated to occupy 20% of the total area of the section [10]. Radiologically, double-contrast barium enema reveals that the boundary range distinguishing these two types is six to nine $polyps/cm^2$ in adults and three to six/cm^2 in children [11].

Small polyps (diameter less than 5 mm) constitute over 80% of the polyps in FAP [10]. A finding of one or more polyps greater than 1 cm in diameter indicates an association of advanced cancer somewhere in the large bowel with a probability of 47% [11]. The malignant potential of the adenomas of FAP seemed to show no significant difference when compared to the usual adenomas of the large bowel [7,8].

Cancer. Advanced cancers of the large bowel were found in 54.0% of the total of 459 cases in the JPC at the time of diagnosis. The frequency was much less in the call-up cases (22.7%) than in the probands (62.4%) [8]. Their subsite dis-

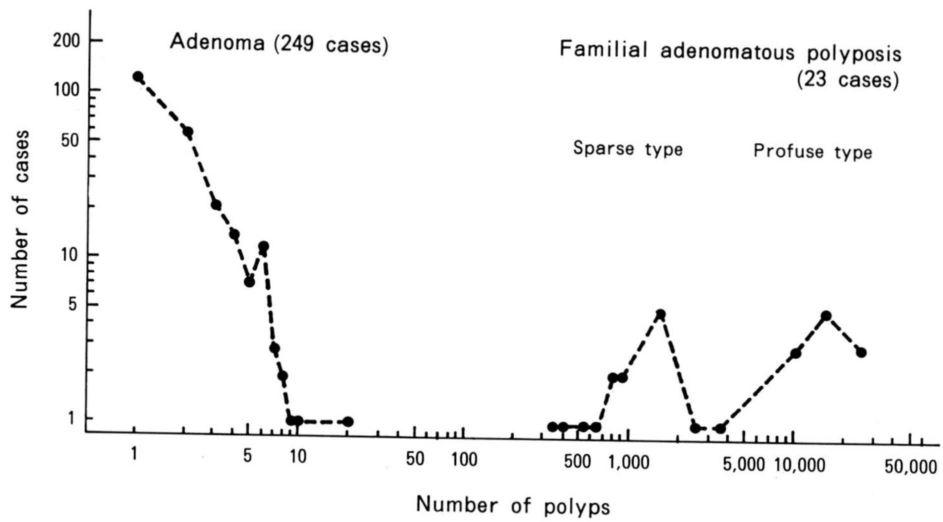

Fig. 1. Case distribution of patients with adenomas regarding number of polyps.

tribution within the bowel was similar to that of the usual colorectal cancers in both Japanese and British series [7,8]. The relative incidence of cancer in the sigmoid colon vs. that in the rectum (S/R ratio) was increased in the FAP patients over that seen in the general colorectal cancer population in Japan [7,8]. This evidence suggests that cancer occurrence in FAP may be affected by environmental factors. Multiple cancers were found in 38.0% of FAP patients with cancer. This is an extremely high frequency compared with the 4.5% occurrence of colorectal cancer in the general population in Japan.

Lesions of the Upper Gastrointestinal (GI) Tract

Polyps. Polyps in the stomach [12,13] as well as in the duodenum [14] were found to be an integral phenotypic expression of the FAP gene. An increasing number of Japanese as well as Western reports suggest that this phenomenon is not specific to Japanese (Table 1). The polyp detection rates are similarly higher in Japanese series for both the stomach (63.1%) and the duodenum (80.3%) than in the Western series (50.8% vs. 64.1%) (Tables 1,2). This suggests that the difference is due to methodological biases among the countries.

There are two types of gastric polyps by histology: 1) adenomatous and 2) hamartomatous polyps of the fundic gland. Neither are specific to FAP [2]. Whereas adenoma was found in 44% of patients with gastric polyps in the Japanese series, the figure was 33% in the Western series. This difference may be related to intestinal metaplasia, which is seen more frequently in the general Japanese population than in the Western populations [13]. Although the fundic gland polyps do not seem to harbor any malignant potential, some evidence of malignant foci associated with the adenomatous lesions has been observed by us.

The duodenal polyps are distributed mainly in the second portion, and adenomatous foci were found in 59% of biopsy specimen obtained from the mucosa around the papilla of Vater and in 25% of accessory papillae in our patients. This finding suggests an increased neoplastic potential around the orifices of the pancreatic duct. Polyps or adenomas were found in the jejunum in eight patients, and the ileum in four patients among a total of 16 patients endoscopically examined at operation [16].

Cancer. The incidence of gastric cancer among Japanese with FAP is estimated to be 2.1%, which is 3.5-fold higher than in Western polyposis (0.6%) (Table 3). In contrast, duodenal

TABLE 1.
Gastric Polyps in Familial Adenomatous Polyposis

		Incidence of polyps				Proportion of adenoma	
		In case		In family			
Report[a]	Place (year)	n	Percent	n	Percent	n	Percent
Japanese literature							
Utsunomiya et al.	Tokyo (1974)	10/15	66.7	6/6	100.0	4/6	66.7
Sugihara et al.	Tokyo (1983)	7/14	50.0			3/7	42.9
Ushio et al.	Tokyo (1984)	25/44	56.8	7/8	87.5	4/25	16.0
Watanabe	Niigata (1986)	23/34	67.8			13/23	56.5
Iida et al.	Kyushu (1987)	29/40	72.5	14/16	87.5	14/29	48.3
Kumatani et al.	Miyagi (1987)	10/23	43.5			6/10	60.0
Utsunomiya et al.	Hyogo (1987)	21/28	75.0	15/21	71.4	10/21	47.6
Total		125/198	63.1			54/121	44.6
Western literature							
Ranzi et al.	Italy (1981)	6/9	66.7	—		4/6	66.7
Jarvinen et al.	Finland (1983)	21/34	61.7	—		4/21	19.0
Burt et al.	U.S. (1984)	7/11	63.6	—		1/7	14.3
Shemesh et al.	Israel (1985)	7/14	50.0	—		7/7	100.0
Tonelli al.	Italy (1985)	6/24	25.0			3/6	50.0
Bülow et al.	Denmark (1985)	13/26	50.0			1/13	7.7
Total		60/118	50.8			20/60	33.3

[a]References can be found in other papers [6–7].

TABLE 2.
Duodenal Polyps in Familial Adenomatous Polyposis

		Incidence of polyps		Proportion of adenoma	
Report[a]	Place (year)	n	Percent	n	Percent
Japanese literature					
Sugihara et al.	Tokyo (1983)	2/12	16.7	1/2	50.0
Ushio et al.	Tokyo (1984)	23/32	71.9	17/23	73.9
Watanabe et al.	Niigata (1982)	25/25	100.0	25/25	100.0
Iida et al.	Kyushu (1987)	34/37	91.9	34/34	100.0
Kumatani et al.	Miyagi (1987)	12/17	70.6	8/12	66.7
Utsunomiya et al.	Hyogo (1987)	22/24	91.7	22/22	100.0
Total		118/147	80.3	107/118	90.7
Western literature					
Ranzi et al.	Italy (1981)	6/9	66.7	6/6	100
Jarvinen et al.	Finland (1983)	20/33	60.6	16/20	80
Burt et al.	U.S. (1984)	8/11	72.3	7/8	89
Shemesh et al.	Israel (1985)	14/14	100.0	14/14	100
Bülow et al.	Denmark (1985)	13/26	50.0	12/10	92.3
Tonelli et al.	Italy (1985)	14/24	58.3	14/14	100
Total		75/117	64.1	69/75	92

[a]References can be found in other papers [6–7].

TABLE 3.
Frequency of Cancer in Various Organs of FAP Patients

Organ	Reporter (year)	Total cases	Cases with cancer n	Percent	Age (years)	Postcolectomy Percent	Year
Large bowel	Japanese						
	Polyposis Center (1986)	788	428	54.3	39.1	—	—
	Western						
	St. Marks Hospital (1975)	410	232	56.6	39.1	—	—
Stomach	Japanese						
	Polyposis Center (1986)	1,564	33	2.1	—	—	—
	Jpn. Soc. L.B.C. Res.[a] (1986)	329	7	2.1	47.7	85.7	5.3
	Literature (~1985)	—	15	—	47.2	76.9	1.9
	Western						
	LCPG Meeting[b] (1987)	1,225	8	0.6	—	—	12.8
	Literature (~1986)	—	8	—	47.7	62.5	15.8
Duodenum	Japanese						
	Polyposis Center (1987)	1,564	10	0.6	—	—	—
	Jpn. Soc. L.B.C. Res. (1987)	319	6	1.9	46.3	100.0	5.7
	Literature (~1985)	—	10	—	41.3	88.9	5.1
	Western						
	LCPG Meeting (1987)	1,255	32	2.5	—	90.6	18.8
	Literature (~1986)	—	48	—	47.5	85.4	13.6
Thyroid gland	Japanese						
	Polyposis Center (1987)	1,564	8	0.5	—	—	—
	Jpn. Soc. L.B.C. Res. (1987)	400	3	0.8	25.2	0.0	0.0
	Western						
	Alm et al. (1973)	340 } 481	2 } 5	0.6 } 1.0	—	—	—
	Sener et al. (1984)	141	3	2.1	—	—	—
	Literature (~1984)	—	17	—	25.2	3.0	3.3

[a]LCPG, Leed Castle Polyposis Group, Second Meeting April, 1987, Washington, DC.
[b]Summed data of the reports at the 26th Meeting of Japanese Society for Large Bowel Cancer Research.

cancer incidence in Japanese polyposis patients (0.6%) is one-fourth that (2.5%) of Western polyposis patients (Table 3). The observation may also indicate environmental modification of the gene action.

Extra-GI Associated Lesions

Gardner's syndrome (GSy). Both of Gardner's stigmata (GSt) (osteoma and fibrous tumor) were observed in about 7% of patients in both of the series we examined personally and in that of the registry, whereas GSy of the incomplete type was found more frequently (35.7%) in the former than in the latter (18.4%) [6,7]. Panoramic X-ray examination of the jaw disclosed the radiopaque lesions ("the occult osteomatous lesion") in 94% of FAP patients [17]. They had a positive relationship to superficial GSt [17]. Complete GSy may prove to be a specific, distinct subtype of FAP, but there may be many clinically indistinguishable, transitional cases between complete GSy and simple FAP. Therefore, these two categories can be grouped as the common subtypes of FAP, whereas Turcot and Zanca syndromes represent the rare subtypes.

Turcot's syndrome. Classical or recessive type of Turcot syndrome is characterized by an association of the central nervous system (CNS), a recessive mode of transmission, younger age of onset, and larger and fewer polyps [18]. Six families have been registered at JPC.

Zanca's syndrome. There are additional case

reports supporting a genetic heterogeneous subtype of FAP, which was proposed by Zanca [19] but failed to be recognized. Miura et al. [20] reported the case of a 41-year-old male who had a typical course of cartilaginous exostosis (MCE) and diffuse adenomatous polyposis of the colon. His father manifested classic MCE and died of colonic cancer associated with polyposis.

The pigmented ocular fundus lesion described by Lewis et al. [21] were found in four of seven cases by Iwama [22] and in seven of our eight cases (73.3%, or 11 of 15 cases in total).

Other neoplastic lesions. Besides the gastrointestinal malignancy, thyroid cancer (0.5–0.8%) (Table 3) and cancer of the uterus (0.5% in JPC) were relatively frequent. Case reports of other neoplasms, such as cancer of the urinary bladder, gall bladder, ovary, accessory testis (bilateral), mammary gland, liver (hepatocellular cancer), and adrenal gland, were each described in a single report.

NATURAL HISTORY AND CANCER RISK

Using well described, registered cases of JPC, age-specific cumulative incidence rate of symptom onset, diagnosis of polyposis, diagnosis of large bowel cancer, and death were calculated [6,7]. From these data, age groups at different risk for the various clinical stages were estimated [6,7], as is shown in Table 4. The age-specific prevalences of large bowel cancer in British patients calculated [6,7] from the data from St. Mark's Hospital [23,24] were similar to those in the Japanese series. However, Japanese males appear to have a slightly slower progression in the natural history compared with the males in the British series (Table 4). By sex, the adenomas as well as cancers were manifested a few years earlier in females than in males (Table 4). Average age of cancer occurrence of the profuse polyp type was 34.0 years. This was about 8 years younger than that of the sparse polyp type (41.8 years) [6,7].

Information has been accumulating increasingly on occurrence of malignancy in diverse organs other than the large bowel. The risks of these are much higher than in the normal population. The frequency of gastric cancer in Japanese polyposis patients (2.1%) is 20–40-fold higher than that of general population [25]. Family studies also showed that the death rate from gastric cancer was significantly higher in family members with FAP than in controls [7]. The majority of patients with these cancers had been colectomized, and the lesion develop many years after colectomy (Table 3). Thyroid cancer, however, occurred at an exceptionally younger age, usually before surgery (Table 3). When the patients live longer as a result of surgical treatment, they may be challenged by diverse malignancies other than of the large bowel. The

TABLE 4.
Ages for Risks or Prevalence of Various Stages of FAP [7]

		Japan		England[a]	
	Risk	Male	Female	Male	Female
Symptom onset	10%	10.3	9.7	10.8	12.3
	50%	22.5	21.3	25.5	25.0
Adenoma diagnosis	10%	12.8	12.1	12.5	11.8
	50%	27.7	24.7	26.7	25.1
Large bowel cancer diagnosis	1%	16.0	13.1	17.5	12.4
	10%	29.5	23.8	27.3	24.6
	50%	42.0	39.8	41.9	40.7
	90%	58.7	65.7	55.1	56.3
Death	10%	32.8	32.8	29.4	29.4
	50%	50.1	49.4	45.4	44.7

[a]Calculated from the data of Veale[23] and Ashley[24].

apparent ability of small bowel adenoma to develop many years after colectomy is one more vexing aspect of the natural history of FAP from the standpoint of surgical management [26].

GENETIC ANALYSIS

The frequency of FAP at birth was estimated to be $0.45 + 0.5 \times 104$ or 1:22,222 [27]. The comparable figures from Western countries were 1:23,930 from England [23], 1:7,437 from the United States [28], and 1:7,646 from Sweden [29].

The male:female ratio was significantly higher for males, being 1.38 or 352:256 in the JPC series [7]. This was similar to the 1.31 ratio at St. Mark's Hospital [23] and the 1.48 in Reed's series [28]. In call-up cases, however, there was no significant sex differences: the ratios were 1.18 or 73.62 in ours, and 1.08 in the St. Mark's series [23]. The decreasing trends in the ratio in the recent JPC series indicated an increased chance of detecting female patients [6,7]. The infant death rate among the siblings of the affected patients was found to be significantly higher than that in controls. This increase in mortality was more predominant in females than in males [30]. This phenomenon indicated that female gene carriers might be less resistant to various diseases in infancy and suggested that it might be related to the earlier manifestation of the disorder in females.

The proportion of nonfamilial cases was 41.5% in the JPC series of 1981 and 45% in the St. Mark's study [23]. The value has been decreasing since the beginning of our study in 1968, when it was 64%, suggesting progress in the ascertainment of family members through the activity of JPC. The relative fitness was calculated to be 0.88 in our series [7]; it was 0.8 in Veale's [23] study and 0.78 in Reed's [28] study.

If parents who were dead of suspected GI malignancy were included in the analysis, the penetrance in our series was 93.7%. The comparable value was 80% in Veale's [23] series and 90% in Reed's [28] series. The observed segregation ratio was 0.427 in our series. The figure from Veale [23] was 0.361 and that from Reed [28] was 0.400.

According to a study of genetic heterogeneity, three major subtypes may present among the common subtypes of FAP: simple FAP with sparse polyps, that with profuse polyps, and GS-type with sparse polyps [7].

CONCLUDING REMARKS

FAP can be subdivided into common and specific rare variants. The former may be further subdivided into the sparse and profuse simple FAP and GSy. The latter includes Turcot's and Zanca's syndromes. Neoplastic involvement of the upper GI tract is the principal phenotypic manifestation of the FAP gene and does not indicate the genetic heterogeneity. Whereas adenomas are generated mainly from genetic factors, cancer may develop under some influence of environmental factors. Genetic backgrounds of the Japanese with FAP were quite similar to those of British and U.S. FAP patients.

References

1. Komatsu I: A clinical genetic study of multiple intestinal polyposes and allied conditions. Jpn J Hum Genet 12:246–297, 1968 (in Japanese with English abstract).
2. Utsunomiya J: Present status of adenomatosis coli in Japan. In Farber E, et al. (eds): "Pathophysiology of Carcinogenesis in Digestive Organs, Tokyo: University of Tokyo Press, Baltimore; University Park Press, 1977, pp 305–321.
3. Utsunomiya J, Iwama T: Studies of hereditary gastrointestinal polyposes. Asian Med J 21:76–96, 1978.
4. Utsunomiya J, Iwama T: Adenomatosis coli in Japan. In Winawer S, Schottenfeld D, Sherlock P (eds): "Colorectal Cancer: Prevention, Epidemiology, and Screening." New York: Raven Press, 1980, pp 83–95.
5. Utsunomiya J, Iwama T: Clinical and Population genetics of the hereditary gastrointestinal polyposis. In Rotter JI, Samloff, Rimoin DL (eds): "Heterogeneity and Genetics of common gastrointestinal disorder". New York: Academic Press, 1980, pp 351–416.
6. Utsunomiya J: Pathology, genetics and management of hereditary gastrointestinal polyposes. In Lynch H, Hirayama T (eds): "Genetic Epidemiology of Cancer". Boca Raton, FL: CRC Press, Inc. (in press).
7. Utsunomiya J: Pathological and genetic aspects of adenomatosis coli in Japan. In Takebe K, Utsunomiya J (eds): "Hereditary Neoplasm". Tokyo: Tokyo University Press (in press).
8. Mishima Y, Yaegashi K: Epidemiology and genetics of colonic polyposis. Clin Gastroenterol 2:1737–1749, 1987 (in Japanese).
9. Bussey HJR: "Familial Polyposis Coli". Baltimore: Johns Hopkins University Press, 1975.
10. Iwama T: Pathological study on adenomatosis coli. J Jpn Surg Soc 79:10–23, 1978 (in Japanese with English abstract).

11. Maeda M, Iwama T, Utsunomiya J, Aoki N, Suzuki S: Radiological features of familial polyposis coli. Grouping by polyp profusion. Br J Radiol 57:217–227, 1984.

12. Utsunomiya J, Maki T, Iwama T, Matsunaga Y, Ichikawa T, Shimomura T, Hamaguchi E, Aoki N: Gastric lesions of familial polyposis coli. Cancer 34: 745–754, 1974.

13. Watanabe H, Enjoji M, Yao T, Ohsato K: Gastric lesions in familial adenomatosis coli. Hum Pathol 9:269–283, 1978.

14. Yao T, Iida M, Ohsato K: Duodenal lesion in familial polyposis of the colon. Gastroenterology 73:1086–1092, 1977.

15. Utsunomiya J, Nakamura T: The occult osteomatous changes in the mandible in patients with familial polyposis coli. Br J Surg 62:45–51, 1975.

16. Nakahara S, Itoh H, Iida M, Iwashita A, Ohsato K: Ileal adenomas in familial polyposis coli: Differences before and after colectomy. Dis Colon Rectum 28:875–877, 1985.

17. Iida M, Nakamura T, Utsunomiya J: Osteomatous changes and tooth abnormalities found in the jaws of patients with adenomatosis coli. Oral Surg 52:2–11, 1981.

18. Itoh H, Ohsato K: Turcot syndrome and its characteristic colonic manifestations. Dis Colon Rectum 28:399–402, 1985.

19. Zanca P: Multiple hereditary cartilaginous exostosis with polyposis of the colon. U.S. Armed Forces Med J 6:116–122, 1953.

20. Miura O, Inoue K, Matsuda S, Adachi Y, Hukutome A, Soga K, Aoki M: A case of familial polyposis coli associated with hereditary multiple cartilaginous exostosis: The so called Zanca's syndrome. Naika [Intern Med] 56:592–597, 1985 (in Japanese).

21. Lewis RA, Crowder WE, Eierman LA, Nussbaum RI, Ferrell RE: The Gardner syndrome: Significance of occular features. Ophthalmology 91:916–925, 1984.

22. Iwama T: Personal communication.

23. Veale AMO: "Intestinal Polyposis". Cambridge: Cambridge University Press, 1965.

24. Ashley DTB: Colonic cancer arising in polyposis coli. J Med Genet 6:376–378, 1969.

25. Segi M, Tominaga S, Aoki K, Fujimoto I: Cancer mortality and mobility statistics: Japan and world. Jpn Sci Soc Press, Tokyo, 1981.

26. Stryker SJ, Carney JA, Dozois RR: Multiple adenomatous polyps arising in a continent reservoir ileostomy. Int J Colorectal Dis 2:43–45.

27. Murata M, Utsunomiya J, Iwama T, Tanimura M: Frequency of Adenomatosis coli in Japan. Jpn J Hum Genet 26:19–30, 1981.

28. Reed TE, Neel JV: A genetic study of multiple polyposis of the colon (with an appendix deriving a method of estimating relative fitness). Am J Hum Genet 7:236–263, 1955.

29. Alm T, Licznerski G: The intestinal polyposes. Clin Gastroenterol 2:577–602, 1973.

30. Utsunomiya J, Iwama T, Suzuki H, Tanaka T, Tonomura A, Sasaki M, Nakamura T, Hamaguchi H, Mori W, Komatsu I: Clinical and genetic studies on familial polyposis coli; Sex ratio. Jpn J Human Genet 20:283, 1976 (in Japanese).

13

Extracolonic Manifestations of Familial Adenomatous Polyposis

Steffen Bülow

Department of Surgical Gastroenterology, Hvidovre Hospital, University of Copenhagen, Copenhagen, Denmark

INTRODUCTION

Familial adenomatous polyposis (FAP) is an autosomal dominant disease; in Denmark, the incidence rate is 1.3 per 1,000,000 inhabitants based on the polyposis register, which is nationwide and nearly complete [1]. The disease is characterized primarily by early development of 100 to several thousand colorectal adenomas, of which one or more will degenerate into carcinoma if colectomy is not performed. The prognosis after early prophylactic colectomy is good.

Until the early 1950s FAP was believed to be an entirely colorectal disease. However, at that time, Gardner reported a polyposis kindred with multiple osteomas and multiple epidermoid cysts [2]. This triad became known as "Gardner's syndrome." During the last decade, it has become clear, however, that the majority of FAP patients have one or more extracolonic manifestations; on this basis, most authors now agree that the term "Gardner's syndrome" has lost its clinical significance and should no longer be used [1].

A large spectrum of diseases and conditions has been reported as being associated with FAP on the basis of casuistic reports, most of them reflecting only accidental coexistence. In the following review, only generally accepted extracolonic manifestations are discussed.

Familial Adenomatous Polyposis, pages 109–114

OSTEOMAS

Osteomas may develop in FAP patients as clinically evident tumors in the facial skeleton and the long bones. They are benign, but their local growth may cause problems [2]. Osteomas preceded the diagnosis of FAP by an average of 17 years in a series of 83 patients [3]. In 1975, Utsunomiya and Nakamura [4] reported the detection by mandibular pantomography of multiple small osteomas in the mandible in 27 of 29 patients (93%), and later studies have shown osteoma frequencies of 76–81% [5–7].

A study of 34 unaffected sibs and children showed that the observed frequency did not differ significantly from the expected frequency, nor from the frequency in the normal population. Therefore, a definite evaluation of the diagnostic value of the method as a screening procedure among unaffected relatives at risk of FAP was not possible on the basis of this study [8]. In a study of seven polyposis kindreds, all affected family members in six kindreds had mandibular osteomas, and seven of twelve children under 16 years old and at risk for FAP had osteomas; all the latter developed colorectal adenomas after a mean interval of 4 years. Five children without osteomas had no colorectal adenomas during a 5–10 year follow-up. Mandibular osteomas thus are good predictors for adenoma development in families that include affected members having mandibular osteomas [9]. In conclusion, mandibular pantomography may be used as a supplementary screening procedure in unaffected first-degree relatives, but, as a consequence of the recent detection of a specific FAP gene [10], a chromosomal test undoubtedly will become the screening method of choice.

EPIDERMOID CYSTS

Epidermoid cysts are benign soft subcutaneous tumors that may be located on the extremities, face, and scalp in FAP patients, whereas in non-FAP patients they are more often found on the back [11]. In a study of 74 FAP patients a mean of four epidermoid cysts (one to twenty) was found in 39 patients (53%) at a mean age of 13 years (range 0–39) [12]. In 13 of the 39 patients with cysts, one or more cysts had been removed during childhood, before FAP was diagnosed [11]. In general, epidermoid cysts, and especially those located on the face or extremities, are very rarely found in children outside FAP families [12].

DESMOID TUMORS

Desmoid tumors are bandlike, fibromatous tumors arising from fasciae, muscles, and aponeuroses. They may be located on the anterior abdominal wall, intraperitoneally, retroperitoneally, or at the periphery, e.g., the shoulder girdle. They show a marked tendency to local growth, but they never metastasize. Desmoid tumors may grow to 20 cm in diameter or even more, and the examination method of choice is computerized tomography (CT) scanning.

Histopathologically, desmoid tumors show two different patterns. One is characterized by fibroblasts surrounded by abundant collagen; this type is characteristic of abdominal wall desmoids. The other type shows activated fibroblasts surrounded by abundant mucopolysaccharide ground substance and little collagen; this pattern is seen in intraperitoneal and mesenteric desmoids. Both types are seen in FAP as well as in nonpolyposis patients [13].

Trauma and hormonal factors have been suggested with regard to the origin of desmoids. The trauma theory is based on the observation that many patients have suffered from earlier trauma, e.g., a previous laparotomy. The hormonal theory is based on the observations that desmoid tumors are often seen in fertile women and that hormonal factors seem to affect the growth of desmoids in women [14].

A study of 201 FAP patients revealed seven (4%) with a desmoid [15]; in the St. Mark's Hospital polyposis series of 617 patients, the development of a desmoid was seen in 26 cases (4%) [16]. Recently, the frequency has been estimated as about 12% in major series [13]. Desmoids constituted only 0.03% among approximately 50,000 cases of neoplastic disease in the general population [17]. Between 70% and 85% of patients with desmoids are women 20–40 years of age [18]. A review of the literature in 1970 revealed 89 FAP patients with desmoid tumors; of these, 45 (51%) tumors were located intraabdominally. The desmoids had been diagnosed, on average, about 2 years after the diagnosis of FAP, but 16 (18%) appeared before FAP had been diagnosed [19]. Among a recent survey of 325 FAP patients, a total of 36 desmoids were found in 29 patients (9%), of whom 22 (76%) were women. The desmoid tumor was diagnosed at a median age of 30 years and colectomy predated the desmoid in 25 of 29 patients at a median interval of 2 years; 26 of 36 desmoids (72%) were located in the small bowel mesentery [20].

With the Danish Polyposis Register, a desmoid tumor was registered in nine of 247 patients (4%). Eight of these patients were women (89%), and the desmoids were diagnosed at a median age of 37 years. In eight of the patients, the desmoids developed after a previous colectomy. Seven desmoids were located at the anterior abdominal wall, and only two were found intraperitoneally. In contrast to the above-mentioned series, this series is based on a national register; consequently, the low Danish incidence of intraperitoneal desmoids may in fact represent the true frequency [21].

The treatment is surgical, and complete excision and atraumatic operative techniques are considered important [14]. However, it was recently stated that, in patients with mesenteric desmoids, surgical removal should be carried out only in selected patients with life-threatening complications, e.g., intestinal or ureteral obstruction, because surgery is very difficult, the complication rate is high, and early recurrence is likely [13,20]. Desmoid tumors have been shown to be highly resistant to radiation therapy and chemotherapy, but ongoing, multicenter, prospective trials show favorable interim results of treatment with a combination of Clinoril and tamoxifen [22]. Several FPC patients with multiple and dense intraperitoneal adhesions have been reported [23], indicating a general "fibroproliferative" tendency in FAP.

GASTRODUODENAL TUMORS

The presence of gastric polyps in FAP was first reported in 1895 [24], but gastroduodenal lesions were considered very rare until fiberendoscopy allowed a more accurate examination and demonstrated gastroduodenal polyps in more than one-half of FAP patients [25,26]. Since the mid-1970s several authors have reported similar findings. The occurrence of polyps is not related to the presence of a colorectal carcinoma, nor to the length of the interval between the endoscopy and a previous colectomy [27]. A questionnaire among members of the international "Leeds Castle Polyposis Group" concerning 1,255 patients showed nine cases of gastric cancer and 41 cases of duodenal cancer, which was nearly a 50-fold difference from the expected frequencies [13].

Stomach

Fundic gland polyposis was first described in 1978 as a nonneoplastic condition. Among a series of 22 FAP patients, six (27%) had several hundred 1–5 mm hemispherical polyps scattered in the fundus of the stomach; histologic examination showed "fundic gland polyposis," i.e., cystic dilated fundic glands, without epithelial dysplasia [28]. Since then, the condition has been diagnosed in 23–56% of FAP patients [27,29–31]. The incidence of fundic gland polyposis does not increase with age [32]. The condition was believed primarily to be specific to FAP, but a recent report showed fundic gland polyposis in 0.09% of ~27,000 non-FAP patients [30].

Hyperplastic polyps are benign and have been found in 8–44% of nine to 26 patients [25,27,33].

Adenomas have been diagnosed in 2–13% in series of 11–100 FAP patients [25,27,29,31–33]. A higher incidence of gastric adenomas was found in one Japanese study (nine of 22); this difference probably reflects the higher frequency of premalignant lesions as compared to the case in the Western hemisphere [34].

Carcinoma is an extremely rare finding in non-Japanese FAP patients. In one Japanese study, three of 22 patients had a gastric carcinoma [28].

Duodenum

Adenomas have been reported in 24–73% in series of 9–100 patients [26,27,29,31–33,35,36]. Usually, 10–50 adenomas are located primarily in the second part of the duodenum and may extend into the upper third part. The papilla of Vater may be affected. The adenomas are most often 3–5 mm in size, irregular, and paler than the surrounding mucosa, and often are located on the mucosal folds. However, larger and even stalked adenomas may be found.

Histologic examination shows adenomas resembling those in the colon. In some patients, biopsies from duodenal mucosa having a normal macroscopic appearance reveal early adenomatous changes at histologic examination [27,32, 33,35]. The incidence of duodenal adenomas seems to increase with age [32].

Carcinomas in the duodenum or periampullary have been reported in 29 FAP patients since the condition was first described in 1935 [37]. A review of 24 of these patients demonstrated a mean age of 46 years (range 18–67) and ten (40%) with synchronous adenomas [38]. In the Danish series, two of 247 patients (1%) developed a periampullary carcinoma [21].

From a cancer-prophylactic point of view, the duodenal adenomas are the most interesting gastroduodenal lesions. As histologic examination of mucosa with a normal appearance has shown early adenomatous changes, the frequency of adenomas may be even higher than is assumed at present. The occurrence of a large number of premalignant polyps in at least one-half of FAP patients, the occasional finding of a duodenal carcinoma, and finally the frequent occurrence of synchronous adenomas in patients with a duodenal carcinoma together indicate that the malignant potential of duodenal adenomas cannot be neglected. The exact risk of malignant degeneration is unknown, but, based on the small number of published cases of duodenal carcinoma, the risk is probably must less than that of the colorectal adenomas. On the other hand, if an adenoma–carcinoma sequence also exists in the duodenum, the recent improvement in the prognosis of FAP patients following prophylactic colectomy [21] may perhaps lead to an increasing number of duodenal carcinomas in the future.

In conclusion, the potential risk of carcinoma development in the duodenum seems substantial enough to justify regular prophylactic surveillance of all FAP patients by gastroduodenoscopy. However, our present knowledge does not permit age limits for this prophylaxis to be determined, nor the length of the intervals between the examinations. Until results of ongoing large studies have been published, it is suggested that gastroduodenoscopy be carried out in all adult FAP patients, e.g., from the age of 20 years. In patients without gastric or duodenal adenomas, the examination may be repeated at 5-year intervals. After radical removal of a gastric adenoma, endoscopy may be repeated at intervals of 1–2 years.

Patients with duodenal adenomas should be followed with annual fiberendoscopy. Biopsies should be taken from several adenomas and from flat, normal-appearing mucosa and the papilla Vateri. The degree of dysplasia may influence the length of the intervals between examinations. Total removal of multiple small adenomas has been attempted by repeated endoscopic bipolar electrocoagulation [32] or by endoscopic laser destruction [39], but these procedures carry a substantial risk of duodenal perforation and should only be used in expert hands and as a part of a controlled trial. Such studies have been planned [32]. Large adenomas may be removed endoscopically by snare or at open surgery, but only carcinoma should lead to pancreaticoduodenectomy.

SMALL INTESTINAL TUMORS

Adenomas have been detected by intraoperative fiberendoscopy in six of seven patients [40]. In St. Mark's Hospital nine patients were found to have ileal adenomas appearing 2–26 years after colectomy [41]. Adenomas may occur in a Kock pouch [42] and in the terminal ileum many years after colectomy and straight ileoanal anastomosis [43].

Carcinomas have been reported in only two patients [44], and the risk thus seems very small.

PANCREATICOBILIARY TUMORS

Adenomas in the common bile duct, gallbladder, and pancreatic duct have been reported in five FAP patients [45–47].

THYROID CARCINOMA

A total of 23 polyposis patients with papillary thyroid carcinoma have been described [48]. Nearly all are women, and the risk of a female FAP patient to develop carcinoma of the thyroid has been estimated to be 100–160 times the risk in the normal population [48,49]. Papillary thyroid carcinoma in FAP therefore represents more than mere coincidence and should be included in the list of extracolonic manifestations that may occur in any FAP patient.

Regular prophylactic examination of the thyroid has been recommended for female polyposis patients [49], but, since the prognosis of papillary thyroid carcinoma is excellent and the surveillance program is already fairly extensive, this author finds that regular thyroid screening is superfluous and even may cause cancerphobia [48].

HEPATOBLASTOMA

Hepatoblastoma has been reported in ten unrelated children with a family history of FAP; six of them survived, and all later developed FAP [50,51]. An international registry of FAP patients with hepatoblastoma is being established [50].

DENTAL ANOMALIES

Among Gardner's original "kindred 109," several family members had dental abnormalities, multiple supernumerary and impacted permanent teeth [52]. In a Danish-Finnish study of 97 FAP patients, 17% had dental abnormalities: 11% had supernumerary teeth, and 9% had impacted permanent teeth. These frequencies are significantly higher than those of the normal population [53].

RETINAL LESIONS

In 1984, an ophthalmoscopic study of three polyposis families demonstrated multiple and bilateral nonpremalignant patches of congenital hypertrophy of the retinal pigment epithelium in all affected family members [54]. In a recent study of 16 polyposis families, 37 of 41 (90%) affected family members had such lesions, which were bilateral in 78%. Among unaffected first-degree relatives at risk, 20 of 43 (47%) had retinal lesions, which occurred in two of 42 (5%) controls [55]. The specificity of bilateral retinal lesions as a marker for FAP was 0.95, and the sensitivity was 0.78. Ophthalmoscopy should therefore be used as a screening method in all first-degree relatives of FAP patients [55].

LYMPHOID POLYPOSIS

Multiple lymphoid polyps are often found in the terminal ileum of FAP patients [56,57] and in rare cases in the colon coexisting with the adenomas [58].

CONCLUSIONS

When the diagnosis of FAP has been confirmed by endoscopy and histology, the patient should have a gastroduodenoscopy to detect possible gastroduodenal adenomas, which are the only premalignant extracolonic manifestations occurring with a frequency that may justify prophylactic examination. Prophylactic examination for an intraabdominal desmoid tumor by CT scanning may be carried out but has little therapeutical consequence; no effective treatment modality has yet been found. Mandibular pantomography and ophthalmoscopy are recommended as screening procedures, because the detection of mandibular osteomas, dental anomalies, and retinal lesions may serve as predictors for future development of FAP in nonaffected first-degree relatives of the proband.

References

1. Bülow S: Familial polyposis coli. A clinical and epidemiological study (thesis). Dan Med Bull 34:1–15, 1987.
2. Gardner EJ, Richards RC: Multiple cutaneous and subcutaneous lesions occurring simultaneously with hereditary polyposis and osteomatosis. Am J Hum Genet 5:139–148, 1953.
3. Duncan BR, Dohner VA, Priest JH: The Gardner syndrome: Need for early diagnosis. J Pediatr 72:479–505, 1968.
4. Utsunomiya J, Nakamura T: The occult osteomatous changes in the mandible in patients with familial polyposis coli. Br J Surg 62:45–51, 1975.
5. Ida M, Nakamura T, Utsunomiya J: Osteomatous changes and tooth abnormalities found in the jaws of patients with adenomatosis coli. Oral Surg 52:2–11, 1981.
6. Järvinen HJ, Peltokallio P, Landtman M, Wolf J: Gardner's stigmas in familial adenomatosis coli. Br J Srug 69:718–721, 1982.
7. Bülow S, Søndergaard JO, Witt IN, Larsen E, Tetens G: Mandibular osteomas in familial polyposis coli. Dis Colon Rectum 27:105–108, 1984.
8. Bülow S, Holm NV, Søndergaard JO, Witt IN, Tetens G: Mandibular osteomas in unaffected sibs and children of patients with familial polyposis coli. Scand J Gastroenterol 21:744–748, 1986.
9. Offerhaus GJ, Levin LS, Giardiello FM, Krush AJ, Welsh SB, Booker SV, Hasler JF, McKusick VA, Yardley JH, Hamilton SR, Luk GD: Occult radiopaque jaw lesions in familial adenomatous polyposis coli and hereditary nonpolyposis colorectal cancer. Gastroenterology 93:490–497, 1987.
10. Bodmer WF, Bailey CJ, Bodmer J, Bussey HJR, Ellis A, Gorman P, Lucibello FC, Murday WA, Rider SH, Scambler P, Sheer D, Solomon E, Spurr NK: Localisation of the gene for familial adenomatous polyposis on chromosome 5. Nature 328:614–616, 1987.
11. Leppard BJ: Epidermoid cysts and polyposis coli. Proc R Soc Med 67:1036–1037, 1974.
12. Leppard BJ, Bussey HJR: Epidermoid cysts, polyposis coli and Gardner's syndrome. Br J Surg 62:387–393, 1975.
13. Jass J: Desmoid disease or fibromatosis. Paper presented at the Leeds Castle Polyposis Group Meeting, Washington, DC, 1987.
14. Dahn I, Jonsson N, Lundh G: Desmoid tumours. Acta Chir Scand 126:305–314, 1963.
15. Smith WG: Multiple polyposis, Gardner's syndrome and desmoid tumors. Dis Colon Rectum 1:323–332, 1958.
16. Bussey HJR: "Familial Polyposis Coli. Family Studies, Histopathology, Differential Diagnosis and Results of Treatment. Baltimore: Johns Hopkins University Press, 1975.
17. Pack GT, Ehrlich HE. Neoplasms of the anterior abdominal wall with special considerations of desmoid tumors. Int Abstr Surg 79:177–198, 1944.
18. Jones EL, Cornell WP: Gardner's syndrome. Review of the literature and report on a family. Arch Surg 92:287–300, 1966.
19. McAdam WAF, Goligher JC: The occcurrence of desmoids in patients with familial polyposis coli. Br J Surg 57:618–631, 1970.
20. Jones IT, Fazio VW, Weakley FL, Jagelman DG, Lavery IC, McGannon E: Desmoid tumors in familial polyposis coli. Ann Surg 204:94–97, 1986.
21. Bülow S: Clinical features of familial polyposis coli. Results of the Danish Polyposis Register. Dis Colon Rectum 29:102–107, 1986.

22. Dozois RR, Berk T, Bülow S, Cohen Z, DeCosse JJ, Hawley PR, Jagelman DG, Järvinen HJ, Macrae FA: Symposium: Surgical aspects of familial adenomatous polyposis. Int J Colorectal Dis 3:1–16, 1988.

23. Watne AL, Core SK, Carrier JM: Gardner's syndrome. Surg Gynecol Obstet 141:53–56, 1975.

24. Hauser G: Ueber Polyposis intestinalis adenomatosa und deren Beziehung zur Krebsentwicklung. Deutsch Arch Klin Med 55:429–448, 1895.

25. Utsunomiya J, Maki T, Iwama T, Matsunaga Y, Ichikawa T, Shimomura T, Hamaguchi E, Aoki N: Gastric lesions of familial polyposis coli. Cancer 34:745–754, 1974.

26. Ushio K, Sasagawa M, Doi H, Yamada T, Ichikawa H, Hojo K, Koyoma Y, Sano R: Lesions associated with familial polyposis coli: Studies of lesions of the stomach, duodenum, bones and teeth. Gastrointest Radiol 1:67–80, 1976.

27. Bülow S, Lauritsen KB, Johansen Aa, Svendsen LB, Søndergaard JO: Gastroduodenal polyps in familial polyposis coli. Dis Colon Rectum 288:90–93, 1985.

28. Watanabe H, Enjoji M, Yao T, Ohsato K: Gastric lesions in familial adenomatosis coli. Hum Pathol 9:269–283, 1978.

29. Järvinen H, Nyberg M, Peltokallio P: Upper gastrointestinal tract polyps in familial adenomatosis coli. Gut 24:333–339, 1983.

30. Iida M, Yao T, Watanabe H, Itoh H, Iwashita A: Fundic gland polyposis in patients without familial adenomatosis coli: Its incidence and clinical features. Gastroenterology 86:1437–1442, 1984.

31. Järvinen HJ, Sipponen P: Gastroduodenal polyps in familial adenomatous and juvenile polyposis. Endoscopy 18:230–234, 1986.

32. Sarre RG, Frost AG, Jagelman DG, Petras RE, Sivak MV, McGannon E: Gastric and duodenal polyps in familial adenomatous polyposis: a prospective study of the nature and prevalence of upper gastrointestinal polyps. Gut 28:306–314, 1987.

33. Burt RW, Berenson MM, Lee RG, Tolman KG, Freston JW, Gardner EJ: Upper gastrointestinal polyps in Gardner's syndrome. Gastroenterology 86:295–301, 1984.

34. Johansen Aa: Early gastric cancer. A contribution to the pathology and to gastric cancer histogenesis (thesis). Copenhagen, University of Copenhagen 1981.

35. Ranzi T, Castagnone D, Velio P, Bianchi P, Polli EE: Gastric and duodenal polyps in familial polyposis coli. Gut 22:363–367, 1981.

36. Kurtz RC, Sternberg SS, Miller HH, DeCosse JJ: Upper gastrointestinal neoplasia in familial polyposis. Digest Dis Sci 32:459–465, 1987.

37. Cabot RC: Case 21061. N Engl J Med 212:263–267, 1935.

38. Sugihara K, Muto T, Kamiya J, Konishi F, Sawada T, Morioka Y: Gardner's syndrome associated with periampullary carcinoma, duodenal and gastric adenomatosis. Dis Colon Rectum 25:766–771, 1982.

39. Herrera-Ornelas L: Endoscopic Nd-YAG laser treatment of gastrointestinal polyps in patients with familial polyposis. Semin Surg Oncol 3:146–148, 1987.

40. Ohsato K, Yao T, Watanabe H, Iida M, Itoh H: Small-intestinal involvement in familial polyposis diagnosed by operative intestinal fiberscopy. Dis Colon Rectum 20:414–420, 1977.

41. Hamilton SR, Bussey HJR, Mendelsohn G, Diamond MP, Pavlides G, Hutcheon D, Harbison M, Shermeta D, Morson BC, Yardley JH: Ileal adenomas after colectomy in nine patients with adenomatous polyposis coli/Gardner's syndrome. Gastroenterology 77:1252–1257, 1979.

42. Stryker SJ, Carney JA, Dozois RR: Multiple adenomatous polyps arising in a continent reservoir ileostomy. Int J Colorectal Dis 2:43–45, 1987.

43. Myrhøj T, Bülow S, Mogensen AM: Adenomas in terminal ileum 25 years after restorative proctocolectomy for familial adenomatous polyposis. Submitted.

44. Ross JE, Mara JE: Small bowel polyps and carcinoma in multiple intestinal polyposis. Arch Srug 108:736–738, 1974.

45. Järvinen HJ, Nyberg M, Peltokallio P: Biliary involvement in familial adenomatosis coli. Dis Colon Rectum 26:525–528, 1983.

46. Walsh N, Qizilbash A, Banerjee R, Waugh GA: Biliary neoplasia in Gardner's syndrome. Arch Pathol Lab Med 111:76–77, 1987.

47. Komorowski RA, Tresp MG, Wilson SD: Pancreaticobiliary involvement in familial polyposis coli/Gardner's syndrome. Dis Colon Rectum 29:55–58, 1986.

48. Bülow S, Holm NV, Mellemgaard A: Papillary thyroid carcinoma in Danish patients with familial adenomatous polyposis. Int J Colorectal Dis 3:29–31, 1988.

49. Plail RO, Bussey HJR, Glazer G, Thomson JPS: Adenomatous polyposis: An association with carcinoma of the thyroid. Br J Surg 74:377–380, 1987.

50. Li FP, Thurber WA, Seddon J, Holmes GE: Hepatoblastoma in families with polyposis coli. JAMA 257:2475–2477, 1987.

51. Garber JE, Finegold MJ, Kingston JE, Krush AJ, Li FP, Strong LC: Familial adenomatous polyposis in hepatoblastoma survivors. Unpublished paper.

52. Gardner EJ, Plenk HP: Hereditary pattern for multiple osteomas in a family group. Am J Hum Genet 4:31–36, 1952.

53. Søndergaard JO, Bülow S, Järvinen H, Wolf J, Witt IN, Tetens G: Dental anomalies in familial polyposis coli. Acta Odont Scand 45:61–63, 1987.

54. Lewis R, Crowder WE, Eierman LA, Nussbaum RL, Ferrell RE: The Gardner syndrome. Significance of ocular lesions. Ophthalmology 91:916–924, 1984.

55. Traboulsi EI, Krush AJ, Gardner EJ, Booker S, Offerhaus GJA, Yardley JH, Hamilton SR, Luk GD, Giardiello FM, Welsh SB, Hughes JP, Maumenee IH: Prevalence and importance of pigmented ocular fundus lesions in Gardner's syndrome. N Engl J Med 316:661–667, 1987.

56. Dorazio RA, Whelan TJ: Lymphoid hyperplasia of the terminal ileum associated with familial polyposis coli. Ann Surg 171:300–302, 1970.

57. Shull LN, Fitts CT: Lymphoid polyposis associated with familial polyposis and Gardner's syndrome. Ann Surg 180:319–322, 1974.

58. Alm T, Licznerski G: The intestinal polyposes. Clin Gastroentrol 2:577–602, 1973.

14

Dental Abnormalities and Bone Lesions in Patients With Familial Adenomatous Polyposis

William Carl, Maureen A. Sullivan, and Lemuel Herrera

Department of Dentistry and Maxillofacial Prosthetics (W.C., M.A.S.), Familial Polyposis Registry and Department of Surgical Oncology (L.H.), Roswell Park Memorial Institute, Buffalo, New York

INTRODUCTION

Adenomatous polyps of the colon in association with multiple soft and hard tissue abnormalities were first described by Gardner and Richards in 1953 [1]. Other features such as mesenteric desmoids, epidermoid cysts, and fibromas have been investigated as well as dental and jaw bone anomalies, which are seen in a high percentage of patients with familial adenomatous polyposis (FAP) [2–4].

The bone abnormalities associated with FAP are areas of bone condensation (osteomas) in the bones of the skull and face, with preference for the maxilla and the mandible. The reported incidences of osteomas range from 11% to 80% [3–6]. Examples of the dental abnormalities associated with FAP are congenitally missing teeth, supernumerary teeth, malformed and malpositioned teeth, aberrant root formations, and impactions. Dental abnormalities appear to be less frequent than osteomas. Some investigators have found the occurrence to be in the 11–38% range, which is significantly higher than the frequency of dental abnormalities in the population not afflicted with any known type of syndrome or pathology [4,5]. To present the various dental and jaw bone abnormalities associated with FAP, we have selected seven cases. The case presentation is followed by an analysis of the data and a discussion of the patients in our study group.

CASE PRESENTATION

Case 1

E.S. is a 39-year-old woman who was diagnosed as having FAP in 1986. She had a laparotomy that year, and a retroperitoneal tumor involving the mesentery and the right colon was found. She underwent a total abdominal hysterectomy, bilateral salpingooophorectomy, right colon and small bowel resection, and a resection of the desmoid tumor.

A panoramic radiograph reveals multiple radiodensities in the mandible (Fig. 1). There are numerous impacted teeth in the anterior right mandible, which appear to involve the secondary cuspid as well as two retained primary incisors. The lower right second molar is impacted and has abnormal root formation. The roots of the lower left second molar and of the upper right first molar appear to be fused.

Case 2

E.W. is a 44-year-old man in whom FAP was diagnosed in 1968. He underwent a subtotal abdominal colectomy, with ileoproctostomy. In 1970, he again had an episode of small bowel obstruction secondary to a desmoid tumor that required resections. In 1979, the patient required an abdominoperineal resection of the rectum for moderately differentiated adenocarcinoma, Dukes

Familial Adenomatous Polyposis, pages 115–120

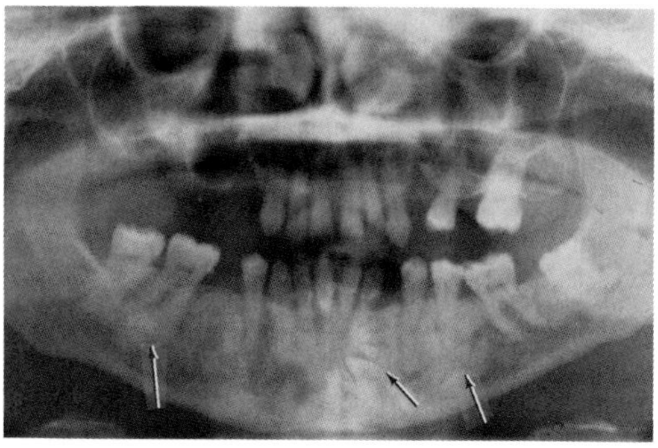

Fig. 1. Dental abnormalities of a patient with FAP consist primarily of a luster of partially formed teeth in the right anterior mandible and impacted mandibular right third molar. Numerous osteomas are present throughout the mandible (arrows).

C (3/2 ×), as well as multiple polyps. An ileostomy was constructed. In 1986, the patient had a right thoracotomy for the removal of a solitary metastatic lesion from colon carcinoma.

In 1986, a firm mass, with expansion, was observed in the left mandible. Small circular radiopacities measuring 4–5 mm in diameter are also present in the body of the mandible. There are impacted left and right mandibular cuspids and retained deciduous cuspids. The remaining right mandibular second and third molars have fused roots (Fig. 2). An occlusal radiograph of the left mandible shows a semicircular radioopaque lateral projection of approximately 2 cm, which appears to be attached to the cortical plate of the mandible (Fig. 3). This boney lesion was removed with the patient under general anesthesia.

Case 3

D.W. is the 9-year-old son of the patient described above (case 2). In 1987, he received a barium enema, which revealed multiple polyps throughout the entire colon. A colonoscopy subsequently revealed multiple polyps throughout the colon, including the rectum. The patient underwent a total abdominal colectomy, mucosalectomy of the rectum, ileoanal anastamosis, creation of a J pouch, and diverting ileostomy in 1987. This patient's father had obstructing carcinoma of the transverse colon at age 21 years and underwent a colectomy, as well as proctocolectomy for cancer of the rectum.

Dental anomalies include missing secondary teeth for mandibular right and left second premolars as well as the maxillary left second premolar. Radiodensities indicate possible developing osteomas in the mandibular anterior region as well as at the apex of the mandibular right second deciduous molar (Fig. 4).

Case 4

S.W. is the 16-year-old sister of the previous patient (case 3). She was born with a bilateral

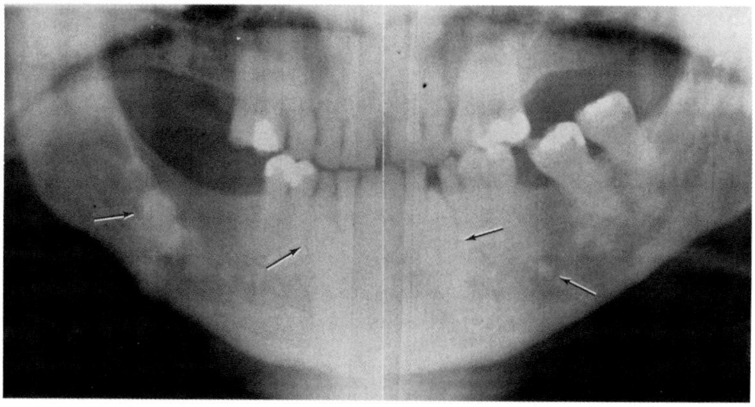

Fig. 2. Dental and bone abnormalities of a patient with FAP are impacted left and right mandibular cuspids, retained deciduous cuspids, fused roots of the right mandibular second and third molars, and osteomas in the body of the mandible (arrows).

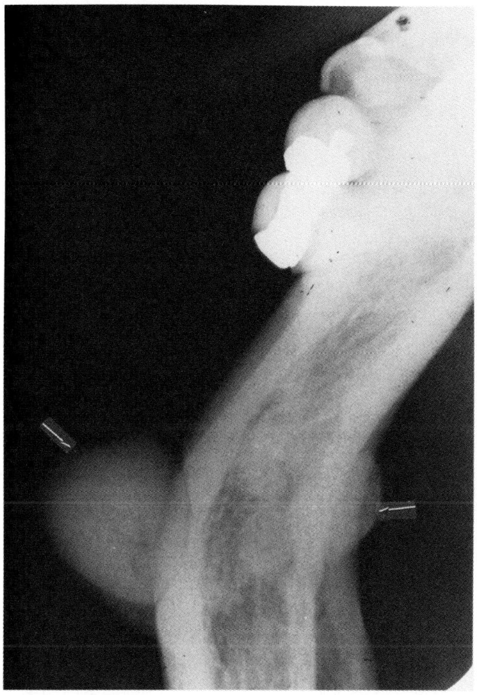

Fig. 3. Occlusal radiograph of the left mandible of the patient shown in Figure 2. The osteoma extends labially and lingually (arrows).

cleft palate and lip and has had multiple episodes of corrective surgery. To date, there is no evidence of adenomatous polyps. Dental anomalies include fused maxillary molar roots as well as fused mandibular second molar roots. There is no evidence of maxillary third molar formations. There are multiple missing teeth in the maxilla, including the right and left second premolars. The parents deny any history of extractions. There is evidence of bone condensation at the apices of the mandibular right cuspid and premolars (Fig. 5).

Case 5

M.D. is a 17-year-old woman with a history of FAP. The disease is present in her father, one sister, an uncle, and some first-degree cousins. At age 13 years, the patient had a subtotal colectomy, with an ileoproctostomy for polyps. Four years later, an adenomatous polyp of the small intestines was found on rigid proctoscopy. She also has been diagnosed with Hashimoto's thyroiditis and papillary carcinoma of the thyroid.

The dental abnormalities include impacted maxillary cuspids and mandibular left second premolar. There is no evidence of toothbud forma-

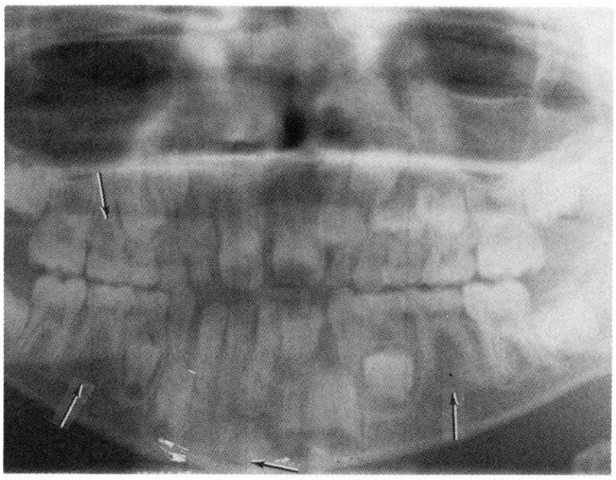

Fig. 4. Panoramic radiograph of a 9-year-old patient with FAP. This is the son of the patient shown in Figures 2 and 3. The dental abnormalities (arrows) consist of missing permanent mandibular left and right second premolars and second left maxillary premolar. One area of bone condensation is present in the anterior mandible.

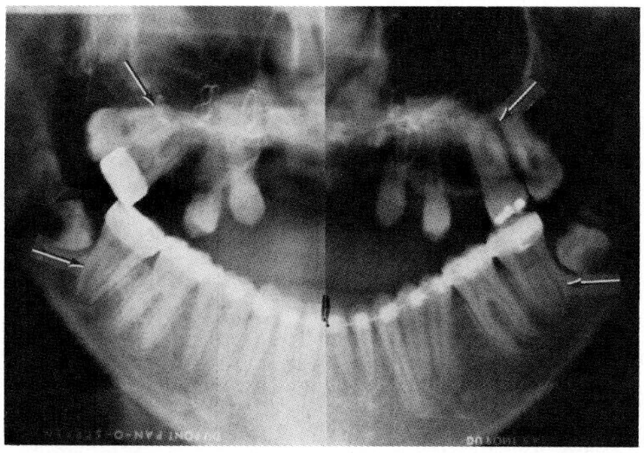

Fig. 5. This patient is the 16-year-old sister of the patient shown in Figure 4. To date, there is no evidence of adenomatous polyps. Dental abnormalities (arrows) consist of fused and tapered roots of the maxillary first and second molars and the mandibular second molars. The maxillary central and lateral incisors and the second premolars are missing. This patient also has bilateral cleft lip and palate.

tion of the left maxillary and mandibular third molars and the right mandibular third molar. The right maxillary third molar has a completely calcified coronal portion. There appears to be a slight cyst formation around the mandibular left second premolar. The maxillary first and second molars and the mandibular second molars have fused roots (Fig. 6).

Case 6

T.D. is the older sister of the previous patient (Case 5). At age 14 years, she had a subtotal abdominal colectomy, with an ileoproctostomy, for polyps. Two years later, additional polyps were removed from the rectum. She developed an unresectable retroperitoneal and mesenteric desmoid tumor, for which she is under treatment with oral tamoxifen (Stuart Pharmaceuticals, Wilmington, DE). She underwent total thyroidectomy for papillary thyroid cancer.

This patient's dental abnormalities include maxillary and mandibular first molars, with fused, long, and tapered roots, which are similar to those of her sister. A narrow radiopacity is present apically and mesially to the root of the mandibular left cuspid. The maxillary and mandibular third molars are impacted. The roots are not yet developed. The patient was 19 years old when the (Fig. 7) radiograph was taken.

Case 7

M.K. is a 26-year-old man who underwent a total abdominal colectomy and ileoproctostomy when he was 11 years old. Dental radiographs show osteomas in the left and right maxilla and in the body of the mandible. The roots of the maxillary left second molar and of the mandibular molars are fused (Fig. 8).

DISCUSSION

FAP is an autosomal dominant condition in which multiple polyps develop in the rectum and colon [7]. Without intervention, carcinomatous changes often occur [8]. FAP is a syndrome in which varied dental and bone abnormalities are distinct features as demonstrated by the cases presented above.

It has been suggested that the atypical tooth formations may be caused by hyperproductivity of the lamina dura as well as by abberations of the mesenchymal tissue adjacent to the lamina [3,9]. This also seems to occur in conditions such as cleidocranial dysostosis and cleft palate.

A recent study by Sondergaard et al. [5] showed that 11% of FAP patients had supernumerary teeth and/or osteomas. In this study, each of the patients had at least one osteoma of the jaw. A study conducted by Utsunomiya and

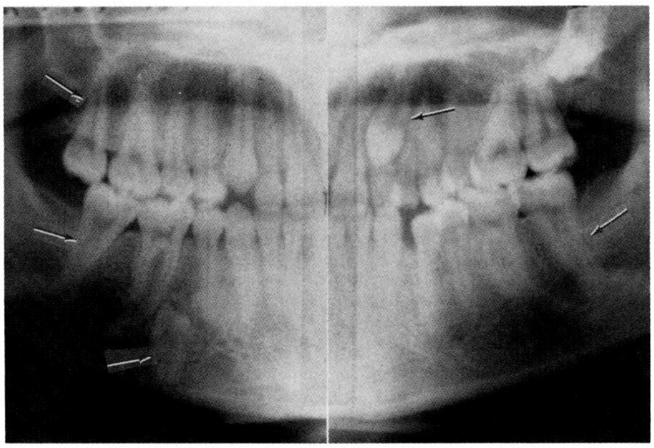

Fig. 6. Panoramic radiograph of a 17-year-old woman with a history of FAP. This patient has impacted mandibular left second premolar and impacted maxillary cuspids (arrows). The roots of the maxillary and mandibular molars are fused.

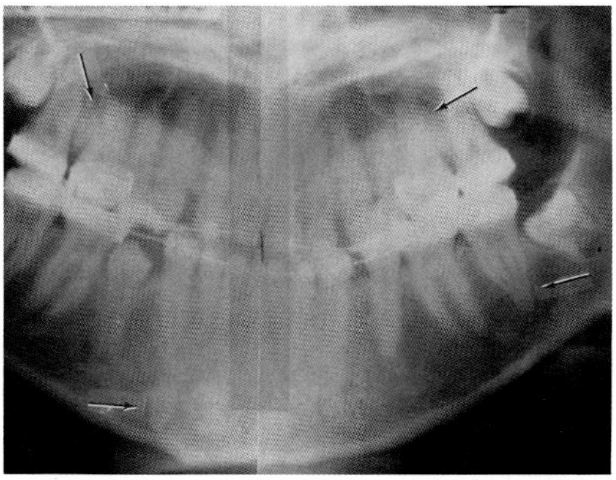

Fig. 7. This patient is the sister of the patient shown in Figure 6. She has the same medical diagnosis. There is one elongated radiopacity in the left mandible, and the maxillary and mandibular molars have fused roots (arrows).

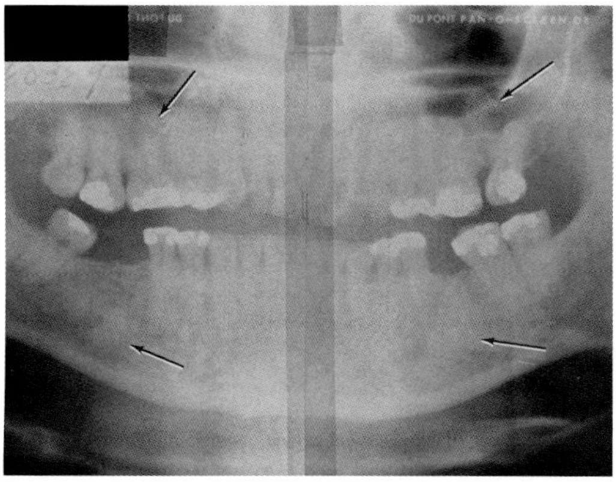

Fig. 8. This 28-year-old man underwent a total abdominal colectomy and ileoproctostomy at age 11 years. He has osteomas in the left and right mandible and in the maxilla, and the roots of the maxillary and mandibular molars are fused (arrows).

Nakamura [9] concluded that 94% of patients with FAP had mandibular osteomas. In our study, which to date has 22 patients, 21 patients had dental and/or bone abnormalities of some type. This is comparable to the findings of Utsunomiya and Nakamura.

Since the frequency of dental abnormalities and bone lesions is significantly higher in FAP patients than in the population not affected by this disease, these abnormalities may serve as markers or diagnostic features similar to the way jaw cysts serve as diagnostic features in the multiple nevoid basal cell carcinoma syndrome [10].

A dental abnormality not very common in the normal population is the fusion of roots of the maxillary and/or mandibular first and second molars. This feature is present in seven of the eight patients described here. Cases 5 and 6 are sisters. Both showed signs of the disease at an early age, and both have unusually long and fused roots of the maxillary and mandibular molars. Case 6 also had an impacted cuspid and mandibular second premolar. Case 7 is a young man with a strong family history of the disease. He had an abdominal colectomy and ileoproctostomy at age 11 years. The patient has osteomas in the maxilla and in the mandible as well as fused roots of the maxillary left second molar and the mandibular molars.

The seven patients described here were selected from a group of 22 with established diagnoses of FAP and/or strong family history of the disease. A summary of the dental abnormalities and bone lesions in these patients is presented in Table 1.

With the exception of one patient, who was totally edentulous, all had several dental and/or bone abnormalities. Seventeen had one or more osteomas, 12 had one or more impacted teeth, and 18 had evidence of abnormal root formation, in most cases fused mesial and distal roots of molars. Since a definite history of dental extractions could not be established in many of these patients, the tabulation of missing teeth is somewhat uncertain.

Considering the number and frequency of dental abnormalities and bone lesions in FAP patients, these are definitely features that should be considered as having diagnostic value. These abnormalities appear early in life and often before the intestinal lesions become a problem. In patients with a familial history of adenomatous polyps, they may well serve as warning signs of future active diseases.

SUMMARY

Dental abnormalities and bone lesions of the maxilla and mandible are present in more than

TABLE 1.
Summary of the Dental Abnormalities and Bone Lesions as seen in Panoramic Radiographs of 22 FAP Patients

Case No.	Sex	Age (years)	Osteomas	Missing teeth	Impacted teeth	Abnormal root formation of teeth
1	M	28	11	?	0	3
2	F	1	1	?	4	8
3	F	17	1	3	4	8
4	F	16	1	8	2	6
5	M	9	1	3	6	?
6	M	44	2+	?	2	2
7	F	39	10+	?	4	1
8	M	57	2	?	0	2
9	M	19	0	0	4	2
10	M	17	0	0	4	2
11	M	33	5+	?	0	0
12	M	40	1	?	1	2
13	F	16	1	0	5	4
14	M	18	2	2	4	4
15	M	39	0	?	0	7
16	M	33	0	3	0	8
17	F	44	2	?	0	?
18	F	23	1	?	0	3
19	M	35	5+	?	0	2
20	M	25	1	?	1	1
21	M	74	6+	?	0	1
22	F	44	0	?	0	0

80% of patients with FAP. The dental abnormalities include impacted teeth (other than third molars), supernumerary teeth, congenitally missing teeth, fused roots of first and second molars, and unusually long and tapered roots of posterior teeth. The bone lesions consist mostly of osteomas, either isolated or in clusters, in the maxilla and mandible. Since dental abnormalities and bone lesions are present early in life, these features might possibly be used for selective screening and for early recognition of FAP.

References

1. Gardner EJ, Richard RC: Multiple cutaneous and subcutaneous lesions occurring simultaneously with hereditary polyposis and osteomatosis. Am J Hum Genet 5:139–147, 1953.
2. Sanchez MA, Zali MR, Khalil AA, Ponce R, Font RG: Be aware of Gardner's syndrome. Am J Gastroenterol 71:68–73, 1979.
3. Ida M, Nakamura T, Utsunomiya J: Osteomatous changes and tooth abnormalities found in the jaws of patients with adenomatosis coli. Oral Surg 52:2–11, 1981.
4. Carl W, Herrera L: Dental and bone abnormalities in patients with familial polyposis coli. Semin Surg Oncol 3:77–83, 1987.
5. Sondergaard JO, Buelow S, Jarvinen H, Wolf J, Witt IN, Tetens G: Dental anomalies in familial adenomatous polyposis coli. Acta Odontol Scand 45:61–63, 1987.
6. Schiffman MA: Familial Multiple Polyposis associated with soft tissue and hard tissue tumors. J Am Med Assoc 179:514–522, 1962.
7. Carr LY, Cohen BA, Goodman JD, Heimann IM, Mendelson DJ: Gardner's syndrome and mesenteric desmoids. Am J Gastroenterol 80:310–312, 1985.
8. Pindborg JJ: "Oral manifestations of systemic disease," Jones JH, Mason DK (eds). Philadelphia: W.B. Saunders Co., 1980, p 47.
9. Utsunomiya J, Nakamura T: The occult osteomatous changes in the mandible in patients with familial polyposis coli. Br J Surg 62:45–51, 1975.
10. Helm F: Multiple nevoid basal cell carcinoma syndrome. In Carl W, Sako K (eds): "Cancer and the Oral Cavity." Chicago: Quintessence Publishing Co., Inc., 1986, pp 69–74.

15

Anthropometric Measurements in Mexican Kindreds With Familial Adenomatous Polyposis

Rafael Padilla-Longoria, E. Cardenas-Gonzalez, Ernestina Peña, Sergio Torres, Sergio Rodriguez-Cuevas, and Lemuel Herrera

Hospital de Oncologia, Centro Medico Nacional IMSS, and Escuela de Antropolgia e Historia, Mexico City, Mexico (R.P.-L., E.C.-G., E.P., S.T., S.R.-C.) and the Familial Polyposis Registry, Division of Surgical Oncology, Roswell Park Memorial Institute, Buffalo, New York (L.H.)

INTRODUCTION

Familial adenomatous polyposis (FAP) is an inherited premalignant disease characterized by the development of gastrointestinal polyps. It is often associated with an array of growth and bone abnormalities. The objective of this study was to obtain anthropometric measures in patients with known FAP and their relatives at risk and to compare them with the "normal," nonaffected population. In this chapter, we present the results of our studies.

PATIENTS, MATERIALS, AND METHODS

We studied 57 subjects who belong to three kindreds documented to have FAP. The list of the anthropometric measurements to be obtained is presented in Figure 1. For purpose of this study, we excluded patients older than 60 years and younger and 20 years of age because of the bone changes normally occurring during these decades. Thus only 31 patients were used for this analysis. They were stratified into the following groups: affected females, ten; affected males, eight; nonaffected females, seven; nonaffected males, six. Four of the affected females had mandibular osteomas and four did not. Only one of the affected males had mandibular osteomas and nine did not. None of the non-affected had maxillar or mandibular osteomas. Controls were selected from a group of patients who had undergone endoscopic examination of the gastrointestinal tract for a variety of symptoms and who were found to be free of polyps. The following are some of the definitions of cephalometric landmarks, used in this study.

Glabella: the smooth area of the frontal bone between the superciliary arches

Opisthion: the midpoint of the lower border of the foramen magnum

Euryon: the point at either end of the greatest transverse diameter of the skull

Gonion: the most inferior posterior and lateral point on the external angle of the mandible

Nasion: the point at which a horizontal line tangential to the highest point on the superior palpebral sulci is intersected by the midsagital plane

Stomiom: pertaining to the mouth

Acromium: lateral extension of the spine of the scapula.

RESULTS

The results obtained are presented in Tables 1–4. They include cranial and extracraneal measurements. The relationship of the results of affected and nonaffected individuals vs. the

Familial Adenomatous Polyposis, pages 121–124

ANTHROPOMETRIC DATA

NAME ______________________________ AGE ________ CHART NO. ______________

DATE OF BIRTH ____________ D/M/Y ______ PLACE ______________

CRANIOFACIAL DATA

1. Cephalic circumference ______ mm
2. Length (glabelle-opisthion) ______ mm
3. Width (euryon) ______ mm
4. Bizygomatic Diameter ______ mm
5. Bigonion Diameter ______ mm
6. Bipalpebral Diameter (Internal) ______ mm
7. Bipalpebral Diameter (External) ______ mm
8. Height (nasion-menton) ______ mm
9. Upper Facial Height (nasion-stomion) ______ mm

EXTRACRANIAL MEASUREMENTS

10. Height (standing-up) ______ mm
11. Height (sitting-down) ______ mm
12. Height (pubic symphysis-floor) ______ mm
13. Height (tibial tuberosity-floor) ______ mm
14. Height (pubic symphysis-tibial tuberosity) ______ mm
15. Height (internal maleolli) ______ mm
16. Height (tibial tuberosity-internal maleolli) ______ mm
17. Foot Length ______ mm
18. Upper extremity length (acromium-Dactylium) ______ mm
19. Arm Length ______ mm
20. Forearm Length ______ mm
21. Hand Length ______ mm
22. Biacromial Diameter ______ mm
23. Biileocrestal Diameter ______ mm

Fig. 1. List of anthropometric measurements to be obtained for FAP Kindreds.

TABLE 1.
Average Craniofacial Parameters Among the Affected Patients

	Female (mm)	Male
Cephalic circumference	547 ±0.42	583.8 ±1.25
Bizygomatic diameter	133.3 ±0.59	129.3 ±0.3
Bigoniac diameter	100.25±0.42	106.10±0.01
Upper face height	69.3 ±0.3	73.10±1.0
Height	109.62±0.1	122.50±0.03

TABLE 2.
Average Extracranial Parameters for the Non-affected Controls

	Female (mm)	Male (mm)
Height	1,530.0	1,643.5
Height sitting down	821.85	854.66
Height from symphysis	776.14	849.83
Biacromial diameter	336.57	366.3
Bicrestal diameter	266.85	268.6
Upper segment		

TABLE 3.
Average Extracranial Parameters Among the Affected Patients

	Female (mm)	Male (mm)
Height	1,517.8 ±0.2	1,682.8±0.1
Height sitting down	803.0 ±0.4	873.0
Height from symphisis	776.4 ±0.03	879.1
Biacromial diameter	352.14±1.60	383.1
Bicrestal diameter	294.85±2.46	281.5
Upper segment	741.42	803.7
Lower segment	51.0 ±0.87	52.1
Ratio upper segment/lower segment	96.1 ±0.8	91.67
Cormic index	52.8 ±0.06	52.0
Index	83.5 ±3.3	73.4

TABLE 4.
Average Craniofacial Parameters Among the Non-affected Controls

	Female (mm)	Male (mm)
Cephalic circumference	543.57	567.83
Bizygomatic diameter	128.57	138.00
Bigoniac diameter	95	106.8
Upper face height	67.42	74.3
Height	108.57	118

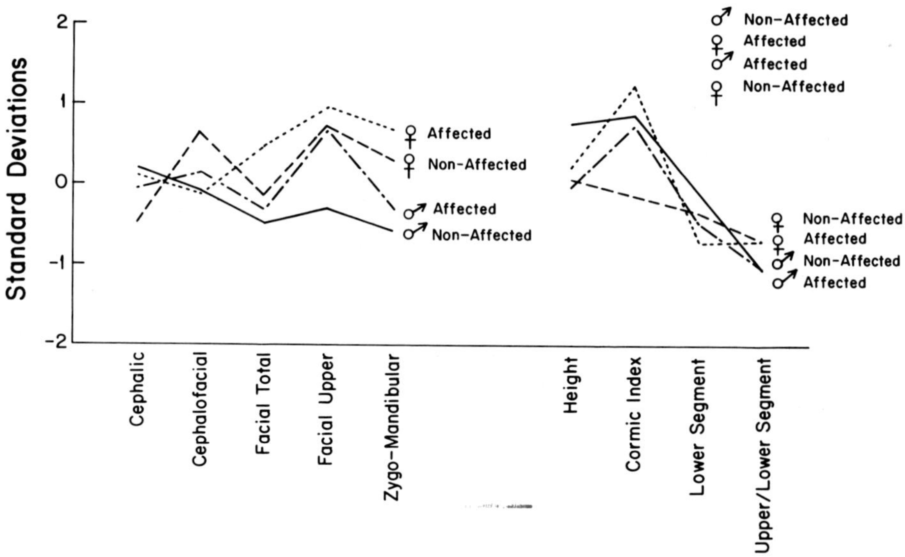

Fig. 2. Anthropometric measurements of affected patients and nonaffected controls.

nonaffected population control is depicted in Figure 2.

Of interest is that four of the affected females and one male had osteomas detectable by Panorex. None of the nonaffected controls had osteomas.

DISCUSSION

FAP is a generalized proliferative disorder of growth. Although the predominant manifestations occur in the gastointestinal tract, bone and retinal abnormalities occur often in affected patients. In fact, since they might precede the appearance of the gastrointestinal symptoms, we hypothesized that they could serve as an early clinical marker in these kindreds.

Our investigation demonstrated that affected females have an upper facial height that is over 1 SD higher than in the control population. Although affected males also had an elevated upper facial index, it did not reach 1 SD. Similarly, we found that the cormic index in affected females was 1 SD standard above that of the controls; in males this was much less pronounced. The ratios upper segment/lower segment were found to be below those of the normal population. In part, this helps to explain the findings of normal growth in the upper segment over the inferior segment.

We found significant differences when comparing the affected individuals to the normal population. However, these differences did not distinguish between the affected and nonaffected within the same kindreds consistently. Thus it is possible that these measurements may represent individual variations of the FAP kindred. They may also be a reflection of the small number of patients and kindreds. Nevertheless, we believe that these physical measures should be included as baseline evaluation of FAP patients, along with others, such as measurements of the width and thickness of the incisor teeth by a special periapical radiologic technique. These measurements are easy to perform, and reproducible, entail minimal cost and effort, and may disclose significant anthropometric parameters of significance in selected and stratified ethnic populations.

16

Ophthalmologic Abnormalities in Patients With Familial Adenomatous Polyposis

Elias I. Traboulsi and Irene H. Maumenee

The Center for Sight, Georgetown University Medical Center, Washington, DC (E.I.T.); The Wilmer Ophthalmologic Institute, The Johns Hopkins Hospitals, Baltimore, Maryland (I.H.M.)

INTRODUCTION

The consistent presence of an ocular abnormality in patients with familial adenomatous polyposis (FAP) was first recognized by Blair and Trempe in a family with Gardner's syndrome in 1980 [1]; these authors observed multiple patches of congenital hypertrophy of the retinal pigment epithelium (CHRPE) in the ocular fundi of three of four patients with Gardner's syndrome. Since their report, several series [2–6] have confirmed the association between CHRPE and Gardner's syndrome and have established multiple patches of CHRPE as reliable clinical markers of the disease.

CHRPE

CHRPE in the normal population is an isolated, dark (light brown to jet black), smooth, sharply demarcated, oval to round lesion located at the level of the retinal pigment epithelium; the lesion is almost always surrounded by a white halo of depigmentation. With time, in some cases, punched-out areas of depigmentation develop in the center of the lesion and coalesce in a cauliflower-like fashion. The size of these lesions varies from 100 μm to 5 mm. They are typically located in the retinal periphery but may occur around the optic nerve head. Histopathologically, retinal pigment epithelial cells are enlarged and contain large round pigment granules instead of the normal football-shaped melanin granules. Overlying retinal photoreceptors are variably to totally degenerated, leading to associated scotomata [7,8]. CHRPE is presumed to be present at birth, and lesions are generally constant in size, although mild enlargement in diameter has been documented in very few cases.

In patients with Gardner's syndrome, the CHRPE lesions are variable in number, size, and configuration. The pigmented lesions are flat, usually well circumscribed, light brown to jet black, with variable degrees of depigmentation in their centers, and often are surrounded by a white, depigmented halo. The lesions are located at the level of the retinal pigment epithelium and take a variety of configurations, as shown in Figures 1–4. Larger lesions may be accompanied by small satellite lesions, and the area of the fundus adjacent to larger lesions may show some disturbance of the retinal pigment epithelium. The pigmented lesions may be as small as one one-twentieth of a disc diameter (0.075 mm) in size, or as large as three disc diameters (4.5 mm). Larger lesions tend to be located closer to the posterior pole area, whereas small lesions occur most frequently in the equatorial region near the vortex veins. In two of our patients, the lesions involved the macular area and led to mild decrease in visual acuity [3]. No histopathologic studies of CHRPE in Gardner's syndrome have yet been performed, but these lesions are presumably identical to other forms of CHRPE [7,8]. In a case-controlled study, Traboulsi et al. [3] showed that none of 42 controls vs. 26 (63%) of

Familial Adenomatous Polyposis, pages 125–131

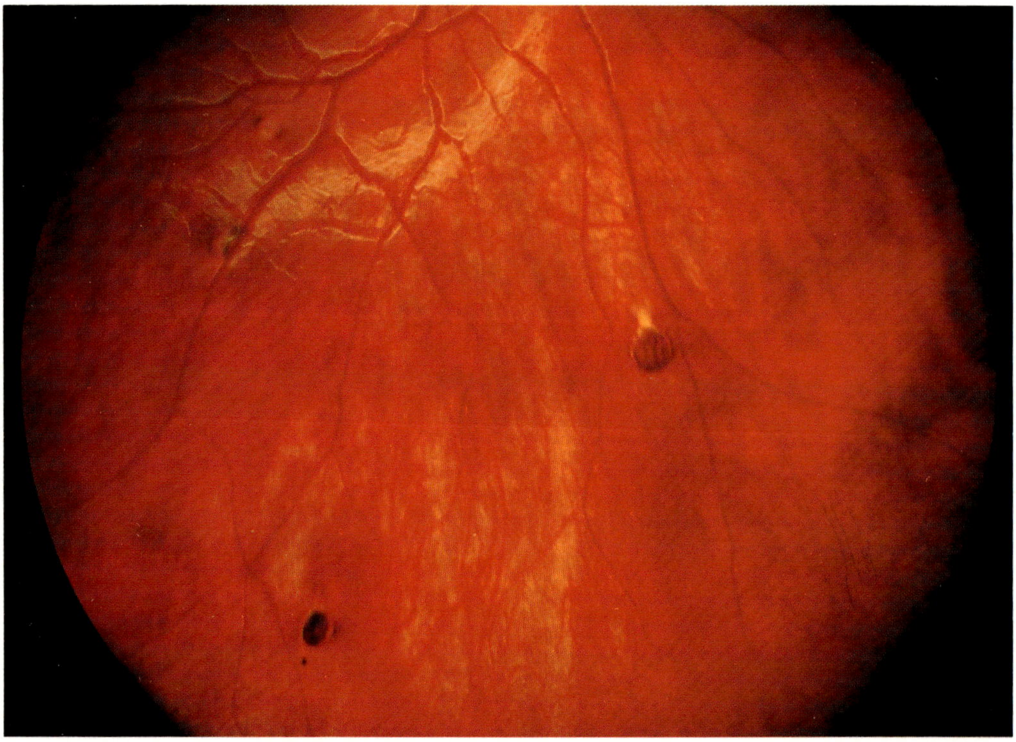

Fig. 1. Four patches of CHRPE of different configurations in the fundus of a 7-year-old girl at risk for Gardner's syndrome. Note two smaller lesions at upper left. (Reprinted by permission of The New England Journal of Medicine 316:661–667, 1987.)

41 patients with Gardner's syndrome had more than a total of four patches of CHRPE; one patient had a total of 38 lesions in both eyes. In a subsequent study, the same group of investigators [6] defined positivity for the ocular trait as a total of three or more patches of CHRPE in one or both eyes. Traboulsi et al. [3] observed the pigmented lesions in a 3-month-old female at risk for Gardner's syndrome; these authors also analyzed the number of lesions as a function of age in patients with Gardner's syndrome and failed to find evidence that lesions increased in number with age.

SIGNIFICANCE OF CHRPE IN GARDNER'S SYNDROME AND FAMILIAL ADENOMATOUS POLYPOSIS

Following the original observations by Blair and Trempe [1], Lewis and coworkers [2], in a study of six families with Gardner's syndrome, found multiple and bilateral patches of CHRPE in affected individuals and in one-half of those at 50% risk for Gardner's syndrome in three of the six families; these authors proposed that multiple bilateral patches of CHRPE may be useful to identify early in life individuals at risk for Gardner's syndrome; they also suggested that Gardner's syndrome may be genetically heterogeneous, with some families showing the ocular trait and others not. Traboulsi et al. [3], in a study of 134 individuals from 16 families with Gardner's syndrome, found the marker ocular lesions in at least one member of all 16 families and suggested not labeling any family as negative for the ocular trait before examining an adequate number of patients and individuals at risk.

In a brief communication published in the Lancet in 1987 [9], Lynch and coworkers reported

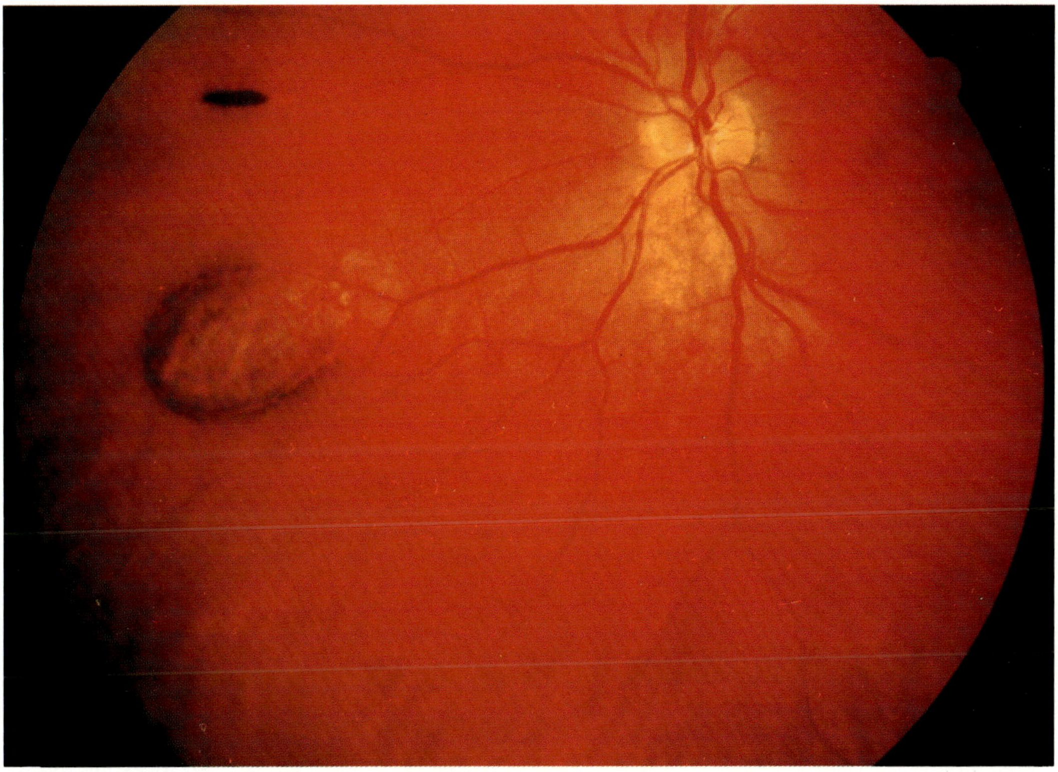

Fig. 2. One large, oval, light brown, mostly depigmented lesion accompanied by a smaller, fusiform, black lesion in the eye of a patient with Gardner's syndrome. (Reprinted by permission of The New England Journal of Medicine 316:661–667, 1987.)

the presence of CHRPE in four members of two families with FAP (adenomatous polyposis without extracolonic manifestations, excluding multiple patches of CHRPE). In another study, Traboulsi et al. [6]—defining FAP families as those among whom patients with adenomatous polyposis had no extracolonic lesions, and Gardner's syndrome families as those among whom at least one affected individual had one or more extracolonic manifestations of the disease—found no CHRPE in five affected members and five individuals at a 50% risk from three families with FAP; these authors also found multiple patches of CHRPE in at least one member of 23 families with Gardner's syndrome and in a total of 70 (86.4%) of 81 patients with Gardner's syndrome.

Because as many as 20% of patients with Gardner's syndrome can be negative for the ocular trait, the absence of the ocular lesions should not be taken as contraindicating a diagnosis of Gardner's syndrome. The presence in significant numbers (three or more, or even two or more) in individuals at risk for Gardner's syndrome should be taken as evidence for inheritance of the abnormal gene, and such individuals should be followed thoroughly for the development of adenomatous polyposis or other extracolonic signs of Gardner's syndrome. We recommend a dilated fundus examination early in life to look for patches of CHRPE. If the examination is unsatisfactory, it should be repeated until the examiner is confident about the results.

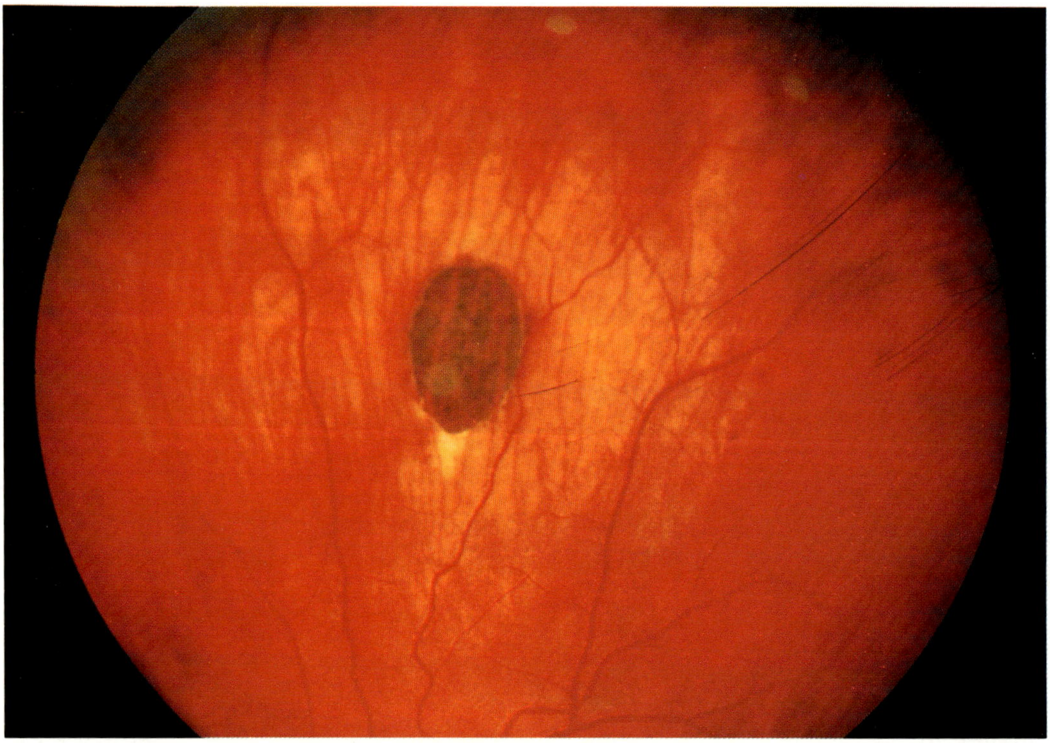

Fig. 3. Single, moderately large, light brown lesion with thin, depigmented, surrounding halo and patch of depigmentation at its tip in the fundus of another patient with Gardner's syndrome. (Reprinted by permission of The New England Journal of Medicine 316:661–667, 1987.)

OTHER OPHTHALMOLOGIC ABNORMALITIES IN GARDNER'S SYNDROME

Orbital osteomas have been reported in a few patients with Gardner's syndrome [10–13]. Orbital osteomas make up less than 2.5% of all orbital mass lesions in adults and most often originate from the bones lining the paranasal sinuses (Fig. 5). Orbital osteomas may lead to orbital or paranasal sinus pain, proptosis, optic nerve head swelling, and extraocular motility deficits with diplopia. Proptosis has been reported to be the initial sign of Gardner's syndrome in one instance [12]. Surgical removal of symptomatic orbital osteomas is indicated, and the surgical approach depends on the location of the tumor [13]. Epidermal cysts of the skin of the eyelid may occur in patients with Gardner's syndrome [14] (also, personal observations) and may result in ptosis. Surgical excision of the cyst may be warranted in selected cases.

OPHTHALMOGIC ABNORMALITIES IN OTHER POLYPOSIS SYNDROMES

Ophthalmologic abnormalities are present in only one other type of familial polyposis: the

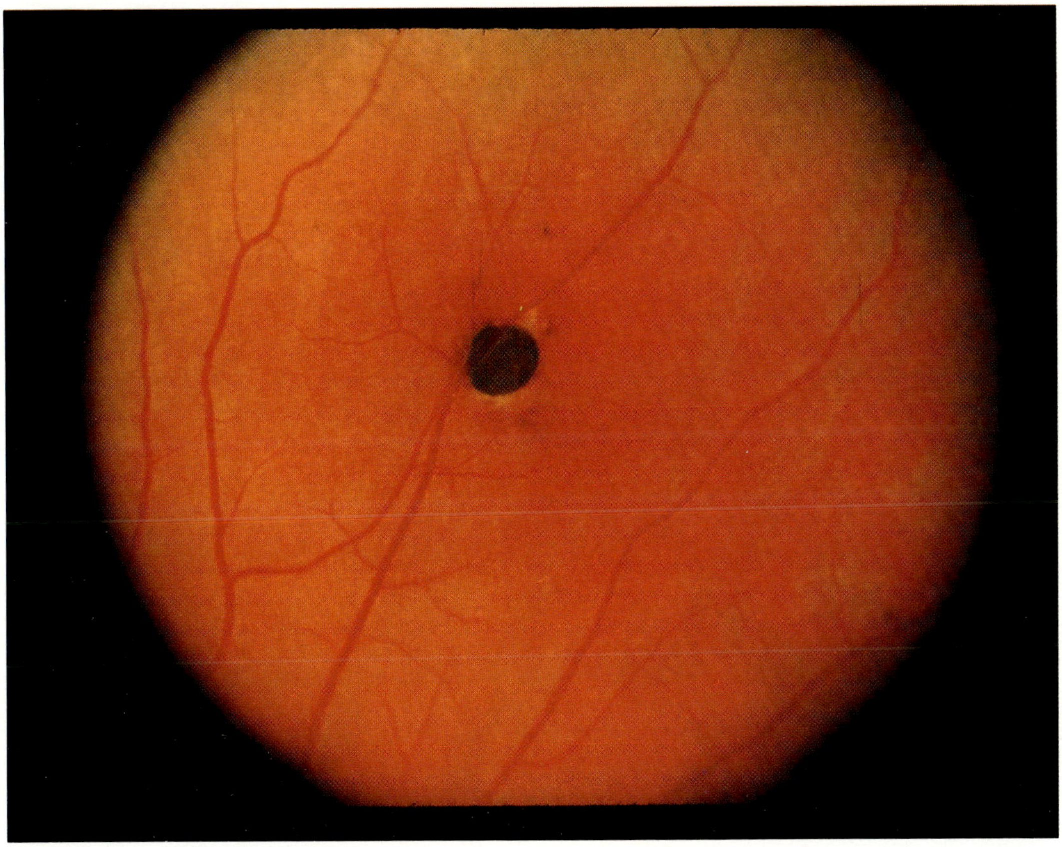

Fig. 4. One-millimeter, black lesion with a few small, satellite lesions in the fundus of another patient with Gardner's syndrome. Note retinal blood vessel coursing over the lesion, indicating its subretinal location at level of the retinal pigment epithelium. (Reprinted by permission of The New England Journal of Medicine 316:661–667, 1987.)

Peutz-Jeghers syndrome (hamartomatous intestinal polyposis and pigmentation of skin and mucous membranes). Melanocytic lesions are present on the eyelids (Fig. 6) and conjunctiva of affected individuals [15]. Patches of CHRPE were not present in nine affected members of three families with the Peutz-Jeghers syndrome examined by Traboulsi et al. [6]. No ophthalmologic abnormalities were present in six affected individuals or in 21 of their first-degree relatives in four families with hereditary nonpolyposis colorectal cancer, excluding the use of the pigmented fundus lesions as markers in this condition [6].

ACKNOWLEDGMENTS

This study was supported by a grant from the Clayton Foundation to E.I.T.

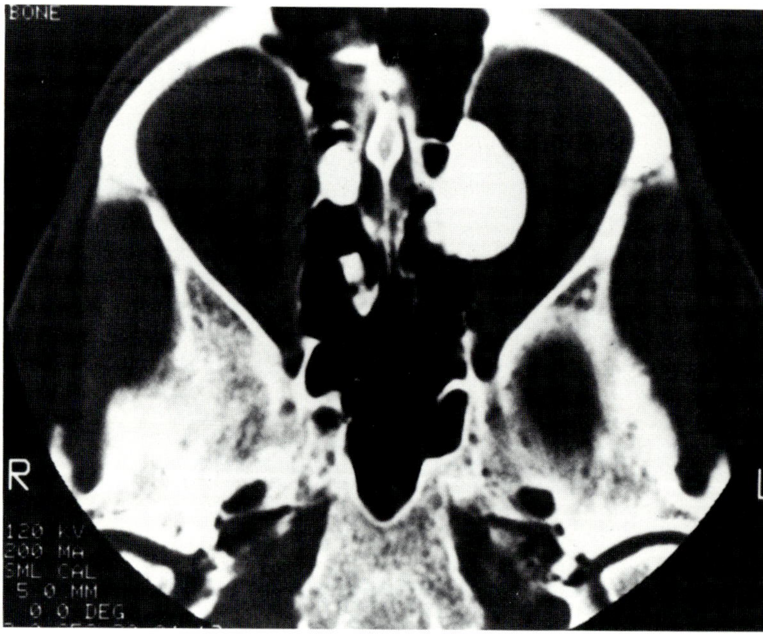

Fig. 5. Orbital osteoma in a 30-year-old woman with Gardner's syndrome. Axial computed tomographic scan cut of the orbits, showing a large, bone-density mass in the left orbit originating from the medial orbital wall. Several small osteomas are present in the ethmoid air cells. (Published with permission from The American Journal of Ophthalmology 101:236– 241, 1986. Copyright by The Ophthalmic Publishing Company.)

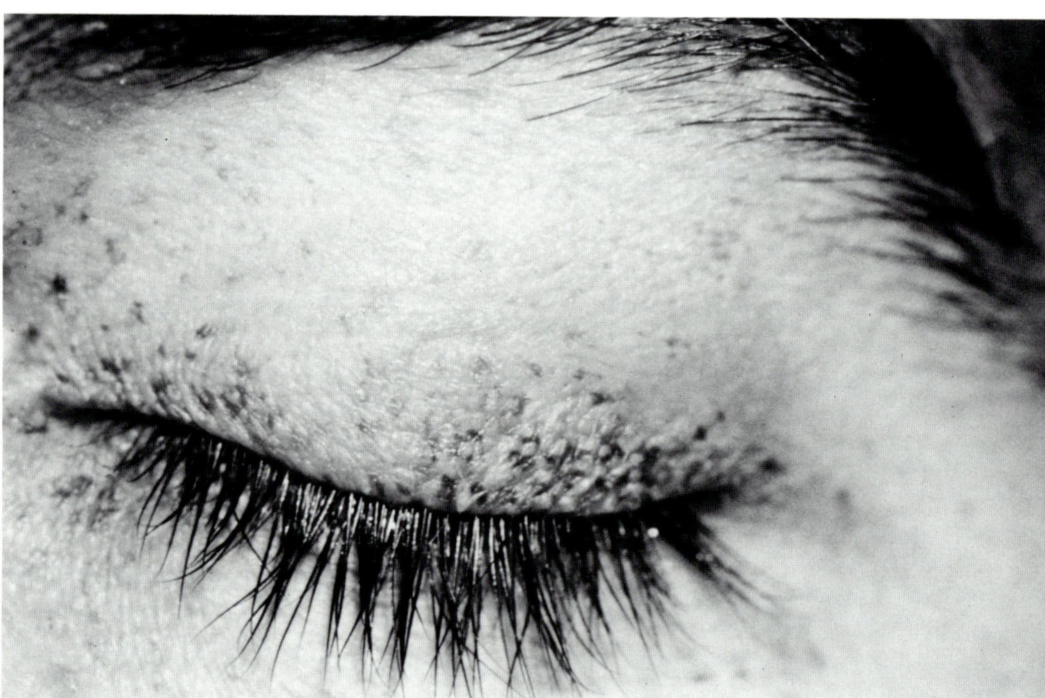

Fig. 6. Cutaneous pigmentation near lid margins in a patient with the Peutz-Jeghers syndrome.

References

1. Blair NP, Trempe CL: Hypertrophy of the retinal pigment epithelium associated with Gardner's syndrome. Am J Ophthalmol 90:661–667, 1980.

2. Lewis RA, Crowder WE, Eierman LA, et al.: The Gardner syndrome. Significance of ocular features. Ophthalmology 91:916–925, 1984.

3. Traboulsi EI, Krush AJ, Gardner EJ, et al.: Prevalence and importance of pigmented ocular fundus lesions in Gardner's syndrome. N Engl J Med 316:661–667, 1987.

4. Diaz Llopis M, Menezo JL: Congenital hypertrophy of the retinal pigment epithelium and familial polyposis of the colon. Am J Ophthalmol 103:235–236, 1987.

5. Berk T, Cohen Z, McLeod RS, Parker JA: Congenital hypertrophy of the retinal pigment epithelium as a marker for familial adenomatous polyposis. Dis Col Rectum 31:253–257, 1988.

6. Traboulsi EI, Maumenee IH, Krush AJ, et al.: Pigmented ocular fundus lesions in the inherited gastrointestinal polyposis syndromes and in hereditary nonpolyposis colon cancer. Ophthalmology 95:964–969, 1988.

7. Kurz GH, Zimmerman LE: Vagaries of the retinal pigment epithelium. Int Ophthalmol Clin 2:441–464, 1962.

8. Buettner H: Congenital hypertrophy of the retinal pigment epithelium. Am J Ophthalmol 79:177–189, 1975.

9. Lynch H, Priluck I, Fritzsimmons ML: Congenital hypertrophy of the retinal pigment epithelium in familial polyposis coli. Lancet 2:333, 1987.

10. Jones EL, Cornell WP: Gardner's syndrome. Review of the literature and report on a family. Arch Surg 92:287, 1966.

11. Bregeat P, Hamard H: Une exophtalmie par osteome. Arch Ophtalmol 28:247, 1968.

12. Jain MR, Mogra HS: Gardner's syndrome presenting as unilateral proptosis. Indian J Ophthalmol 29:55, 1981.

13. Whitson WE, Orcutt JC, Walkinshaw MD: Orbital osteoma in Gardner's syndrome. Am J Ophthalmol 101:236– 241, 1986.

14. Gardner EJ, Richards RC: Multiple cutaneous and subcutaneous lesions occurring simultaneously with hereditary polyposis and osteomatosis. Am J Hum Genet 5:139, 1953.

15. Traboulsi EI, Maumenee IH: Periocular pigmentation in Peutz-Jeghers syndrome. Am J Ophthalmol 102:126–127, 1986.

17

Current Treatment of Desmoids in Familial Adenomatous Polyposis Patients

Raul Ramos, Aaron Carrel, and Lemuel Herrera

Department of Surgery, University of Texas Health Sciences Center at San Antonio (R.R.), State University of New York at Buffalo, School of Medicine (A.C.), Department of Surgery, State University of New York at Buffalo and Familial Polyposis Registry, Department of Surgical Oncology, Roswell Park Memorial Institute, Buffalo, New York (L.H.)

DEFINITION

The term desmoid is derived from Greek and means band-like appearance. Desmoid tumors are nonmetastatic, fibrous tumors of slow growth. Nonencapsulated, they seem to arise from musculoaponeurotic tissues. They proliferate by local invasion and may produce intractable obstruction from pressure in adjacent structures. The first description of these tumors was in 1832 by John Macfarlane of Glasgow, however, it was Muller who introduced the term in 1838 [1]. In 1923, Nichols reported the association of desmoids and gastrointestinal polyposis, however, the significance of the hereditary trait, was apparent only after the publication of a classical paper by Gardner in 1953 [2].

INCIDENCE

It is difficult to determine the true incidence of desmoids. The incidence varies with the population under study, also the referral center bias needs to be taken into consideration to assess the validity of the sample. In the general population, the incidence is about 3.5% of all fibrous tumors, or 0.03% of all neoplasms; however, in familial adenomatous polyposis (FAP) the incidence varies from 6% to 13%. For instance, among the 111 patients reported by Sener, 21 had desmoid tumors (13 intraabdominal, 6 abdominal wall, 2 extraabdominal). There also appears to be some clustering of these tumors within selected FAP families (kindreds) [3,4]. Often, reported series do not distinguish between desmoids associated with FAP and those who are not—"sporadic" type—allowing for some confusion.

PATHOLOGY

Grossly, desmoids have a hard rubbery consistency. Their surface is glistening white. They are hard to cut. In large tumors, areas of cystic degeneration can be found in the center. Tumors may cross fascial planes infiltrating the surrounding muscle and bone, but not the skin; occasionally they infiltrate the wall of the bowel, but they seldom perforate it. Histologically, they consist of bundles of spindle cells with various amounts of collagen. Formation of sarcolemmic gigantic cells is very characteristic, although not exclusive. The center of the tumor is usually acellular, but in the periphery the cellularity is so rich that it may resemble a low-grade fibrosarcoma. No true capsule is identified. A lymphocytic infiltrate is often seen at the tumor margins. The presence of normal mitosis and the fact that they never metastasize distinguishes desmoids from fibrosarcomas.

Herrera et al. [5] used slide cytometric analysis and cytophotometric analysis to identify the degree of ploidy in desmoid tumors of patients with and without FAP. Results demonstrated that there were no differences in the ploidy value of

Familial Adenomatous Polyposis, pages 133–146

desmoids associated or not to FAP. Ploidy number was not useful for predicting the aggressiveness of clinical behavior.

Occasionally, desmoids undergo mucoid or cystic degeneration. Then, they increase in size by fluid sequestration, or by hemorrhage into the substance of the tumor. These changes may also produce pain. Another eventuality is that the cystic degeneration is secondarily infected and the patient may develop fever and tenderness characteristic of an abscess (Fig. 1). At surgery, with or without associated inflammation, it is often difficult to define clearly the limits of the tumor.

Most desmoids associated with FAP are located in the abdomen, retroperitoneum, and mesenterium of the bowel. Only occasionally, they occur in other anatomical locations such as the neck, extremities, and thoracic and pelvic girdle. This is just the opposite to ''sporadic'' desmoids and it is well exemplified in the population from Roswell Park Memorial Institute (Tables 1 and 2). Successful surgical treatment of desmoids is related to the ''sporadic'' type and not to the desmoid associated with FAP. However, these findings may be a reflection of our previous vigorous surgical approach and autopsy frequency. Fibromatosis, in general, are categorized according to their anatomic distribution. Mesenteric fibromatosis defines a type of desmoid that infiltrates the mesenterium as a single tumor sheet or multiple whitish ''plaque-like'' lesions. This is often associated with unresectability and is seen more frequently in our FAP than in those patients without FAP.

CLINICAL PICTURE

Because of the usual slow growth of the desmoid, symptoms are few or nonexistent. At times, these tumors can reach a very large size before noticed by the patient and the physician. The tumor may grow intraabdominally or retroperitoneal producing intestinal obstruction or ureteral obstruction. This may lead to cachexia, hydronephrosis, and ultimate death by mechanical

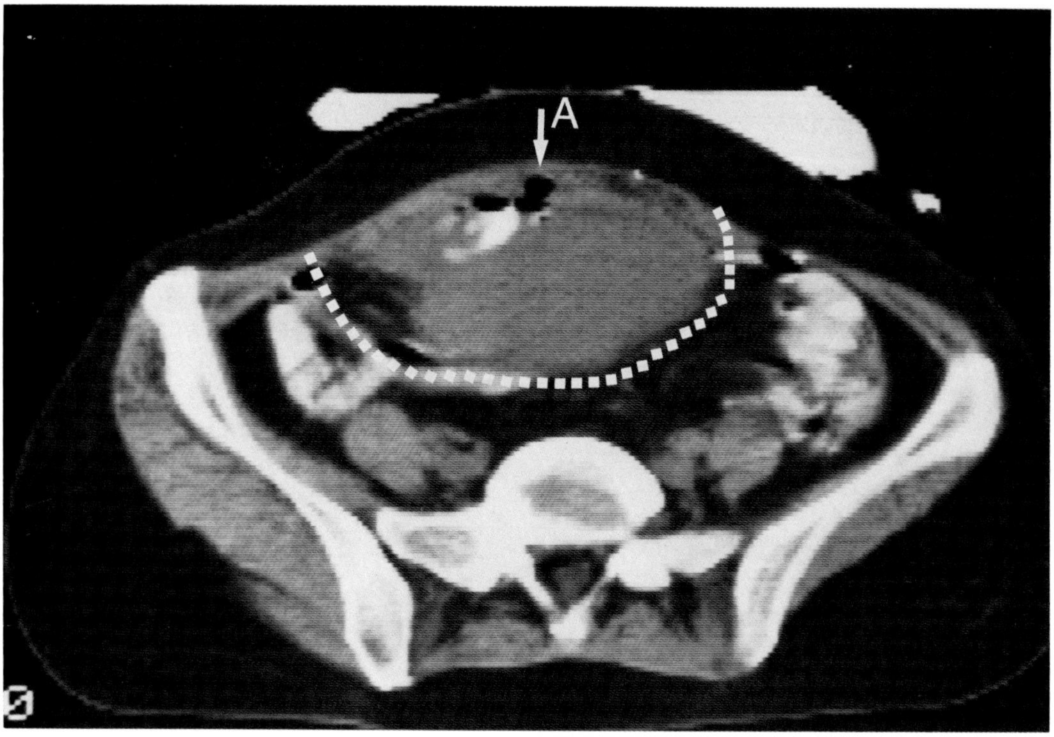

Fig. 1. Cystic degeneration of a desmoid, secondarily infected in presenting as an abscess. (A)

TABLE 1.
Desmoids Associated With FAP

Patient	Date of birth	Sex/race	Date of diagnosis of FAP	Assn to cancer	Surgical TX/Date	Desmoid: Date of diagnosis	Desmoid: Location	Desmoid: Treatment and dates	Outcome	Comment
CL	2/68	F W	7/76	No	STC/IP 8/76	2/80	Mesentery of small bowel	Incomplete surgical removal 2/80	Progression	
								Testolactone 7/80–7/82	Development of epigastric tumor	
								Removal of egigastric tumor 11/83		
								On Tamoxifen since 1/84	Alive with disease	
LE	3/61	F W	10/74	No	STC/IP 8/76	8/81	Retroperit	Unresectable at surgery 9/81		Mandibular osteoma before G.I. polyps
								Testolactone × 12 mos, progesterone × 12 mos.	Progression	
									Died of urosepsis and Hydroureter secondary to desmoid compression, 8/84	Autopsy-yes
LM	10/41	M W	7/79	Yes Colon (1) Rectum (1)	TPC 5/80	4/84	Retroperit	Refused	Died of cachexia secondary to desmoid compression	5 q deletion Autopsy-yes

(continued)

TABLE 1.
Desmoids Associated With FAP (continued)

						Desmoid				
Patient	Date of birth	Sex/race	Date of diagnosis of FAP	Assn to cancer	Surgical TX/Date	Date of diagnosis	Location	Treatment and dates	Outcome	Comment
PF	8/51	F W	10/74	No	STC/IP 1/78	2/79	Retroperit	Surgery, incomplete removal 3/79		Lost to FU 1984
								Adriamycin Vincristine × 12 mos.	Stable disease	Villous adenoma in rectal remnant
JM	8/28	F W	8/79	No	STC/IP 10/79	1975	R Groin	Incomplete excision 9/83		Short bowel syndrome Home TPN
						1981	Mesentery of small bowel	On Tamoxifen and Testolactone × 12 mos.	Stable disease	
PY	10/55	M W	1/72	No	STC/IP 3/72	7/79	Mesentery of small bowel	Incomplete resection		
						7/86	Mesenteric progression	Testolactone Indomethacin	Progression	
						4/87	Retroperit	Small bowel resection & ileostomy	Attempted resection	Short bowel syndrome, Home TPN
								External radiation (PR)	Stable disease	

CB	2/55	F	W	1/60	No	TPC/ Illeostomy 7/67	7/69	Abdominal wall	Resected	Recurred at retroperit	
							7/73	Retroperit	None	Lost to FU, 1974	
AL	10/30	M	W	7/67	No	TPC/ Ileostomy 9/67	8/73	Mesentery small bowel and Retro- perit	Unresectable, Vincristine Adriamycin 1973–1977	Died of liver metastases from adeno- carcinoma unknown origin, 1985	No autopsy
TD	10/65	F	W	6/81	No	STC/IP 7/81	8/82	Retroperit	Unresectable Tamoxifen since 3/82	Stable, Alive with disease	
RW	8/58	M	W	6/76	No	STC/IP 6/76	2/78	Abdominal wall	Resected	Polyps in rectal remnant	
								Mesentery small bowel	Resected	On oval calcium	

Abbreviations: STC, subtotal colectomy; IP, Ileoproctostomy; TPC, total protocolectomy; PR, partial response.

TABLE 2.
"Sporadic" Desmoids (Not Associated With FAP)

Patient	Date of birth	Sex	Race	Assn of cancer	Date and type of surgery	Adjuvant treatment	Subsequent treatments			Outcome
1. PF	2/24/60	M	Black	7/84 Possible fibrosarcoma	(3/82) Resection of right inguinal mass	None	(3/85) Exploratory laparotomy, desmoid anterior abdominal wall extension to pelvis			Died 4/20/85 septicemia and renal failure secondary to tumor compression Autopsy-yes
2. JMM	1/15/65	M	White	No	(8/84) Resection of desmoid at neck	External Radiation	—		—	NED
3. JR	2/4/64	M	Hispanic	No	(8/75) Resection of desmoid on back (r. scapula)	External Radiation	(8/76) Recurrence re-exised by partial scapulec-tomy		External radiation treatment started and discontinued —wound breakdown 8/79	Lost to FU on 2/84 NED
4. SH	3/7/36	F	White	No	(11/75) Resection of desmoid-lower chest and abdominal wall	None	(7/76) Re-excision of abdom-inal wall desmoid	(1/78) Abdominal wall re-section	(11/79) Tumor recurrence in wall	Died 7/27/80 No autopsy
5. RT	11/17/40	F	White	No	(11/84) Resection of abdominal wall desmoid	None	(6/85) Wide excision desmoid abdominal wall reconstruction with marlex mesh			Lost to FU on 3/86, NED

6. VR	2/14/31	F	White	No	(3/86) Resection of left infra-clavicular desmoid	External Radiation			Lost to FU on 7/86, NED
7. AW	5/11/36	F	White	No	(11/86) Resection of desmoid from right buttock	None			NED
8. NVM	1956	F	White	No	(3/83) Resection of desmoid from back	None	(3/85) Recurrent desmoid excised from back	(5/87) Re-currence desmoid on back, re-resected	NED

Abbreviations: NED, No evidence of disease; FU, Follow-Up

compression. In at least one of our patients (L.M.), it produced a clinical significant hypoglycemia. However, it is important to emphasize that in some patients desmoids may have a lenient clinical course.

Desmoids may precede to the development of the gastrointestinal polyps, so it is suggested that the gastrointestinal tract is thoroughly examined for polyposis in any patient presenting with "sporadic" abdominal desmoids and who has not already been diagnosed with FAP. It is also important to establish a schedule for periodic and methodic evaluations in these patients.

If an abdominal mass is detected in a patient with FAP, the first diagnostic test to be ordered is a Computerized Tomographic (CT) scan of the abdomen and pelvis. The scan will provide information about the tumor density, its relation to the abdominal wall, mesenterium, retroperitoneal structures, and the presence or absence of intestinal obstruction, hydronephrosis, as well as the number of tumors [6] (Figs. 2,3). An arteriogram may provide valuable information, useful for inoperative decisions as the desmoid is often intimately attached to major vessels (Fig. 4).

Surgical trauma appears to be one of the factors that trigger the growth of desmoid tumors, as a number of desmoids are seen within 1 or 2 years following colectomy for polyps or cancer [7]. Since the slow growth produces few symptoms, it is not unusual that the tumor may be first discovered by the surgeon upon palpation of the adbominal wall or next to a surgical scar.

Hormonal factors have been found associated to desmoid tumor growth, this is especially true in the "sporadic" type. Experimentally, Lipschitz induced desmoids of the abdominal wall in animals by administering high doses of estrogens, whereas Geschikter and Lewis [8] reported high concentrations of gonadotrophic hormones in desmoid tumors. A high incidence of desmoids in females after parturition, and cases of tumor regression after menopause, have been also reported. In addition, Reitamo et al. [2] found

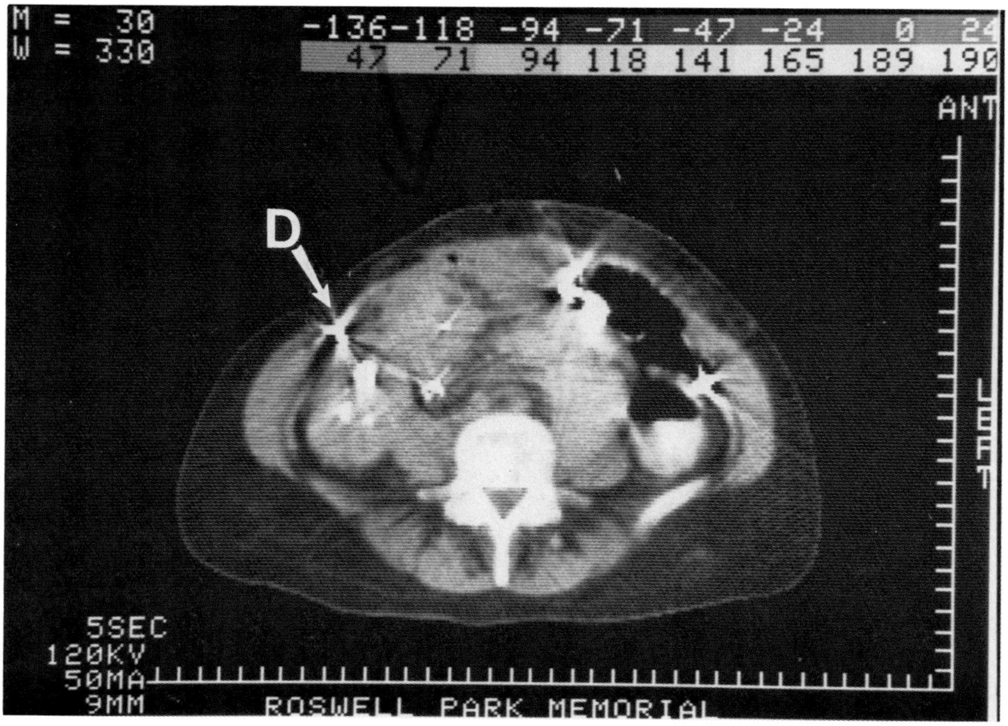

Fig. 2. Desmoid involving the abdominal wall. It begins at the hemoclip at the liver margin and extends towards the midline.

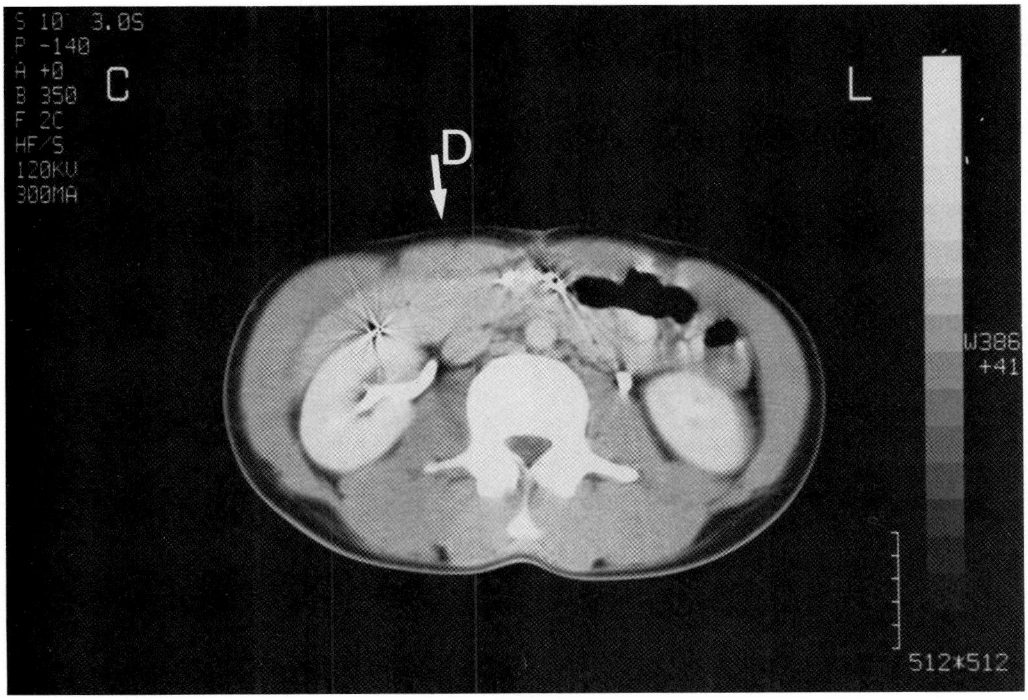

Fig. 3. Desmoid involving the head of the pancreas and the area of the superior mesenteric vessels.

significant levels of estrogen receptors in 33% of the resected desmoid tumors, however, no clear distinction between those desmoids associated or not to FAP, was made. Thus, the possible clinical significance remains inconclusive.

SURGICAL TREATMENT

In general, the recommended treatment for the desmoids is complete resection with a normal margin (1-2 inches) of tissue around it [7]. This particular therapy is more applicable for tumors of the abdominal wall, for small intraabdominal tumors and extraabdominal desmoids a condition more often seen with the "sporadic" type. "Recurrences" of the tumor may be indicative of incomplete resection, a missed desmoid, or a true recurrence. Frozen section and microscopic examination of the margins or resection, may be helpful in deciding amount of tissue to be resected.

"En bloc" resections of the abdominal wall may result in large defects. They may require the use of marlex mesh, gortex fabric, or complicated plastic surgical reconstruction [9,10] for which the patient and the surgeon must be prepared. Even at extensive surgery, one must attempt to preserve the blood supply of the bowel; however, this may not be possible in diffuse mesenteric fibromatosis (Fig. 5). In selected individuals, massive small bowel resection may be necessary for appropriate local control (Fig. 6). "Complete" resections have been taken to the point of creating short bowel cripples requiring parenteral nutrition. Not only is this not associated with preservation of the quality of life, but even after "complete" excisions, the local recurrence

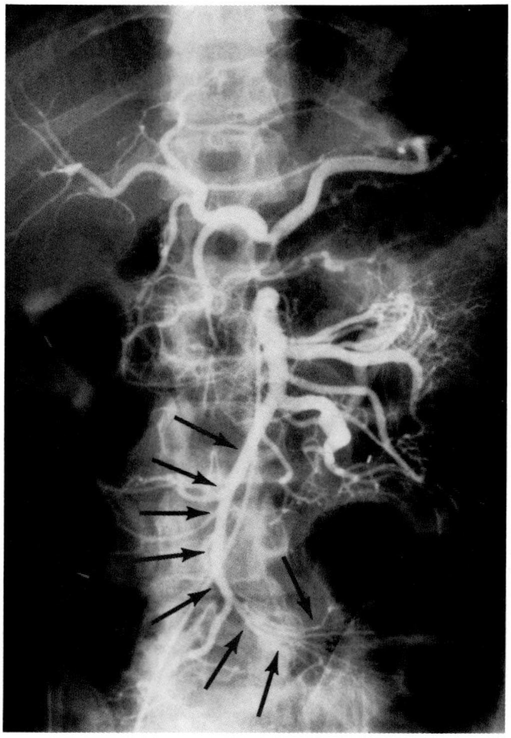

Fig. 4. Vessel displacement by the desmoid tumor.

rate of those tumors has been quoted at 27 to 57% [7,11,14].

A more consecutive approach has recently been advocated by Dozois [12]. The rationale is that radical extirpative surgery leads to many failures, complications, and sequelae. Benefit is difficult to predict, as many of these tumors are symptomless. The plan is to manage mesenteric and retroperitoneal fibromatosis desmoids without surgery until they become symptomatic. Only then, surgical attempts are indicated for limited resection, bypass for signs and symptoms of impending obstruction, ureteral stents for hydronephrosis. One should pursue non-surgical treatment for control of the tumor growth.

MEDICAL TREATMENT

The disappointment created by the high rate of recurrence and the difficulty in applying the principles of wide local excision especially in FAP patients with retroperitoneal and mesenteric desmoids has encouraged investigators to look at a variety of agents capable of slowing or controlling tumor growth; although the basic mechanisms for disorder remains unknown. Waddell et al. in 1983 [13] reported on a patient with a large sternal desmoid. The patient received indomethacin for treatment of pericarditis and experienced as an unexpected side effect; significant decrease in the size of the desmoid. Further observations by the same author confirmed the effect of nonsteroidal antiinflammatory drugs (NSAID) in the control of desmoid tumor growth, especially if they were used in association with oral administration of tamoxifen and ascorbic acid. The side effects in the gastric mucosa remains a problem.

The rationale for the use of NSAID for inoperable tumors is based on the importance of prostaglandins in growth and proliferation and the prostaglandin synthesis inhibition produced by NSAID compounds with a consequent effect believed to promote an immunologic attack on tumor cells.

Ornithine decarboxylase, the first and rate-limiting enzyme in polyamine biosynthesis, is an enzyme associated with tumor proliferation. It has been shown to be inhibited by indomethacin.

Another reported agent is [(Clinoril) Merck, Sharp and Dohme], a nonsteroidal anti-inflammatory agent (fluorinated indene acetic acid) Belliveau and Graham [14] used it to treat a patient with a desmoid tumor of the abdomen, with significant reduction in the patient's symptoms. Nevertheless, severe adverse reactions such as: hepatocellular dysfunction, hepatitis, or cholangitis, may have a negative impact in the extended use of this medication [15].

Hormonal manipulation, utilizing estrogen blockers, appears to be another alternative in the management of desmoid tumors [9]. The clinical use has gained impetus following the observation that desmoid tumor growth seems stimulated by estrogens. Support is given specially by a higher incidence of "sporadic" desmoids in women of child-bearing age and the association of significant growth of desmoids while pregnant. Reitamo et al. [2] reported that the rate of desmoid growth in 89 patients roughly

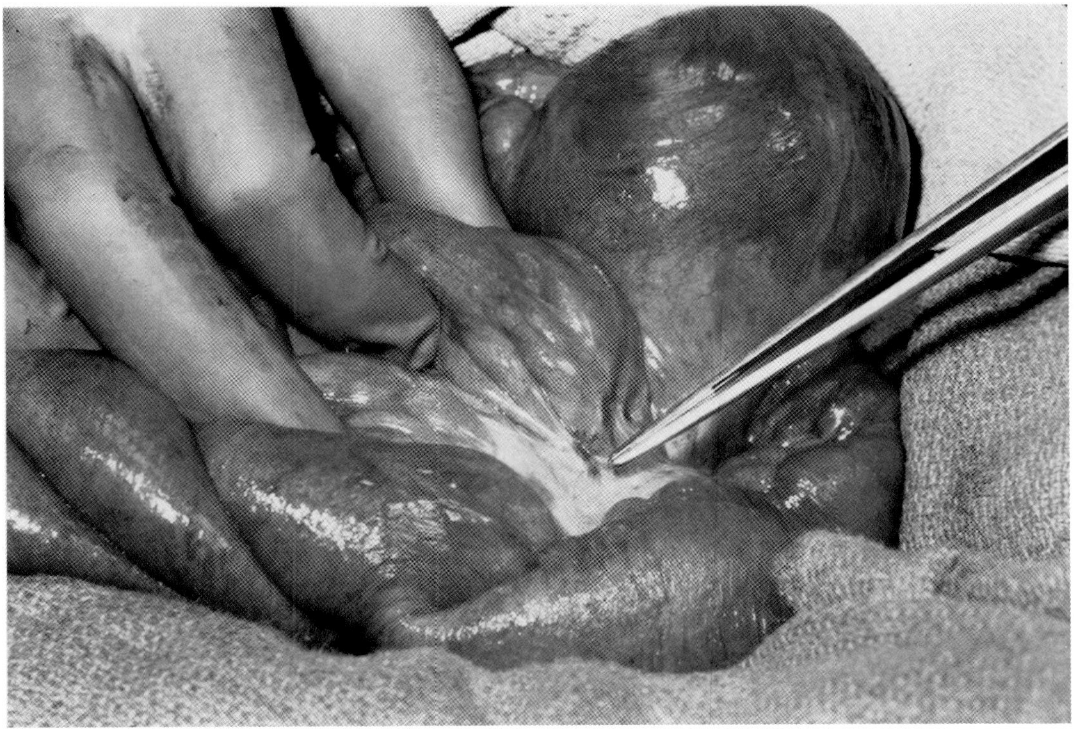

Fig. 5. Diffuse mesenteric fibromatosis.

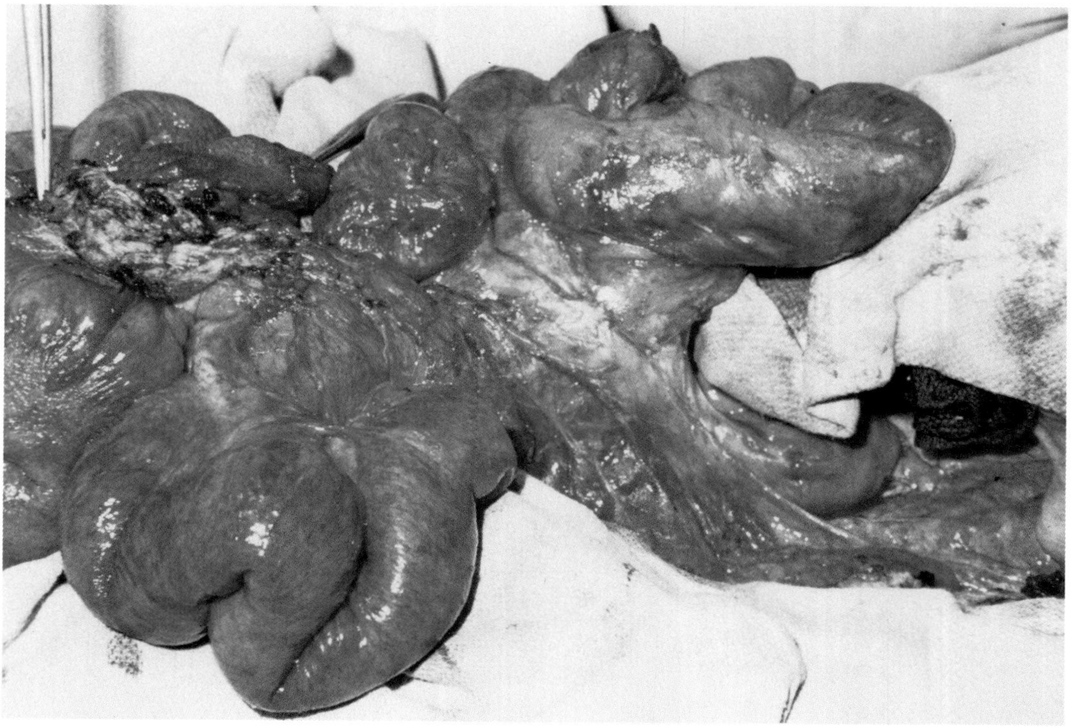

Fig. 6. A small bowel resection with its mesenteric vessels in wall by desmoid tumor resected with healthy surgical margins.

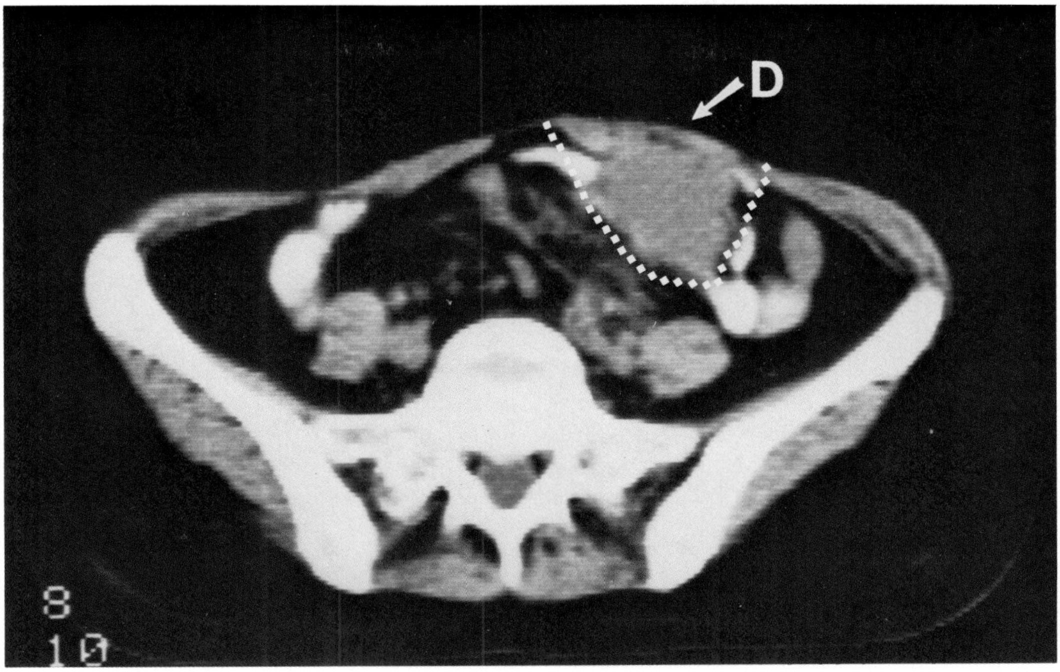

Fig. 7. Abdominal wall desmoid in patient with FAP before treatment with Tamoxifen and Sulindac.

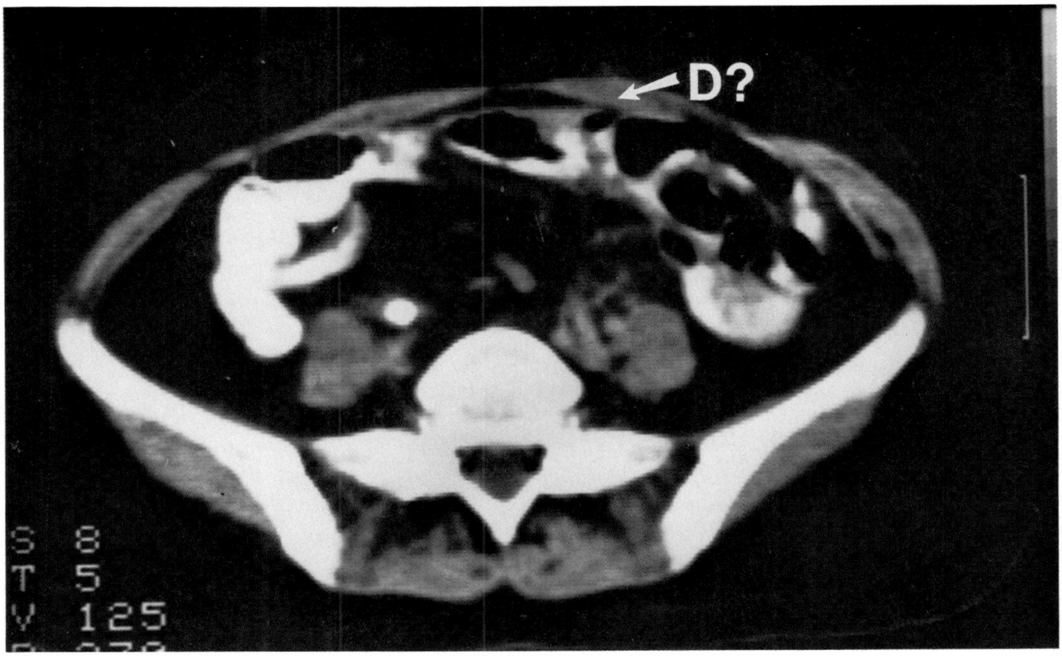

Fig. 8. Disappearance of a desmoid after one year of Tamoxifen and Sulindac.

followed their levels of endogenous estrogens. Tamoxifen has been used alone or in combination with NSAID treatment for patients with desmoids with apparent good results (Fig. 7,8). The effect of tamoxifen appears to be the result of the inhibition of desmoid growth by restricting RNA synthesis and by alterations in the transcription of genes necessary for tumor growth and possibly by also interfering with polyamine metabolism [16,17].

Many other treatments have been tried and abandoned due to their ineffectiveness, among them radiation therapy, chemotherapeutics agents such as 5-fluorouracil, Adriamicin, and Vincristine. Other medications such as Theophylline, Chlorothiazide, testolactone; have been tried as an effort to manipulate cyclic AMP attempting the inhibition of tumor cells [14] but without consistent success.

Clearly, much more knowledge related to the basic control mechanisms of this tumor is necessary for a logical and intelligent use of intervention that may affect desmoids' appearance, growth and possible malignant progression.

References

1. Hayry P, Scheinin T: The desmoid (Reitamo) syndrome: Etiology, manifestations, pathogenesis, and treatment. Curr Prog Surg 25:225–320, 1988.
2. Reitamo JJ, Scheinin TM, Hayry P: The desmoid syndrome. New aspects in the cause, pathogenesis and treatment of the desmoid tumor. Am J Surg 151:230–237, 1986.
3. Jones IT, Jagelman DG, Fazio VW, Lavery IC, Weakley, FL, McGannon E: Desmoid tumors in familial polyposis coli. Ann Surg 204:94–97, 1986.
4. Sener SF, Miller HH, DeCosse JJ. The spectrum of polyposis S G & O 159:525–532, 1984.
5. Herrera L, Carrel A, Petrelli N. DNA in desmoid tumors Am J of Surg (In Press).
6. Magid D, Fishman EK, Jones B, Hoover HC, Feinstein R, Siegelman SS: Desmoid tumors in Gardner syndrome: use of computed tomography. Am J Roentgenol 142:1141–45, 1984.
7. Khorsand J, Karakousis CP: Desmoid tumors and their management. Am J Surg 149:215–218, 1985.
8. Gesschikter CF, Lewis D: Tumors of connective tissue. Am J Cancer 25:630–635, 1935.
9. Kinzbrunner B, Ritter S, Domingo J, Rosenthal CJ: Remission of rapidly growing desmoid tumors after Tamoxifen therapy. Cancer 52:2201–2204, 1983.
10. Sheridan R, D'Avis J, Seyfer AE, Quispe G: Massive abdominal wall desmoid tumor. Treatment by resection and abdominal wall reconstruction. Dis Colon Rectum 29:518–520, 1986.
11. Jarvinen HJ: Desmoid disease as part of familial adenomatous polyposis coli. Acta Chir Scand 153:379–83, 1987.
12. Dozois, RR: Surgical aspects of familial. Int J Col Rect Dis 3:1–16, 1988.
13. Waddell WR, Gerner RE, Reich MP: Nonsteroid anti-inflammatory drugs and Tamoxifen for desmoid tumors and carcinoma of the stomach. J Surg Oncol 22:197–211, 1983.
14. Belliveau P, Graham AM: Mesenteric desmoid tumor in Gardner's syndrome treated by sulindac. Dis Colon Rectum 27:53–4, 1984.
15. Daniele B, Pignata S, D'Agostino L, Vecchione R, Mazzacca G: Sulindac-induced severe hepatitis. Am J of Gastroenterology, 83:1429–1432, 1988.
16. Itoh H, Ikeda S, Oohatay, Iida M, Inove T, Onitsuka H: Treatment of desmoid tumors in Gardner syndrome. Dis Colon Rectum 31:459–461, 1988.
17. Kelin WA, Miller HH, Anderson M, DeCosse JJ: The use of indomethacin, sulindac, and Tamoxifen for the treatment of desmoid tumors associated with familial polyposis. Cancer 60:2863–2868, 1987.

18

Decision-Making Process in Kindreds With Familial Adenomatous Polyposis

Lemuel Herrera, Nicholas Petrelli, and Victoriano Saenz

From the Department of Surgical Oncology (N.P., L.H.), Roswell Park Memorial Institute, and Department of Surgery (L.H., N.P.), State University of New York at Buffalo, Buffalo, New York; Department of Surgery, Hospital Universitario "Angel Leano," Universidad Autonoma de Guadalajara, Guadalajara, Mexico (V.S.)

Of the premalignant conditions, Familial Adenomatous Polyposis (FAP) is considered a classic prototype for the study of human neoplastic development. FAP is inherited in an autosomal dominant pattern, and its clinical behavior is predictable once phenotypical manifestations have appeared. These phenotypical manifestations are protean and affect a variety of organs and systems. Each of these manifestations may in turn require the expertise of a specialist. However, once the specialist has finished the evaluation and made recommendations for the care of the patient, the patient usually is sent back to the referring physician for continued medical care. The primary physician, usually a family practicioner, internist, surgeon, gastroenterologist, or pediatrician, is not likely to be versed in every one of the earliest manifestations and complications of this relatively rare disease.

In this chapter, we present an algorithm for the management of kindreds with FAP. It is intended to serve as a quick reference to busy clinicians. This algorithm is a flow scheme representing a graphic description of the thought process of a a group of physicians who have had experience with multiple facets and stages of FAP. This algorithm has stemmed from the need to provide a methodical approach to the disease, with maximal conceptual clarity for physicians at various levels of education and training. It should be expected that modifications will occur in the future.

Crucial to the management of these kindreds is the ascertainment of all benign and malignant phenotypical manifestations of the disease prior to definitive recommendations. Identification of relatives at risk will be of benefit to them for advice about screening, early detection and prevention of cancer, whereas understanding as to how these kindreds are predisposed and affected by the disease may prove to be significant for clinical research. Without accurate demographic data, it would not be possible to obtain an adequate overall picture or to identify informative pedigrees. A good rapport between a member of every family and the polyposis registry is mandatory, since one has to rely on the informant to keep current new additions to the family, changes in address and surnames, and deaths. This is especially true in kindreds potentially suitable for genetic linkage, where a single misclassification is tantamount to a disaster.

Most clinicians will agree that any symptomatic patient coming from a FAP kindred must undergo a complete evaluation. Regardless of age, symptoms must be explained. Controversy exists regarding the age at which one should evaluate asymptomatic family members. We have seen children as young as 9 years of age with the large bowel carpeted with adenomatous polyps; however, they were symptomatic. We recommend screening to begin at about 15 years of age. Screening includes in addition to the careful his-

Familial Adenomatous Polyposis, pages 147–149

ALGORITHM FOR FAMILIAL ADENOMATOUS POLYPOSIS KINDREDS

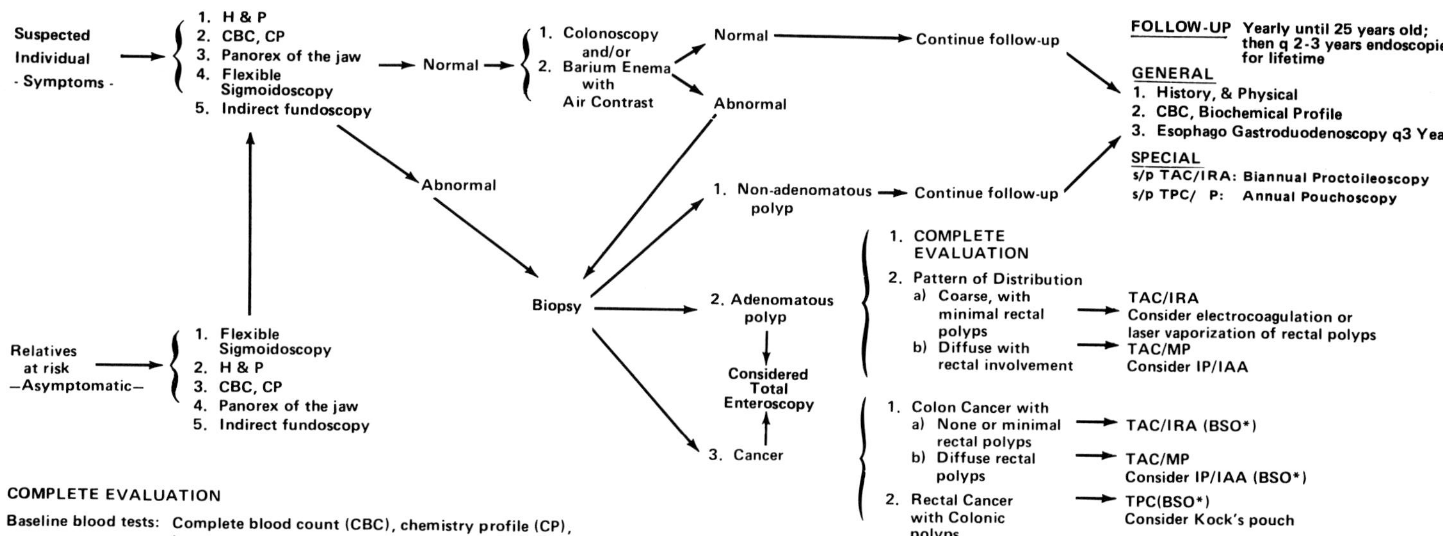

COMPLETE EVALUATION

Baseline blood tests: Complete blood count (CBC), chemistry profile (CP), karyotype, establishment of lymphoblastoid line

Baseline X-rays: Bone survey to include long bones, skull, Panorex of the jaw Intravenous pyelogram, Enteroclysis

Baseline Endoscopy: Esophagogastroduodenoscopy (Fore and side view), Colonoscopy

H & P = History and Physical to include digital examination of rectum and test for occult blood in feces.

P = Pouch

MP = Mucosal proctectomy
IRA = Ileorectal anastomosis
TAC = Total abdominal colectomy
IP = Ileal pouch
IAA = Ileoanal anastomosis
TPC = Total proctocolectomy
BSO* = Bilateral salpingoophorectomy

*BSO may be considered complementary to cancer operation.

tory and physical, specific digital rectal examinations, testing the stool for occult blood, sigmoidoscopy, panorex views of the jaw and ocular fundoscopy. The screening evaluation must accommodate the time constraints imposed by daily school activities and the availability of parents.

We recommend the use of flexible sigmoidoscopy for screening. This procedure is not time-consuming, requires minimal bowel preparation, produces minimum discomfort, and reveals polyps proximal to the rectal ampulla. One must carefully inspect the mucosa, as polyps may be minute (1–2 mm). For members with symptoms, total colonoscopy must be performed. Ileoscopy in search of polyps should be attempted when at the cecum. The introduction of routine baseline esophogogastroduodenoscopy has disclosed that as many as one-third of patients may have asymptomatic polyps in the proximal gastrointestinal tract synchronous to those in the colon and rectum. Duodenal adenomatous polyps seem to have the same significant malignant potential as those located in the large bowel. Enteroclysis consists of the introduction of a column of barium through the tip of a nasogastric tube placed into the duodenum under X-ray or endoscopic guidance. The bolus of barium is followed by fluoroscopy and affords a thorough view of possible polys in the small bowel mucosa. Clearly, abnormal findings may alter the treatment options. At times, diagnostic and/or therapeutic small bowel endoscopy may be needed.

Extracolonic manifestations may precede the appearance of the gastrointestinal polyps serving as a useful clinical marker in some kindreds. Therefore, we recommend that all members of the kindred undergo a baseline Panorex examination of the jaw and an opthalmologic examination. The former will disclose osteomas in the jaw and teeth abnormalities; the latter may show the multiple, bilateral congenital ocular retinal patches associated with subsequent development of epithelial gastrointestinal polyps in some kindreds. Bone surveys that include long bones are a time-honored investigation. However, we place significant reliance on the actual palpation of the patient's skull, bony prominences, and skin because a thorough physical examination may detect small osteomas and epidermal inclusion cysts not seen with X-rays or other diagnostic methods.

All phenotypical manifestations must be clearly documented and if possible measured since they will form the morphologic basis for correlation to available genetic markers. It is through the combination of accurate clinical descriptions and identification of coinherited, closely linked genetic markers to the "bad gene" that the biological risk of a specific individual for FAP will be defined. In the future, these tests may help to reassure those family members without the "bad gene" that they will not develop polyps early in life, that they have the same risk as the general population of developing colonic polyps and cancer, and that they will not pass the family "bad gene" to their future generations.

When females with FAP have been diagnosed preoperatively with cancer, we often consider the possibility of a bilateral salpingoophorectomy at the time of surgical treatment. The removal of the ovaries is a staging procedure, since ovarian metastases from colorectal cancer signals an extremely poor prognosis. Oophorectomy does not add to the morbidity or mortality of the primary surgical procedure and is the best possible means of ensuring that an unwanted pregnancy will not occur. This acquires special significance in patients who are of child-bearing age and are sexually active. Some of them unfortunately develop intrabdominal desmoid tumors postoperatively. Also, some patients will require potentially teratogenic chemotherapy regimens as adjuvant or as definitive therapy. Under these circumstances pregnancy may not be a welcomed event.

For patients who previously have undergone an abdominal colectomy and ileoproctostomy, and later present with recurrent rectal adenomatous polyps, we recommend local control of these polyps. Although we prefer to biopsy and then follow with Nd-YAG laser vaporization, one can also use the approach of biopsy and electrocoagulation. Surgical options presented to patients with benign colorectal polyps should aim to preserve anal continence, prevent rectal submucosal scarring, and allow for unimpaired surveillance for the early detection of gastrointestinal malignant and premalignant lesions.

19

Counseling Families With Familial Adenomatous Polyposis

Anne J. Krush

Division of Medical Genetics, Department of Medicine, The Johns Hopkins University School of Medicine, Baltimore, Maryland

The following is a hypothetical history of a family, a composite of many families in the polyposis registry at the Johns Hopkins Hospital, their psychosocial and other problems, and some of the ways that their problems were met. At the time of referral to the polyposis clinic, Family J consisted of Mrs. J, a 42-year-old woman with familial adenomatous polyposis (FAP); her husband; one brother, aged 30 years; and four children; a son, D, aged 20 years; a daughter, C, aged 16 years; a son, B, aged 14 years; and a daughter, A, aged 11 years (Fig. 1). Mrs. J had been having intermittent rectal bleeding and alternating diarrhea and constipation for about 1 year before she decided to have a colon examination. At first, she believed that these were flulike symptoms, but, when they persisted, she knew that "something was wrong."

A flexible sigmoidoscopy was performed, and Mrs. J was told by the gastroenterologist that she had FAP. He explained the hereditary nature of the condition, drew a picture of the colon with a polyp outlined, and explained the risk of developing cancer of the colon. He asked about her family history, but the shock of learning that she had a serious hereditary disorder was so great that she could not think about family illnesses at that time.

The family investigator then talked briefly with Mrs. J and learned that she had four children, who should soon have colon examinations, but decided not to broach that subject just then. Instead, she listened while Mrs. J talked about how healthy she felt, but at the same time expressed fear of cancer, fear of surgery, and fear of loss of part of her body. In fact, Mrs. J could not even consider the next steps in medical planning but left the clinic carrying a medical and genealogical questionnaire to be filled out and a booklet describing FAP. She said that she would be in touch with the investigator after she had "had time to think."

In a few days, Mrs. J phoned the family investigator, saying that she had read through the booklet and started to fill in the questionnaire, but she had questions about it. She wanted to know how it would be used and she wondered about confidentiality. She was reassured that the information she shared with us was, indeed, confidential. It would be placed on the computer, but access to the computer was limited only to our clinic personnel. The information would be used to construct a "working" pedigree and would give us information concerning which side of the family had the FAP gene and which members should be made aware of their risk of having or of developing FAP.

Mrs. J said that, when she had begun to investigate illnesses in her family, one relative had told her that only women in the family could have FAP. That relieved her because she has two sons. She was asked to take out the booklet, and turn to the description of hereditary factors and the pedigree drawing. From that she saw that each

Familial Adenomatous Polyposis, pages 151–154

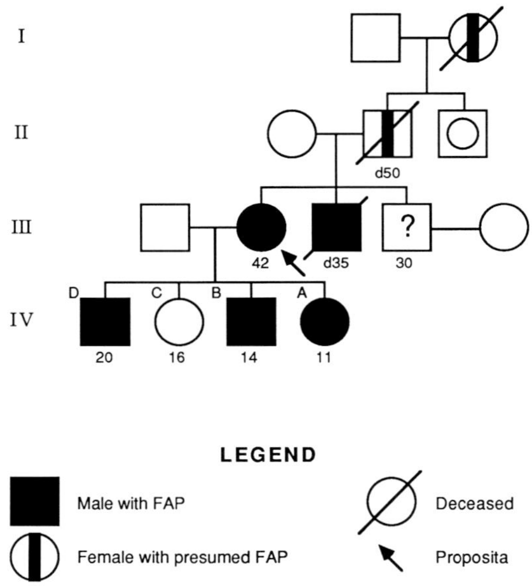

Fig. 1. Pedigree of Family J.

of her children has a 50% chance of having the gene for FAP. That was another shock, but she said that she was not going to make appointments for her children until after she had come to some decision concerning her own medical plan. She was assured that no pressure would be put on her at this time.

Mrs. J said that her father had died of colon cancer at age 50 years. Her paternal grandmother had also died of "stomach" cancer in middle age. Mrs. J. said that her older brother had died eight years ago at age 35 years, but she was unsure of his diagnosis. She later learned that he died of colon cancer with metastasis to the liver. Although he had had symptoms that were similar to those of their father, with rectal bleeding and abdominal pain, he refused to go for a colon examination until he began to lose weight and the abdominal pain became severe. Their younger brother, now aged 30 years, observed his brother's physical decline and death from FAP and for this reason has adopted a "head-in-the-sand" approach, and ignores his sister's urging that he go for a colon examination.

Later, both the gastroenterologist and the family counselor tried to persuade the young man to have a colon examination. When he refused, the counselor talked with his wife, who attempted persuasion also. However, this almost caused a rift in the marital situation. Perhaps, later, when he observes good results from early treatment and surgery in other family members, or develops symptoms, himself, he may accept the need for medical surveillance.

Some of Mrs. J's aunts, uncles, and cousins on her father's side of the family have also had "bowel problems," some dying of colon cancer. This is information that requires histopathologic confirmation. She said that she would help us obtain authorizations for release of medical information. In fact, she has now become the medical genealogist for her father's side of the family, or the "key" person for the study.

When Mrs. J returned a month later to the polyposis clinic for a complete physical examination and an upper endoscopy, she talked with both the gastroenterologist and the surgeon. She said that she had been depressed for some time after learning her diagnosis but has now accepted what would "have to be," i.e., surgical removal of her colon. The different kinds of surgery were explained to her and she elected to have the ileoanal pull-through procedure. She then talked with the family counselor, expressing fear of what her husband's reaction would be to her surgery. Would he be repelled by it? Would it affect their marital relationship? What if her children have FAP? Will he blame her for passing this condition on to them? She was already blaming herself, even before the children were examined.

Arrangements were made for both Mr. and Mrs. J to talk with the gastroenterologist and the family counselor, at which time both had a chance to discuss the whole problem and it was clear that Mr. J was going to be understanding and completely supportive. Plans were made for surgery, and all four children rose to the occasion and assigned themselves duties for the time their mother would be in the hospital. Mrs. J had the two-stage surgery and was not depressed during the 3 months that she had a temporary ostomy. She handled the situation very well, and set a good example for any of her children who might have to undergo the same procedures. Her recovery was uneventful.

Several months later, the four children underwent flexible sigmoidoscopies. At first they were frightened at the idea of the scope, but Mrs. J could tell them in all honesty that the procedure would not be as painful as they anticipated. All were upset, however, when it was learned that only daughter C, aged 16 years, was unaffected. Son D, aged 20 years had had no symptoms, and it was difficult for him to accept the fact that he must undergo surgery. About 1 month after his first surgery, he became depressed and threatened his mother, blaming her for his FAP and all the pain it entailed. When Mr. J could not reason with him, it was necessary to seek psychiatric help. Long afterward he still referred to his family as "death family"; when his first child was born, she had the rare condition of hepatoblastoma (that we now know can be associated with FAP) and lived only a few months. His second child, however, was born without complications or medical problems, though of course D and his wife are aware that this child has a 50% risk of developing FAP. Counseling was offered betewen the two births, but decisions concerning future pregnancies, of course, were left up to D and his wife. One of the physicians who attended the birth of the first child was unaware of the association (though rare) with FAP and told the family that the liver tumor was not hereditary and would not occur in a later pregnancy. D and his wife were informed that in all the families known to our polyposis registry to this date as well as in the medical literature, no later pregnancy had resulted in another child with hepatoblastoma, but this did not preclude its happening. We felt that honesty was best in this case.

Son B and daughter A then underwent surgery over a period of 1 year with no apparent medical or emotional problems resulting. Two years later, Mrs. J developed an abdominal wall desmoid that was successfully resected. She has continued to be followed by her gastroenterologist at 3–4 year intervals with upper endoscopies and flexible sigmoidoscopies. She wondered why she had not been told prior to her first surgery that she should continue under medical surveillance for the rest of her life. We told her that, in our opinion, that information would have been too much to bear, having just learned the FAP diagnosis and the need for surgery. By this time, however, she could accept the fact that she was still at risk for extracolonic cancer and desmoids and had bowel habits that were not back to normal. She and Mr. J discussed the matter with the children and those affected agreed to remain under medical surveillance.

One might surmise that, all this time, daughter C, having no problems with polyps, would be well adjusted and happy to know that she had little chance of developing polyps and would not pass the condition on to her children later on. However, this was not the case. She developed psychosomatic problems that were directly related to the fact that she felt left out and different from her siblings. Both parents took special pains to assure her of their love and caring even though they had to attend to the medical and psychological problems of the other chidlren. She was helped to see that she could also be helpful in many ways to her affected siblings and was reminded that the others might envy her because she did not have to be under medical surveillance for FAP for the rest of her life. She realized then that she was loved and needed.

At age 18 years, daughter A developed an intramesenteric desmoid. The family had group health insurance at Mr. J's place of work, but the company refused, at first, to pay for chemotherapy or hormonal or radiation therapy for the desmoid that could not be removed surgically. Both surgeon and family counselor listened to the concerns of the family. After the surgeon explained the situation to the insurance agent, the payments were allowed. This worried the family; they realized that, if Mr. J did not have group insurance at work, the affected members of the family would not be able to obtain health nor possibly life insurance. Mr. J. realized, too, that, were he to consider a change of jobs or be dismissed from his present job, he would have to make certain that health insurance for his family would be available at the new job. This might limit his choice of occupation.

As son B reached his late teens and still had

problems with bowel continence, he wondered if a girl would ever like him, if he would ever marry, and, if so, would his wife want a child who would be at 50% risk for FAP? Would she blame him if the child *did* develop symptoms? Could he stand to see his child go through all the examinations, surgery, and follow up that had befallen him? The gastroenterologist prescribed a new medication that relieved the continence problem and with the family counselor discussed the sexual and marital problems, suggesting strongly that before marriage the matter should be discussed thoroughly with his bride-to-be and that she be given an opportunity to discuss the matter with a physician. Prevention was stressed; knowing of the risk to their child, the parents would be prepared for early detection and prevention of colon cancer through surgery.

Unfortunately, several years later, when daughter A married, her first child developed a brain tumor at age 3 years. The family could hardly believe that so many serious extracolonic conditions could occur in one family; but they all pulled together to stand behind A and her husband. They accepted supportive help from members of the polyposis team and from members of the support organization, IMPACC (Intestinal Multiple Polyposis And Colorectal Cancer). Surgery was performed, and the tumor was entirely removed. A and her husband realize, however, that the tumor indicates that polyps will almost certainly develop in a few years.

Hidden strengths abound in this family. The more that adverse physical conditions appeared, the more they banded together to help each other. They also accepted outside help when needed. When we first started to counsel FAP families, we had no idea how many problems might arise. We have admiration for those who, like this family, have withstood the stress, have made the best of many difficult situations, and, for the most part, continue to follow medical surveillance plans with their physicians.

ACKNOWLEDGMENTS

I thank all the families in the polyposis registry at the Johns Hopkins Hospital who have expressed their thoughts and feelings and helped me to understand many of the problems they have faced. I thank Miss Joanna Strayer, Research Assistant at the Johns Hopkins University School of Medicine, for technical assistance; and Mrs. Susan Booker, Coordinator of the Polyposis Clinic at the Johns Hopkins Hospital, for reviewing the manuscript.

20

The Leed's Castle Polyposis Group

Lemuel Herrera

Familial Polyposis Registry, Division of Surgical Oncology, Roswell Park Memorial Institute, and Department of Surgery, State University of New York at Buffalo, Buffalo, New York

The rarity of Familial Adenomatous Polyposis (FAP) makes it difficult for any single clinical unit to develop experience with the wide spectrum of manifestations of this disease. In June of 1985, 30 people from 11 countries, met at Leed's Castle, Kent, United Kingdom to consider some of the problems associated with FAP. They agreed to cooperate in the collation of clinical data from their patients' populations. Four proformas were subsequently developed and circulated to cover several specific clinical aspects [1]. The group is now known as the Leeds Castle Polyposis Group.

These thirteen registries from around the world have recorded 3,243 members of families with FAP. Of these, 1,136 (54%) were affected members. Six hundred twenty-two deaths were reported: 432 (69%) from colorectal cancer and 51 (8%) from other cancers. Of the latter 51 deaths, 36 (21%) were secondary to upper gastrointestinal malignancies; the other 15 were secondary to heaptoblastoma or adrenal, thyroid, or brain tumors. It is likely that in subsequent reports there may be a relative decline in deaths related to colon cancer.

Incidence of FAP in Denmark was reported as being 1 per 10,000 births and in Japan 1 per 22,000. In both Denmark and Japan, about 40% of the cases were "sporadic," the remainder coming from families with more than one affected member. This was reported by Dr. J.M.A. Northover, Chair for the demographic data [2]; most researchers feel that the incidence of new "mutants" is above 20%.

Nine hundred sixty patients underwent surgical treatment. Total colectomy with ileorectal anastomosis was performed in 55% (morbidity rate: 7.8%; mortality rate: 1.1%), restorative proctocolectomy in 9.8% (morbidity rate: 34%; mortality rate: 0%), and proctocolectomy and ileostomy in 19.7%.

Twenty-nine cases of rectal cancer occurred among the 535 patients who survived total abdominal colectomy and ileoproctostomy, an incidence of 5.5%. Seven of the 29 had the rectal cancer diagnosed within 2 years after the initial surgery. The presence of a colon cancer in the surgical specimen of FAP patients may be a predictive risk factor for the development of subsequent cancer in the rectal remnant, thus the importance of careful examination of *all* the polyps. However, the risk is higher for the development of upper gastrointestinal malignancies and desmoid tumors than from rectal cancer. Dr. J.P.S. Thomson concluded that the preferred operative procedure in asymptomatic polyposis patient without distal rectal cancer was a total abdominal colectomy with ileoproctostomy [2].

One of the most serious complications of FAP; desmoid disease was covered by P. Hawley and J. Jass [2]. At St. Mark's Hospital, London, clinically significant desmoid disease occurred in about 10% of polyposis patients. These were mainly intrabdominal and retroperitoneal. Among the 20 patients at St. Mark's Hospital with intrabdominal desmoids, six have died. Desmoid

Familial Adenomatous Polyposis, pages 155–158

tumors do not metastasize, but they kill. There is no current therapy of predictable benefit for these patients. The lethal course of the tumors is exemplified in the Roswell Park Registry series of causes of death [3] whereas a preferential localization at the retroperitoneum in patients with FAP is emphasized in the chapter for desmoids.

Sixty-nine instances of upper gastrointestinal cancer were found in 60 of 1,255 patients. Eleven tumors were in the ampulla of Vater, nine in the stomach, and the rest were scattered throughout the duodenum. Dr. Jagelman emphasized at the groups' meeting in Washington, DC, that these tumors seemed to have been preceded by an adenoma [2]. Approximately 50% of asymptomatic patients with FAP will have multiple gastric or duodenal adenomatous polyps; thus a recommendation was made for baseline upper gastrointestinal endoscopy at the initial evaluation for a possible premptive breakage of the adenoma–carcinoma sequence. Recently, Fausa has reported a frequency of close to 100% for duodenal adenomas in FAP patients. The gastric polyps are usually gland hyperplasia and dilatation. Surveillance for gastric polyps in asymptomatic patients is usually recommended on a 2–3 year basis and for patients with documented adenomas every 6–12 months. The latter is performed in search of possible lesions amenable to endoscopic treatment, sequential biopsies or determination of a surgical resection.

Indirect fundoscopy detects retinal pigmentation and it seems to be an important subclinical marker segregating into patients who have inherited the FAP gene. S. Baba reported that only 6/1984 non-affected control individuals had unilateral, solitary retinal spots, whereas 35/44 patients with FAP had multiple and bilateral lesions.

Significant advances in the understanding of genetics have occurred in the last 3 years. To understand these, it is important to review some basics of genetic linkage. Genetic linkage relies on the shuffling of genes occurring between each generation in the meiotic divisions leading to the production of the sperm and ova. In the course of meiosis, chromosomal fragments repeatedly recombine; they "cross over" and exchange segments of equal length. As a result, every chromosome transmitted in a germ cell represents a patchwork of segments from the two original parental chromosomes. Two genes that are structurally closely together on a given chromosome region are likely to remain together throughout the shuffling (linked), so they will be coinherited together, whereas genes that are farther apart are likely to be separated. The extent of coinheritance of an associated marker gene to a diseased gene exceeding that expected by chance, is in direct relation to the distance that separates the diseased gene known from the marker gene in the chromosome.

Closely linked gene markers may consistently be coinherited with the diseased gene and therefore potentially helpful for diagnosis [4]. Recombination is the phenomenon that enables one to find linkage between a DNA marker and a disease. Recombinant DNA technology has permitted the identification of many specific sequences of DNA (gene markers) that are physically close to genes of interest (linked sequences).

This technological achievement has been possible through the understanding of the actions of restrictions endonucleases. Endonucleases are a specialized set of enzymes found in microorganisms such as *Escherichia coli* and other primitive forms of life. These enzymes recognize sequences of four to six base pairs of specific, short oligonucleotides. They cleave (cut) DNA at all such sites (restriction sites) when the sequence is recognized. The name of the particular restrictive enzyme is derived from its identification in the bacteria of origin, i.e., ECol; HindI, Taq1, HpaII, etc. The function of these enzymes is to destroy (restrict) the incoming DNA foreign to the bacteria. Another enzyme system protects the bacterial own DNA from cleavage by modifying it at or near each potential cleavage site. This is accomplished by adding a methyl group. This restriction modification system that protects the host DNA while destroying foreign DNA provides of a pattern that can be traced to a progenitor to obtain a point of reference in the genome of interest. Following the identification of this reference point, the short stretches of polymorphic DNA, whose inheritance pattern is now known, become a unique genetic marker useful to trace inheritance. If in addition, a restriction site is identified close to a diseased gene in question, then a powerful tool has been developed. With the use of the allele of interest identified by restriction fragment length polymorphism (RFLP) techniques, the diseased, coinherited gene may be then traced through the offspring; it will lie in the same chromosomal region as the DNA marker of the affected progenitor. Although the marker DNA will not reveal the physical position of the gene itself, it is a crucial step towards its identification and is potentially clinically useful. Botstein proposed a scheme for constructing a complete linkage map of the human genome by using RFLPs. Such polymorphisms can be detected by hibridizing a DNA segment probe to blots containing genomic DNA, from different individuals, digested with various restriction enzymes. DNA sequence alterations involving changes in restriction enzyme recognition sites or deletion of DNA within the restriction fragments can be detected by the change in hybridization band patterns. If a probe is found to exhibit different band patterns after testing in several individuals using several restriction enzymes, it is considered reasonably polymorphic for use in linkage analysis [5]. The usefulness of these techniques is exemplified by the cooperative work with the Center for the Study of Human Polymorphism (CEPH) in Paris. The CEPH has undertaken to collect, store, and distribute DNA from 40 families. Investigators from around the world get complete sets of DNA from the collection; in return, they report their markers and inheritance patterns to the CEPH, providing the basis for a single but continuously enlarging human genetic map.

Finding a marker whose inheritance is correlated with the appearance of disease is a task of staggering proportions with unmarked chromosomes. The first clue to the chromosomal location of the FAP gene came from the examination of the karotype chromosomes of an individual with colonic polyps, colon cancer, and desmoid tumor [6]. Karyotype study of the patient showed that a portion of chromosome 5 was missing. This finding focused the attention of molecular biology researchers on this segment of the chromosome. An RFLP that revealed polymorphism, previously assigned by hybridization to chromosome 5, showed close linkage to FAP, with a maximum LOD score (likelihood recombination fraction in a set of progeny chromosomes) of over 3 at a recombination fraction of 0. This corresponds to odds of more than 1,000 to 1 in favor of close linkage between the probe and the FAP gene. Insitu annealing showed that the probe localized to the long arm of chromosome 5, 5q21–q22, which had been shown to be missing in the multiply abnormal reported sporadic case of FAP [7]. Sir W. Bodmer, one of the Leed's Castle group's members, reported that the chromosomal region for the polyposis gene had been found; however, it was recessive at the cellular level [2]. Although the actual gene responsible for FAP has not been identified, I have previously mentioned that the localization of the polyposis gene to a specific chromosomal region is a substantial step towards the eventual identification and isolation of the gene. Localization of the gene to a particular chromosomal region has been compared to knowing the correct state, city, and street but not knowing the particular house in which the gene resides. More recently, Sasazuki has reported the introduction of a single human chromosome 5 into carcinoma cell lines using a microcell technique. He concluded that a tumor suppression gene is located at the long arm of chromosome 5, whereas Miyaki and others have suggested that the inactivation of suppression genes on chromosomes 5, 17, 18, and 22 contributes to the progression of tumors from benign to malignant.

The Leed's Castle Polyposis Group has proved its leadership in optimizing the clinical management of patients with FAP, and it is now considering the initiation of prospective multidisciplinary studies. The group is in a position of significant advantage to explore the possibility of banking tissues and serum and even lymphobastoid cell lines from well studied patients for the sharing of scientific and clinical data for the interpretation of molecular biology results, as it seems that flanking markers to the diseased gene have been identified. Furthermore, the combination of data from pedigree, bowl, eye, bone, and DNA, currently allows for a probability of 95% prediction of FAP gene carriers. These efforts may eventually result in the genetic diagnosis and possible manipulation of this disease, and are the object of discussion following the Third meeting of The Leed's Castle Polyposis Group at Worcestershire, U.K., in June, 1989.

References

1. Northover MD JMA: Activities of the Leed's Castle Polyposis Group. Semin Surg Oncol 3:118–119, 1987.
2. Thomson JPS: Leed's Castle Polyposis Group meeting. Dis Colon Rectum 31:613–616, 1988.
3. Herrera-Ornelas L, Elsiah S, Petrelli N, Mittelman A: Causes of death in patients with familial polyposis coli (FPC). Semin Surg Oncol 3:109–117, 1987.
4. Ponder BAJ: Familial cancer: Opportunities for clinical practice and research. Euro J Surg Oncol 13:463–473, 1987.
5. Fa-Ten Kao: Somatic/Cell genetics and gene mapping. Int Rev Cytol 85:109–146, 1983.
6. Herrera L, Kakati S, Gibas E, Pietrzak, Sanberg A: Brief clinical report: Gardner syndrome in man with an interstitial deletion of 5q. Am J Med Genet 25:473–476, 1986.
7. Bodmer W, Bailey CJ, Bodmer J, et al.: Localization of the gene for familial adenomatous polyposis on chromosome 5. Nature 328:614–616, 1987.

APPENDIX A

Any interested clinical or basic researcher may contact, for further information,

The Honorary Director
ICRF Colorectal Cancer Unit
St. Mark's Hospital, City Road
London ECIV 2PS, England

or any of the following clinicians/scientists:

Dr. T. Alm, Karolinska Hospital, Sweden
R. Audisio, National Cancer Institute, Milan, Italy
S. Baba, Hamamatsu University, Japan
Miss T. Berk, Toronto General Hospital, Canada
Prof. Bergen, Rikshospitalet, Oslo, Norway
Sir W. Bodmer, I.C.R.F., United Kingdom
Dr. S. Bülow, University of Copenhagen, Denmark
Dr. H.J.R. Bussey, St. Mark's Hospital, United Kingdom
Dr. Z. Cohen, Toronto General Hospital, Canada
Dr. J.J. DeCosse, Cornell Medical Center, United States
Dr. F. den Hartog Jager, Amsterdam, Holland
Dr. H. Gordon, Mayo Clinic, United States
Mr. A. Gunn, Ashington Hospital, Northumberland, United Kingdom
Dr. S. Hamilton, Johns Hopkins University, United States
Mr. P. Hawley, St. Mark's Hospital, United Kingdom
Dr. L. Herrera, Roswell Park Institute, United States
Dr. M.J. Hill, Porton Down, United Kingdom
Dr. J. Hognestad, Oslo, Norway
Ms. L. Hruska, Mayo Clinic, United States
Dr. T. Iwama, Tokyo, Japan
Dr. D. Jagelman, Cleveland Clinic, United States
Dr. H.J. Jarvinen, Helsinki, Finland
Dr. J. Jass, University of Auckland, Auckland, New Zealand
Prof. M. Khan, University of Leiden, Leiden, The Netherlands
Prof. A.J. Krush, Johns Hopkins Hospital, United States
Dr. S. Levitt, West Perth, Australia
Dr. F. Macrae, Royal Melbourne Hospital, Victoria, Australia
Ms. E. McGannon, Cleveland Clinic, United States
Ms. H. Miller, Cornell Medical Center, United States
Dr. T. Muto, University of Tokyo, Tokyo, Japan
Miss K. Neale, St. Mark's Hospital, United Kingdom
Mr. J.M.A. Northover, St. Mark's Hospital, United Kingdom
Dr. S. Quan, New York, United States
Dr. S. Ritchie, St. Mark's Hospital, United Kingdom
Dr. L. Ritter, Budapest, Hungary
Dr. M. Sizak, Cleveland Clinic, United States
Mrs. K. Skullerud, Norwegian Radium Hospital, Norway
Dr. J. Slak, St. Mark's Hospital, United Kingdom
Mr. J.P.S. Thomson, St. Mark's Hospital, United Kingdom
Dr. J. Utsunomiya, Hyogo College Medicine, Japan
Dr. R. van Stolk, Cleveland Clinic, United States
Dr. H.F.A. Vasen, Utrecht, The Netherlands

21

Anatomy of Anal Sphincters

Ahmed Shafik

Department of Surgery, Faculty of Medicine, Cairo University, Cairo, Egypt

INTRODUCTION

During the last decades, there was greater interest in research into the anatomy and physiology of rectal sphincters and pelvic floor musculature. Commonly accepted anatomic entities were confirmed, altered, or negated, and new ones were revealed. These findings have improved our understanding of functional relations within the anorectum. They also led to new etiologic concepts of rectal pathologies as well as to new approaches for surgical treatment. This chapter reviews the anatomy of the anal sphincters.

EXTERNAL ANAL SPHINCTER

The external anal sphincter is a triple loop system [1], consisting of top, intermediate, and base loops. Each loop is separated from the other by a fascial septum (Fig. 1) and has its individual attachment, direction of muscle bundles, and innervation.

The top loop comprises the deep part of the external sphincter and puborectalis, which are intimately fused together. Its muscle bundles loop around the upper part of the rectal neck and are attached to symphysis pubis. A downward prolongation descends along the rectal neck and shares in the formation of the longitudinal muscle (Figs. 1, 2). It is supplied by the inferior hemorrhoidal nerve. The intermediate loop embraces the midportion of the rectal neck and is innervated by the perineal branch of the fourth sacral nerve. The base loop encloses the lower rectal neck and is supplied by the inferior hemorrhoidal nerve.

Familial Adenomatous Polyposis, pages 159–167

Mechanism of Action

The external sphincter induces voluntary continence by a double-fold action [2]: 1) prevention of internal sphincter relaxation on destrusor contraction, which I termed *voluntary inhibition action*; and 2) direct compression of the rectal neck, or the *mechanical action*.

Voluntary inhibition action. As stools enter the rectum, the detrusor contracts and the internal sphincter relaxes reflexly to open the rectal neck. The latter does not open unless the external sphincter relaxes voluntarily. However, if there is no desire to defecate, the external sphincter contracts, mechanically preventing relaxation of the internal sphincter. Failure of the latter to relax reflexly inhibits contraction of the rectal detrusor, which relaxes and dilates to accomodate the new contents (Fig. 3). Voluntary external sphincter contraction to inhibit reflex internal sphincter relaxation is the *voluntary inhibition action* [2]. This is the main action responsible for voluntary continence. The internal sphincter integrity is thus necessary not only for involuntary continence but also for voluntary continence, the voluntary inhibition action being mediated through it. For this reason, internal sphincter reconstruction should be considered an essential step in rectal incontinence repair [3].

Voluntary mechanical action. Besides the voluntary inhibition action, external sphincter contraction firmly seals the rectal neck by mechanical compression. Being striped, the external sphincter cannot contract for a long period to maintain continence mechanically. The mechanical compression action is thus momentary and serves to occlude the rectal neck by the time the

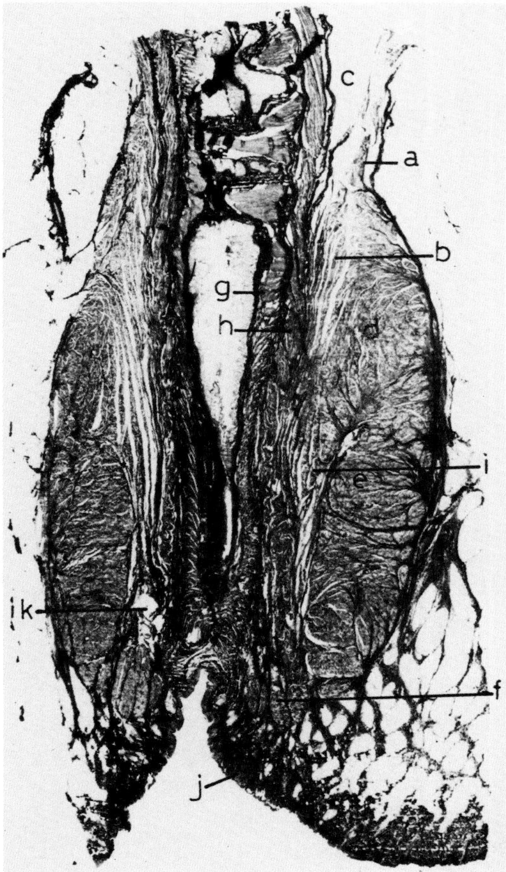

Fig. 1. Coronal section of the rectal neck showing muscles and perirectal spaces. a, Levator plate; b, suspensory sling (intermediate longitudinal muscle); c, pelvirectal space; d,e,f, top, intermediate, and base loops, respectively, of external sphincter; g, internal sphincter; h, medial longitudinal muscle; i, lateral longitudinal muscle; j, subcutaneous space; k, central space. Verhoeff-van Gieson stain. × 19. (Reprinted with permission from Shafik [5], Copyright by Williams & Wilkins, 1975.)

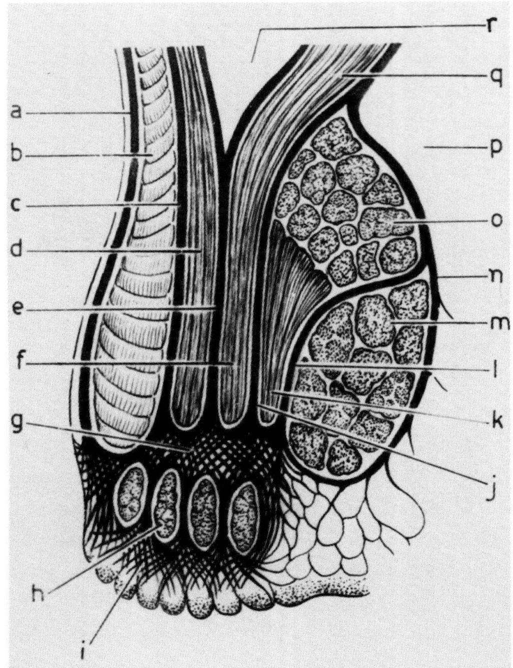

Fig. 2. Diagram illustrating the rectal neck musculature and perirectal spaces. a, Submucous space containing internal fascial septum; b, internal sphincter; c,e,j,1, four inter-sphincteric spaces; d,f,k, medial, intermediate, and lateral longitudinal muscles, respectively; g, central space occupied by central tendon; h,m,o, base, intermediate, and top loop of external sphincter, respectively; i, subcutaneous space containing corrugator ani cutis; n, external fascial septum; p, ischiorectal space; q, levator plate; r, pelvirectal space. (Reprinted with permission from Shafik [4], Copyright by Williams & Wilkins, 1976.)

detrusor relaxes as a result of the voluntary inhibition action.

Stress Defecation

In conditions of internal sphincter damage, voluntary continence is induced only by the mechanical action of the external sphincter. The voluntary inhibition action is lost. Being stripped, the external sphincter cannot contract long enough to withstand the noninhibited prolonged contraction of the loaded detrusor. Detrusor contraction continues despite external sphincter contraction till the latter fatigues and relaxes and the detrusor evacuates itself. Hence, in cases of internal sphincter damage, once the desire to defecate is initiated, evacuation should occur. This condition, which I named *stress defecation* [2], is observed in patients after internal sphincterotomy for anal fissure. It could also explain the impaired control of feces and flatus after internal sphincterotomy.

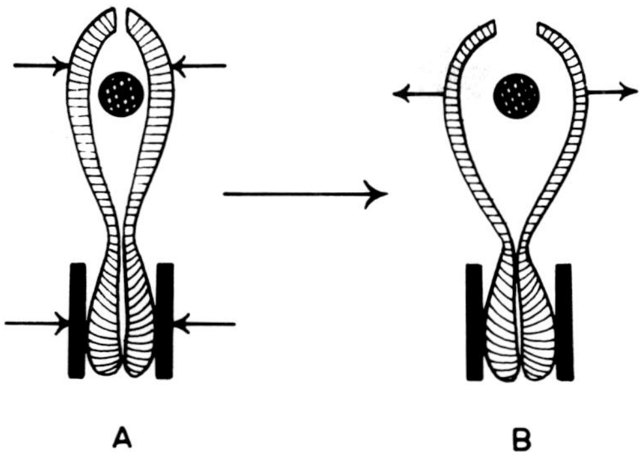

Fig. 3. Mechanism of voluntary inhibition action to oppose a call to stool. **A:** Detrusor contraction with failure of internal sphincter relaxation because of voluntary external sphincter contraction. **B:** Reflex detrusor relaxation because of failure of internal sphincter relaxation (voluntary inhibition action). (Reprinted from Shafik [2], with permission of the J.B. Lippincott Co.)

Single Loop Continence

As a result of the separate arrangement of the three external sphincter loops and since each loop has its own separate and bilateral innervation, any single loop can function as a sphincter. The external sphincter continent action can be achieved by a single loop contraction and not necessarily by the three loops. This constitutes the basis of the *single loop continence* [2]. On contraction, a single loop induces continence by both voluntary inhibition action and mechanical occlusion. The latter action is significantly tight in loop contraction, being effected not only by direct compression but also by rectal neck kinking [1].

LONGITUDINAL MUSCLE

The longitudinal muscle consists of three layers: medial, intermediate, and lateral [4] (Figs. 1, 2). The medial longitudinal muscle is a continuation of the longitudinal rectal muscle coat. The intermediate muscle is the suspensory sling of the levator ani [5], whereas the lateral muscle is the longitudinal extension of the top loop of the external anal sphincter [1].

The fleshy longitudinal muscle ends at the level of the lower border of the internal sphinter by giving rise to a fascial condensation called *central tendon*. The latter splits into multiple fibrous septa. The medial septum attaches to the rectal neck lining, whereas the lateral passes into the ischiorectal fossa. The intermediate septa penetrate the external sphincter base loop, decussate to form the corrugator cutis, and insert in the perineal skin (Fig. 2).

The longitudinal muscle plays an important role in the mechanism of defecation [4]. On contraction at stool, it shortens and widens the rectal neck. Furthermore, it helps to fix the rectal neck during straining at defecation, thus preventing rectal prolapse [4]. Subluxation of the longitudinal muscle shares in rectal prolapse genesis [6].

Six perirectal spaces could be identified [7]: subcutaneous, central, intersphincteric, pelvirectal, ischiorectal, and submucous (Figs. 1, 2). The subcutaneous space was found to be continuous with the ischiorectal space. The central space lies in the lower rectal neck and is occupied by the central tendon. It is the main perirectal space; it communicates with all of the other spaces along the central tendon septa.

LEVATOR HIATUS AND TUNNEL

The levator ani consists essentially of the pubococcygeus, the iliococcygeus being rudimentary in humans. The puborectalis is not a part of the levator; both differ in morphology, innervation, and function [5]. The pubococcygeus is funnel shaped, with a transverse portion called the *levator plate* and a vertical portion called the *suspensory sling* [5] (Figs. 1, 2).

The levator plate is an oval cone that stretches across the pelvis; the levator hiatus occupies its anterior portion and the rectococcygeal raphe exists posteriorly. Two patterns of the rectococcygeal raphe could be identified: single and triple decussation patterns [5]. The "hiatal ligament" connects the medial border of the levator plate to the rectum at the rectal neck inlet [5]. The levator plate consists of two "crura" that bound the levator hiatus and two "lateral masses" [8]. Three crural patterns were identified: classic, crural overlap, and crural scissor.

The levator ani is the principal muscle of defecation. On contraction at defecation, it opens the rectal neck for the stools to descend. Any interference with levator function results in disturbance of the defecation act, e.g., in levator dysfunction syndrome [9] and rectal prolapse. The different patterns of the rectococcygeal raphe and levator crura play an important role in rectal neck support; their subluxation may eventually lead to rectal prolapse [5,6].

The "levator tunnel" is a muscular tube that surrounds the intrahiatal organs (rectal neck, prostate in males or vagina and urethra in females) along their way down from the levator hiatus to the perineum [8]. The posterior tunnel wall (3–4 cm) is longer than the anterior (2.5–3 cm). The tunnel is double sheathed with an inner coat of the suspensory sling and an outer of the puborectalis. Both coats are of striped muscle bundles. The inner coat is a tunnel "dilator," which opens the rectal neck at defecation, whereas the outer coat is a tunnel "constrictor" [8]. The "tunnel septum," a greyish-white membrane, lines the inner aspect of the levator tunnel and separates it from the fascis propria of the intrahiatal organs [8]. It separates the voluntary from the involuntary components of the levator tunnel. It serves as an important landmark during mobilization of the intrahiatal organs from within the levator tunnel as in the operation of anorectal mobilization [10–12].

Hiatal Ligament

The levator plate is connected to the intrahiatal organs by a fascial condensation called the *hiatal ligament* [5] (Fig. 4). It arises from the inner edge of the levator plate and splits fanwise into multiple septa to insert into the rectal and vesical neck as well as into the upper vaginal end. Anteriorly, the ligament fills the gap between the two levator crura at their origin, forming the puboprostatic or pubovesical ligament [8]. The hiatal ligament plays a vital role in harmonizing the action between the levator plate and the intrahiatal organs during evacuation of their contents (defecation and urination). Hiatal ligament subluxation would not only interfere with the act of evacuation but also lead to prolapse of the intrahiatal organ [6,13].

Puborectalis and the Double-Sphincter Control

The puborectalis, as it proceeds backward from its origin in symphysis pubis, gives off muscle bundles to each intrahiatal organ, forming "individual" voluntary sphincters for these organs [8] (Fig. 4). It gives rise to the external urethral sphincter and deep external anal sphincter in both sexes, as well as to the vaginal sphincter in the female and prostatic sphincter in the male. However, the puborectalis and deep external anal sphincter were found fused together; the conjoint muscle is given the name *top loop* [1].

Each intrahiatal organ is thus provided with a double voluntary sphincteric apparatus: 1) an "individual" organ sphincter derived from the puborectalis and is specific for the organ and 2) a "common" tunnel sphincter, the puborectalis itself, which acts on the intrahiatal organs collectively. This separate sphincteric activity for the individual organs under the control of a common continent muscle secures not only an immune sphincteric function to the organ but also a harmonized action among the structures enclosed within the levator tunnel. Further, the double sphincteric mechanism provided to each organ could be a guarantee of functional maintenance in case either of the two sphincters is damaged. Injury of either sphincter alone does not induce incontinence of the concerned organ. Unless both sphincters, the individual and common, are destroyed, continence could be maintained by either [8].

THE MALFORMED RECTUM

The embryologic basis of the correlation of the anatomical features with the clinical appearance of rectal anomalies was studied [14]. Under normal developmental conditions, the hindgut enters the levator hiatus and migrates through the levator tunnel to the perineum, where its blind end is invaginated by the proctodeal dimple. The levator tunnel guides the hindgut to its normal perineal location and seems to initiate proctodeal dimpling. It could be that a delay in tunnel development or mal-tunnel formation would dis-

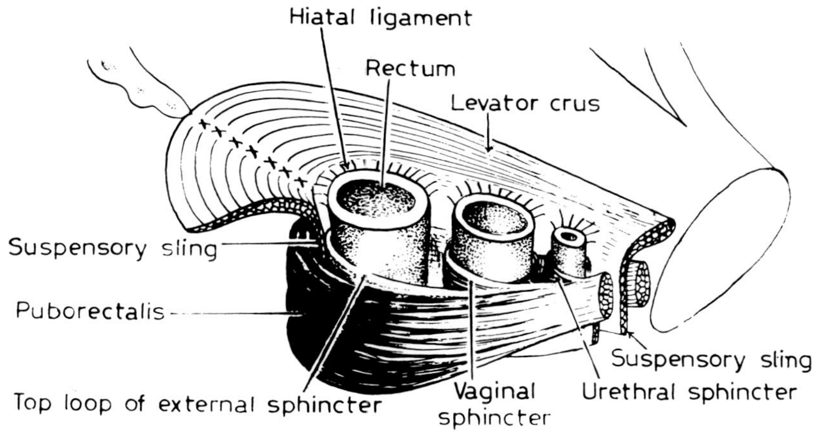

Fig. 4. Diagram illustrating the "individual" sphincters arising from the puborectalis, which acts as a "common" sphincter for the intrahiatal structures. (Reprinted from Shafik [8], with permission of the J.B. Lippincott Co.)

turb such a process and be responsible for the mal-developed rectum. This constitutes the basis of the "tunnelization theory," which explains the embryologic origin of the different rectal anomalies [14].

Two main types of rectal anomalies could be identified in a series of 95 patients: suprahiatal and infrahiatal. This classification is based on the relation of the rectal stump to the levator hiatus, which lies at the level of the pubococcygeal line about 1.5 cm from the perineal skin.

Suprahiatal Anomalies

Forty-four cases were studied. Hindgut does not enter the levator tunnel, and lies above its upper end, probably because of delayed or mal-tunnel formation. It ends blindly or fistulizes.

Infrahiatal Anomalies

Fifty-one cases were studied. Hindgut enters levator tunnel but fails to run normal development. Four types were encountered.

Proctodeal agensis. Thirty-seven cases were studied. Hindgut reaches the perineal skin but is not invaginated by the proctodeum, leaving the hindgut imperforate with or without fistulization.

Imperforate rectal membrane. One case was studied. Hindgut is invaginated by proctedeum but without rectal membrane rupture.

Rectal neck stenosis. Ten cases were studied. Rectal membrane ruptures, but rectal neck fails to remodel.

Rectal neck atresia. Three cases were studied. Hindgut is invaginated, perforated, and remodelled, but shows atresic segment about the rectal neck midportion, probably from intrauterine vascular accident.

MECHANISM OF DEFECATION

Muscles of Defecation

The muscles that act on the rectal neck are the external and internal sphincters and the puborectalis, levator ani, and longitudinal muscles. The external and internal sphincters and the puborectalis are muscles of continence. Their role at stool is that they contract to interrupt or terminate the act of defecation [1,15]. However, the principal muscles of defecation are the levator ani and the longitudinal muscle [4,5]. They act jointly to open the rectal neck at defecation. The two muscles are interrelated because the suspensory sling, a part of the levator, constitutes the middle layer of the longitudinal muscle [4,5] (Figs. 1, 2).

Mechanism of Defecation

With the knowledge of the physioanatomical aspects of the rectal neck muscles, and assisted by pressure, electromyogram (EMG), and barium enema studies, the precise mechanism of defecation could be explored [16]. As stools enter the rectum, reflex detrusor contraction and internal sphincter relaxation occur. The continuation of defecation depends on two factors 1) external sphincter relaxation and 2) straining. If defecation is acceded, the external sphincter is voluntarily relaxed. Straining is necessary to maintain defecation as it raises the intra-abdominal pressure. This serves a double purpose: It compresses the detrusor, which helps evacuation, and it stimulates levator contraction. Although the intra-abdominal pressure compresses the detrusor, the rectal neck is spared because of its protected location below the levator plate.

When the levator plate contracts, it moves from the cone to the flat position and is elevated and laterally retracted [5,16] (Fig. 5). This results in pulling the hiatal ligament, which in turn pulls open the rectal neck inlet and partially opens the rectal angle. Simultaneously, the suspensory sling contracts and not only pulls up the base loop to unseal the rectal neck outlet but also partially opens the rectal neck (Fig. 5).

The longitudinal muscle joins the detrusor in contraction, which results in the shortening and opening of rectal neck as well as in complete straightening of the rectal angle. This brings the rectal neck into alignment with the detrusor so that efficient fecal pumping occurs. The final result of the joint contraction of the detrusor, longitudinal muscle, and levator ani is the opening of the rectal neck, with its inlet and outlet for the rectum to evacuate its contents.

Rectal Continence

Continence is a function of the internal sphincter and the voluntary sphincter complex (puborectalis and its external sphincter derivative). The internal sphincter normally contracts involuntarily and is responsible for involuntary continence. On the other hand, the voluntary sphincter complex (VSC) normally is relaxed and responsible for voluntary continence.

Although the internal sphincter maintains involuntary continence, its damage may not lead to incontinence. This is ascribed to the resting tone of the VSC, which helps to keep the rectal

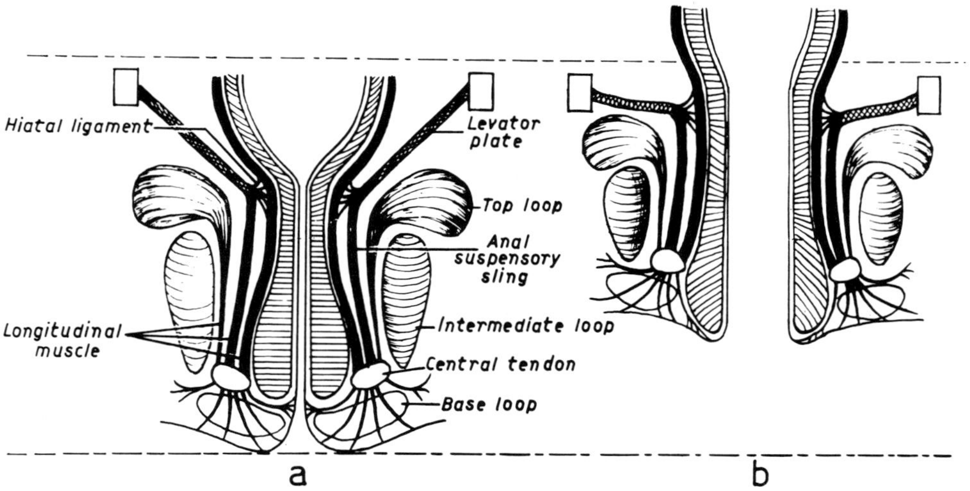

Fig. 5. Mechanism of defecation. **a:** At rest. **b:** At defecation: flattening of levator cone and suspensory sling contraction results in opening of rectal neck. (Reprinted from Shafik [16], with permission of Edition Nymphenburg.)

neck involuntarily closed. The VSC resting tone, measured by EMG, was found to be augmented after internal sphincter excision in anorectal mobilization operation for rectal cancer [10–12]. It was responsible for the involuntary control in these patients. The increased tone makes up for the lost internal sphincter involuntary continent action.

The function of the VSC is to resist, interrupt, or terminate the act of defecation. Injury to this complex destroys these functions. To ''resist'' a call for evacuation, the VSC contracts. It occludes the rectal neck mechanically by the time the voluntary inhibition action relaxes the detrusor [2]; the mechanism of action has already been described.

Rectal Incontinence

Incontinence results from damage of either the internal sphincter or VSC or both. Four types of rectal incontinence have been identified [17]: 1) Stress defecation: This condition results from internal sphincter damage; mechanism is described above. 2) Stress incontinence: There is detrusor leak of fluid stools or flatus with sudden increased intra-abdominal pressure from coughing or sneezing. It is due to a weakened VSC. 3) Urgency incontinence: The VSC is completely damaged, whereas the internal sphincter is intact. Evacuation occurs rather simultaneously with the desire. It is different from stress defecation in which the patient, after feeling the desire, can hold evacuation for 40 to 60 seconds. 4) Total incontinence: All sphincters, voluntary and involuntary, are damaged. Patient is incontinent with fecal soiling, whether or not there is a desire to evacuate.

The Rectal Neck

A preceeding study has shown that the anal canal does not exist either embryologically or anatomically and that the rectum extends down to the perineal skin [18]. As the lower blind end of the hindgut reaches the perineal skin, it is invaginated by the proctodeal dimple, with a resulting rectal membrane rupture, opening of the rectum to the exterior, and fusion of the ectodermal with the endodermal lining. The lower narrow part of the hindgut, which I named the *rectal neck,* extends downard and slightly backward from the levator plate level to the perineal skin, whereas the part above is the *rectum proper* [18] (Fig. 6). The only share the proctodeum has in the rectum is the skin lining of the rectal neck termination, which occurs in the course of fusion of the hindgut mucosa with the perineal skin.

Anorectal Sinus and Band

As the proctodeal dimple invaginates the lower end of the hindgut, it pushes up the rectal membrane and enfolds the lower end of the hindgut mucosa (Fig. 7). Invagination continues until the rectal membrane ruptures. Two spaces result from proctodeal ''invagination'' of the hindgut [19]: 1) an outer space that I call the *anorectal sinus,* and 2) an inner space that I call the *para-anal space* (Fig. 7). The anorectal sinus represents the enfolded part of the hindgut mucosa, and it is that structure termed by investigators as the *anal glands*.

The anorectal sinus is normally obliterated and forms a fibroepithelial tube called the *anorectal band,* which is absorbed and disappears completely (Fig. 7). This is followed by rectal neck remodelling, with a resulting para-anal space obliteration [19].

The anorectal sinus may persist or is partially obliterated, resulting in the formation of the epithelium-lined structures in the submucosa of the lower rectal neck. Sinus obliteration may be

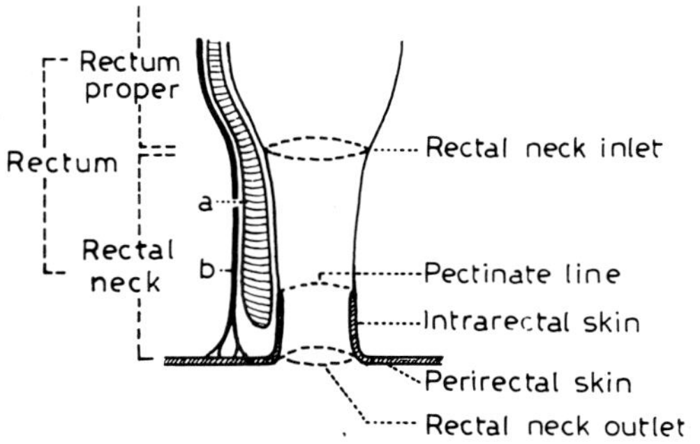

Fig. 6 The anatomical features of the rectum. **a:** Internal rectal sphincter. **b:** Longitudinal rectal muscle. (Reprinted from Shafik [18], with permission of the McMahon Group.)

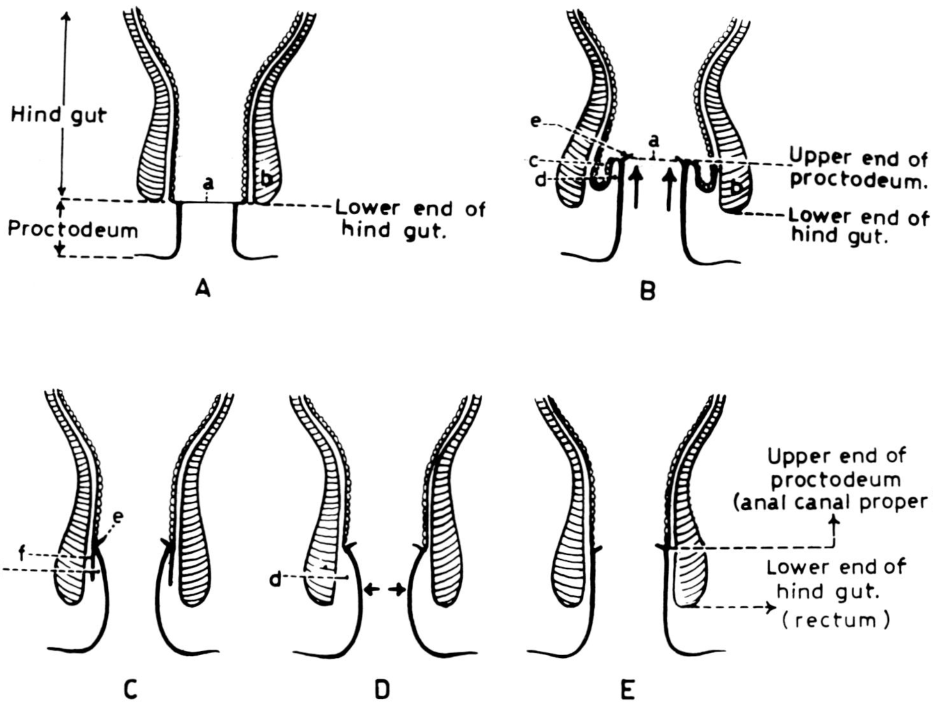

Fig. 7. Diagram illustrating embryonic proctodeum–hindgut invagination. a, Rectal membrane; b, internal sphincter; c, anorectal sinus; d, para-anal space; e, anal valves; f, anorectal band. **A:** Proctodeum and hindgut separated by rectal membrane. **B:** Proctodeum invaginating hindgut with resultant anorectal sinus and para-anal space formation, as well as rectal membrane rupture. **C:** Anorectal sinus obliteration leaving anorectal band. **D:** Disappearance of anorectal band with persistent para-anal space. **E:** Remodelling of proctodeum so that it comes into alignment with the hindgut, thus obliterating the para-anal space. (Reprinted from Shafik [19], with permission of the J.B. Lippincott Co.)

complete but leaves an "anorectal band" or "epithelial debris" that marks the anorectal sinus position [19]. Failure of rectal neck remodelling results in "congenital rectal neck stenosis."

Persistence of the anorectal sinus or its epithelial elements (anorectal band and epithelial debris) could explain the pathogenesis of some idiopathic rectal neck lesions, e.g., perirectal abscess and fistula [20–22], chronic fissure [23], pruritus ani [24], hemorrhoids [25–27], cysts, and rectal neck adenocarcinoma.

ACKNOWLEDGMENT

The valuable assistance of Mrs. Margot Yehis in revising the manuscript is highly appreciated.

References

1. Shafik A: A new concept of the anatomy of the anal sphincter mechanism and the physiology of defecation. I: The external anal sphincter: A triple loop system. Invest Urol 12:412, 1975.
2. Shafik A: A new concept of the anatomy of the anal sphincter mechanism and the physiology of defecation. IX: The single loop continence. A new theory of the mechanism of anal continence. Dis Colon Rectum 23:37, 1980.
3. Shafik A: A new concept of the anatomy of the anal sphincter mechanism and the physiology of defecation. XI: Anal incontinence: A technique for repair. Am J Proctol Gastroenterol Colon Rectum 32:8, 1981.
4. Shafik A: A new concept of the anatomy of the anal sphincter mechanism and the physiology of defecation. III: The longitudinal anal muscle: Anatomy and role in anal sphincter mechanism. Invest Urol 13:271, 1976.

5. Shafik A: A new concept of the anatomy of the anal sphincter mechanism and the physiology of defecation. II: Anatomy of the levator ani muscle with special reference to puborectalis. Invest Urol 18:175, 1975.
6. Shafik A: A new concept of the anatomy of the anal sphincter mechanism and the physiology of defecation. XIII: Rectal prolapse: A new concept of pathogenesis. Am J Proctol Gatsroenterol Colon Rectum 32:6, 1981.
7. Shafik A: A new concept of the anatomy of the anal sphincter mechanism and the physiology of defecation. IV: Anatomy of the perianal spaces. Invest Urol 13:424, 1976.
8. Shafik A: A new concept of the anatomy of the anal sphincter mechanism and the physiology of defecation. VIII: Levator hiatus and tunnel: Anatomy and function. Dis Colon Rectum 22:539, 1979.
9. Shafik A: A new concept of the anatomy of the anal sphincter mechanism and the physiology of defecation. XVIII: The levator dysfunction syndrome. A new syndrome with report of 7 cases. Coloproctology 5:158, 1983.
10. Shafik A: A new concept of the anatomy of the anal sphincter mechanism and the physiology of defecation. XII: Anorectal mobilization: A new surgical access to rectal lesions. Am J Surg 142:629, 1981.
11. Shafik A: A new concept ofthe anatomy of the anal sphincter mechanism and the physiology of defecation. XXV: Anorectal mobilization in the treatment of rectal lesions. Further study. Coloproctology 7:107, 1985.
12. Shafik A: A new concept of the anatomy of the anal sphincter mechanism and the physiology of defecation. XXIX: Reversion to normal defecation after combined excision operation and end colostomy for rectal cancer. Am J Surg 151:278, 1986.
13. Shafik A: A new concept of the anatomy of the anal sphincter mechanism and the physiology of defecation. XXVIII: Complete rectal prolapse: A technique for repair. Coloproctology 9:345, 1987.
14. Shafik A: A new concept of the anatomy of the anal sphincter mechanism and the physiology of defecation. XIX: The malformed rectum: A new theory of pathogenesis with simplified classification. Am J Proctol Gastroenterol Colon Rectum 34:16, 1983.
15. Shafik A: A new concept of the anatomy of the anal sphincter mechanism and the physiology of defecation. V: The rectal neck: Anatomy and function. Chir Gastroenterol 11:319, 1977.
16. Shafik A: A new concept of the anatomy of the anal sphincter mechanism and the physiology of defecation. XVII: Mechanism of defecation. Coloproctology 4:49, 1982.
17. Shafik A: A new concept of the anatomy of the anal sphincter mechanism and the physiology of defecation. XX: The pelvic double-sphincter control complex. Theory of pelvic organ continence with clinical application. Urology 23:313, 1984.
18. Shafik A: A new concept of the anatomy of the anal sphincter mechanism and the physiology of defecation. XIV: Anal canal: A fallacious anatomical and embryological entity. Am J Proctol Gastroenterol Colon Rectum 33:14, 1982.
19. Shafik A: A new concept of the anatomy of the anal sphincter mechanism and the physiology of defecation. X: Anorectal sinus and band: Anatomic nature and surgical significance. Dis Colon Rectum 23:170, 1980.
20. Shafik A: A new concept of the anatomy of the anal sphincter mechanism and the physiology of defecation. VI: The central abscess: A new clinicopathologic entity in the genesis of anorectal suppuration. Dis Colon Rectum 22:336, 1979.
21. Shafik A: A new concept of the anatomy of the anal sphincter mechanism and the physiology of defecation. VII: Anal fistula: A simplified classification. Dis Colon Rectum 22:408, 1979.
22. Shafik A: A new concept of the anatomy of the anal sphincter mechanism and the physiology of defecation. XXVI: Fistula-in-ano: A new theory of pathogenesis. Coloproctology 10:148, 1988.
23. Shafik A: A new concept of the anatomy of the anal sphincter mechanism and the physiology of defecation. XV: Chronic anal fissue: A new theory of pathogenesis. Am J Surg 144:262, 1982.
24. Shafik A: A new concept of the anatomy of the anal sphincter mechanism and the physiology of defecation. XVI: Pruritus ani: A new theory of pathogenesis. Coloproctology 3:239, 1981.
25. Shafik A: A new concept of the anatomy of the anal sphincter mechanism and the physiology of defecation. XXII: The pathogenesis of hemorrhoids and their treatment by anorectal bandotomy. J Clin Gastroenterol 6:129, 1984.
26. Shafik A: A new concept of the anatomy of the anal sphincter mechanism and the physiology of defecation. XXVII: Treatment of hemorrhoids: Report of a technique. Am J Surg 148:393, 1984.
27. Shafik A, Mohi M: A new concept of the anatomy of the anal sphincter mechanism and the physiology of defecation. XXIV: Hemorrhoidal venous plexuses: Anatomy and role in hemorrhoids. Coloproctology 5:291, 1985.

22

Anatomical Considerations Relevant to Fecal Continence

Alberto Peña

Schneider Children's Hospital, Long Island Jewish Medical Center, Clinical Campus of SUNY, Stony Brook, New Hyde Park, New York

INTRODUCTION

The following discussion is not an exhaustive review of the anatomy of the anorectal area. Rather, it represents a description of anatomical operative findings considered relevant to fecal continence. These findings were learned during the surgical exploration of the pelvis of patients (mainly children) through a posterior sagittal incision [1–7]. This series includes mainly patients with anorectal malformations, but we were also able to treat, through a posterior sagittal approach, individuals of different ages with rectal prolapse, trauma sequellae, rectal stenosis of different origins, pelvic tumors, and rectourethral or rectovaginal fistula. The specific skin incision is not new, since venerable pioneers have used it in the past [8–10]. There are also some contemporary reports [11–14] of surgeons who use a very similar incision. However, these reports do not include detailed anatomical descriptions of the area, and for an unknown reason the approach has not been very popular.

All of the author's surgical explorations were carried out with special emphasis on meticulous dissection and hemostasis, using an electrical stimulator and magnifying glasses. Simultaneously, the author has been exposed to the treatment of a series of patients with Hirschsprung's disease, which also constitutes the basis of this experience. Thus, this review represents a limited view of the anatomy of this crucial region. Normal defecation requires the integrity of the 1) nerve supply, 2) involuntary smooth muscle (bowel wall and internal sphincter), and 3) voluntary striated muscle.

NERVE SUPPLY

Sensation

The classic paper of Duthie and Gairns [15] is still valid for the description of the sensation of the anus and rectum. The pectinate line seems to be a good landmark for the distribution of sensitive terminals. An important transition seems to exist approximately 0.5 to 1.5 cm cranial to this line (in adults). Above this line, the rectal mucosa has an autonomic nerve supply and is thus insensitive to cutting and pricking. The distention of the rectum in this area represents a nonspecific stimuli, and it is felt and described as ''fullness'' with pain in the lower abdomen. Stephens and Smith [16], based on clinical observations, assume that there are sensory receptors located in the puborectalis muscle and surrounding pelvic muscles (proprioceptive reflex mechanisms). Rectal distention provokes stimulation of visceral afferents and dorsal root ganglia, which connect with spinal segments, conveying its messasge to the sensory cortex through ascending tracts. It is assumed that they also have connections with neurons dorsal to the ventral horn cells to mediate reflex of relaxation of the external sphincter. Below the above-mentioned line (anal canal) there is exquisite sensation, and Duthie and Gairns [15] were able to correlate these with specific struc-

Familial Adenomatous Polyposis, pages 169–174

tures. They then described free intraepithelial corpuscles related to pain, Meissner corpuscles related to sensation to touch, Krause end bulbs sensitive to cold, Paccini and Golgi Mazoni sensitive to pressure or tension, and genital corpuscles sensitive to friction. All of these structures convey sensory afferent messages to the brain, which are essential for the integration of control mechanisms of continence.

Somatic Innervation

Branches of the ventral rami of second, third, and fourth sacral segments integrate the pudendal nerve. This leads to the inferior rectal nerve, which innervates the external sphincter, anal canal, and perianal skin, as well as the levator muscles (ileococcygeus, pubococcygeus, and puborectalis muscles). This nerve runs on the cranial surface of the levator muscle. A perineal nerve, also a branch of the pudendal, will innervate the labia, scrotum, and urogenital diaphragm [16,17]. Also a sensitive branch from the pudendal is a dorsal nerve of the clitoris and penis.

Sympathetic Innervation

Sympathetic innervation is basically represented by connections between hypothalamus, splanchnic nerves, and sympathetic trunks. Second, third, and fourth lumbar segments unite in the preaortic plexus and form the hypogastric plexus in front of L5. Sacral sympathetic chain joins the pelvic ganglion, which seems to be located anterior and lateral to the rectum [16]. The effect of sympathetic stimulation seems to activate the internal sphincter and inhibits the rectal motility.

Parasympathetic Innervation

Parasympathetic innervation is given by the anterior division of the third and fourth sacral nerves, which forms the nervi erigenti and gives branches to the rectum. All of these are preganglionic fibers that synapse to ganglion cells (Auerbach's plexus) in the rectal wall. The postganglionic fibers are distributed in the smooth muscle of the rectal bowel, including the internal sphincter [18]. These nerves are considered to be motor to the bowel and inhibitors to the internal sphincter.

There are very obvious practical and surgical implications related to the nerve distribution of this area. It is very important to preserve the mucosa below the pectinate line if one wants to maintain the integrity of the sensory mechanism [19]. We have been exposed to patients in whom this important mucosa was resected, and they sufffered from different degrees of fecal incontinence in spite of the fact that they had normal voluntary muscles and intact pelvic innervation. They do not seem to be completely incontinent, but they are particularly unable to control liquid stools. They also seem to be unable to discriminate gas from liquid and solid material inside the rectum. Endorectal dissections used for the treatment of Hirschsprung's disease and polyposis must, therefore, be done carefully, preserving that area of sensitive mucosa [15,19].

The distribution of all the nerves thus described is bilateral and symmetric; therefore, the most conspicuous surgical implication is obvious. Any procedure done through the midline sagittal plane will preserve the nerves intact. Another important implication is that sacral and other spinal abnormalities, either congenital or acquired, are frequently associated with different degrees of fecal incontinence because of defective innervation.

Remaining exactly in the midline and even going through the rectum dividing this structure into two lateral halves is a precondition to preserving rectal innervation. One must resist the temptation to dissect lateral to the rectum to approach structures located anterior to the rectum. At least theoretically, such perirectal dissection risks nerve injury. What the author has done in cases of pelvic tumors or other urologic problems is open the posterior rectal wall in the midline; the anterior rectal wall is then also opened to expose the prerectal space and to repair there whatever is necessary. This approach of course makes a colostomy a mandatory protective measure, which must be done prior to the main operation. Surgical dissection and mobilization of a high rectal pouch during the treatment of anorectal malformations provoke most likely a dennervation of the rectum and sometimes of the sigmoid. These patients then behave as individuals with megarectum and may suffer different degrees of disturbance of rectosigmoid peristalsis, encopresis, and constipation.

VOLUNTARY MUSCLES

Two main voluntary muscle structures have been described in anatomy books in an exhaustive way [18]. These are the external sphincter and the levator muscle. The latter structure comprises the iliococcygeus, pubococcygeus, and puborectalis subdivisions. The external sphincter has been described as "an admixture of circular and elliptical fasciculi with its cranial extremity contiguous to the caudal portion of the puborectalis muscle" [16]. It is also described in three parts: a subcutaneous, a superficial, and a deep one [18]. It is the author's conviction that all of these subdivisions are rather artificial and perhaps irrelevant. The external sphincter and levator muscle constitute a single structure integrated by muscle fibers running in different directions (Figs. 1, 2). This concept originated from surgical exploration through a posterior sagittal approach, and seems to be consistent with images seen in dissections of cadavers [20]. This has also been observed by others [21,22].

The entire striated muscle mechanism has the form of a funnel. It inserts into the pubic bone and the pelvis, as well as the lowest part of the anterior aspect of the sacrum. This funnel-like muscle structure has central orifices for the urethra, vagina, and rectum. The stimulation of the upper portion of the funnel elicits a contraction aimed to push the rectum forward, toward the pubic bone. An electrical stimulation of the lower part of the funnel muscle structure elevates the anus, indicating the presence of vertical fibers that run in a cephalocaudal manner parallel to the rectum and reaching the skin. We could not find a clear reference to this muscle structure in the literature, but we have evidence of its presence. Perhaps what has been called *puborectalis muscle* is represented by a concentration of hor-

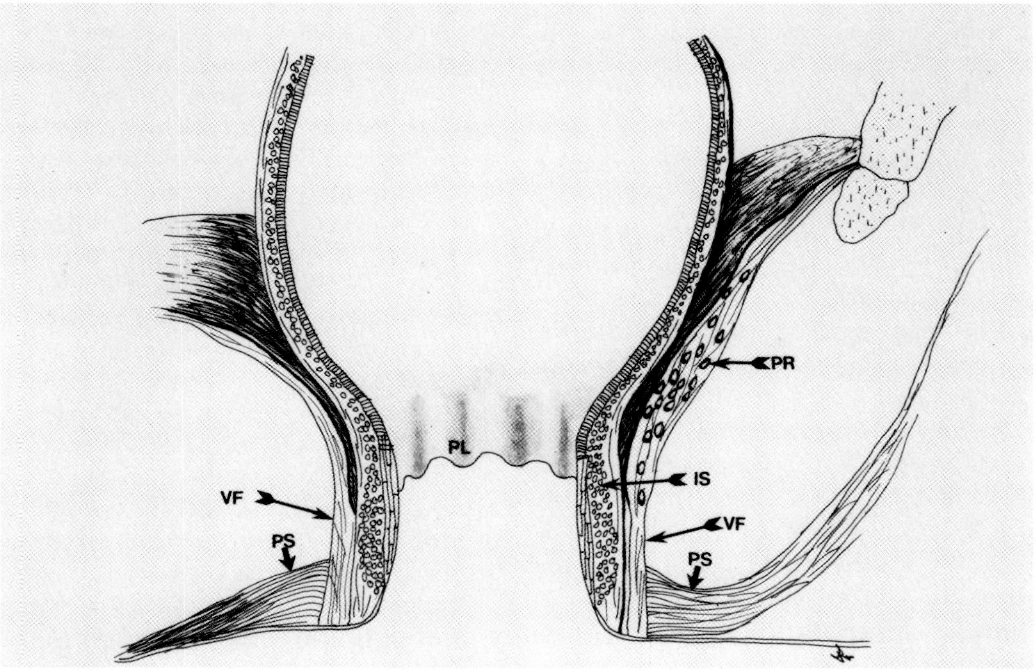

Fig. 1. Anorectal anatomy, sagittal view. PR, puborectalis (levator); IS, internal sphincter; VF, vertical fibers (levator); PS, parasagittal fibers (external sphincter); PL, pectinate line.

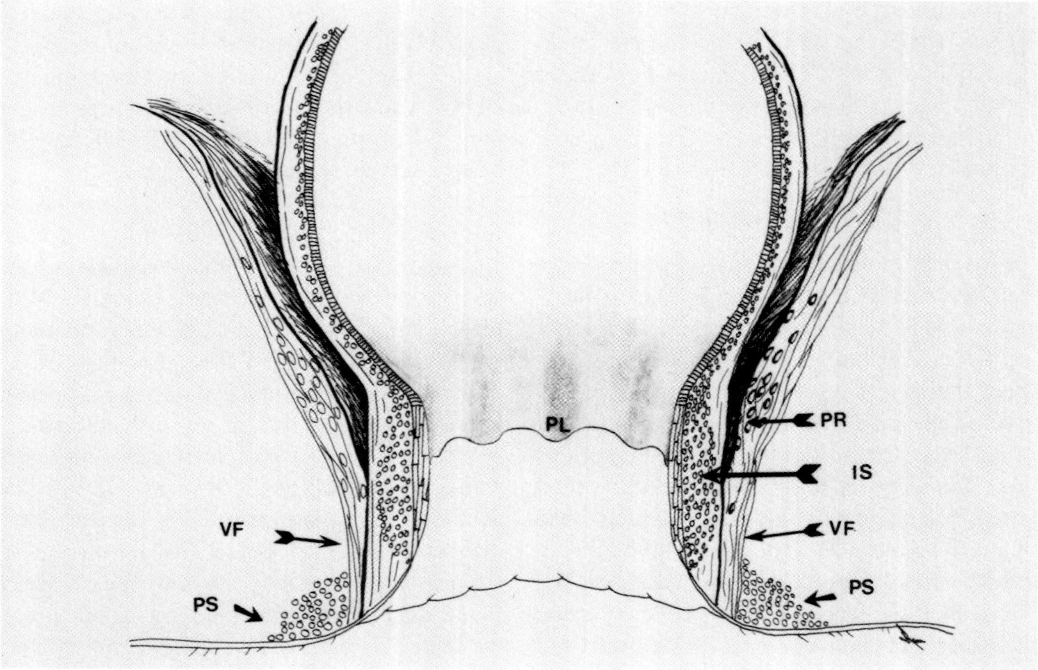

Fig. 2. Anorectal anatomy, coronal view. PR, puborectalis (levator); IS, internal sphincter; VF, vertical fibers (levator); PS, parasagittal fibers (external sphincter); PL, pectinate line.

izontal fibers in the middle portion of the levator muscle that pushes the rectum forward during its contraction (Figs. 1, 2).

The electrical response of this entire muscle mechanism does not permit the consideration that one part of it is more important than another. One rather gets the impression that the preservation of the entire muscle mechanism is what counts for fecal continence. The vertical or cephalocaudal fibers of the muscle funnel run medial to the parasagittal or paramedial fibers of the external sphincter (Figs. 1, 2).

The lowest part of this muscle structure represents the external sphincter, and we have been unable to identify the deep and superficial portions of it. The external sphincter seemed to be formed by striated muscle fibers running in a paramedian fashion, one side meeting with its corresponding opposite group anterior and posterior to the anus, without really crossing the midline. The contraction of these paramedian fibers of the external sphincter tends to shorten the length of these fibers, and because these fibers from one side seem to be anchored to the one on the opposite side, such contraction could erroneously be considered to be due to circular fibers around the anus. We do not think that such circular fibers actually exist.

The description of this structure by Changyul and Kark [21] seems to be very accurate. However, they describe the presence of decussating fibers (circular) mainly in the posterior aspect of the anus. The posterior sagittal incision allows the surgeon to be directly exposed to the muscles posterior to the rectum; the appearance of the muscles seen from behind do not allow one to affirm that they cross the midline. The stimulation of the paramedian fibers of the external sphincter close to the skin provokes a contraction aimed to close the anal orifice.

The direct exposure to the anatomy of patients with anorectal defects led us to understand that we are dealing with a spectrum of conditions. Within the range of this spectrum, there are patients with almost no muscles and patients with musculature whose strength and characteristics are very similar to that of a normal person's. Obviously, those with very poor muscles have poor continence. Unfortunately, we cannot determine in a precise way how much of that poor fecal continence is due to poor innervation, which usually coincides with patients with poor muscles. It is obvious that the voluntary striated muscle structures are important for fecal control. From the surgical point of view, the best way to preserve the voluntary striated muscles includes endorectal dissections or midsagittal incisions. However, personally, I feel that the importance of voluntary muscle in bowel control has been overestimated. Most publications dealing with the problem of fecal incontinence discuss only voluntary muscles and different ways to bring muscle structures from neighboring or distant areas around the rectum to provide bowel control. There is, in contrast, very little written about sensation and bowel motility, which I personally believe are at least equally important for fecal continence.

SMOOTH MUSCLE (BOWEL WALL AND INTERNAL SPHINCTER)

The smooth muscle of the sigmoid, rectum, and anal canal is responsible for the bowel motility and the sphincter-like action of the lowest part of the rectum and anal canal. The internal sphincter has been defined as a thickening of the circular layer of the smooth muscle of the lowest part of the intestine (Figs. 1, 2). However, its precise limits in different ages have not been defined.

The upper rectum and the sigmoid act as a reservoir, and therefore their motility seems to be very different from the rest of the gastrointestinal tract. At a certain point of fullness, the rectosigmoid initiates a series of contractions that increase the intrarectal pressure and represent the sensory stimuli for the person to know the need of evacuating the intestine. The sensory stimuli may be represented by the rectal distention (vague sensation) and by a mechanism of brief sampling, during which part of the rectal content is voluntarily exposed to contact with the mucosa of the anal canal (below the pectinate line), which has an exquisite sensation. This allows the individual to discover the nature of the bowel content (gas, solid, or liquid). At that point, the person can use voluntary muscles to hold the bowel movement until it is socially convenient to release it. In the event of a voluntary bowel movement, the person relaxes the voluntary muscles, and the involuntary contraction of the rectosigmoid then will empty the rectal ampulla and part of the sigmoid colon. The coordination of these movements is a sophisticated function, not very well understood. Some surgical procedures used in the past for the treatment of anorectal malformations included the resection of the rectum, which then obligated the surgeon to bring a portion of colon from inside the abdomen down to the perineum. These patients do not suffer from constipation, but rather have constant bowel movements since they lost the reservoir of a normal person and they now have something similar to what could be considered a perineal colostomy.

We do not know the precise role of the internal sphincter in fecal continence, although there is one study that suggests that the internal sphincter plays an important role in the maintenance of the pressure zone in the anal canal [23]. There is some evidence [24] that suggests that children with high anorectal malformations also have an internal sphincter, and our own studies also suggest this. Most likely, the distal part of the blind rectal pouch, or else that part of the rectum that communicates with the urinary tract or with the vagina (fistula), has a thickening of the smooth muscle layer consistent with the existence of an internal sphincter. This reinforces our belief that the most distal part of the rectum must be preserved and pulled down during the repair of an anorectal defect. We do not know, however, how efficient and functional this sphincter is, after one of these pullthroughs.

In the past, patients with high anorectal malformations frequently underwent procedures in which the most distal part of the rectum was resected, and therefore we assumed they did not have internal sphincters. It is interesting to find that the degree of continence varies from one patient to another. The difference between one patient and another seems to be more related to the degree of sacral abnormality, voluntary muscle development, and height of the malformation and does not necessarily seem to depend on the presence or absence of the potential internal sphincter located in the most distal part of the blind rectal pouch. We conclude that although the internal sphincter must play a role in fecal continence, it does not seem to be a crucial one.

The manometric evaluation of the rectal function frequently includes the so-called anorectal reflex. This has been described as the "relaxation of the internal sphincter" consecutive to the inflation of an intrarectal balloon located high inside the rectum. A normal individual has a normal reflex, whereas the reflex is absent in patients with Hirschsprung's disease. Looking carefully to the distribution and location of muscle fibers in this area (Figs. 1, 2), it is difficult to conclude that the internal sphincter is the only one that is relaxing during the evaluation of such a reflex, since the internal sphincter is overlapped with the striated muscle (both external sphincter and levator mechanism). Perhaps it would be more appropriate to describe this reflex as a drop of pressure in the lowest part of the rectum, consecutive to the inflation of a balloon in its upper part, without mention of specific muscle structures.

References

1. deVries PA, Peña A: Posterior sagittal anorectoplasty. J Pediatr Surg 17:638–643, 1982.
2. Peña A, deVries PA: Posterior sagittal anorectoplasty: Important technial considerations and new applications. J Pediatr Surg 17:796–811, 1982.
3. Peña A: Posterior sagittal anorectoplasty as a secondary operation for the treatment of fecal incontinence. J Pediatr Surg 18:762–773, 1983.
4. Peña A: Surgical treatment of high imperforate anus. World J Surg 9:236–243, 1985.
5. Peña A: Posterior sagittal approach for the correction of anorectal malformations. Adv Surg 19:69–100, 1986.
6. Peña A: Surgical management of anorectal malformations: A unified concept. Pediatr Surg Int 3:82–93, 1988.
7. Peña A: Posterior sagittal anorectoplasty: Results in the management of 332 cases of anorectal malformations. Pediatr Surg Int 3:94–104, 1988.
8. Amussat JJ: Anus artificiel cree par un nouveau procede. Gas Med (Paris) 654–655, 1835.
9. Kraske P: Zur exstirpation hochsitzender mastdarmkrebse. Verh Dtsch Ges Chir 14:464–474, 1985.
10. Matas R: The surgical treatment of anorectal imperforation. In the light of modern operative procedures. Trans Am Surg Assoc 1897.
11. Westbrook KC, Lang NP, Broadwater JR: Posterior surgical approaches to the rectum. Ann Surg 195:677–683, 1982.
12. Henderson DJ, Middleton RG, Dahl DS: Single stage repair of rectourinary fistula. J Urol 125:592–593, 1981.
13. Hargrove WC, Gertner MH, Fitts WT: The Kraske operation for carcinoma of the rectum. Surg Gynecol Obstet 148:931–933, 1979.
14. Mason AY: Trans-sphincteric surgery of the rectum. Prog Surg 13:66–97, 1974.
15. Duthie HL, Gairns FW: Sensory nerve-endings and sensation in the anal region of man. Br J Surg 206:585–595, 1960.
16. Stephens FD, Smith ED: Anatomy and function of the normal rectum and anus. In Stephens FD, Smith ED (eds): Anorectal Malformations in Children. Chicago: Year Book Medical Publishers, Inc., 1971, pp 14–32.
17. Decker GA, du Plessis DJ: Surgical Anatomy, ed 12. Bristol: Wright, 1986, pp 41–78.
18. Gardner E, Gray DJ, O'Rahilly R: Anatomy, ed 3. Philadelphia: W.B. Saunders, 1966, 506 pp.
19. Martin LW: The critical level for preservation of continence in the ileoanal anastomosis. J Pediatr Surg 20:664–667, 1985.
20. McMinn RMH, Hutchings RT: Color Atlas of Human Anatomy. Chicago: Year Book Medical Publishers, Inc., 1977, 248 pp.
21. Changyul OH, Kark AE: Anatomy of the external anal sphincter. Br J Surg 59:717–723, 1972.
22. Goligher JC, Leacock AG, Brossy JJ: The surgical anatomy of the anal canal. Br J Surg 43:51–55, 1955.
23. Duthie HL, Watts JM: Contribution of the external anal sphincter to the pressure zone in the anal canal. Gut 6:64–68, 1965.
24. Lambrecht W, Lierse W: The internal sphincter in anorectal malformations: Morphological investigations in neonatal pigs. J Pediatr Surg. 12:1160–1168, 1987.

23

Anorectal Physiology and Pathophysiology

Arnold Wald

Department of Medicine, Montefiore Hospital, University of Pittsburgh School of Medicine, Pittsburgh, Pennsylvania

INTRODUCTION

The principal functions of the anorectum are to maintain continence and to evacuate fecal material in a controlled and socially acceptable fashion. To accomplish these tasks, the individual must sense rectal filling; discriminate between liquids, solids, and gas; accommodate and store fecal material comfortably for variable periods of time; and defecate at appropriate times.

The physiology of continence and defecation and the pathophysiology of disorders that impair these vital functions have become better understood since the development of techniques that can more accurately measure anorectal physiology in health and disease. This chapter describes the important anorectal structural components, the functions that they serve, and the techniques that are currently available to assess anorectal physiology. In addition, it reviews recent advances in our understanding of the pathogenesis of disorders of continence and defecation.

RECTAL RESERVOIR FUNCTION

The rectum (Fig. 1) and colon act as a reservoir for fecal material until defecation becomes socially convenient. The rectum does so through adaptive compliance in which intraluminal pressures increase by only small amounts in response to increases in rectal content [1]. This phenomenon is due to the viscoelastic properties of the rectum and can be measured by constructing pressure-volume (compliance) curves in response to stepwise filling of a rectal balloon (Fig. 2). Since the walls of the latex balloon contribute to the overall pressures recorded, it is necessary to measure pressures when the balloon is inflated outside the body and to subtract these values from the pressures recorded in the rectum [2]. In our laboratory, mean compliance for rectal volumes of 50 to 250 ml is 12.1 ml/mm Hg (range 4.0 to 25.0 ml/mm Hg).

Abnormalities of rectal storage capacity have been observed in a variety of disorders of defecation and continence. Decreased rectal compliance may be associated with ulcerative proctitis [3,4], rectal ischemia [5], radiation proctitis and fibrosis [6]., colorectal surgery to correct congenital disorders such as imperforate anus [7], and rectal trauma. Conversely, increased compliance is seen in patients with megarectum associated with chronic constipation and fecal impaction [8]. The presence of these disorders may be suggested by rectal compliance studies (Fig. 2). Patients with disorders associated with reduced compliance may complain of rectal urgency and tenesmus, increased frequency of defecation, and urgent incontinence; those with megarectum may have fecal impaction, diminished perception of rectal distension, and, occasionally, overflow soiling.

RECTAL AND ANAL SENSATION

In contrast to the epithelium of the anal canal, which is richly supplied with sensory nerve endings [9], the rectum is insensitive to painful stimuli. However, through the activation of mechanoreceptors, a sensation of rectal fullness with an urge to defecate can be elicited by rectal dis-

Familial Adenomatous Polyposis, pages 175–183

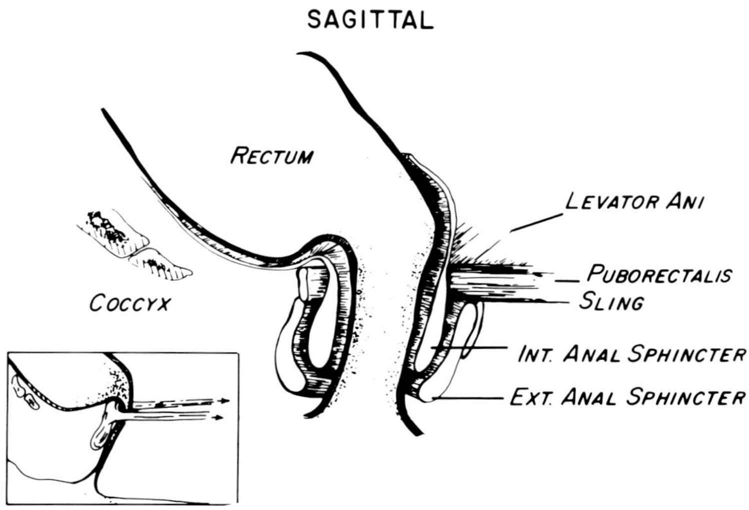

Fig. 1. Sagittal view of the anorectum illustrating the important structural components. Inset illustrates the anterior pull of the anorectum during contraction of the puborectalis muscle, with narrows the anorectal angle. (Reproduced from Wald [31], with permission of Churchill Livingstone, Inc.)

tension of as little as 5 ml of air [10]. The exact location of these mechanoreceptors is unknown; they may lie in the seromuscular layers of the rectum or in the perirectal tissues. The sensation of rectal fullness appears to be transmitted by parasympathetic fibers of the second, third, and fourth sacral nerves and can be abolished by their transection [11].

Rectal sensation can be determined by positioning a latex balloon in the rectum 5 cm above the anal verge. The balloon is connected by tubing to a 60 ml syringe, which is used to inflate and deflate the balloon rapidly with different volumes of air. The best technique is to distend the rectum initially with 50 ml to insure that the patient identifies the stimulus and then to reduce the volume in 5 to 10 ml amounts until the patient can no longer detect the distension. The smallest

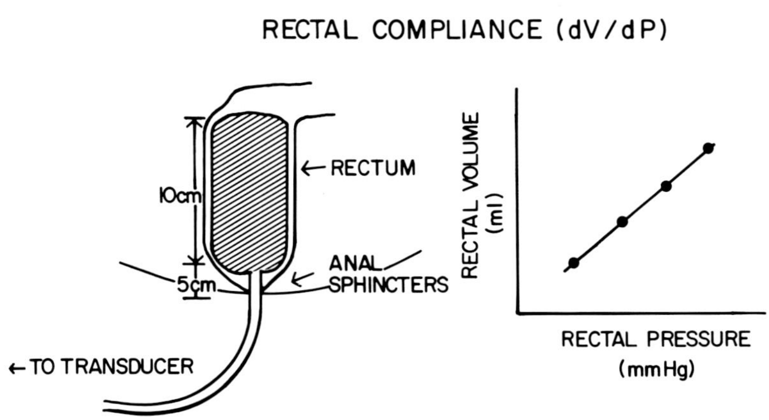

Fig. 2. Rectal compliance apparatus shown in place in the rectum. At right is a representative pressure-volume curve.

volume that is reproducibly detected is the threshold of rectal sensation [12]; in our laboratory, the mean threshold is 10.8 ml (range 5 to 25 ml).

There are several potential pitfalls when measuring rectal sensation. Since the speed with which the rectal balloon is inflated influences whether it will be felt, it is important to be consistent with respect to speed of inflation [13]. Some patients consciously or unconsciously listen for auditory cues such as injection of air or movement of the syringe; occasionally use of sham distensions can detect these individuals. Finally, some patients may be inattentive or only report sensation when they are completely certain; in such patients, use of the forced-choice technique [12] has been successful. In this technique, the balloon will always be inflated in one of two intervals and the patient *must* state in which interval distension was sensed.

Impaired rectal sensation is common in patients with diabetes mellitus and fecal incontinence [2], meningomyelocele [14], neurogenic disorders involving the colon and rectum, elderly patients with fecal impaction [15], and chronic constipation with or without megarectum [16–18].

Since the anal epithelium can discriminate between liquids, solids, and gas, it has been thought to play an important role in maintaining continence [19]. This concept was challenged by demonstrating that the application of a topical anesthetic to the anal canal of normal volunteers did not impair their ability to retain saline infused into the rectum [20]. However, this study was unphysiologic since subjects were aware that they must retain the saline during the infusion period, in contrast to the episodic uncertainties encountered in everyday life. A recent report provides supporting evidence concerning the potential contributions of anal sensation in helping to maintain continence [21].

PUBORECTALIS MUSCLE AND THE ANORECTAL ANGLE

Perhaps the most important continence mechanism is the sharp anteroposterior angulation of the anorectum (Fig. 1). This is maintained by the puborectalis muscle, a striated muscle that forms a sling around the anorectum and inserts anteriorly to the symphysis pubis. At rest, the anorectal angle is approximately 85° to 95°; with voluntary contraction of the puborectalis the rectum is pulled anteriorly, which further narrows the anorectal angle (Fig. 1), whereas when the puborectalis relaxes the angle becomes more obtuse, thereby decreasing the resistance to passage of stool. Although it was previously thought that the motor supply to the puborectalis was via the pudendal nerves, a recent study indicates that innervation comes from the third and fourth sacral nerves which lie above the pelvic floor [22]. Thus, neurogenically induced changes in external sphincter function (see below) may not be reflected in changes in puborectalis function and vice versa, a finding consistent with clinical observations [23].

Although the strength of contraction of the puborectalis muscle can be assessed on digital examination, it cannot be reliably measured by manometric techniques. A validated technique to do so is the chain proctogram in which the rectum is filled with a small amount of barium, and the axis of the anal canal is determined by a beaded chain attached to a small sphere inserted into the distal rectum (Fig. 3). Lateral X-rays are obtained with the patient at rest, during voluntary contraction of the puborectalis, and during defecatory straining [24]. In addition to puborectalis function, an assessment of the pelvic floor muscles can be made by determining the location of the anorectal angle with respect to the normal position of the pelvic floor, indicated by a line drawn from the tip of the coccyx to the symphysis pubis.

Normally, the anorectal angle lies close to the plane of the pelvic floor; when it is significantly lower, it indicates weakness of the pelvic floor muscles, a condition termed *perineal descent*.

Weakness of the puborectalis muscle and external and sphincter (see below) are associated with the syndrome of perineal descent [25], a condition seen frequently in women with increasing age, obstetric injury, or with chronic constipation or straining at defecation. The anorectal angle is also more obtuse in patients with spinal cord injuries that paralyze the pelvic floor muscles [13].

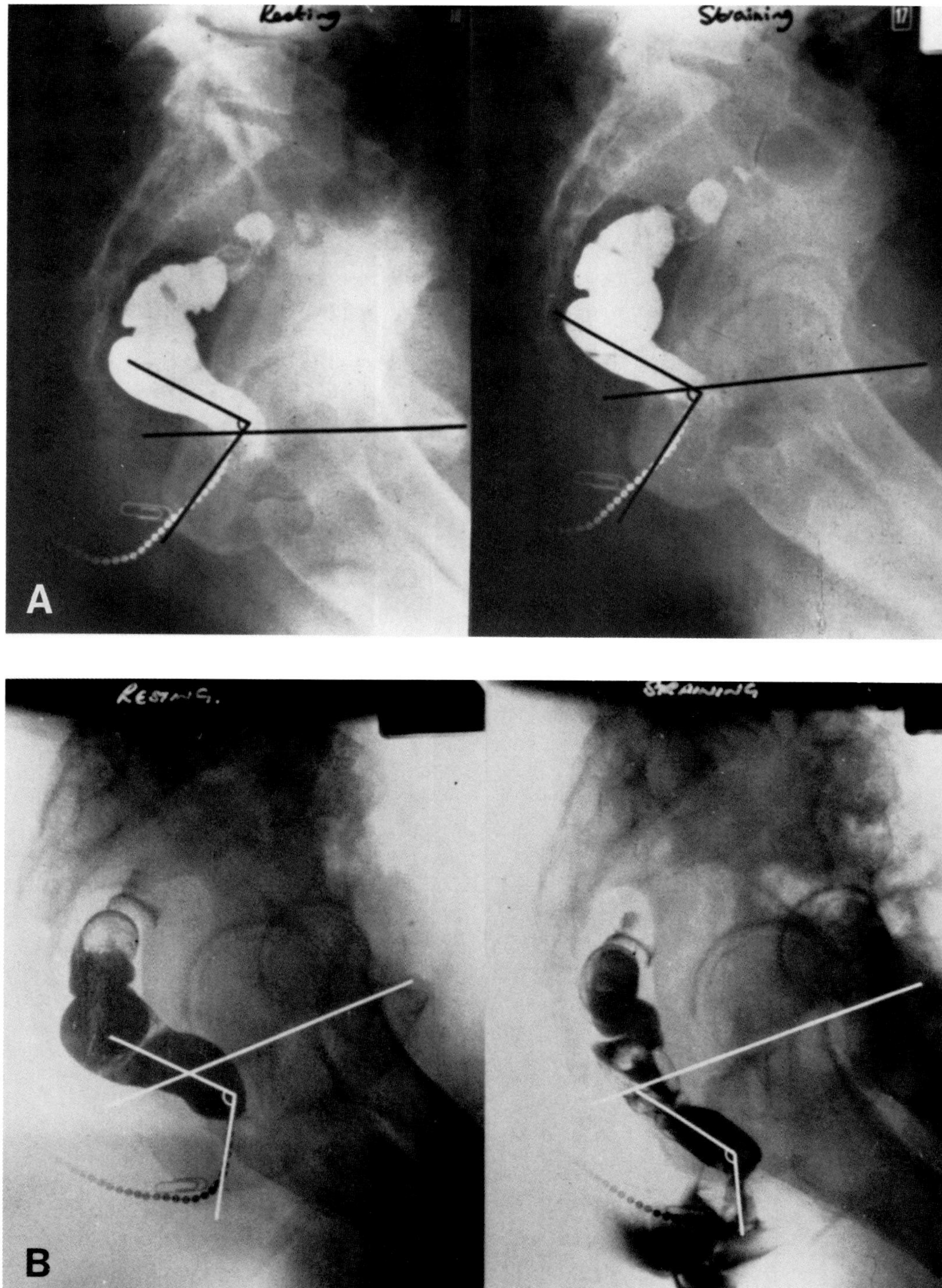

Fig. 3. A: Lateral radiographs of the anorectum in a normal subject at rest (left) and while straining (right). The anorectal angle is defined by intersecting lines drawn along the inferior border of

Modifications of the standard chain proctogram have recently been introduced and are currently under investigation. In patients with defacatory complaints, a dynamic proctogram (also called a *defecogram*) utilizes a mixture of barium and potato starch or psyllium to achieve a consistency similar to that of stool [24]. The thickened barium is injected into the recrum, and the patient sits on a specially constructed chair in the radiology suite. Lateral X-rays of the anorectum are obtained at rest, with contraction of the puborectalis, and during attempted expulsion of the barium mixture. In addition to assessing pelvic floor structure, anatomical abnormalities such as rectoceles, intussusceptions, rectal prolapse, and failure of puborectalis relaxation can be detected. The importance of such abnormalities remains to be clarified, since they are not uncommon in a control population [26]. It is also important to emphasize that many patients may be embarrassed by the nature of the procedure and may consciously inhibit expulsion of the barium; thus, the significance of failure to relax the puborectalis must be interpreted in the context of the study setting.

Another modification of the proctogram is the use of a balloon inserted into the anorectum, which can then be filled with contrast material [27,28]. This technique permits assessment of anorectal angulation and pelvic floor structures but does not allow the detection of anatomical abnormalities.

INTERNAL ANAL SPHINCTER

The internal anal sphincter arises from a thickening of the circular smooth muscle layer of the rectum at the dentate line (Fig. 1). Internal sphincter tone normally accounts for 80–85% of the resting pressure of the anal canal based on manometric studies done before and after denervation of the external anal sphincter [29]. Resting pressure can be assessed by a perfused, multilumen catheter withdrawn stepwise from the rectum through the anal canal when the patient is completely relaxed; it is important that the patient be totally relaxed so as not to overestimate resting pressures because of external sphincter contraction.

It is widely believed that the internal sphincter is chiefly responsible for continence of liquid stools and gas during resting conditions. However, the internal sphincter is reflexly inhibited during defecation and also following rectal distension with volumes greater than 20 ml of air. This relaxation can be assessed with balloon manometry (Fig. 4) or with perfused catheters. Failure to elicit internal sphincter relaxation occurs with Hirschsprung's disease, a congenital disorder associated with loss of ganglion cells in the myenteric plexus of the distal colon [30]. It can also be seen in patients with idiopathic acquired megacolon [31] and various other disorders such as amyloidosis [32]. Reduced resting anal canal pressures have been reported in disorders associated with fecal incontinence such as diabetes mellitus [33] as well as in patients with idiopathic fecal incontinence [34].

EXTERNAL ANAL SPHINCTER

The external anal sphincter consists of three striated muscle bundles that surround the internal anal sphincter and act as a single unit. It is innervated by the pudenal nerves, which contain fibers from the second, third, and fourth sacral nerves. Unlike most other striated muscles, the external anal sphincter displays continuous tonic activity [35] but can be stimulated to contract further in response to rectal distension, postural changes, cough, lifting, perianal pinprick, and by voluntary efforts [36]. In contrast, external anal sphincter tone is normally inhibited during defecation.

the rectum and a beaded chain that lies in the anal canal. The pelvic floor is defined by a line drawn from the symphysis pubis to the tip of the coccyx. **B.** A female patient with idiopathic fecal incontinence associated with perineal descent. Compared with the normal subject, the anorectal angle is more obtuse and lies below the pubococcygeal line. Also, barium is expelled during straining. (Reproduced from Wald [31], with permission of Churchill Livingstone, Inc.)

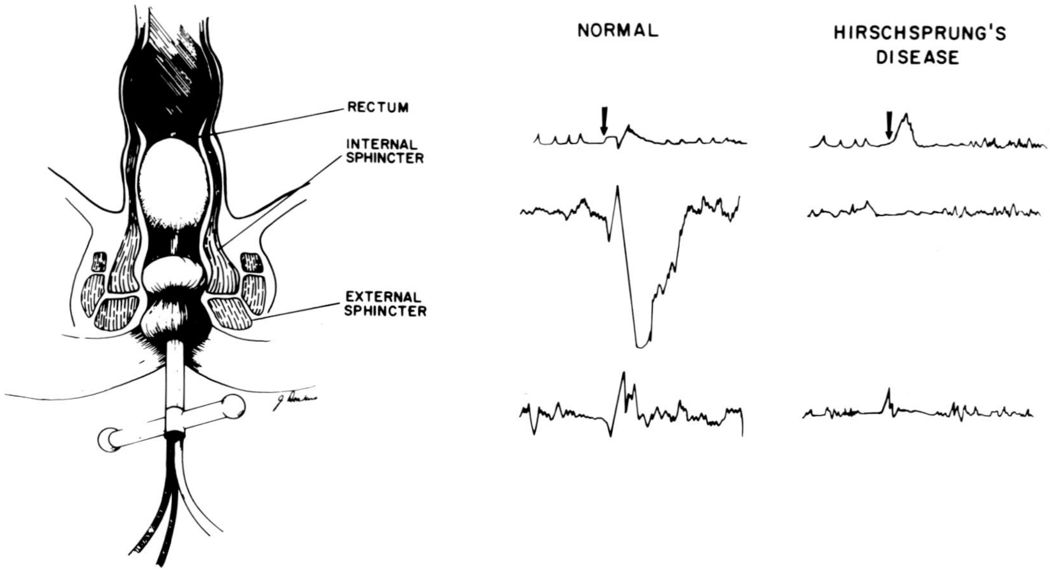

Fig. 4. Anorectal manometer is shown positioned in the anorectal canal so that the middle balloon is surrounded by the internal anal sphincter and the distal balloon is partially surrounded by the external anal sphincter. In a normal subject, rectal distension (arrow) results in reflex relaxation of the internal sphincter and phasic contraction of the external sphincter. In a subject with Hirschsprung's disease, there is no relaxation of the internal sphincter in response to distension (arrow) of any volume.

Although the transient contraction of the external anal sphincter, which occurs following rectal distension, has been called a *reflex*, recent studies suggest that it is a learned voluntary response that can be modified by conditioning techniques [37]. The precise importance of the external anal sphincter to continence is debated. It has been suggested that the simultaneous contraction of the external sphincter and relaxation of the internal sphincter following rectal distension allow rectal contents to come into contact with anal epithelium; this permits the subject to identify liquids, solids, or gas, which allows appropriate decisions concerning retention or expulsion to be made [38]. Another reason for believing that the external sphincter is important for continence is that voluntary contractions are often weak or absent in many patients with fecal incontinence. These responses are dependent on the integrity of the different pathways from the anorectal structures to the cerebral cortex as well as the motor pathways from the brain and spinal cord [39,40].

In addition to assessment of external sphincter tone and strength by digital examination, the integrity and function of the anal sphincters can be measured manometrically or by electromyographic (EMG) techniques. The strength of external sphincter contractions is best measured by perfused catheters or by on-line pressure transducers [13]. Although normal values range widely and sphincter contractions decrease with age [41] and are lower in women than in men [42], patients with rectosphincteric incontinence have significantly lower pressures than do continent subjects [13].

The three-balloon probe [43] has a number of methodologic shortcomings compared with perfused catheters. However, it is useful in evaluating expulsion patterns during attempted defecation; in some patients with constipation, there is inappropriate contraction of the external sphincter (Fig. 5), and thus the puborectalis muscle as well, which may hinder effective explusion of rectal contents [44,45]. This is probably an acquired, learned response, since it can be successfully normalized using operant conditioning techniques [46].

Another means of assessing sphincter function is by integrated EMG recordings made from surface electrodes [12], an anal plug with stainless steel plates in its surface [47], or by electrode wires embedded into the muscle with tiny needles. The relative ease and noninvasiveness of the surface recording techniques is somewhat offset by the loss of specificity concerning the source of EMG activity. A recently described highly sophisticated technique utilizes ultrathin needle electrodes inserted into the sphincter muscle to quantify the number of different motor units firing at one site to determine reinnervation of the muscle following nerve injury [48,49]. This has been combined with techniques to measure pudendal nerve conduction velocity to quantify efferent nerve damage and to determine if the injury lies in the proximal or distal portion of the pudendal nerve [50].

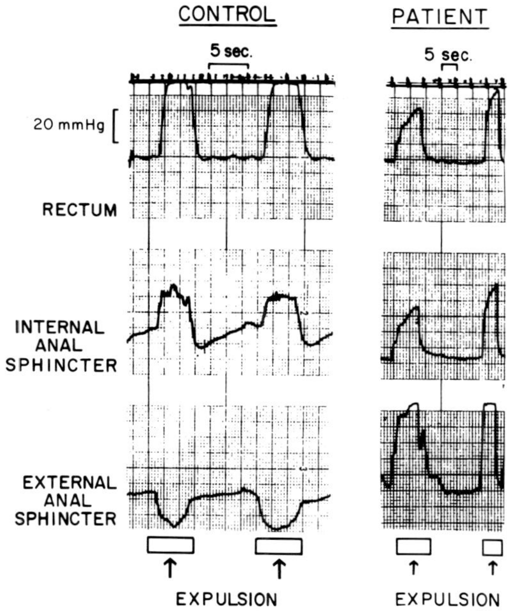

Fig. 5. Anorectal expulsion dynamics in a control subject and in a child with encopresis. Normally, expulsion attempts are associated with an increase in intrarectal pressures (reflected in the rectal and internal sphincter balloons) and a decrease in external sphincter pressures. In the child with encopresis, expulsion attempts were associated repeatedly with inappropriate increases in external sphincter pressures. (Reproduced from Wald et al. [45], with permission of Raven Press, Inc.)

MAINTENANCE OF FECAL CONTINENCE

Fecal continence is maintained by a variety of different mechanisms working in concert. These include 1) the ability to perceive and identify rectal distension (*rectal sensation*); 2) the ability to identify the nature of rectal contents (*anal sensation*); 3) the ability of the rectum to serve as a reservoir for fecal material through adaptive compliance and accommodation (*reservoir function*); 4) voluntary contraction of the puborectalis, external anal sphincter, and/or gluteal muscles at appropriate times and with sufficient strength (*contraction ability*); and 5) *motivation* to make the appropriate responses. Most patients with fecal incontinence have demonstrable abnormalities of one or more of these mechanisms (Table 1).

RECOMMENDED EVALUATION OF CONTINENCE MECHANISMS

Physical examination

The anal and perianal areas should be inspected for deformity, fistulae, hemorrhoids, and other anatomic abnormalities. The patient should be requested to bear down to check for mucosal prolapse. Digital examination should test for resting tone of the anal canal; contraction of the puborectalis, which is estimated by a finger hooked over the posterior rim of the rectum during voluntary squeeze; strength of the external anal sphincter, estimated by a finger inserted approximately 1 cm into the anal canal and asking the patient to squeeze; and "gaping" of the anal canal after the finger is removed. In addition, estimation of perianal sensation should be performed as well as observation for transient contractions of the anal sphincter in response to perianal pinprick ("anal wink").

TABLE 1.
Abnormalities in Patients With Fecal Incontinence

Categories of Patients	Continence Mechanisms: Reservoir	PRM	Sphincters	Sensation	Motivation
Adults					
Anal trauma/surgery	−	−	+	−	−
Idiopathic (adult)	−	+	+	−	−
Diabetes mellitus	−	−	+	+	−
Proctitis	+	−	−	−	−
Ileoanal anastomosis	+	−	−	−	−
Neurogenic (spinal cord)	−	+	+	+	+
Neurogenic (frontal cortex or subcortical)	−	−	−	−	+
Associated with constipation	−	−	−	−	Variable
Children					
Encopresis	−	−	−	Some	Variable
Meningomyelocele	−	+	+	+	Variable
Imperforate anus repair	+	+	+	−	Variable

+, Abnormal; −, normal; PRM, puborectalis.

Anorectal Sensorimotor Evaluation

The threshold of rectal sensation should be performed in all patients. Sphincter tone and strength should be assessed with station pullthrough of a perfused, miltilumen catheter. Anal sphincter responses can be assessed with balloon or perfusion manometry. Expulsion pattern is best assessed with the three-balloon manometer and should be done in all patients with constipation or defecatory difficulties. Rectal compliance should be correlated with sensory thresholds and with assessment of anorectal anatomy.

Structural and Functional Evaluation

This can be readily accomplished with chain or balloon proctography or, if defecatory dynamics and anatomic abnormalities must be assessed, by defecography. These studies are usually done following manometry or on a separate day. Thus it is possible to do a comprehensive evaluation of defecation and continence mechanisms in the course of a half day of testing.

References

1. Arhan P, Faverdin C, Persoz B, et al.: Relationship between viscoelastic properties of the rectum and anal pressure in man. J Appl Physiol 41:677–682, 1976.
2. Wald A, Tunuguntla AK: Anorectal sensorimotor dysfunction in fecal incontinence and diabetes mellitus. N Engl J Med 310:1282–1287, 1984.
3. Farthing MJ, Lennard-Jones JE: Sensibility of the rectum to distension and the anorectal distension reflex in ulcerative colitis. Gut 19:64–69, 1978.
4. Denis P, Colin R, Galmiche JP, et al.: Elastic properties of the rectal wall in normal adults and in patients with ulcerative colitis. Gastroenterology 77:45–48, 1979.
5. Devroede G, Vobecky S, Masse S, et al.: Ischemic fecal incontinence and rectal angina. Gastroenterology 83:970–980, 1982.
6. Touchais J-Y, Paillot B, Denis P, et al.: Severe rectal urgency and fecal incontinence following pelvic irradiation. Gastroenterol Clin Biol 6:1003–1007, 1982.
7. Heppell J, Kelly KA, Phillips SF, et al.: Physiologic aspects of continence after colectomy, mucosal proctectomy, and endorectal ileo-anal anastomosis. Ann Surg 195:435–443, 1982.
8. Meunier P, Mollard P, Marechal JM: Physiopathology of megarectum. The association of megarectum with encopresis. 17:224–227, Gut 1976.
9. Duthie HL, Gairns FW: Sensory nerve endings and sensation in the anal region of man. Br J Surg 67:585–595, 1960.
10. Goligher JC, Hughes ESR: Sensibility of the rectum and colon. Lancet 1:543–547, 1951.
11. Devroede G, Lamarche J: Functional importance of extrinsic parasympathetic innervation to the distal colon and rectum in man. Gastroenterology 66:273–280, 1974.
12. Whitehead WE, Schuster MM: Manometric and electromyographic techniques for assessment of the anorectal mechanism for continence and defecation. In Hoelzl R, Whitehead WE (eds): Psychophysiology of

the gastrointestinal tract: Experimental and clinical applications. New York, Plenum, 1983, pp321–309.

13. Whitehead WE, Schuster MM: Anorectal physiology and pathophysiology. Am J Gastroenterol 82:487–497, 1987.

14. Wald A: Biofeedback for neurogenic fecal incontinence: Rectal sensation is a determinant of outcome. J Pediatr Gastroenterol Nutr 2:302–306, 1983.

15. Read NW, Abouzekry L, Read MG, Howell P, Ottewell D, Donnelly TC: Anorectal function in elderly patients with fecal impaction. Gastroenterology 89:959–966, 1985.

16. Meunier P, Marechal JM, DeBeaujeu MJ: Rectoanal pressures and rectal sensation studies in chronic childhood constipation. Gastroenterology 77:330–336, 1979.

17. Baldi F. Ferrarini F, Corinaldesi R, Balestra R, Cassan M, Fenati GP, Barbara L: Function of the internal anal sphincter and rectal sensitivity in diagnostic constipation. Digestion 24:14–22, 1982.

18. Kamm MA, Lennard-Jones JE: Evidence for a rectal sensory neuropathy in severe slow transit constipation. Gastroenterology 94:A214, 1988.

19. Duthie HL, Bennett RC: The relation of sensation in the anal canal to the functional anal sphincter. A possible factor in anal continence. Gut 4:179–182, 1963.

20. Read MG, Read NW: Role of anorectal sensation in preserving continence. Gut 23:345–347, 1982.

21. Miller R, Bartolo DCC, Cervero F, Mortensen NJM: Anorectal sampling: A comparison of normal and incontinent patients. Br J Surg 75:44–47, 1988.

22. Henry MM, Swash M: Assessment of pelvic floor disorders and continence by electrophysiological recordings of the anal reflex. Lancet 1:1290–1291, 1978.

23. Percy JP, Swash M, Neill ME, Parks AG: Electrophysiological study of motor nerve supply of pelvic floor. Lancet 1:16–17, 1980.

24. Mahieu P, Pringot J, Bodart P: Defecography: I. Description of a new procedure and results in normal patients. Gastrointest Radiol 9:247–251, 1984.

25. Parks AG, Porter NH, Hardcastle JD: The syndrome of the descending perineum. Proc R Soc Med 59:477–482, 1968.

26. Turnbull GK, Bartram CL, Lennard-Jones JE: Radiologic studies of rectal evacuation in adults with idopathic constipation. Dis Colon Rectum 31:190–197, 1988.

27. Preston DM, Lennard-Jones JE, Thomas BM: The balloon protogram. Br J Surg 71:29–32, 1984.

28. Lahr CJ, Rothenberger DA, Jensen LL, Goldberg SM: Balloon topography: A simple method of evaluating anal function. Dis Colon Rectum 29:1–5, 1986.

29. Frenckner B, Euler CV: Influence of pudendal block on the function of the anal sphincters. Gut 16:482–489, 1975.

30. Tobon F, Reid NCRW, Talbert JL, et al.: A nonsurgical diagnostic test for Hirschsprung's disease. N Engl J Med 278:188–193, 1968.

31. Wald A: Abnormalities of anorectal function. In Cohen S, Soloway RE, (eds): Functional Disorders of the GI Tract. London: Churchill, Livingstone, Inc., 1987 pp 121–138.

32. Wald A, Kichler J, Mendelow H: Amyloidosis and chronic intestinal pseudoobstruction. Dig Dis Sci 26:462–465, 1981.

33. Schiller LR, Santa Ana CA, Schmulen AC, et al.: Pathogenesis of fecal incontinence in diabetes mellitus. Evidence for internal-anal-sphincter dysfunction. N Engl J Med 307:1666–1671, 1982.

34. Read NW, Haynes WG, Bartolo DCC, et al.: Use of anorectal manometry during rectal infusion of saline to investigate sphincter function in incontinent patients. Gastroenterology 85:105–113, 1983.

35. Floyd WF, Walls EW: Electromyography of the sphincter ani externus in man. J Physiol (Lond) 122:599–609, 1953.

36. Hill JR, Kelly ML, Schlegel JF, et al.: Pressure profile of the rectum and anus of healthy persons. Dis Colon Rectum 3:203–209, 1960.

37. Whitehead WE, Orr WC, Engel BT, et al.: External anal sphincter response to rectal distension: Learned response of reflex. Psychophysiology 19:57–62, 1982.

38. Schuster MM, Hendrix TR, Mendeloff AI: The internal anal sphincter response: Manometric studies on its normal physiology, neural pathways and alteration in bowel disorders. J Clin Invest 42:196–207, 1963.

39. Read NW, Harford WV, Schmulen AC, et al.: A clinical study of patients with fecal incontinence and diarrhea. Gastroenterology 76:747–756, 1979.

40. Bartolo DCC, Read, NW, Jarratt JA, et al.: Differences in anal sphincter function and clinical presentation in patients with pelvic floor descent. Gastroenterology 85:68–75, 1983.

41. Bannister JJ, Abouzekry L, Read NW: Effect of aging on anorectal function. Gut 28:353–357, 1987.

42. McHugh SM, Diamant NE: Effect on age, gender and parity on anal canal pressures: Contribution of impaired anal sphincter function to fecal incontinence. Dig Dis Sci 32:726–736, 1987.

43. Alva J, Mendeloff AI, Schuster MM: Reflex and electromyographic abnormalities associated with fecal incontinence. Gastroenterology 53:101–106, 1967.

44. Preston DM, Lennard-Jones JE: Anismus in chronic constipation. Dig Dis Sci 30:413–418, 1985.

45. Wald A, Chandra R, Gabel S, Chiponis D: Anorectal function and continence mechanisms in childhood encopresis. J Pediatr Gastroenterol Nutr 5:346–351, 1986.

46. Wald A, Chandra R, Gabel S, Chiponis D: Evaluation of biofeedback in childhood encopresis. J Pediatr Gastroenterol Nutr 6:554–558, 1987.

47. MacLeod JH: Biofeedback in the management of partial anal incontinence. Dis Colon Rectum 26:244–246, 1983.

48. Snooks SJ, Barnes PR, Swash M: Damage to the innervation of the voluntary anal and periurethral sphincter masculature in incontinence: An electrophysiological study. J Neurol Neurosurg Psychiatry 47:1269–1273, 1984.

49. Snooks SJ, Henry MM, Swash M: Anorectal incontinence and rectal prolapse: Differential assessment of the innervation to puborectalis and external anal sphincter. Gut 26:470–476, 1985.

50. Kiff ES, Swash M: Normal proximal and delayed distal conduction in the pudendal nerves of patients with idiopathic (neurogenic) faecal incontinence. J Neurol Neurosurg Psychiatry 47:820–823, 1984.

24

Enteric Continence and the Ileal Pouch-Anal Anastomosis Operation

Andrew M. Bell, John H. Pemberton, and Roger R. Dozois

Section of Colon and Rectal Surgery and Gastroenterology Unit, Mayo Medical School, Mayo Foundation and Mayo Clinic, Rochester, Minnesota

INTRODUCTION

The influence of ileal pouch-anal anastomosis (IPAA) procedures on the surgical management of patients with familial adenomatous polyposis has been profound. Previously, a choice had to be made between eliminating the premalignant potential of the colonic and rectal mucosa entirely by employing proctocolectomy and Brooke ileostomy or eliminating "most" of the risk by performing an ileorectostomy. Proponents of each approach were persuasive [1–3]. However, with the introduction of a procedure that concomitantly eliminates cancer risk *and* preserves continence, the alternate choices now are ileorectostomy and ileal pouch-anal anastomosis. The IPAA procedure would appear to be an ideal surgical approach for patients with familial adenomatous polyposis (FAP) because the colorectal disease and its intrinsic cancer risk are eliminated.

Despite removal of the rectum and its replacement by an ileal reservoir, patients retain a satisfactory degree of enteric continence after IPAA. This clinical observation has prompted renewed interest in the mechanisms whereby continence is maintained and defecation facilitated. These mechanisms include the anal sphincters; the anorectal angle; anorectal sensation and reflex mechanisms; the capacity, distensibility, motility, and evacuability of the rectum; and the quality and volume of the enteric content itself and its transit through the more proximal bowel. This new operation has indeed confirmed the importance of some of the more well-accepted tenets of anorectal continence but has challenged the physiological relevance of others. The aims of this chapter are to detail the effects of ileal pouch-anal anastomosis on the mechanisms of continence and defecation. Moreover, the relative importance of each of the mechanisms to each other will be discussed.

THE ILEAL POUCH-ANAL ANASTOMOSIS OPERATION

Rationale

The rationale for the operation is that abdominal colectomy, proximal proctectomy, and distal mucosal resection remove all potentially premalignant mucosa but preserve the anal sphincter apparatus, while the addition of an ileal pouch restores reservoir capacity. Moreover, because the distal mucosal resection is performed endorectally, normal bladder and sexual function should be better protected.

The Operation

The operation is performed in two stages. The abdominal colectomy, proximal proctectomy, distal rectal mucosal resection, and diverting ileostomy are performed as the first stage. At a second stage, usually 2 to 3 months later, the diverting ileostomy is closed.

The abdominal colectomy is performed in standard fashion except that the ileocolic vessels

Familial Adenomatous Polyposis, pages 185–197

are preserved and the ileum is transected close to the cecum. The attachments of the ileal mesentery are divided to the level of the pancreas, providing more mesenteric mobility. When mobilizing the rectum, the nerves at the sacral promontory are swept away from the superior hemorrhoidal vessels. The dissection is carried down to the level of the coccyx posteriorly, to the midvagina or midprostate anteriorly, and to the levators laterally.

The mobility of the terminal ileum is next determined; if a point on the antimesenteric aspect of ileum approximately 12 to 15 cm from the transected end of the ileum reaches comfortably beyond the symphysis pubis, then it is likely that the apex of the future ileal pouch will reach the anus without tension. Sometimes the ileocolic vessels must be divided to provide adequate mobility. The pouch is constructed from the distal 24 to 30 cm of ileum using either the linear stapling device [4] or a hand-sewn technique [5].

The surgeon then moves to the perineum. The anus is effaced by placing two Gelpi retractors at right angles to each other at the dentate line. The mucosal dissection is begun posteriorly. At the dentate line, a submucosal plane is developed circumferentially for a distance of 3 to 5 cm above the dentate line. The specimen is removed, and the apex of the pouch is delivered through the rectal muscular cuff to the dentate line. The pouch is anchored to the puborectalis muscle. The apex of the pouch is then incised, and the IPAA is constructed using an absorbable suture (Fig. 1).

The loop ileostomy is next constructed in the right lower quadrant at a premarked site. The stoma is matured immediately.

Closure of the ileostomy is planned for a convenient time, 8 to 12 weeks following the oper-

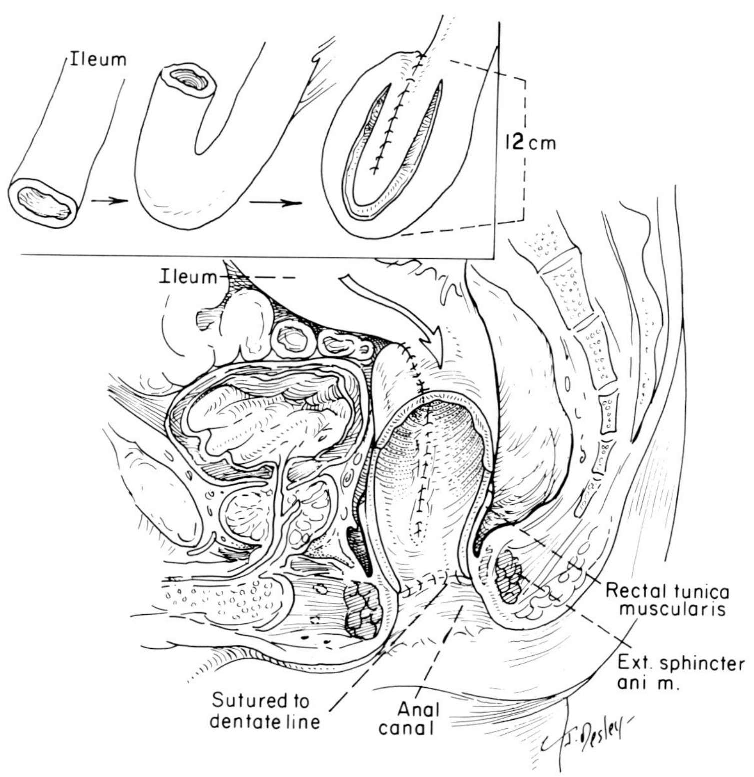

Fig. 1. Diagram of completed ileal J pouch anastomosed to the internal sphincter and the anoderm. (Reproduced from Kelly [50], with permission of Blackwell Scientific Publications.)

ation. Patients undergo preclosure manometric and radiographic studies. A resting anal canal pressure of more than 40–50 mm Hg and a voluntary squeeze pressure that is double the resting pressure is desirable. The capacity of the pouch is then measured with a balloon; a volume in excess of 100–120 ml is ideal. Finally, an ileal pouch radiograph is obtained to ensure the integrity of the anastomosis and of the pouch. Closure may be accomplished in one of two ways: "folding over" of the stoma or resection with end-to-end ileoileostomy.

In summary, the *technical* goals of the operation are to preserve the innervation of the bladder and genitalia, the anal sphincter, and the puborectalis muscles and to construct a leak-proof pouch and tension-free anastomosis. If these goals are achieved, complications are minimized and functional results will be predictably good.

THE CLINICAL RESULTS

It has been our observation [6–8] as well as that of others [9,10] that patients undergoing IPAA for FAP achieve a better functional result (fewer stools and episodes of incontinence during the day and night) than do patients operated on for chronic ulcerative colitis. Reports detailing functional results of the operation only in patients with FAP, however, are nonexistent. Table 1 summarizes the results that several investigators have achieved in a *mixture* of chronic ulcerative colitis and FAP patients.

Deaths following IPAA have been few (approximately 0 to 0.1%) [10–12], probably because patients are usually operated on electively, are young, and are selected carefully. Rates of morbidity, however, have been moderate, varying between 13 and 30% in most reports [9–12]. Failure of the operation occurs in about 5% of the patients [11,12] and necessitates permanent ileostomy.

IMPACT OF ILEAL POUCH-ANAL ANASTOMOSIS ON MECHANISMS OF CONTINENCE AND DEFECATION

Anal Canal High Pressure Zone

The anal canal high pressure zone in healthy people is about 4 cm in length, being slightly longer in men than in women (4.6 cm vs. 3.7 cm) [13].

Resting Pressure

The external anal sphincter (EAS) and internal anal sphincter (IAS) envelop the anal canal and are responsible for maintaining resting pressures. The IAS contributes about 80% of total resting tone [14]. Resting pressures can be detected using a variety of devices, but we have relied on a water-perfused four-channel rigid probe [15]. By pulling the probe through the anal canal high pressure zone in a stepwise fashion, a gradual increase in resting pressure from proximal to distal is recorded (Fig. 2). Highest pressures are measured about 1 to 2 cm from the anal verge. The mean resting anal canal pressure in healthy adults was approximately 65 ± 5 mm Hg [15,16]. There may be radial variations of resting pressure in the anal canal [17], but this is controversial [18]. In addition, there were small oscillations in resting pressure, which occurred at a frequency of about 14 cycles per minute with an amplitude of about 7 mm Hg [16], the importance of which is unknown.

After IPAA, the length of the anal canal did not differ from controls [16]. However, although resting pressures were generally maintained, they were lower than in corresponding healthy controls (patients, 56 ± 3 mm Hg vs. controls, 65 ± 3 mm Hg; $P < 0.05$) [16]. Moreover, patients with impaired continence had significantly lower resting pressures than did patients who were continent (45 ± 4 mm Hg vs. 64 ± 3 mm Hg; $P < 0.001$) [15]. This decrease after operation may be due to stretching of the anal canal when performing the rectal mucosal dissection. In addition, Stryker et al. [19] have shown that the EAS may be damaged during the operation in some patients. Oscillations of resting pressures recorded after IPAA differed markedly from recordings performed in controls; the frequency was less (8.6 ± 0.4 vs. 13.8 ± 0.5 cpm) but the amplitude was greater (28 ± 4 mm Hg vs. 7 ± 1 mm Hg) [16]. Furthermore, large fluctuations in pressure ("giant slow waves") were recorded in patients after IPAA but not in controls. These large fluctuations in the resting pressure, however,

TABLE 1.
Functional Results of Several Investigators in Patients With CUC or FAP

Investigators	No. of patients (indications)	Type of reservoir	Follow-up (months) Mean	Range	No. of stools/day (mean)	Incontinence (%) Never	Occasionally	Gross
Fonkalsrud [47] (1984)	38 (CUC and FAP)	Lateral	N.S.	(4–46)	4–7	87	N.S.	N.S.
Nicholls and Pezim [48] (1985)	70 (CUC)/18 (FAP)	J 12	12	(5–28)	6	75	25	0
		S 58	24	(3–65)	4	67	28	5
		W 18	4	(2–12)	4	89	11	0
Metcalf et al. [6] (1985)	177 (CUC)/11 (FAP)	J 183	12	(3–30)	D, 6 (CUC)	81	19	0
		S 5			N,1 (CUC)	52	44	4
					D,4 (FAP)	91	9	0
					N,0 (FAP)	73	27	0
Becker and Raymond [10] (1986)	78 (CUC)/22 (FAP)	J	N.S.	(1–24)	5	75	25	0
Harms et al. [49] (1987)	10 (CUC)/5 (FAP)	W	14	(6–24)	5	D 100	0	0
						N 80	20	0
Fleshman et al. [9] (1988)	163 (CUC)/11 (FAP)	S 107	N.S.	(12–60)	6 (CUC)	D 83 (CUC)	17	0
		J 72			5 (FAP)	N 78 (CUC)	22	0
						D 78 (FAP)	22	0
						N 67 (FAP)	33	0

CUC, chronic ulcerative colitis; FAP, familial adenomatous polyposis; J, two-limb pouch; S, three-limb pouch; W, four-limb pouch; D, day; N, night; N.S., not stated.

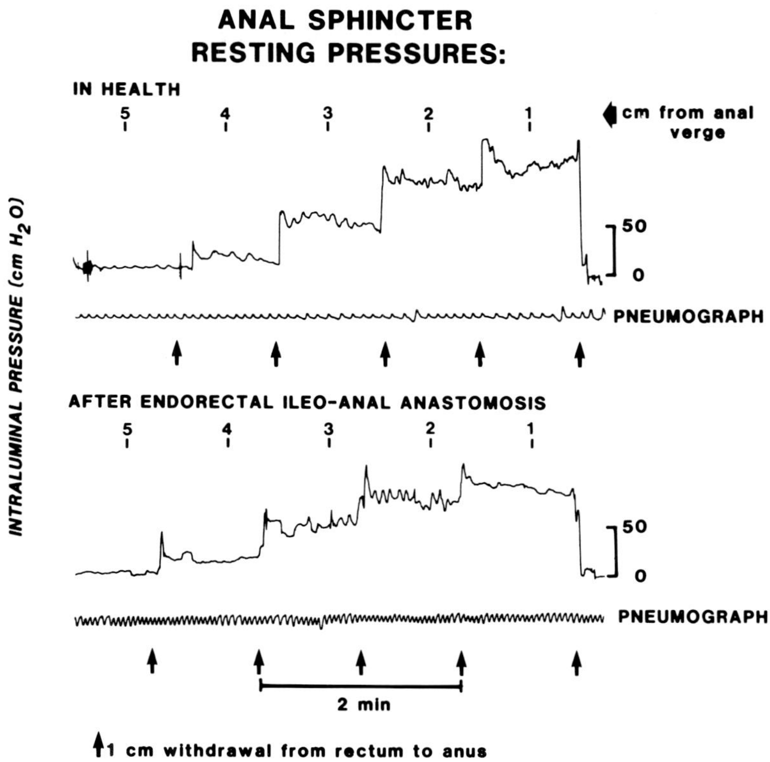

Fig. 2. Single channel pullthrough pressure profile of anal canal high pressure zone in health and after ileoanal anastomosis. (Reproduced from Kelly and Pemberton [51], with permission of Elsevier Science Publishers, Biomedical Division.)

did not seem to be associated with disturbed continence in any of the patients [16].

Squeeze Pressures

Voluntary contractions of the EAS and the puborectalis muscle generate squeeze pressures within the anal canal. With maximum effort, such pressures are twofold greater than resting pressures (Fig. 3). However, the duration of maximal elevation of intracanal pressure lasts only 40 to 60 seconds because the EAS tires rapidly [20]. Because this voluntary increase in anal canal pressure is so brief, the squeeze mechanism may act simply as an emergency mechanism that prevents leakage of content at inopportune times.

After IPAA, squeeze pressures were maintained (patients, 126 ± 6 mm Hg vs. controls, 131 ± 9 mm Hg; $P > 0.05$) as was the duration of the squeeze effort [16]. However, *patients who had impaired continence postoperatively* had lower maximum squeeze pressures than patients who did not (104 ± 7 mm Hg vs. 143 ± 7 mm Hg; $P < 0.05$) [16]. In some patients with incontinence after IPAA, electromyographic (EMG) evidence of EAS damage was also detected [19].

In summary, the IPAA technique preserves the integrity of the anal canal high pressure zone, although in slightly altered form; resting pressures were lower in patients after IPAA, but squeeze pressures were not. Patients who had problems with continence after the operation, however, had lower resting *and* squeeze pressures than those who did not. Moreover, anal canal motility changed dramatically, but with-

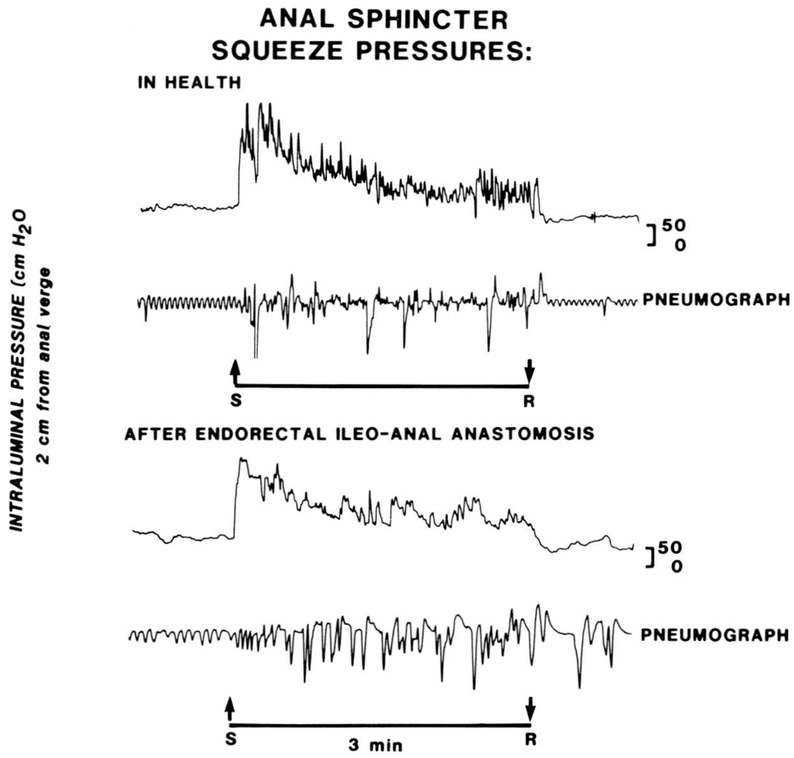

Fig. 3. Single channel squeeze pressure profile of the anal canal high pressure zone in health after ileoanal anastomosis. S, start of squeeze effort; R, relaxation of squeeze effort. (Reproduced from Kelly and Pemberton [51], with permission of Elsevier Science Publishers, Biomedical Division.)

out apparent functional significance. These observations have confirmed the importance of the IAS and EAS as primary factors maintaining enteric continence, but they cannot act alone.

The Anorectal Angle

The result of the anatomic configuration of the pelvic floor, in which the junction of the rectum and anal canal is enveloped by the puborectal muscle, is termed the *anorectal angle* (Fig.4). In health, this angle varies between 60° and 105° [21,22]. At rest, the puborectal muscle, which pulls the anorectal junction anteriorly, thus accentuating the anorectal angle, is continuously active. The anorectal angulation contributes to fecal continence probably in one of two ways (or a combination of both): Parks [23] has ascribed a ''flap valve'' function to the angle, but Bartolo et al. [24] dispute this and instead assert that the puborectal muscle acts as a sphincter at the anorectal junction. Whatever the mechanism, during times of rapidly increasing intra-abdominal pressure (cough, Valsalva's maneuver, laughing), fecal content is kept from entering the anal canal by the action of the puborectal muscle. In contrast, the anorectal angle must open for defecation to proceed. This is accomplished by squatting and flexing the hips to 90° (the angle opens to >110°) and by straining, at which time the puborectal muscle often becomes electrically silent and relaxes.

Barkel et al. [22], using a new low-dose radiation technique for imaging of the anorectal angulation, found that in 13 healthy adult controls

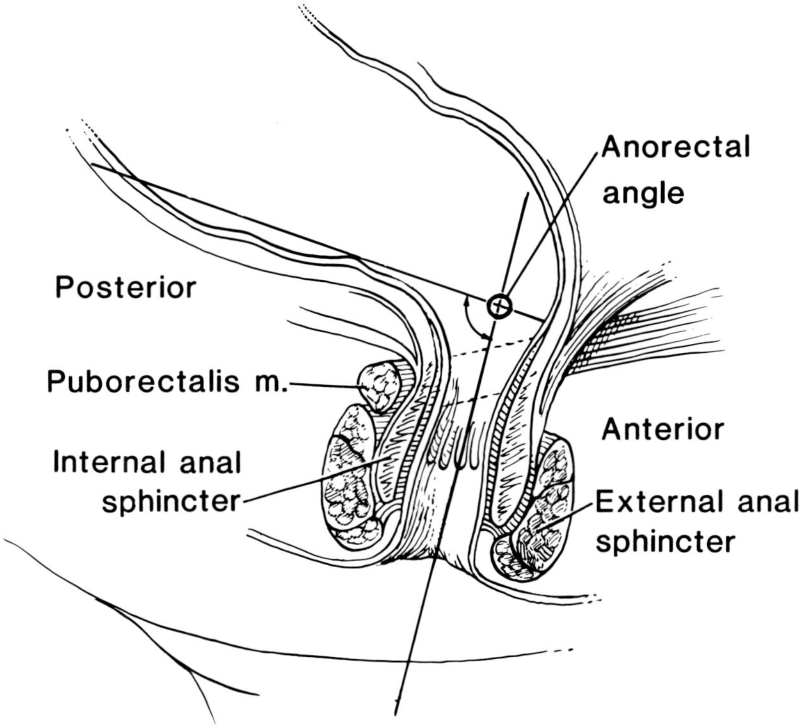

Fig. 4. Diagram of anorectal angle. The angle is formed at the level of the rectal-anal junction by the puborectal muscle.

the mean (± SD) anorectal angle was 102 ± 18°. The angle did not change with standing but did increase to a mean (± SD) of 119 ± 17° upon sitting. Maneuvers that favored continence (squeezing) or stressed it (Valsalva's maneuver), rendered the angle more acute. In six patients after IPAA, an anopouch angle was present in each and movements of the angle resembled movements of the anorectal angle in health (Fig. 5). (However, patients could not sharpen the angle significantly while lying on their side, which may help to explain why some patients have more problems with incontinence of pouch contents during the night.)

In summary, IPAA preserves the anatomic relationships of the pelvic floor such that an anoneorectal angle is reconstructed, which, in general, functions as in health. Subtle differences from the situation in health do remain and may explain why some patients have problems with continence postoperatively.

ANORECTAL SENSATION AND REFLEX MECHANISMS

The anorectal sensory mechanism allows discrimination of the character of the enteric content as well as its presence within the rectal lumen.

Rectum

Balloon distension of the rectal ampulla produces a sensation of pelvic fullness and the desire to defecate. The site of the receptors for this sensation may lie in the rectal muscularis and/or in the pelvic floor musculature surrounding the anorectal ring [25]. These receptors are likely *not* in the rectal mucosa or more proximal rectal muscularis, because discrimination persists after oper-

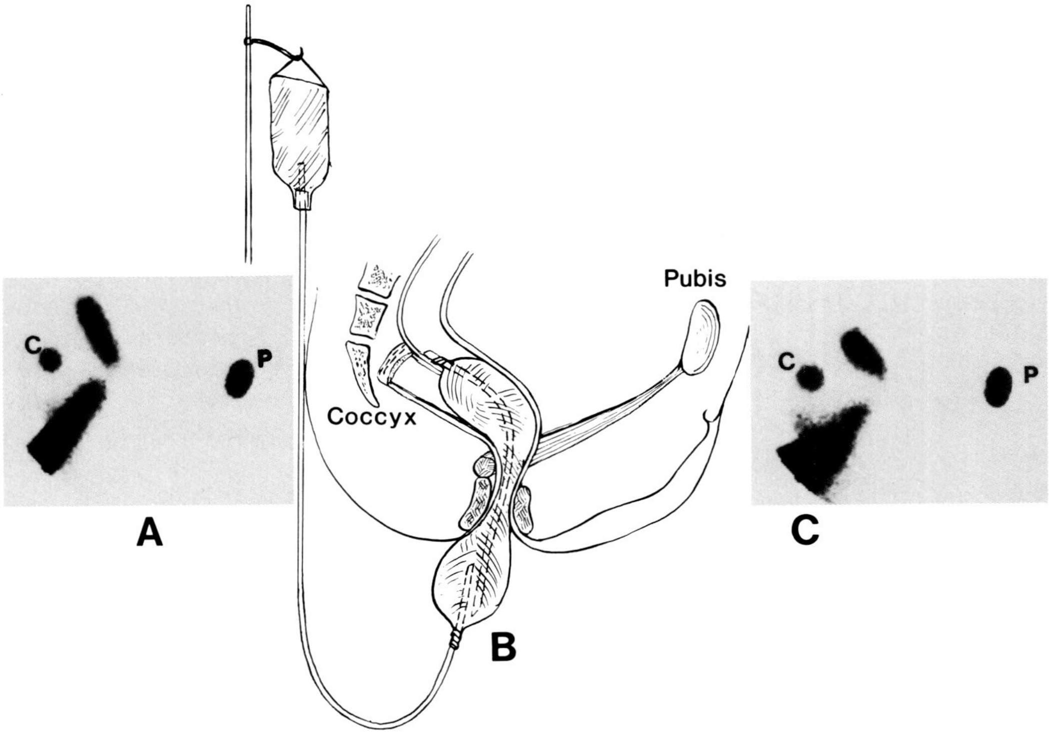

Fig. 5. Scintigraphic assessment of the anal-neorectal angle after IPAA. **A:** Scintigraphic image of the anoneorectal configuration at rest. **B.** Imaging balloon in position. The imaging medium is 99 TcM-labeled water. **C.** Scintigraphic image showing anoneorectal angle becomes more acute during squeeze. C, coccyx; P, pubis. (Modified from Pezim et al. [8].)

ations that remove these areas, such as coloanal anastomosis and low anterior resection. Indeed, sensory fibers have been identified in the levator ani muscle complex [26].

Anal Canal

The cephalad half of the anal canal is lined by mucosa, the distal 1.5 to 2 cm of which contains sensory nerve endings [27]. Roe et al. [28] have found this area of the transition zone (which includes the columns of Morgani) to be sensitive to electrical stimulation. This zone of mucosal sensitivity may supplement receptors present in the rectal and/or pelvic floor musculature at the anorectal junction and be responsible for "fine tuning" of the continence mechanism.

After IPAA, patients are still able to detect the need for evacuation of the pouch and can discriminate between gas and stool [12, 29]. These observations support previous suspicions that the rectal mucosa is not needed for rectal sensation. The 3 to 4 cm cuff of in situ rectal muscularis and the intact pelvic floor musculature must be responsible, therefore, for discrimination after IPAA. There is little question, however, that sensory mechanisms are not completely intact, as some patients do leak small amounts of mucus and stool and sometimes mistake gas for stool.

An interesting physiologic argument has recently appeared in the literature concerning the necessity for sparing the distal 2 to 3 cm of the transitional zone mucosa. It is claimed by Johnston et al. [30] that improved sensation and better rates of perfect continence were obtained in patients in whom the transitional zone was spared. Keighley et al. [31], while agreeing that sensation was somewhat diminished after excision of the transition zone, found no demonstrable improvement in continence in patients in whom the zone was retained. What may make the argument somewhat moot, however, is the report of Wolfstein et al. [32] of recurrence of polyposis in two patients in whom the transition zone was not excised at the time of IPAA. It may be that retaining perfectly intact distal sensory mechanisms after IPAA may have to be sacrificed to ensure extirpation of all premalignant mucosa. Nonetheless, sensation does persist after IPAA and complete rectal mucosal resection, but in a somewhat blunted form.

Rectal Anal Sphincter Inhibitory Response

The most readily identifiable and reproducible reflex present in the anorectum is the rectal anal sphincter inhibitory response (RASIR) (Fig. 6). Upon distending a balloon in the rectal ampulla acutely, the proximal portion of the anal canal (IAS) relaxes while the distal portion (EAS) contracts transiently [33,34]. This response is present in all healthy adults, but is absent in patients with Hirschsprung's disease. The threshold for the response is about 5 to 10 ml of balloon distension. The hypothesized role of the RASIR is that it would allow rectal contents to come into contact with the sensitive transitional zone mucosa transiently while the contracted EAS would prevent leakage [34].

After IPAA, the response is abolished [15,35], (Fig. 6) but discrimination and recognition of the urge to evacuate are retained [29]. The response, however, has been demonstrated in some patients with a long rectal muscular cuff (10 to 12 cm) [10]. The response, therefore, is likely mediated by receptors in the more proximal rectal muscular wall and carried intramurally or submucosally to the IAS [8]. Another reason why the response may not be demonstrable after operation is that the full thickness of the ileal pouch rests against the IAS; even if the IAS relaxed, the relaxation would be damped by the juxtaposed full thickness of the ileal wall and thus not recorded.

In summary, the RASIR cannot be demonstrated in most patients after IPAA, yet discrimination and the urge to defecate remain intact. The role assigned traditionally to the response, therefore, may be disputed.

NEORECTAL CAPACITY AND DISTENSIBILITY

In health, the rectum accommodates passively to distension. The maximum tolerable capacity is approximately 350 to 400 ml, yet even at these

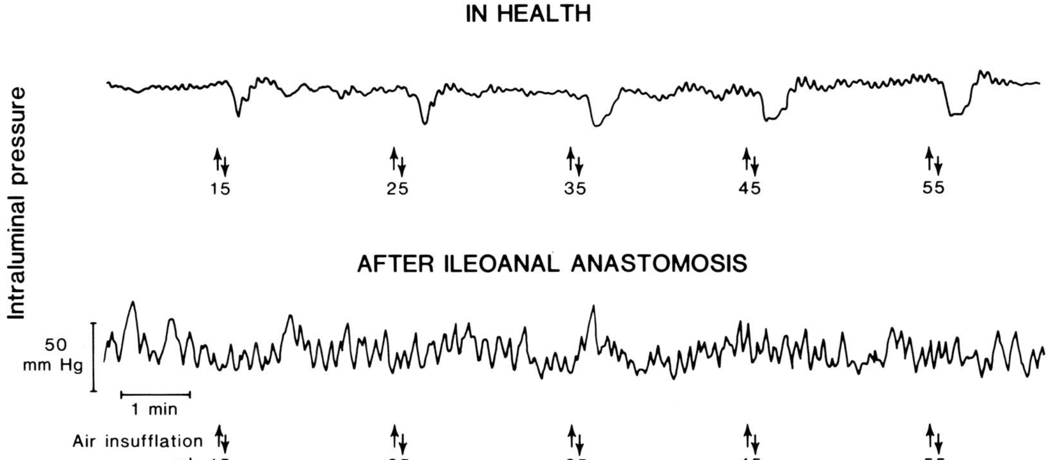

Fig. 6. The graded increase in the rectal anal sphincter inhibitory response to increasing volumes of distension in health cannot be documented in a patient after ileoanal anastomosis. (Reproduced from O'Connell et al. [16], with permission of Seminars in Surgical Oncology 3:92–98, 1987.)

volumes intraluminal pressures rarely exceed 15 to 20 mm Hg. Resting intraluminal pressure is approximately 5 mm Hg. By plotting the slope of $\Delta P/\Delta V$ (i.e., change in pressure vs. change in volume) and taking its reciprocal, distensibility (or "compliance") of the rectum can be calculated. In health, the distensibility of the rectum is 16.8 ± 2 ml/cm H_2O [15]. By comparison, distensibility of the ileum is 1.9 ± 0.05 ml/cm H_2O [36].

The capacity of the J pouch 6 months or more after IPAA is similar to the capacity of the healthy rectum [37]. Likewise, the distensibility of a well-functioning J pouch is approximately 15 ml/cm H_2O, which is similar to healthy rectal compliance. If an ileal pouch is *not* constructed and a segment of ileum anastomosed directly to the anus instead, capacities are tiny (less than 70 ml), and distensibility is 1.3 ± 0.4 ml/cm H_2O [38]. Clinically, the effects of constructing a pouch are even more dramatic; over one-third of adult patients failed the operation if no pouch was constructed [39], while only 5% of *pouch* patients have failed [12].

In summary, well-functioning ileal pouches are as distensible and capacious as are healthy rectums; the rationale for incorporating such pouches in this operation, therefore, seems sound. In addition, we have found that the more distensible the pouch, the lower the frequency of stooling postoperatively [38].

Neorectal Motility

Motor events in the rectum are characterized by infrequent small-amplitude contractions, which usually do not exceed 10 cm H_2O no matter the volume to which the rectum is distended. Connell [40] found a frequency gradient for contractile activity that *increased* from the sigmoid colon to the rectum; this would tend to impede the aboral flow of content.

Motor events in the ileum differ markedly from those in the rectum. There are two types of ileal contractions [41,42]; one type is a wave of small amplitude and short duration (<10 mm Hg, 3–6 seconds) while the other is a wave of high amplitude and long duration (>25 mm Hg, 40–60 seconds). These latter waves are termed *high pressure waves* (HPW or Code type IV [41]). They are propulsive and are associated with the passage of content [42]. The apparent stimulus for such waves is luminal distension.

After construction of the ileal pouch, the typical patterns of ileal motility persist but the onset of the propulsive HPWs is delayed; storage of content can, therefore, occur. Neorectal filling triggers the HPWs when a "threshold volume" of distension is reached. The threshold volume is approximately 45% of maximum capacity [43]. Interestingly, the HPWs are associated with the urge to evacuate. Upon evacuation, the HPWs are abolished until the pouch fills and the threshold volume is reached once again [35] (Fig. 7). This pattern of motility clearly contrasts with the pattern of motility present in the normal rectum and may be another reason why perfect continence after IPAA is not achieved in all patients.

Neorectal Emptying

Not only must the ileal pouch store content effectively, it must also evacuate that content efficiently. J-shaped pouches do empty spontaneously and nearly completely; in health, about 73 ± 7% of instilled artificial stool is evacuated compared with 57 ± 3% in patients with J pouches [44]. The rate of content evacuation approximates 11 ml/second, which, together with the observation that defecation can be willed, suggests that raised intra-abdominal pressures and not pouch contractions are responsible for defecation after IPAA.

Proximal Small Bowel Motility

The normal fasting pattern of small bowel motility is not disrupted by IPAA [37]. Importantly, the abnormalities in patterns of small bowel motility seen by Summers et al. [45] in typical mechanical small bowel obstruction are *not* seen in patients after IPAA [45]. This may be due to the fact that obstruction of aboral flow of ileal content is *intermittent*. The HPWs that are recorded in the ileal pouch as it fills can also be recorded from the ileum and distal jejunum proximal to the pouch. These HPWs, however, are not associated with the urge to defecate and may occur in re-

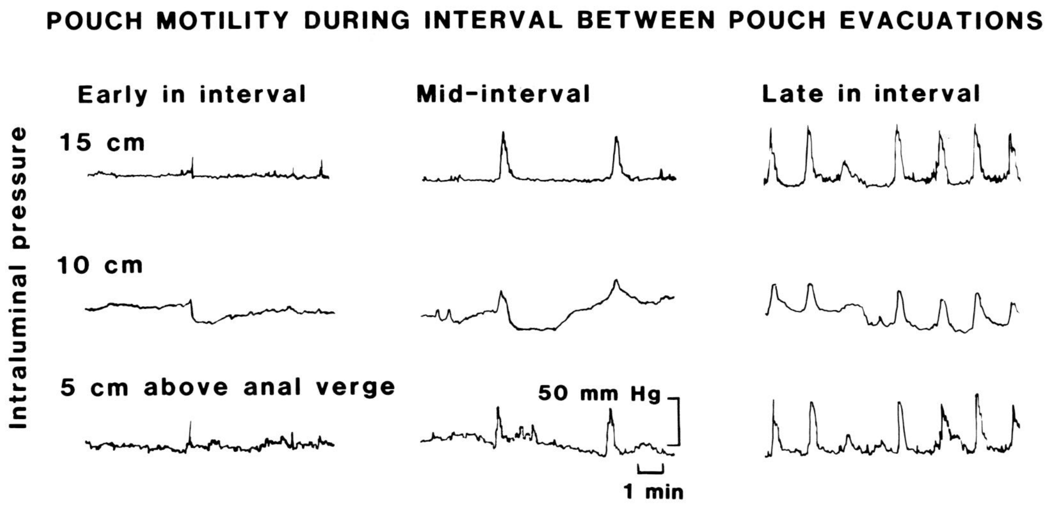

Fig. 7. Recording of high pressure waves from an ileal pouch after ileal pouch-anal anastomosis. As the pouch fills (late in interval), the frequency of these waves increases. The waves are associated with the urge to evacuate. (Reproduced from Stryker et al. [35], with permission of Annals of Surgery 203:55–61, 1986.)

sponse to filling of the pouch. This may further stress the continence mechanism.

Content

In healthy persons, the colon absorbs more than 90% of the 1,000 to 1,500 ml of fluid presented to it each day; the resulting fluid volume of 100 to 150 ml [46] is then passed with a frequency of between three stools per day and three stools per week.

After IPAA, the volume excreted each day increases to between 400 and 800 ml [43]. Storage of content in the pouch does not of itself lessen or increase these amounts, as 400–800 ml is the normal volume output from standard well-functioning Brooke ileostomies. We have recently confirmed that the most important determinant of stool frequency after IPAA may well be the total content output for 24 hours [37]. Maneuvers aimed at moderating this volume output usually fail, but do slow transit of content (Loperamide hydrochloride) and bulk the stools (Metamucil) such that the stool is less liquid, less irritating, and perhaps more easily perceived and retained voluntarily. Measures that would increase absorption and thus reduce net output would be welcome.

COMMENTS

More than 90% of patients achieve continence after IPAA. This occurs because adequate reservoir function is restored by constructing an ileal pouch and because a functioning pelvic floor and anal canal continence mechanisms are preserved. These mechanisms function as an efficient barrier to outflow yet perform relatively normally during defecation.

Some patients, however, have episodes of fecal spotting, urgency, and frequent stools. Entirely normal patterns of enteric continence cannot be restored by the operation. This is not surprising given the observations that pelvic ileal pouches possess motility characteristics distinctly different from the normal rectum and that the character and consistency of enteric content is likewise wholly different from the situation in health. Moreover, after IPAA, the RASIR is abolished and resting anal canal pressures are lower than in health. If the EAS is also damaged during the operation, then patients are even more likely to have episodes of incontinence. Furthermore, new signals of impending defecation (the HPWs) must be recognized and acted upon.

Nevertheless, the overall success of the procedure illustrates that some mechanisms of continence may not be as important as others. These include an intact rectal muscular wall, the RASIR, and proximal anal canal sensation. It is certainly possible that although these mechanisms are not needed for *gross* fecal continence, subtle problems with continence occur if they are destroyed.

If it is accepted, however, that enteric continence is the ability to *willfully* defer defecation until a suitable time and place is found, then patients after IPAA *are* continent. By studying the various mechanisms that act together to maintain enteric continence after IPAA, knowledge of their interactions will improve. This may in turn prompt changes and modifications in the operative technique that may facilitate better long-term function. We have learned thus far that efforts in the future will need to be directed toward increasing stool consistency, decreasing stool volume, ensuring complete pouch evacuation, and minimizing postoperative complications.

There is little doubt that this new operation is demanding, that complications occur, that not all patients are candidates, and that stool habits are changed rather dramatically for patients with FAP. Nevertheless, given the fact that the only other surgical option that *eliminates* colorectal cancer risk is proctocolectomy and Brooke ileostomy, IPAA must be seen as an important advance in the management of patients with familial adenomatous polyposis.

ACKNOWLEDGMENTS

This work was supported in part by USPHS NIH grant DK 37990 and by the Mayo Foundation.

References

1. Moertel CG, Hill JR, Adson MA: Surgical management of multiple polyposis. Arch Surg 100:521–526, 1970.
2. Bess MA, Adson MA, Elveback LR, Moertel CG: Rectal cancer following colectomy for polyposis. Arch Surg 115:460–467, 1980.
3. Bussey HJR, Eyers AA, Ritchie SM, Thomson JPS: The rectum in adenomatous polyposis: The St. Mark's policy. Br J Surg [Suppl] 72:529–531, 1985.
4. Ballantyne GH, Pemberton JH, Beart RW Jr, Wolff BG, Dozois RR: Ileal J pouch-anal anastomosis: Current technique. Dis Colon Rectum 28:197–202, 1985.
5. Kelly KA: Ileal pouch-anal anastomosis after proctocolectomy. Surgical Rounds 8:48–47, 1985.
6. Metcalf AM, Dozois RR, Kelly KA, Beart RW Jr, Wolff BG: Ileal "J" pouch anal anastomosis: Clinical outcome. Ann Surg 202:735–739, 1985.
7. Taylor BA, Dozois RR: The J ileal pouch-anal anastomosis. World J Surg 11:727–734, 1987.
8. Pezim ME, Pemberton JH, Dozois RR: Enteric continence and the ileal pouch-anal procedure. Semin Surg Oncol 3:92–98, 1987.
9. Fleshman JW, Cohen Z, McLeod RS, Stern H, Blair J: The ileal reservoir and ileoanal anastomosis procedure—Factors affecting technical and functional outcome. Dis Colon Rectum 31:10–16, 1988.
10. Becker JM, Raymond JL: Ileal pouch-anal anastomosis: A single surgeon's experience with 100 consecutive cases. Ann Surg 204:375–383, 1986.
11. Williams NS, Johnston D: The current status of mucosal proctectomy and ileoanal anastomosis in the surgical treatment of ulcerative colitis and adenomatous polyposis. Br J Surg 72:159–168, 1985.
12. Pemberton JH, Kelly KA, Beart RW Jr, Dozois RR, Wolff BG, Ilstrup D: Ileal pouch-anal anastomosis for chronic ulcerative colitis: Long-term results. Ann Surg 206:504–513, 1987.
13. Nivatvongs S, Stern HS, Fryd DS: The length of the anal canal. Dis Colon Rectum 24:600–601, 1981.
14. Freckner B, Euler CV: Influence of pudendal block on the function of the anal sphincters. Gut 16:482–489, 1975.
15. Heppell J, Kelly KA, Phillips SF, Beart RW Jr, Telander RL, Perrault J: Physiologic aspects of continence after colectomy, mucosal proctectomy and endorectal ileoanal anastomosis. Ann Surg 195:435–443, 1982.
16. O'Connell PR, Stryker SJ, Metcalf AM, Pemberton JH, Kelly KA: Anal canal pressure and motility after ileoanal anastomosis. Surg Gynecol Obstet 166:47–54, 1988.
17. Taylor BM, Beart RW Jr, Phillips SF: Longitudinal and radial variation of pressure in the human anal sphincter. Gastroenterology 86:693–697, 1984.
18. Miller R, Bartolo DCC, Roe AM, Mortensen NJM: Assessment of microtransducer in anorectal manometry. Br J Surg 75:40–43,1988.
19. Stryker SJ, Daube JR, Kelly KA, Telander RL, Phillips SF, Beart RW Jr, Dozois RR: Anal sphincter electromyography after colectomy, mucosal rectectomy and ileoanal anastomosis. Arch Surg 120:713–716, 1985.
20. Phillips SF, Edwards DAW: Some aspects of anal continence and defecation. Gut 6:396–406, 1965.
21. Hardcastle JD, Parks AG: A study of anal incontinence and some principles of surgical treatment. Proc R Soc Med [Suppl] 63:116–118, 1970.
22. Barkel DC, Pemberton JH, Phillips SF, Kelly KA, Brown ML: Scintigraphic assessment of the anorectal

angle in health and following ileal pouch-anal anastomosis. Ann Surg 208:42–49, 1988.

23. Parks AG: Anorectal continence. Proc R Soc Med 68:681–690, 1975.
24. Bartolo DCC, Roe AM, Locke-Edmunds J, Virjee J, Mortenson NJM: Flap valve theory of anorectal continence. Br J Surg 73:1012–1014, 1986.
25. Pemberton JH, Kelly KA: Achieving enteric continence: Principles and application. Mayo Clin Proc 61:586–599, 1986.
26. Winckler G: Remarques sur la morphologie et l'innervation du muscle relevent de l'anus. Arch Anat Histol Embryol (Strasb) 41:77–95, 1958.
27. Duthie HL, Gairns FW: Sensory nerve endings and sensation in the anal region of man. Br J Surg 47:585–595, 1960.
28. Roe AM, Bartolo DCC, Mortenson NJM: New method for assessment of anal sensation in various anorectal disorders. Br J Surg 73:310–312, 1986.
29. Beart RW Jr, Dozois RR, Wolff BG, Pemberton JH: Mechanisms of rectal continence: Lesions from the ileoanal procedure. Am J Surg 149:31–34, 1985.
30. Johnston D, Holdsworth PJ, Nasmyth DG, Neal DE, Primrose JN, Womack N, Axon ATR: Preservation of the entire anal canal in conservative proctocolectomy for ulcerative colitis: A pilot study comparing end-to-end ileoanal anastomosis without mucosal resection with mucosal proctectomy and endoanal anastomosis. Br J Surg 74:940–944, 1987.
31. Keighley MRB, Winslet MC, Yoshioka K, Lightwood R: Discrimination is not impaired by excision of the anal transition zone after restorative proctocolectomy. Br J Surg 74:1118–1121, 1987.
32. Wolfstein IH, Bat L, Neumann G: Regeneration of rectal mucosa and recurrent polyposis coli after total colectomy and ileoanal anastomosis. Arch Surg 117:1241–1242, 1982.
33. Gowers WR: The automatic action of the sphincter ani. Proc R Soc 26:77–84, 1963.
34. Duthie HL, Bennett RC: The relation of sensation in the anal canal to the functional anal sphincter: A possible factor in anal continence. Gut 4:179–182, 1963.
35. Stryker SJ, Kelly KA, Phillips SF, Dozois RR, Beart RW Jr: Anal and neorectal function after ileal pouch-anal anastomosis. Ann Surg 203:55–61, 1986.
36. Pemberton JH, van Heerden JA, Beart RW Jr, Kelly KA, Phillips SF, Taylor BM: A continent ileostomy device. Ann Surg 197:618–626, 1983.
37. O'Connell PR, Pemberton JH, Kelly KA: Motor function of the ileal J pouch and its relation to clinical outcome after ileal pouch anal anastomosis. World J Surg 11:735–741, 1987.
38. Heppell J, Taylor BM, Beart RW Jr, Dozois RR, Kelly KA: Predicting outcome after endorectal ileoanal anastomosis. Can J Surg 26:132–134, 1983.
39. Telander RL, Dozois RR: The endorectal ileoanal anastomosis. Prob Gen Surg 1:39–50, 1983.
40. Connell AM: The motility of the pelvic colon. Motility in normals and in patients with asymptomatic duodenal ulcers. Gut 2:175–186, 1961.
41. Code CF, Rogers AG, Schlegel J, Hightower NC Jr, Barge JA: Motility patterns in the terminal ileum: Studies on two patients with ulcerative colitis and ileal stomas. Gastroenterology 32:651–665, 1957.
42. Heppell J, Pemberton JH, Kelly KA, Phillips SF: Ileal motility after endorectal ileoanal anastomosis. Surg Gastroenterol 1:124–127, 1982.
43. O'Connell PR, Pemberton JH, Brown ML, Kelly KA: Determinants of stool frequency after ileal pouch anal anastomosis. Am J Surg 153:157–164, 1987.
44. O'Connell PR, Pemberton JH, Brown ML, Kelly KA: Neorectal emptying after "J" pouch-anal anastomosis. Br J Surg 72:1026, 1985.
45. Summers RW, Anuras S, Green J: Jejunal manometry patterns in health, partial intestinal obstruction and pseudo-obstruction. Gastroenterology 85:1290–1300, 1983.
46. Phillips SF, Giller J: The contribution of the colon to electrolyte and water conservation in man. J Lab Clin Med 81:733–746, 1973.
47. Fonkalsrud EW: Endorectal ileoanal anastomosis with isoperistaltic ileal reservoir after colectomy and mucosal proctectomy. Ann Surg 199:151–157, 1984.
48. Nicholls RJ, Pezim ME: Restorative proctocolectomy with ileal reservoir for ulcerative colitis and familial andenomatous polyposis: A comparison of three reservoir designs. Br J Surg 72:470–474, 1985.
49. Harms BA, Hamilton JW, Starling JR, Yamamoto MD: Quadruple-loop ileal pouch reconstruction after proctocolectomy: Analysis and functional results. Surgery 102:561–567, 1987.
50. Kelly KA: Ulcerative colitis: Advances in Surgical Management. In Jewell DP, Gibson PR (eds): Topics in Gastroenterology. Oxford: Blackwell Scientific, 1985 pp 163–177.
51. Kelly KA, Pemberton JH: Mechanisms of Fecal Continence: Alterations with ileal pouch-anal anastomosis. In Szurzewski JH (ed): Cellular Physiology and Clinical Studies of the Gastrointestinal Smooth Muscle. Amsterdam: Elsevier Science Publishers B.V., pp 399–418, 1987.

25

Surgical Alternatives in the Treatment of Familial Adenomatous Polyposis

Robert W. Beart, Jr. and David R. Welling

Section of Colon and Rectal Surgery (R.W.B.) and Section of Gastroenterologic and General Surgery (D.R.W.), Mayo Clinic and Mayo Foundation, Rochester, Minnesota

INTRODUCTION

Consider the plight of the patient who has polyposis. In its early stages, it is a disease without symptoms, but polyposis is inevitably lethal if allowed to evolve without surgical intervention. The surgical options involve a major, perhaps even mutilating, operation, difficult to accept for both the patient and the surgeon.

This chapter explores the various treatment options available. Each option offers advantages and disadvantages.

In 1925, P. Lockhart-Mummery [1] drew attention to the idea that polyposis was a premalignant condition, and others since then (Dukes [2] and later Bussey [3]) have emphasized the point. There is no longer a discussion on whether these patients will develop cancer; the question now seems to be when the cancer will occur. Surgical intervention has always been planned around the idea that polyps appear at puberty, and, in the average case, symptoms begin to appear at around age 20 years. Cancer usually develops 15 years after the onset of symptoms. Ideally, family members of a patient who has polyposis should begin having screening with proctoscopy at around age 10 years [4]. When polyposis is discovered, the patient should be considered for surgery. It is possible for patients younger than age 10 years to develop polyposis [5]. There is one report of a 13-month-old infant with polyposis [6]. Leggett et al. [7] reported on four children, two of whom were 7 and 8 years old, who had total abdominal colectomy, mucosal proctectomy, and ileoanal anastomosis for polyposis.

Why not wait for symptoms to occur prior to surgery? Symptoms can be the harbinger of cancer. Waugh et al. [8] reported in 1964 that there was invasive cancer in 32% of patients coming to colectomy. Bussey [3] found that up to 66% of his 293 patients who had symptoms of bleeding also had cancer. Alm and Licznerski [9] found that 65% of symptomatic individuals had developed cancer. Although the symptomatic patient is more likely to appreciate surgery more fully, delay is generally not recommended; one cannot afford to wait.

In considering the surgical alternatives, one should first identify the features of the ideal procedure for the management of the patient who has polyposis. First, it would completely eradicate all colonic mucosa, thereby eliminating the colonic manifestations of the disease and its risks of malignancy. Second, normal or near-normal bowel function would be preserved and a stoma avoided. Third, the operation should be accomplished with little risk. Fourth, sexual function should remain normal.

HISTORY OF THE TREATMENT OF POLYPOSIS

Although Cripps, Virchow, Sir Astley Cooper, and Corvisart [6] had written about polyposis, it was Lockhart-Mummery [1], in 1925, who noted that there was a high incidence of cancer of the

Familial Adenomatous Polyposis, pages 199–208

colon in polyposis and that this cancer was more likely to occur in younger patients compared with patients without polyposis. In 1927, Cockayne [10] showed that polyposis was inherited as a mendelian dominant trait. Dukes [2] published an accoount in 1930 of a series of families with the disease and emphasized its inheritance. Over the years, there were scattered reports of extracolonic pathology existing in patients who had polyposis. In 1950, Gardner and Stephens [11] described the so-called ''Gardner's syndrome,'' a collection of extracolonic manifestations of polyposis, including fibromas, desmoid tumors, sebaceous cysts, and osteomas. In 1955, Cronkhite and Canada [12] described two patients with polyposis, gastrointestinal dysfunction, alopecia, atrophy of the nails, and skin pigmentation. Turcot et al. [13], in 1959, described two patients with central nervous system tumors and polyposis. More recent reports of Gardner's syndrome emphasize malignant periampullary tumors, gastric and duodenal polyps, and the need for upper gastrointestinal monitoring for neoplasia [14].

The initial surgical treatment for polyposis was reserved for the patient who developed cancer. Elective, prophylactic colectomy was not used until after 1925. In 1939, McKenney [15] reported performing total colectomy with ileostomy or ileosigmoid anastomosis. He favored ileosigmoid anastomosis and fulgurated the remaining rectal polyps. In 1957, Hubbard [16] reported spontaneous resolution of rectal polyps after ileorectal anastomosis. This idea popularized ileorectal anastomosis and is still used today as one justification for that operation. Dunphy et al. [17] also reported a case of complete regression of all polyps and speculated about whether there was a polyp-clearing factor, either produced by or activated by the mucosa. In 1961, Cole et al. [18] reported that in a patient with ileoproctostomy without colectomy there was polyp regression in the rectal segment and progression in the defunctionalized colon.

Ravitch and Sabiston [19] reported three patients who had undergone ileoanal anastomosis without creation of a pouch. Sphincter function was preserved. Evidently these patients were not totally rehabilitated, and the operation was not advocated or pursued. A short account of a similar type of operation in one patient was reported in 1933 by Nissen [20].

In 1954, Everson and Allen [21] found that 5.2% of their patients developed cancer of the rectal stump. Bacon et al. [22] found a 17% incidence in their patients. In 1967, Lockhart-Mummery [23] reported cancer in the rectal stump in two of 65 patients. He also noted polyps initially regressed after ileorectal anastomosis, but after awhile they re-formed at the preoperative rate. Moertel et al. [24] reported rectal cancer developing in 59% of patients followed for 23 years after ileorectal anastomosis. They advocated proctocolectomy and ileostomy for polyposis. In contrast, reports from St. Mark's Hospital [3] identified a cumulative risk for cancer of only 3.6% at 25 years. Gingold et al. [25] from The Cleveland Clinic also reported a low incidence of rectal carcinoma after ileorectal anastomosis, and since their paper in 1979, Dr. Jagelman [4,14] has written as an advocate of the ileorectal operation. Bess et al. [26] reviewed the Mayo Clinic experience in 1980; again, an unacceptably high rectal cancer rate was reported. However, of 35 patients who had no rectal polyps preoperatively, 26 developed them after ileorectal anastomosis, but none of these patients developed cancer. Forty-six (32%) of 143 patients who preoperatively had rectal polyps developed cancer in the retained rectum postoperatively. There was an interval of from 1 to 32 years (mean, 15 years) from colectomy to discovery of cancer. The mean age at colectomy was 36 years. In this Mayo series, lower rectal anastomosis was actually associated with a higher incidence of rectal cancer than was higher anastomosis. Twenty-three patients had ileorectal anastomosis at 15 cm or closer to the dentate line. Eight had a higher anastomosis, but a lower incidence of rectal cancer. This finding refuted the argument that cancer risk was due to the level of the anastomosis.

In patients unsuited for ileorectal anastomosis, or at institutions where that operation was not performed, ileostomy with proctocolectomy became the procedure of choice. The Brooke ileostomy is still the standard against which all other procedures should be compared; it was developed in 1949 and reported in 1952 [27]. Although most patients with an ileostomy have a high quality of life, for those who desire to be rid of the bag, several surgical options have been developed. In the 1960s, Dr. Kock [28] developed the continent ileostomy operation. A large series of patients who had this operation was reported from the Mayo Clinic. The continent ileostomy valve was also developed at the Mayo Clinic [29].

While the great debate on the pros and cons of ileorectal anastomosis continues, scattered reports of ileoanal anastomosis began appearing again in the later 1970s. Martin, Parks, Utsunomiya, Fonkalsrud, Dozois, Goldberg, Becker, and many others have made great contributions to the procedure. At the Mayo Cllinic, this is now the most frequently performed procedure for familial polyposis.

SURGICAL ALTERNATIVES IN PERSPECTIVE

Brooke Ileostomy

The advantage of the Brooke ileostomy is its simplicity (Fig. 1); each of the other options we will discuss involves a mechanical device or an anastomosis—something more complex that might fail. For the elderly or debilitated patient who presents with polyposis, a Brooke ileostomy is the procedure of choice. For the patient who desires the simplest procedure with the lowest chance of associated complications, the Brooke ileostomy is a good choice.

The disadvantages of a Brooke ileostomy are mostly cosmetic and relate to the presence of the appliance bag and the stoma. In addition, Roy et al. [30] found that up to 14% of patients with Brooke ileostomies required reoperations for complications of the ileostomy, and about 26% had peristomal skin difficulties. Because the ileostomy is incontinent, a large percentage of patients (Roy and associates estimated 25%) had difficulty accepting the abdominal route of excretion and had psychological problems as a result. Aylett [31] speaks in strong terms about the severe psychological problems he observed in children with ileostomies and tells of the dramatic improvement brought about by subsequent creation of an ileorectal anastomosis in patients who had the rectum left in place after ileostomy.

The residual small bowel is not without potential difficulties; polyposis is a generalized disease, not always confined to the colon. Berry et al. [32] described a patient who had polyposis

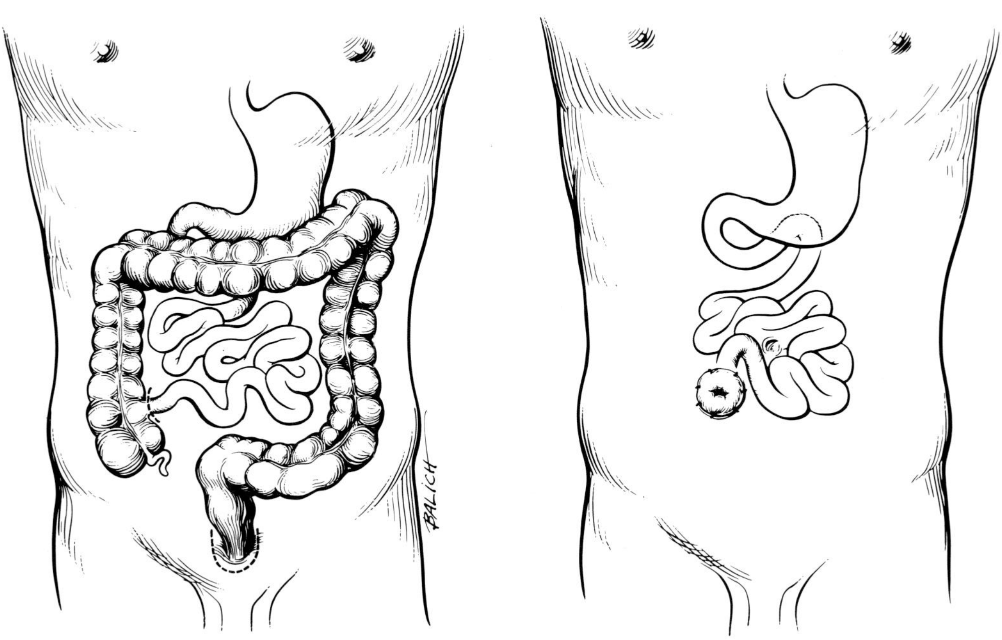

Fig. 1. Brooke ileostomy.

and developed tubular adenomas in the peristomal skin 15 years after proctocolectomy and ileostomy. Roth and Logio [33] reported a patient who had a prolonged and complicated course and who eventually developed a carcinoma in the ileal stoma.

Brooke [27] pointed out that this operation is within the capabilities of a general surgeon; its attractiveness is its simplicity. Certainly, it will continue to be used in the case of a failed ileoanal anastomosis or other more complex procedure. It will remain a safety net and, in some cases, the primary procedure for polyposis.

Continent Ileostomy

There are two procedures that render an abdominal ileostomy continent. First is the continent ostomy valve (Fig. 2). This has been devel-

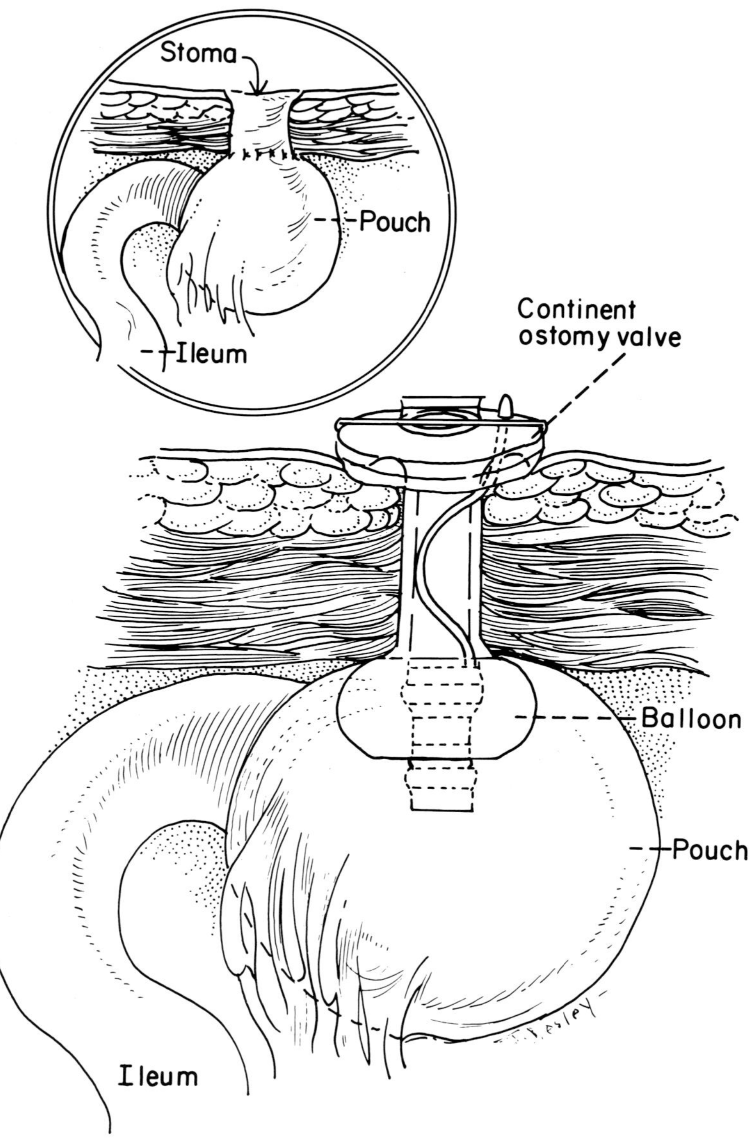

Fig. 2. Continent ileostomy valve.

oped and reported by Pemberton et al. [29] and is used in patients with a Brooke ileostomy or a failed Kock pouch. The device is made of molded Silastic and occludes the ileostomy by inflating the balloon tip, which rests snugly against the inner abdominal wall. After development in dogs, it has been used clinically in a series of patients. When used experimentally in dogs with simple ileostomy without pouch, the ileum gradually dilated and formed a reservoir. When used clinically in a small series of patients who had a prestomal reservoir constructed, increased reservoir capacity was noted, and generally these patients did well initally, although their long-term results are not as encouraging. Four of seven patients discontinued use of the device at 1 year or more after operation. One patient required emergency laparotomy after perforation of the pouch during insertion and irrigation of the valve.

The main use of the continent ileostomy valve seems to be in patients who have failed Kock pouch operations. At the Mayo Clinic, from some 450 patients who have had creation of a Kock pouch, 50 with failed operations were offered the valve instead of revision surgery. All of these patients achieved complete continence, although some complained of peristomal pain, bulkiness of the appliance, and mucus discharge from beneath the device. Forty-two patients have continued to use the device, and the others either have had pouch revision or simply wear a bag. This valve technique has been used in a limited number of patients. Perhaps future modifications will make it less bulky and more acceptable to patients. Its use avoids another surgical procedure and is simple.

The Kock pouch (Fig. 3) enjoyed relative popularity from the early 1970s until the early 1980s. The goal of the continent ileostomy was to improve the quality of life of the patient. A well-functioning Kock pouch eliminates the bag, restores the patient to a more normal lifestyle, and allows the patient to wear clothing that is more fashionable. Patients who have had a Brooke ileostomy converted to pouch virtually always seek pouch revision if it fails, attesting to the perceived advantages of the pouch. Since the first reports of the Kock operation, most series

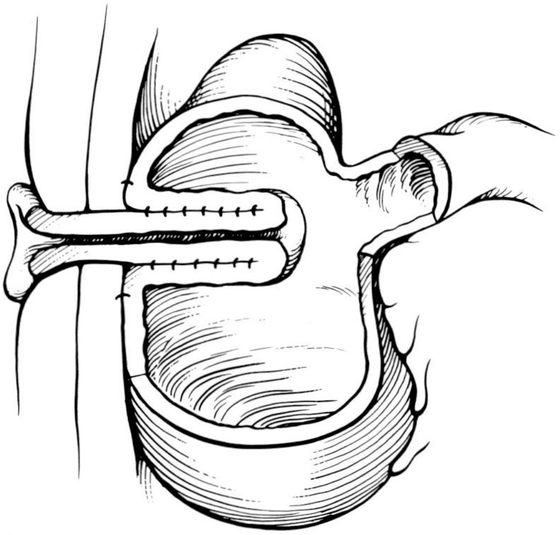

Fig. 3. Kock pouch.

have reported 10–30% revision rates. Beahrs [34] described this as a "technically difficult operation," and it probably should be performed only in large centers where there are surgeons experienced in the technique.

Besides the usual reported difficulties of valve extrusion, incontinence, skin breakdown, and difficulties with intubation, some unusual reports also exist. Beart et al. [35] had a patient who developed tubulovillous adenomas in a Kock pouch: a reminder that polyposis is not necessarily limited to the colon.

Ileorectal Anastomosis

Were it not for a few centimeters of colonic mucosa left in place, ileorectal anastomosis (Fig. 4) would be the ideal operation for polyposis. It is technichally an easy anastomosis to accomplish, it can be done safely by the trained general surgeon, and it can be accomplished in a rapid and safe fashion. The pelvic autonomic nerves should remain untouched during the dissection, and the sphincter mechanism is not harmed. Several large medical centers have advocated ileorectal anastomosis for patients who have polyposis coli, including the St. Mark's group and The Cleveland Clinic. We have mentioned the differences in their rates of cancer formation

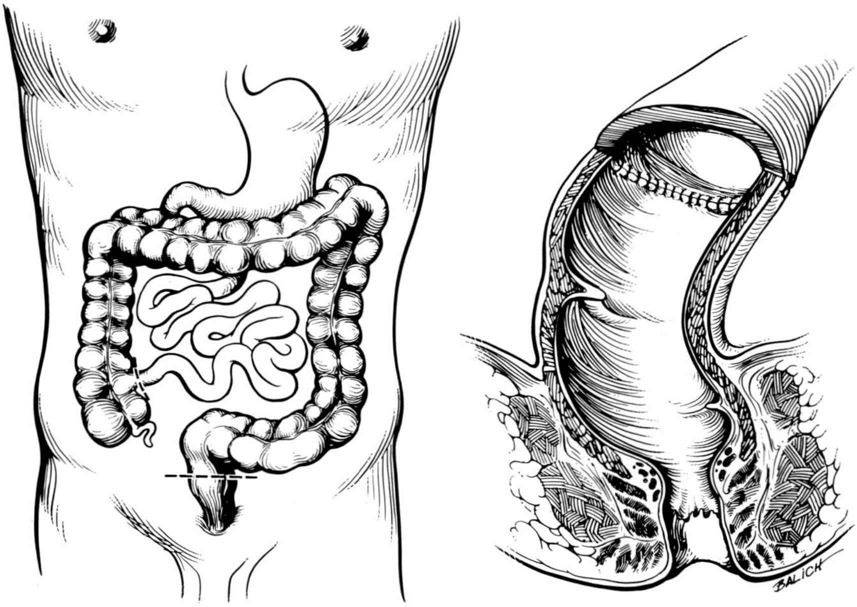

Fig. 4. Ileorectal anastomosis.

as opposed to the Mayo Clinic experience. Jagelman [14] pointed out that the operation should be done in young patients, and the anastomosis should be performed in the true rectum. Postoperative proctoscopic examinations every 6–12 months, with electrocoagulation of any polyps seen, is of utmost importance. Lifelong follow-up is necessary, and the patient needs to be reliable for such a program to be successful.

Several concerns about the operation remain, although the majority of patients will, initially, have a satisfactory result. A number of patients (5–40%) will develop rectal cancer.

Most investigators seem to agree on one point: When the patient with polyposis has no or few rectal polyps preoperatively, ileorectal anastomosis is a satisfactory operation. The Mayo Clinic series indicated that such a patient should have a low risk of developing cancer later. Although St. Mark's and the Mayo Clinic have been pictured as being at opposite extremes of management of this disease, this difference is probably more in emphasis than in practice. Both institutions offer an ileorectal procedure to 60–75% of their patients [36].

Ileoanal Anastomosis

Our final option is considered by many to be the procedure of choice, especially in the polyposis patient. Ileoanal anastomosis certainly combines many of the advantages of the other procedures (Fig. 5). First, it eliminates virtually all of the colonic mucosa. There has been a report [37] of one patient who had a 1 cm strip of mucosa just above the dentate line left in place for supposed better postoperative continence. This patient had regeneration of colonic mucosa. Most surgeons no longer leave this strip of tissue in place, but make a point of removing all the mucosa from the dentate line upward. Second, the patient who has successful creation of the pouch eliminates per anus in a natural fashion. Bowel demands are generally reasonable; most patients have five or six movements daily, with minimal urgency, and few if any at night. Third, these patients usually have good sphincter con-

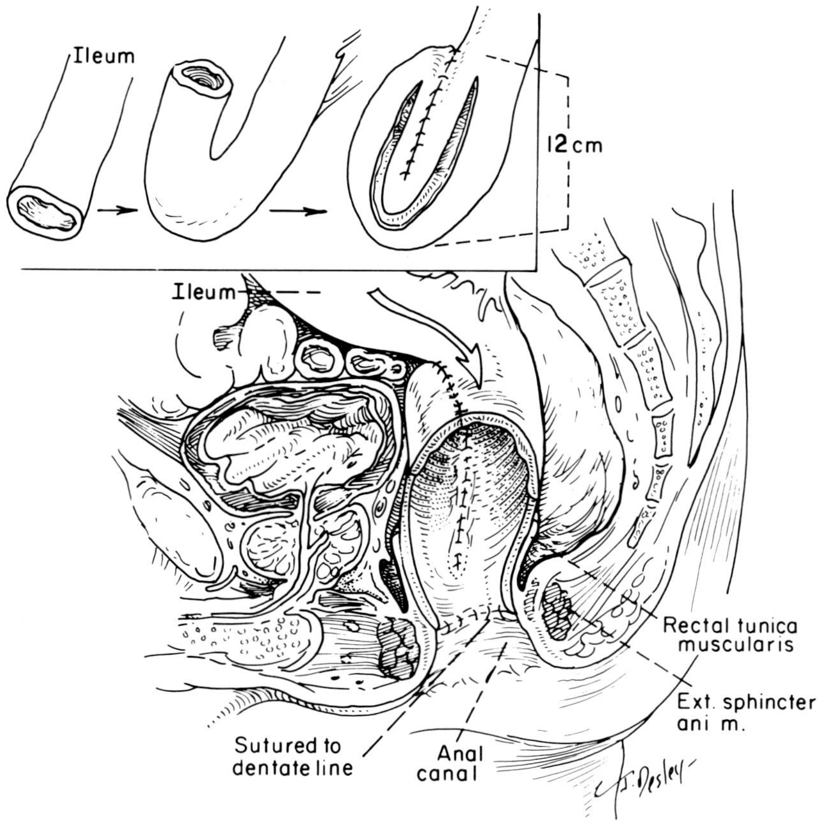

Fig. 5. Ileoanal anastomosis.

trol. Leakage of liquid or gas is seldom a problem, and control improves with time. Stool can be thickened by judicious use of bulk-forming agents or by dietary changes. Fourth, most patients report that sexual function has not suffered because of surgery. A small number of patients became pregnant and successfully delivered or underwent cesarean section after the anastomosis. In general, rehabilitation is good, patients are pleased with the final outcome, and the worry about subsequent cancer is all but eliminated.

There are, of course, complications associated with this procedure, including pelvic sepsis, anastomotic breakdown, obstruction, and wound infection. Like the Kock pouch, this operation is technically difficult and requires an expert surgeon for creation of the pouch, lengthening the mesentery to be able to create the anastomosis, and, finally, creating the ileoanal anastomosis. Usually a diverting loop ileostomy completes the procedure; this is left in place for several months and then taken down. By then, in most patients, the anastomosis is well-healed and anal elimination begins. Unlike the usual patient who has colitis and has been chronically ill, the patient who has polyposis can be expected to weather this operation with fewer difficulties.

From January 1981 through March 1986, 55 patients with familial adenomatous polyposis had an ileoanal anastomosis at the Mayo Clinic. All but four of the patients had a pouch created. Forty-eight of the 55 patients had ileostomies at the same time; of the seven who were not diverted, no postoperative difficulties were noted. None of the 55 had postoperative pelvic sepsis, but there was postoperative small bowel obstruction in eight of the 55, and three of the eight required reoperation. Only one patient developed "pouchitis," a much lower incidence than in the colitis group. Thus far, there is no evidence of polyps forming in the ileal pouch in any of these patients.

Carcinomas were found in four of the 55 patients at the time of surgery. One patient has postoperative impotence. Two patients had desmoid tumors at surgery, and a third patient developed a desmoid postoperatively. There is a high degree of satisfaction among these patients, and most of them are fully rehabilitated and lead normal lives after the ileostomy takedown.

References

1. Lockhart-Mummery P: Cancer and heredity. Lancet 1:427–429, 1925.
2. Dukes C: The heredity factor in polyposis intestini, or multiple adenomata. Cancer Rev 5:241–256, 1930.
3. Bussey HJR: Familial Polyposis Coli: Family Studies, Histopathology, Differential Diagnosis, and Results of Treatment. Baltimore: Johns Hopkins University Press, 1975, p 69.
4. Gebert HF, Jagelman DG, McGannon E: Familial polyposis coli. Am Fam Physician 33:127–137, 1986.
5. Reed TE, Neel JV: A genetic study of multiple polyposis of the colon (with an appendix deriving a method of estimating relative fitness). Am J Hum Genet 7:236–263, 1955.
6. Watne AL: Syndromes of polyposis coli and cancer. Curr Prob Cancer 7:1–31, 1982.
7. Leggett PL, Arensman RM, Falterman KW: Familial polyposis in children: Early detection and preferred treatment. South Med J 77:462–464, 1984.
8. Waugh JM, Harp RA, Spencer RJ: The surgical management of multiple polyposis. Ann Surg 159:149–154, 1964.
9. Alm T, Licznerski G: The intestinal polyposes. Clin Gastroenterol 2:577–602, 1973.
10. Cockayne EA: Heredity in relation to cancer. Cancer Rev 2:337–347, 1927.
11. Gardner EJ, Stephens FE: Cancer of the lower digestive tract in one family group. Am J Hum Genet 2:41–48, 1950.
12. Cronkhite LW Jr, Canada WJ: Generalized gastrointestinal polyposis: An unusual syndrome of polyposis, pigmentation, alopecia and onychotrophia. N Engl J Med 252:1011–1015, 1955.
13. Turcot J, Després J-P, St Pierre F: Malignant tumors of the central nervous system associated with familial polyposis of the colon: Report of two cases. Dis Colon Rectum 2:465–468, 1959.
14. Jagelman DG: Familial polyposis coli. Surg Clin North Am 63:117–128, 1983.
15. McKenney DC: Multiple polyposis: Congenital, heredofamilial, malignant. Am J Surg 46:204–216, 1939.
16. Hubbard TB Jr: Familial polyposis of the colon: The fate of the retained rectum after colectomy in children. Am Surg 23:577–586, 1957.
17. Dunphy JE, Patterson WB, Legg MA: Etiologic factors in polyposis and carcinoma of the colon. Ann Surg 150:488–496, 1959.
18. Cole JW, McKalen A, Powell J: The role of ileal contents in the spontaneous regression of rectal adenomas. Dis Colon Rectum 4:413–418, 1961.
19. Ravitch MM, Sabiston DC Jr: Anal ileostomy with preservation of the sphincter: A proposed operation in patients requiring total colectomy for benign lesions. Surg Gynecol Obstet 84:1095–1099, 1947.
20. Nissen: Demonstrationen aus der operativen Chirurgie Zunächst einige Beobachtungen aus der plastischen Chirurgie. Zentralbl Chir 60:883–888, 1933.
21. Everson TC, Allen MJ: Subtotal colectomy with ileosigmoidostomy and fulguration of polyps in retained colon: Evaluation as method of treatment of polyposis (adenomatosis) of colon. Arch Surg 69:806–817, 1954.
22. Bacon HE, Giambalvo GP, Sauer I, Fleming JP, Villalba G: Intestinal polyposis. J Int Coll Surg 28:346–356, 1957.
23. Lockhart-Mummery HE: Intestinal polyposis: The present position. Proc R Soc Med 60:381–388, 1967.
24. Moertel CG, Hill JR, Adson MA: Surgical management of multiple polyposis: The problem of cancer in the retained bowel segment. Arch Surg 100:521–525, 1970.
25. Gingold BS, Jagelman D, Turnbull RB: Surgical management of familial polyposis and Gardner's syndrome. Am J Surg 137:54–56, 1979.
26. Bess MA, Adson MA, Elveback LR, Moertel CG: Rectal cancer following colectomy for polyposis. Arch Surg 115:460–466, 1980.
27. Brooke BN: Historical perspectives. In Dozois RR (ed): Alternatives to Conventional Ileostomy. Chicago: Year Book Medical Publishers, 1985, pp 19–28.
28. Kock NG: Intra-abdominal "reservoir" in patients with permanent ileostomy: Preliminary observations on a procedure resulting in fecal "continence" in five ileostomy patients. Arch Surg 99:223–230, 1969.
29. Pemberton JH, Kelly KA, Beart RW Jr: Achieving ileostomy continence with a prestomal ileal pouch and a stomal occlusive device. Surgery 94:72–77, 1983.
30. Roy PH, Sauer WG, Beahrs OH, Farrow GM: Experience with ileostomies: Evaluation of long-term rehabilitation in 497 patients. Am J Surg 119:77–85, 1970.
31. Aylett S: Comments. In Dozois RR (ed): Alternatives to Conventional Ileostomy. Chicago: Year Book Medical Publishers, 1985, pp 122–125.
32. Berry AR, Thomson D, Macintyre IMC, McNair TJ: Peristomal cutaneous tubular adenomas following proctocolectomy for polyposis coli. J R Coll Surg Edinb 28:108–111, 1983.
33. Roth JA, Logio T: Carcinoma arising in an ileostomy stoma: An unusual complication of adenomatous polyposis coli. Cancer 49:2180–2184, 1982.
34. Beahrs OH: Comments. In Dozois RR (ed): Alterna-

tives to Conventional Ileostomy. Chicago: Year Book Medical Publishers, pp250–251, 1985.

35. Beart RW Jr, Fleming CR, Banks PM: Tubulovillous adenomas in a continent ileostomy after proctocolectomy for familial polyposis. Dig Dis Sci 27:553–556, 1982.

36. Beart RW Jr: Familial polyposis. Br J Surg [Suppl] 72:31–32, 1985.

37. Wolfstein IH, Bat L, Neumann G: Regeneration of rectal mucosa and recurrent polyposis coli after total colectomy and ileoanal anastomosis. Arch Surg 117:1241–1242, 1982.

APPENDIX A

Editorial Comments

James P.S. Thomson

The Polyposis Registry, St. Mark's Hospital for Diseases of the Rectum and Colon, London, England

The St. Mark's Hospital Polyposis Registry values the opportunity of adding a postscript to the excellent chapter by Robert Beart and David Wellings. The debate will clearly continue as to which of the three options, colectomy with ileorectal anastomosis, restorative proctocolectomy with ileoanal anastomosis, or proctocolectomy with Brooke ileostomy is appropriate in a given individual for the proplylectic management of the large intestine. If a cancer has developed by the time of treatment, its position may dictate the operation required. It is important to emphasize that familial adenomatous polyposis is not confined to the large intestine; it is a generalised disorder affecting other parts of the gastrointestinal tract and other tissues such as fibrous tissue (desmoid tumours) and the thyroid gland (papillary adenocarcinoma), to give two examples. This factor will also influence the final choice concerning the management of the large intestine.

It was on 8 December 1948 that the late O.V. Lloyd-Davies carried out the first colectomy with an ileorectal anastomosis at St. Mark's Hospital. Over the next 40 years 197 similar operations were performed, representing 75% of all primary operations for patients with familial adenomatous polyposis (10% of whom had a colonic malignancy). Between 1983 and 1987 87% of the patients had this procedure, indicating that it is still regarded as the treatment option of choice.

The most recent analysis of our data, which supersedes that reported in 1985 [1] indicates that there has been one postoperative death (in 1953) and that 176 (89.3%) have had an uneventful postoperative course. The incidence of anastomotic leakage was 2.5% and of prolonged postoperative obstruction 6.5%. It is thus a relatively safe operation, and with a bowel function of between three to four stools per 24 hours, it can confidently be recommended to asymptomatic patients. However, it must be understood that follow-up is essential.

The rectum is screened every 3–6 months and polyps 5 mm or more in size are treated, usually by diathermy fulguration. The original practice of clearing the rectum of polyps was abandoned about 20 years ago, mainly because postoperative polyp regression was noted. The cumulative risk of developing carcinomas in the rectal stump is about 10% at 25 years after the operation, with a cumulative mortality of about 5%. It is noteworthy that the risk of developing an upper gastrointestinal malignancy is also about 10% but that the cumulative mortality is 10%, indicating the poor prognosis of these tumours. The only factor that has emerged as a pointer to the development of malignancy in the rectal stump is the presence of malignancy in the original colectomy specimen—the incidence is increased four-fold.

Common with the Leeds Castle Polyposis Group [2], those at St. Mark's Hospital still feel that colectomy with ileorectal anastomosis is the first option. However, there are patients with dense rectal polyps or large sessile polyps in whom restorative proctocolectomy would be more appropriate. Proctocolectomy with Brooke ileostomy should only be considered in those with malignancy in the lower rectum. Finally, the complex nature of the treatment of these patients and the assessment of those at risk suggests that they are best treated at centres with a special interest in this fascinating disorder.

References

1. Bussey HJR, Eyers AA, Ritchie SM, Thomson JPS: The rectum in adenomatous polyposis: The St. Mark's policy. Br J Surg 72:S29–S31, 1985.
2. Thomson JPS: Leeds Castle Polyposis Group meeting. Dis Colon Rectum 31:613–616, 1988.

26

Timing of Prophylactic Surgery for Patients With Familial Adenomatous Polyposis

Heikki J. Järvinen

Second Department of Surgery, Helsinki University Central Hospital, Helsinki, Finland

IDENTIFICATION OF DESCENDANTS AFFECTED

Of the several premalignant conditions of the colon and rectum, familial adenomatous polyposis (FAP) offers the best opportunity for secondary cancer prevention by screening examinations of the asymptomatic descendants of FAP patients. The appropriate screening method is rigid rectosigmoidoscopy (25 to 30 cm), or preferably flexible sigmoidoscopy (60 cm), because this is more comfortable for the subjects and allows a wider area of the colon to be inspected. All children of an affected FAP patient, and also his siblings and the descendants of other close relatives known to have died of cancer, should be called up for such screening examinations beginning at the age of 10 to 15 years. Even if the findings are negative, the examination should be repeated at 1 to several year intervals, perhaps up to the age of 40 years.

The exact time table of the development of colonic adenomatosis in FAP is not known, but data from the relatively few cases investigated adequately both before and after the development of the first adenomas suggest that the mean time of their appearance is between 12 and 16 years of age, and practically all cases can be identified before the age of 34 to 40 years [1,2]. In addition to the colorectal adenomas, there are other indicators of the disease, which may present useful hints in the screening program of descendants at risk, because these extracolonic signs, or Gardner's stigmas, may be detectable before the adenomas appear. These include, e.g., osteomatous jaw lesions demonstrable in panoramic X-ray examination of the mandible [3,4] and a characteristic retinal pigmentation [5]. Furthermore, increased activity of ornithine decarboxylase in ''normal looking'' colonic mucosal biopsy material seems to antedate the development of visible adenomas [6].

The sensitivity and specificity of the indicators of FAP other than colonic adenomas remain, however, uncertain. There is perhaps not so urgent a need for a very early diagnosis, because the greatest risk of the disease is bound to the colonic adenomas and the risk of colorectal carcinoma involved. Thus systematic sigmoidoscopies are essential in every case in spite of other possible signs of the disease.

CENTRALIZED POLYPOSIS REGISTRIES

The principal aim of screening is to detect and treat surgically all FAP patients before colorectal carcinoma has developed. An effective and continuous screening is best realized in a centralized call-up organization, for which purpose special polyposis registries have been established in many countries on a national basis or in larger regional units, e.g., in all Nordic countries, England, many other European countries, Japan, Canada, Australia, and the United States [7–11].

Familial Adenomatous Polyposis, pages 209–214

Such registries have clearly shown that the frequency of colorectal carcinoma has decreased to about 3 to 9% in the call-up group as compared with the frequency of 60 or 70% observed in the probands, i.e., in those FAP patients detected on the basis of symptoms. That the frequency of cancer in the call-up patients is greater than 0%, which could be the optimum in an ideal world, is due to the fact that new cases and families with FAP emerge continually, and in such families many members at risk have already passed the optimal age for beginning screening examinations. There are also sometimes difficulties in contacting all the family members at risk because of changing addresses, immigration, or lack of cooperation despite repeated attempts to motivate the risk subjects in question.

PLANNING OF TIMING FOR SURGERY

The most important determinant of the possibilities for preventive surgery in FAP is a well-organized call-up system capable of identifying the disease between 10 to 20 years of age, as seems to be possible in most cases. When the diagnostic criteria for FAP have been fulfilled, i.e., endoscopic and histological demonstration of multiple colorectal adenomas, it is time to make plans for the prophylactic operation. The extent of the disease, the age of the patient and his attitudes, and his current situation of life all influence the evaluation. The safest action in the face of the threat of colorectal carcinoma may be an undelayed operation at the nearest convenient time, and this course of action is self-evident in all patients already having symptoms, such as prolonged diarrhea, peranal bleeding episodes, or anemia. The operation also cannot be postponed in patients in whom histological examination reveals advanced dysplasia in biopsy material, or in whom there are several adenomas larger than 5 to 10 mm in diameter. In such patients even very close endoscopic surveillance may fail to detect early cancers.

In totally asymptomatic patients with multiple but very small adenomas the question may arise concerning whether surgery could be postponed to a more convenient time. According to the theory of the adenoma–carcinoma sequence, the evolution of a single, small adenoma to an invasive carcinoma takes perhaps 10 to 15 years [12], and it is also known that adenomas of less than 5 mm in size very rarely exhibit carcinomatous change [13]. Young patients with newly diagnosed FAP may have considerable difficulty in understanding the cancer risk, and they often require some time for motivation. In addition, these asymptomatic patients often have some unfinished personal matters like schooling, which they want to manage before surgery. In the Finnish polyposis registry the timing of operation has been conducted liberally, taking into account the patients' wishes as far as possible. We have analyzed our data to determine at least some age limits beyond which the operation cannot be safely postponed even under close endoscopic surveillance.

AGE VARIATION IN CANCER ONSET

The Finnish polyposis registry at present contains data on 73 FAP families, with nearly 200 affected patients, whose disease history is adequately documented. As has been repeatedly shown earlier, the risk of colorectal carcinoma increases progressively depending on age [7–9], and practically all FAP patients will ultimately develop cancer unless a prophylactic operation is performed. The cumulative incidence of colorectal carcinoma was calculated on the basis of 185 Finnish FAP patients, with the following risk figures: 0.6, 4, 13, 23, and 37% at ages 20, 25, 30, 35, and 40 years, respectively (Fig. 1). There were only a few patients (5.8% of 185 patients) who had the cancer diagnosed after the age of 65 years [14].

The above figures are in accordance with those presented by Bussey on the basis of the St. Mark's polyposis registry. He observed a cancer incidence of 0.5% before age 20 years, and the risk figure was 6.9% at age 25 years [8]. According to studies by Alm [7], carcinoma had developed before age 25 years in 9 of 180 patients (5%) with FAP and cancer in Sweden, and Bülow [9] documented one case of cancer in a 17-year-old among more than 300 Danish FAP patients. Even younger patients with FAP and colorectal carcinoma are known, e.g., Coleman and Eckert

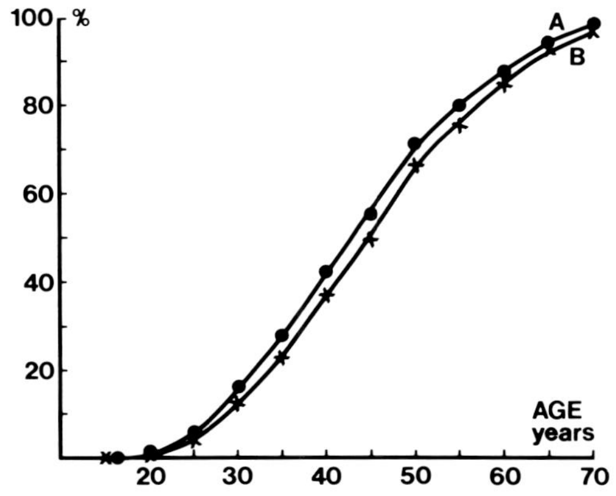

Fig. 1. Cumulative occurrence of colorectal carcinoma in FAP as related to age: **A:** Patients with cancer only (N = 105). **B:** All patients (N = 185). (Reproduced from Järvinen [14], with permission of Lippincott/Harper & Row.)

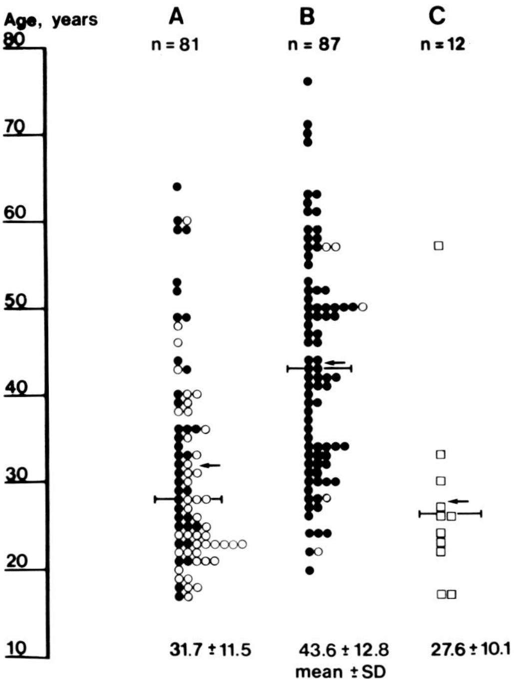

Fig. 2. Age distribution of FAP patients: **A:** Without colorectal carcinoma at operation. **B:** With carcinoma. **C:** Age at operation of patients with postoperative desmoid tumors. ●, Proband; ○, call-up patient; arrow, mean; grossline, median.

[15] described a 13-year-old boy with five synchronous colorectal carcinomas complicating FAP, but such young cancer patients seem to be extremely rare even in FAP.

The variable time scale of the development of colorectal carcinoma in FAP is clearly demonstrated also in Figure 2. When the ages of those FAP patients who had no cancer at the time of colectomy or proctocolectomy are compared with those who already had colorectal carcinoma, a significant overlapping can be seen. The mean age of patients with no cancer was 31.7 years at the time of surgery (median, 28 years), while in those with cancer it was 43.6 years (median, 43 years). The figures are also in good accordance with those from the Swedish, Danish, and St. Mark's polyposis registries, in which the mean ages at the time of cancer diagnosis has varied from 34.5 to 43 years [7–9].

Because of the great variation in the time scale of adenoma development, progression, and malignant transformation, there is perhaps some place for an individual assessment of the most suitable operation time in single cases. In the Finnish registry an evaluation of the whole colon has always been performed at the time of a new diagnosis to see the distribution and size of adenomas, using either colonoscopy or double-contrast barium enema. An expectant attitude has been taken in asymptomatic cases in which the polyp size has been less than 5 mm and the number of polyps has been relatively small. The patients have been examined yearly, at least, by fiberoptic sigmoidoscopy (60 cm) to detect any progression of the adenomas, and colonoscopy or repeated barium enema has been performed every second year. Thus far, no unexpected cases of colorectal carcinoma have been observed even though expectant follow-up has continued as long as nearly 10 years in some cases (Fig. 3).

At present, 19 FAP patients await the operation and come to yearly check-ups, and another 20 patients have been operated on with no cancer after variable observation. In 29 patients diagnosed by family screening examinations, the operation was performed without delay within 6

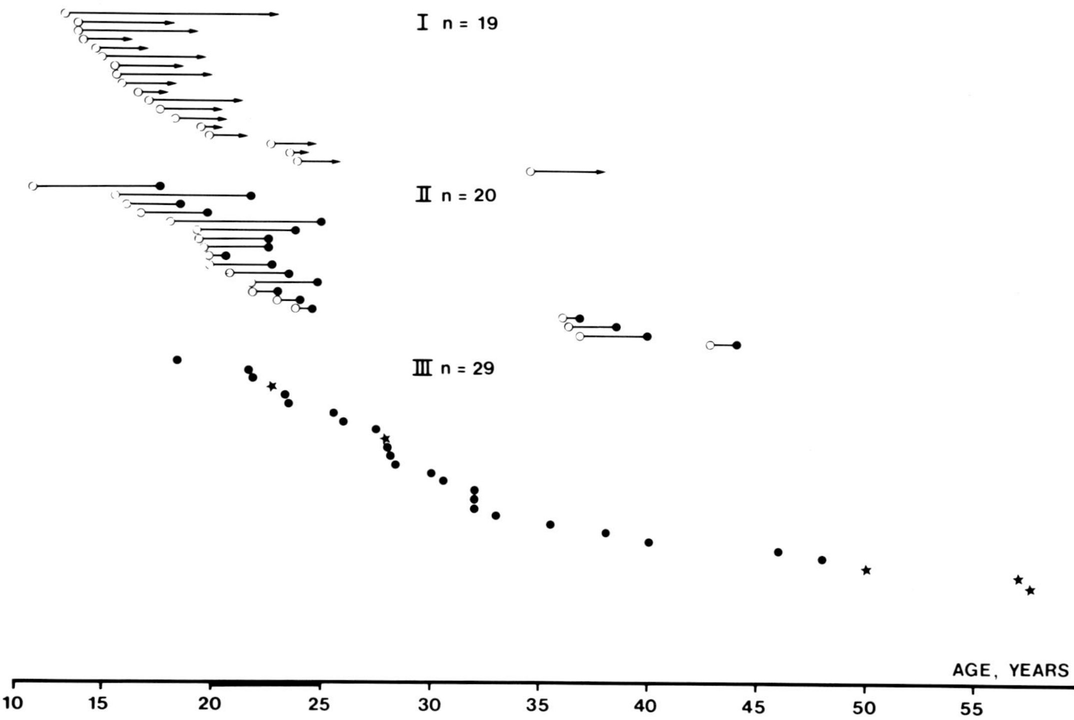

Fig. 3. Timing of operation in 68 call-up patients: ○, age at diagnosis; ●, age at operation; ★, cancer at operation. Lines indicate the length of follow-up, and the thickened baseline the recommended time for prophylactic operation.

months of the diagnosis. In this latter group many patients already had symptoms and the ages were more advanced; five patients with colorectal carcinomas were included in this group at ages 57, 57, 50, 27, and 22 years. The youngest of these patients was asymptomatic, but was operated on immediately on the basis of large polyp size and was found to have a sigmoid carcinoma of Dukes' class C_1.

On the basis of our experience, we have come to a thumb rule that a prophylactic operation should be performed as soon as any clear symptoms develop (bleeding, diarrhea, anemia) or when the age approaches 20 years. The operation has to be done earlier if the adenoma size begins to be more than 5 mm as observed in endoscopic surveillance, and, as a rule, the operation cannot be postponed beyond 25 years of age. Thus far, we have been able to follow this policy with only few exceptions and without great mistakes.

Postponing the prophylactic operation is by no means necessary, and it may be asked what can be gained by delaying the operation, which has to be done later in every case. It seems, however, likely that following the rules delineated above the fear of unexpected colorectal carcinoma can be minimized and the contacts with all family members of the FAP families can be maintained easily. The danger of cancer is greater in those family members who refuse to come for screening visits at all.

INFLUENCE OF OPERATION TYPE AND OF DESMOID TUMORS

While the risk of colorectal carcinoma is by far the most important determinant in considering the time of operation in FAP, other factors, such as choice of operation type and the presence or risk of other manifestations of this disease, especially the possible risk of desmoid tumors after surgery, may also influence the timing of the operation. Colectomy and ileorectostomy with a relatively short rectal stump (about 10 cm) was the most feasible type of operation until recent years and was also more acceptable for the patient than was proctocolectomy. There remained, however, an undeniable risk of rectal stump cancer increasing over the years even under the closest follow-up. As the newest operative alternative, the restorative proctocolectomy with an ileal reservoir and pouch-anal anastomosis can now obviate the problems of rectal stump cancer risk, and the results of this restorative operation are promising [16]; there may be time to change attitudes regarding type of operation. The risk of postoperative complications may still be somewhat higher after restorative proctocolectomy than after ileorectostomy, and this certainly requires centralization of these operations to centers with adequate experience.

That the operation type is changing from colectomy to restorative proctocolectomy favors an earlier timing of operation than would be absolutely necessary because of the cancer risk. The younger the patient is, the quicker the recovery from the operation, and also the better the functional results. As fecal continence and frequency of defecation are always somewhat changed after the ileoanal procedures, any unnecessary delay may only make the functional outcome more unpredictable.

The threat of postoperative desmoid tumors may, on the other hand, also influence both the timing of the operation and the operative method chosen. Desmoid tumors are very rare in the general population, but patients with FAP have a special predisposition to develop these fibromatous lesions. The frequency of desmoid tumors is around 10% in FAP, and their development is in association with the operation trauma, which is unavoidable. Even though presenting histologically benign lesions, desmoids are locally invasive, and their surgical treatment may be very difficult and hazardous. This is especially true in the case of mesenteric desmoids, which account for nearly one-half of those occurring in FAP [17]. Mesenteric desmoids may prove fatal by causing untreatable bowel and/or ureteric obstruction or by surgical complications during their treatment.

Parks et al. [18] believed that, at least in those FAP patients with clear signs of Gardner's syndrome in the family, an unnecessarily early operation should be avoided, because young FAP patients in such families have an unusually high tendency to develop postoperative desmoid tumors. Similar observations were also made by Jones et al. [17] in a series of 29 FAP patients with desmoids. In an analysis of 19 Finnish FAP patients with desmoid tumors, it was observed that the age of patients at the time of colectomy was significantly lower in cases with desmoids than in those without: 26 vs. 38 years, respectively (Fig. 2). In our experience, the cumulative frequency of postoperative desmoids approached 16% within 10 years after surgery [19]. Even though no deaths caused by desmoid tumors have thus far occurred in our patients, these tumors form a serious aspect in the follow-up after surgical treatment. It is clear that even a higher risk of desmoids after surgery at a young age does not allow postponing the prophylactic operation beyond the age of 25 years. Thus, only a limited hope of influencing the frequency of desmoids is attained by means of surgical timing.

When the restorative proctocolectomy gains more favor as the procedure of choice in FAP, questions may arise whether this operation leads to a higher risk of mesenteric desmoid formation. The technique requires more preparation of the ileal mesenterium in order to give sufficient reach of the ileal pouch to the anus. Until more experience with this operation in FAP is gained, the possible risk of an increased desmoid formation cannot be evaluated.

SUMMARY

A well-organized call-up system for the family members at risk of FAP is the most important prerequisite for carcinoma prophylaxis in these families. Preventive surgery becomes possible after a reliable diagnosis, which is possible between 12 to 16 years of age in most cases. The development of cancer in one or more of the adenomas is highly age-dependent, but the time scale varies widely. In large series the risk of colorectal carcinoma has been less than 1% at 20 years of age and about 5% at 25 years. Correspondingly, prophylactic surgery is rarely absolutely necessary before age 20, but the operation cannot be postponed beyond age 25 years. If the operation is postponed, great care must be placed on the surveillance of the whole colon, and adenomas should not be allowed to grow much larger than 5 mm. Besides the cancer risk, the choice of operation type and the possible risk of postoperative desmoid tumors must also be considered in planning the timing of operation. Restorative proctocolectomy eliminates the risk of rectal stump cancer, but may have more complications than colectomy with ileorectostomy. The functional results after restorative proctocolectomy are possibly better, the younger the patient. On the other hand, a very early age at operation may increase the risks of desmoid tumor formation, which sometimes causes significant problems after the operation. It is not clear whether the operation type influences the tendency of desmoid formation.

References

1. Dozois R: Symposium—Surgical aspects of familial adenomatous polyposis. Int J Color Dis 3:1–16, 1988.
2. Bülow S: Clinical features of familial polyposis coli. Results of the Danish Polyposis Register. Dis Colon Rectum 29:102–107, 1986.
3. Bülow S, Søndergaard JO, Witt IN, Larsen E, Tetens G: Mandibular osteomas in familial polyposis coli. Dis Colon Rectum 27:105–108, 1984.
4. Wolf J, Järvinen HJ, Hietanen J: Gardner's dentomaxillary stigmas in patients with familial adenomatosis coli. Br J Oral Maxillofac Surg 24:410–416, 1986.
5. Traboulsi EI, Krush AJ, Gardner EJN et al.: Prevalence and importance of pigmented ocular fundus lesions in Gardner's syndrome. N Engl J Med 316:661–667, 1987.
6. Luk GD, Baylin SB: Ornithine decarboxylase as a biologic marker in familial colonic polyposis. N Engl J Med 311:80–83, 1984.
7. Alm T: Hereditary Adenomatosis of the Colon and Rectum in Sweden. Thesis, Karolinska Institutet, Stockholm, Sweden, 1974.
8. Bussey HJR: Familial Polyposis Coli. Family Studies, Histopathology, Differential Diagnosis, and Results of Treatment. Baltimore: The Johns Hopkins University Press, 1975.
9. Bülow S: Familial Polyposis Coli. A Clinical and Epidemiological Study. Thesis, Odense Universitet, Laegeforeningens Forlag, Copenhagen, Denmark, 1986.
10. Cohen Z, Berk T: Treatment and follow-up of affected family members with familial polyposis. In Ingall JRF, Mastromarino AJ (eds): Prevention of Hereditary Large Bowel Cancer. New York: Alan R. Liss, 1983, pp 157–166.
11. Järvinen HJ, Husa A, Aukee S, Laitinen S, Matikainen M, Havia T: Finnish registry for familial adenomatosis coli. Scand J Gastroenterol 19:941–946, 1984.
12. Morson BC: Evolution of cancer of the colon and rectum. Cancer 34:845–849, 1974.
13. Muto T, Kamiya J, Sawada T, Morioka Y: Morphogenesis of human colonic cancer. Dis Colon Rectum 26:257–262, 1983.
14. Järvinen HJ: Time and type of prophylactic surgery for familial adenomatosis coli. Ann Surg 202:93–97, 1985.
15. Coleman S, Eckert C: Preservation of rectum in familial polyposis of the colon and rectum. Arch Surg 73:635–664, 1956.
16. Heimann TM, Gelernt I, Salky B, Bauer J, Greenstein A, Beck AR: Familial polyposis coli. Results of mucosal proctectomy with ileoanal anastomosis. Dis Colon Rectum 30: 424–427, 1987.
17. Jones IT, Jagelman DG, Fazio VN, Lavery IC, Weakley FL, McGannon E: Desmoid tumors in familial polyposis coli. Ann Surg 204:94–97, 1986.
18. Parks TG, Bussey HJR, Lockhart-Mummery HE: Familial polyposis coli associated with extracolonic abnormalities. Gut 11:323–329, 1970.
19. Järvinen HJ: Desmoid disease as a part of familial adenomatous polyposis coli. Acta Chir Scand 153:379–383, 1987.

27

Nd-YAG Laser Treatment of Gastrointestinal Polyps in Patients With Familial Adenomatous Polyposis

Lemuel Herrera, Nicholas J. Petrelli, and Ghassan Farah

Familial Polyposis Registry, Department of Surgical Oncology, Roswell Park Memorial Institute, Buffalo, New York and Department of Surgery, State University of New York at Buffalo, New York (L.H., N.J.P.); Jordan University Hospital, Amman, Jordan (G.F.)

INTRODUCTION

Of the nonsurgical treatments for intestinal polyps such as endoscopic electrocoagulation, surgery, cryotherapy, and photoresection with the Nd-YAG (neodymium-yttrium aluminum garnet) laser, the latter is at present a favored modality of treatment for scattered benign gastrointestinal polyps [1]. This chapter reports on selected cases of patients with familial adenomatous polyposis (FAP) who were managed by this modality of treatment, reviews the physical principles related to the laser, and gives details of the treatment technique as utilized at Roswell Park Memorial Institute.

CASE REPORTS

Patient 1

M.K., a 30-year-old white male, underwent a total abdominal colectomy and ileoproctostomy for FAP at age 11 years. During the following 19 years, regular and periodic evaluations failed to disclose any abnormalities. At 28 years of age, five adenomatous polyps were found in the remaining 7–8 cm of rectal mucosa and several more in the mucosa of the distal ileum just proximal to the anastomosis. He had good anal sensation, sphincter tone, and solid stool continence, with six to seven bowel movements per day. There was no perianal dermatitis. A mucosal proctectomy and ileoanal anastomosis was proposed at another hospital, but he refused it following an explanation of the possible complications. After further evaluation at Roswell Park, adenomatous polyps in the distal small bowel were also discovered. He also had evidence of extraintestinal manifestations of FAP such as trichilemmal cysts of the skin, face, and leg. His upper gastrointestinal endoscopy was normal.

We recommended biopsy followed by vaporization of the polyps in the small and large bowel to be performed with the Nd-YAG laser via a flexible endoscope. Two treatments have been necessary to control his polyps. He continues to be followed with proctoileoscopy every 3 months and esophagogastroduodenoscopy (EGD) every 2–3 years. We plan to continue with polyp vaporization as needed. The patient continues to have good nocturnal continence and a full-time occupation as a mechanic.

Patient 2

J.B., a 33-year-old white male diagnosed with FAP at age 11 years, underwent a subtotal colectomy and ileosigmoid anastomosis. Seven years later, the sigmoid colon was removed to the level of the peritoneal reflection because of recurrent adenomatous polyps. A mucosal proctectomy and ileoanal anastomosis was performed. Since then,

Familial Adenomatous Polyposis, pages 215–221

he has continued to be followed at regular intervals.

Because of upper abdominal pain, he underwent an EGD during which an 8–10 mm duodenal polyp was found. Enteroclysis disclosed another polyp in the proximal jejunum just distal to the ligament of Treitz. The patient has refused to undergo surgical treatment as he remains asymptomatic. At EGD, a 10 × 20 mm sessile friable polyp was found in the first portion of the duodenum, and there were additional multiple 1–2 mm polyps in the first and second portions of the duodenum. The latter were diagnosed as villous adenomas. The polyps were biopsied and treated with Nd-YAG laser photoresection. He continues to be followed at regular intervals with EGD and enteroclysis.

Patient 3

H.B., a 37-year-old white male, underwent total proctocolectomy and a Brooke's ileostomy at age 17 years for FAP. Postoperatively, he developed an episode of intestinal obstruction that resolved without surgery. Five and 15 years later epidermal inclusion cysts from the eyelid and the thigh were removed, respectively. His clinical course has been characterized by repeated episodes of small bowel obstruction secondary to postoperative adhesions. Two episodes have required surgical intervention.

An EGD performed in July 1986 showed multiple 1–4 mm adenomatous polyps with mild atypia in the duodenum. It was thought that vaporization and photoresection of these polyps with the Nd-YAG laser would have been less lengthy and more effective than removal with the cold biopsy forceps and electrocoagulation. The patient tolerated the former procedure well. He continues to be followed with EGD and enteroclysis at 4–6 month intervals.

Patient 4

J.M., a 59-year-old white female, underwent the removal of an abdominal desmoid in 1975. A subtotal colectomy and an ileorectal anastomosis were performed in 1979 for colonic adenomatous polyps. Recurrence of the desmoid tumor led to a major resection of the small bowel, which resulted in a short bowel syndrome and has required long-term parenteral nutrition for metabolic support. She is incontinent for mucous discharge. Frequent small meals triggered several loose bowel movements. In 1988, a large villous adenoma of the rectum containing intramucosal carcinoma was diagnosed. After anal dilation, the adenoma was visualized and biopsied (Fig. 1). Application of the Nd-YAG laser beam was directed by a single hand-held fiberoptic (Fig. 2 and 3). Approximately four sessions with doses as high as 4,700 joules have been necessary for local control of the villous adenoma. She continues with her baseline anal continence and is able to travel and enjoy her life with minimal impairments.

THE LASER

We utilized an Nd-YAG solid state constant wave laser, with a wavelength of 1.06. The power is a maximum of 100 w at the laser head, continuously adjustable down to 15 w. The pilot light is He-Neon laser 2 mW wavelength 0.63. The laser pulse length is adjustable from 0.1 to 9.9 seconds in 0.1 second steps and from 1 to 99 seconds in 1 second steps. The power meter is provided by photoelectric 0–150 w. The transmission system utilizes a Teflon-coated 0.6 mm core diameter quartz fiberglass. A constant coaxial flow of CO_2 is used when in operation. The weight and the dimensions of the basic unit are 180 kg and 510 × 830 × 410 mm, respectively. The light laser head is 185 × 135 × 540 mm (Coagulation laser, MediLas 2, Endo-Lase, Inc., New York, NY).

THE PROCEDURE

Most patients can undergo endoscopy and laser treatment on an outpatient basis. They are encouraged to start a low residue diet 48 hours before the procedure and a clear liquid diet the day before. If they still have a substantial length of large bowel and no medical contraindications, an oral mechanical cleansing with colon electrolyte lavage preparation such as Colyte™ (Reed & Carnrick) is used. This method of cleansing can accomplish a satisfactorily clean bowel in 3–5 hours. One or two Fleets enema are usually sufficient to prepare the distal bowel, for patients needing work only in the rectum. Selected patients may be clean with only a minimal preparation while those with ileorectal anastomosis may be very difficult to clean. Thirty minutes prior to laser treatment, an intramuscular injection of atropine and meperidine is given if there are no contraindications.

The patient is brought into the endoscopy suite. An intravenous solution is started with D_5W. The patient is asked to wear protective goggles. For insertion of the endoscope we prefer to place them in the left lateral position (SIMS). An automatic blood pressure monitor is used, the cuff is usually placed in the right forearm. For an EGD, a topical anesthetic for the oropharynx is used and diazepam at a dose of 0.02 mg/kg is given. If colonoscopy needs to be performed, then meperidine 0.5 mg to 1 mg/kg may be added. The endoscopic suite is equipped to handle the respiratory problems that will occasionally ensue following the use of these medications. Occasionally, glucagon 1 mg i.v. is given to diminish the contractions of the duodenum in order to obtain a still target for biopsies and accurate guidance and positioning of the laser beam.

Prior to insertion of the colonoscope, a gentle digital rectal examination will relieve the pressure in the anal sphincter and will get the patient used to having a foreign body in the anus. The top of the scope is thoroughly lubricated. Its insertion proceeds at a slow and deliberate pace. The lumen is seen at all times before advancing. Scope torquing and minimal tip deflection are techniques often used for insertion and advance. The quartz fiber is then passed through the biopsy channel of a Pentax endoscope (Pentax Precision Instrument Corporation, Orangeburg, NY) (Fig. 1). The laser machine is retested and recalibrated at the time of the procedure transmitting the pilot light and the laser. Eye protector goggles are used by all individuals in the endoscopy suite. The laser light is positioned with the aid of the red pilot light (Fig. 2). The laser fiber tip is held approximately 1 cm away from the tumor, and

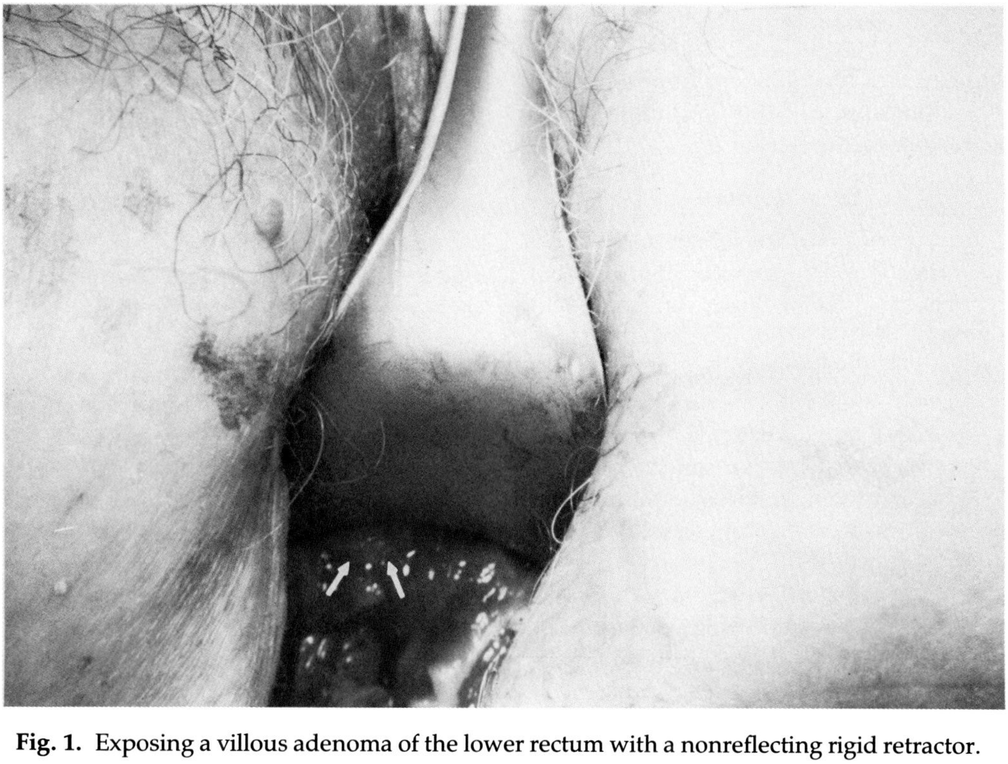

Fig. 1. Exposing a villous adenoma of the lower rectum with a nonreflecting rigid retractor.

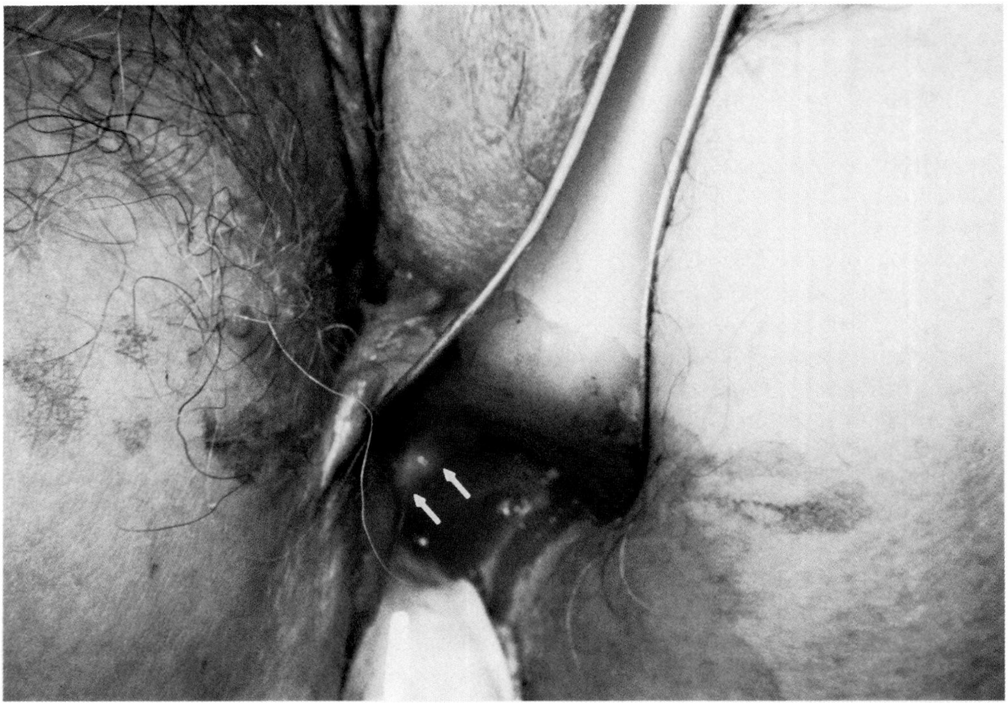

Fig. 2. Aiming the laser beam with the help of the pilot light.

multiple 2 to 3 second bursts of 60–80 w are directed to the tissue. Polyp tissue is then coagulated and/or vaporized (Fig. 3).

DISCUSSION

Until recently, treatment options for scattered gastrointestinal neoplasias were limited to surgery, electrocoagulation, and cryotherapy. With the introduction of lasers in clinical practice, vaporization and photoresection of polyps has now become an option. This may be of special relevance to familial adenomatous polyposis patients who have polyps in the rectum following a subtotal colectomy. For these patients there are clear advantages of local control with laser over electrocoagulation. Laser treatment not only is time efficient but also produces good healing without the submucosal scarring associated with electrocoagulation. Scarring will increase significantly the technical difficulties of a subsequent mucosal proctectomy and may preclude the construction of an ileal pouch and an ileoanal anastomosis. Laser vaporization may also be a very good option for patients who have isolated benign polyps elsewhere in the gastrointestinal tract within reach of an endoscope. Control of the polyps with laser vaporization should be carefully considered in those FAP patients with a familial or a personal history of desmoids, in patients with repeated bouts of intestinal obstruction and in those in whom the potential risks of surgery clearly outweigh its possible benefits.

As more polyps are being discovered in the asymptomatic state with the use of baseline endoscopic evaluations of the whole gastrointestinal tract in FAP patients, we have gradually come to recognize that FAP is not a disease limited to the colon, but that proliferative manifestations of the whole gastrointestinal mucosa, are common. These patients may require multiple and repeated therapeutic interventions, and, therefore, preservation of tissue and function should be an important pre-eminent concern throughout their care.

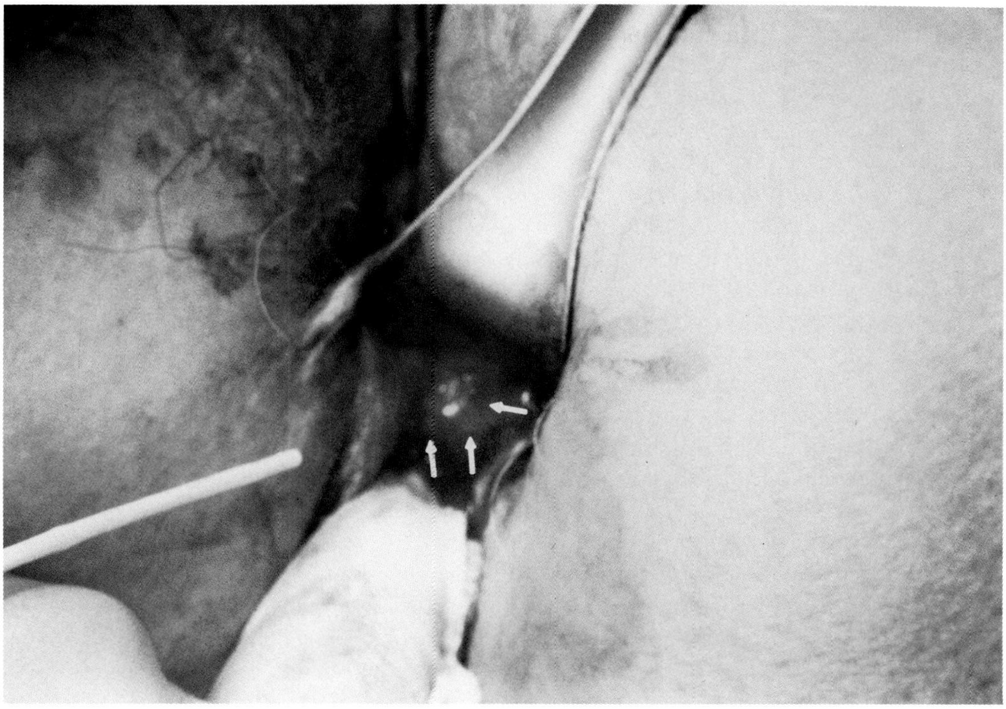

Fig. 3. Beginning of the vaporization of the polyp.

Although there seems to be a tendency for polyps in the proximal gastrointestinal tract to be fewer in number as compared with those found in the colon, these polyps also have shown a propensity for malignant transformation following the appearance of adenomas [2]. Thus the importance of trying new methods for local control of these neoplasias and interruption of the adenoma–carcinoma sequence without having to resort to a formal surgical exploration could maximize preservation of function.

Albert Einstein conceived the basis of the laser energy. He understood the interaction of atoms, ions, and molecules with electromagnetic radiation in terms of absorption and spontaneous emission of energy. Applying thermodynamic principles, he concluded that a third process of interaction, which is induced or stimulated emission, existed. In this electromagnetic radiation would be produced by an atomic process. In 1954, Townes achieved the stimulated emission of radiation in the microwave range of the spectrum (*m*icrowave *a*mplification by *s*timulated *e*mission of *r*adiation, MASER). In 1960, Maiman reported on the first light amplification by stimulated emission of radiation action with synthetic ruby crystals. A 0.69 μm wavelength beam was obtained.

Atoms are the smallest complete amount of any substance. An atom has a heavy nucleus containing positively charged particles called *protons* and far from the nucleus a whirl of negatively charged electrons. These electrons orbit at several discreet distances from the nucleus. This is specific and different to each atom. The more the distance of the electrons from the nucleus, the greater the energy associated with a change of levels and, therefore, the greater is the overall potential energy of the atom. The ''ground state'' is the lowest energy state of the atom. In this state, the electrons are closest to the nucleus. The electrons in an atom can change orbits or energy levels; however, energy from outside the atomic system is required to move the electron. When the electron is ''kicked'' to a more distant orbit and the atom achieves a higher overall energy, the atom is now described as *excited.* These electrons do not stay excited very long. The natural ground level, called *thermal equilibrium,* is intrinsically sought. As electrons are spontaneously dropped from higher to lower levels, the energy that was initially absorbed is given off. Einstein felt that if an atom in the excited state was impinged upon by a proton of the same energy as the one absorbed, then the decay to ground state would be accelerated. Two identical photons (one incident and one produced by the decay) would be exiting the atomic system. Both photons would have equal frequency and energy; they would travel in the same direction and in perfect spatial and temporal phase. This is what in turn is called *stimulated emission of radiation,* and it is the physical basis of the laser effect [3].

Photons given off by atomic systems can be described in terms of the length of the electromagnetic wave (expressed in metric units) or frequencies of oscillation (measured in Hertz). Various atomic and molecular substances in different physical states have been used to create laser action. The laser effect can only be created when the majority of the atom population of the laser medium is in the excited state. To maintain this state, energy must be constantly ''pumped'' into the atom population of the laser medium and confined to a chamber called the *optical* or *resonant cavity.* Diffferent laser media and instrument design use different types of pumping: i.e., electrical discharges, flashes of light, radio frequency excitation, or other laser stimulation.

Atoms in the excited state spontaneously emit photons within the optical chamber. However, with helpful mirrors, one can direct these photons into a preferred direction. They finally are made to emerge through a partially reflecting mirror, a laser beam is then produced. The first laser, which utilized the synthetic ruby crystal of the laser media, used flashes from a xenon lamp as the pumping source. Today, mixtures of helium and neon gases, combinations of neodymium, yttrium-aluminum and garnet; argon and crypton gases; various dyes; and CO_2, helium, and nitrogen gases; are all used as laser media. These lasers produce beams of various wavelengths and physical characteristics.

First of all, laser (*l*ight *a*mplification-*s*timulated *e*mission of *r*adiation) produces the brightest existing light. This light has the properties of uniformed wavelength (coherent), collimated (parallel ray directions), single color (monochromatic), and can be accurately focused to deliver high levels of energy into small areas under precise visual control. All of these characteristics have made lasers a useful addition to the medical armamentarium.

Of the several types of lasers mentioned, the Nd-YAG laser has become the popular choice for photoresection because of its penetrance into tissues and its ability to be transmitted via fiberoptics through the channel of an endoscope.

Yttrium-aluminum garnet (YAG) is widely used as a fake diamond substance. It has crystalline strength able to withstand the stress of continuous wave laser light formation [4]. The pink-colored rare earth neodymium (Nd) ''doped'' into the crystal lattice structure is the active lasing medium. It has a suitable wavelength in the near infrared range (1,064 nm) and appropriate tissue-ablating properties. At low power it can shrink and coagulate tissue without vaporization, whereas at higher power it will vaporize the tissues mechanically deaggregating into small fragments [5]. It is well carried through fiberoptic material, and it is best absorbed by the dark colors. It is also diffusely absorbed by body tissue permitting deep penetration of the laser energy. However, it is poorly absorbed by hemoglobin. This is an advantage, if one is working close to major vessels. Interaction between laser and tissue is a function of the power density and duration of the exposure. Suggested power setting for laser therapy are 80–95 W when vaporizing polyps. However, if the tip of the endoscope is close to the target, then it is advised to begin with 4–50 W as this may be sufficient. The duration of the energy delivered should be given in bursts of 2–3 seconds, with a total energy to the target lesion ranging between 3,000 and 10,000 joules [6].

The laser energy must be directed at the polyp by aiming the collimated light in a tangential manner. Hence, the energy should not be directed to the wall of the bowel but to the polyp and its base, while the time of exposure should be kept limited to avoid thermal damage to healthy surrounding tissue. Otherwise, complications such as hollow viscus perforation or bleeding are more likely to occur. The latter may apply especially to those polyps close to major vessels [7]. Herein, the dissipation of energy may not produce readily visible changes in the lesion until significant damage has ensued.

We also believe that with proper orientation of personnel, training in the care of handling the laser [8], and careful patient selection [9], the alternative of vaporization and photoresection of residual and recurrent scattered gastrointestinal polyps is a safe, practical and effective option. However, more experience and a longer follow-up of FAP patients and treated lesion are needed before definitive therapeutic recommendations can be made, regarding this modality of therapy.

References

1. Mathus-Vliegen EM, Tytgat GN: Nd-YAG laser photocoagulation in colorectal adenoma. Gastroenterology 90:1865–1873, 1986.
2. Herrera-Ornelas L, Elsiah S, Petrelli N, Mittelman A: Causes of death in patients with FPC. Semin Surg Onc 3:109–117, 1987.
3. Wright VC, Riopelle MA: Laser Physics for Surgeons. Houston: Biomedical Communications, 1982.
4. Joffe SN: The Neodymium: YAG Laser in General Surgery Contemporary Surgery, Vol 27, 1985, pp 17–26.
5. Mathus-Vliegen EMH, Tytgat GNJ: Laser ablation and palliation in colorectal malignancy. Gastrointest Endosc 32:393–396, 1986.
6. Beth Israel Laser Institute Course: Laser treatment for gastrointestinal illness. Endosc Rev 46–48, 1986.
7. Ross JS, O'Donovan PB, Mehta A: Magnetic resonance and computed tomography evaluation of tracheobronchial lesions prior to laser photoresection. Cleve Clin Q 53:335–344, 1986.
8. Bendick PJ: Laser safety in the operating room. ACS Bull 71(7):10–12, 1986.
9. Unger SW, Arroyo P, Barkin JS: Nd-YAG laser applications in surgical endoscopy: A single center comprehensive experience. Am Surg 54(2):89–92, 1988.

Introduction

Milton M. Weiser

Division of Gastroenterology, Department of Medicine, State University of New York at Buffalo, Buffalo General Hospital, Buffalo, New York

The organization of this book on familial adenomatous polyposis differs from the usual sequence: The more basic science section is placed at the end of the volume. This appears to have two effects. One, it allows readers to begin the book by first reviewing progress on the clinical aspects of familial adenomatous polyposis without feeling guilty over not reading the preceding obligatory ''basic'' chapters found in most review texts. Two, and more importantly, the clinical observations of the earlier chapters frame and orient the research that has to be addressed by immunology, biochemistry, cell biology, molecular biology, and genetics. Another important feature of this basic science section is that it is a review of current research by those doing the research. This section illustrates the wide variety of questions that have been asked regarding intestinal polyps, intestinal differentiation, and the multiplicity of factors needed to induce cancer. The investigators are careful to emphasize the complexities of interpreting their findings; research first uncovers the paradoxes before revealing their solutions.

The chapters in this section fall into four groups. The first group discusses research related to dietary or environmental factors that may interact with inherited susceptibilities and thus to enhancement in the formation of colon cancer. Martin Lipkin and his colleagues begin by reviewing the proliferative and differentiation properties and phenotypic expressions of normal mucosal epithelial cells, cells from possible premalignant diseases, and cancer cells. In many ways they preview the research presented in the other chapters of this section. Their major point, however, is to relate this research to possible therapeutic approaches. The emphasis is on those ''natural'' agents that may inhibit cancer formation. They try to organize and classify these ''chemopreventive'' agents. One discussed particularly is dietary calcium.

A number of experiments have shown that supplementary dietary calcium in animal tumor models decreased epithelial cell proliferation and increased cell maturation. Appleton and Williamson present data demonstrating this effect of calcium, but emphasizing the effects of calcium as a chelator of fatty acids and bile acids, with obvious implications on the presumed role of bile acids as promotors of colon cancer. This subject is discussed further by Michael Hill in his chapter on fecal bile acids and bacteria in familial adenomatous polyposis. Hill reviews bile acid and cholesterol catabolism by gut flora and describes the unexpected finding that patients with familial adenomatous polyposis show decreased deconjugation and dehydroxylation of bile acids and decreased reduction of cholesterol despite the lack of differences from normal controls of fecal flora composition or fecal bacterial metabolism. The chapter by Eileen Friedman extends these observations to familial adenomatous polyposis by demonstrating that most of the cells from colonic biopsy specimens have lost their normal calcium responsiveness; that is, cancer cells show no effects of calcium on cell proliferation or maturation. More work needs to be done to show that this calcium unresponsiveness is a characteristic

Familial Adenomatous Polyposis, pages 223–226

feature of all types of cancer cells and to define the stage of malignant development during which this unresponsiveness first becomes manifest. The precise mechanisms whereby calcium exerts these effects on normal cells and how premalignant and malignant cells become resistant are not known, but most readers will be aware of the second messenger concept of cell calcium and the critical involvement of calcium in many controls of cell responsiveness to hormones and growth factors.

John Bertram (chapter 30) also uses the term *chemoprevention* when discussing the use of agents such as retinoids, ascorbic acid, and calcium and other dietary manipulations such as increased dietary fiber in the prevention of cancer or its recurrence. The theoretical bases for these controversial concepts are discussed, as well as the problems in evaluating studies on the effects of "chemotherapeutic" agents. The line between holistic medicine, nutritional fads, and conclusions based on science well done has always been difficult to define in this field; one can feel the frustration from those who want quick and unequivocal results from what have to be complicated and long-term studies.

The second group of chapters in this section contains discussions of research related to phenotypic changes in familial adenomatous polyposis, other presumed premalignant conditions, and colon cancer. These changes are related to possible markers of the premalignant and malignant state some of which may have possible clinical usefullness. Professor Kopelovich's chapter tries to present a theoretical basis for the similarity of phenotypic expressions among different cancers: ". . . while distinct forms of cancer may represent a *single* and *specific* gene defect, additional genes can pleiotropically modulate the expression of these cancer predisposing genes." His studies on skin fibroblasts from patients with neurofibromatosis or familial adenomatous polyposis demonstrated that not all cells are equally able to express the transformed phenotype, a finding consistent with the heterogeneity of clinical expression of inherited cancer syndromes. In addition, relatively few cells actually become tumorigenic, promotion appearing to be the most important step in the development of cancer. Trosko and Chang want to emphasize one phenotypic change characteristic of many cancers (but not all) to propose ". . . a completely different approach to cancer prevention and treatment . . ., based on newer concepts of carcinogenesis." They review data that suggest that maintenance of intercellular communication, particularly through gap junctions, is an essential feature for normal growth. The postulate is that tumors have a defect in intercellular communication through their gap junctions. They discuss how these findings fit with current theories on initiation and promotion of cancer and propose that a new approach to cancer therapy might be directed toward agents that would promote normal gap junction formation and function, agents still, as yet, to be defined. As with many theories based on one phenotypic change, it is probably too all inclusive to explain the behavior of tumor cells and metastases. As with theories centered around plasma membrane glycoproteins, it may lead to disappointments, but it is well argued and should lead to further experiments that will ultimately better define the intercellular controls of growth, development, and differentiation and thereby aid in understanding cell relationships in cancer.

Specific phenotypic changes that may predict or characterize cancer and be used as clinically useful markers are discussed in a series of chapters by A.L. Silverman et al., T. Muto, C.R. Boland, S. Sakamoto et al., J.G. Guillem and I.B. Weinstein, and A. Quaroni. A.L. Silverman et al. describe their findings that ornithine decarboxylase activity was a marker that identified those persons who would later express a phenotype of familial adenomatous polyposis, that is, a true prediction marker. Stepwise increases in ornithine decarboxylase activity were reported to be associated with progression from flat mucosa to polyps to dysplasia to cancer. C.R. Boland reviews studies (such as those of Y. Kim and of D. Podolsky) and presents new data that attempt to define the changes in mucin structure and synthesis that might herald premalignant changes in polyps and characterize colon cancer. He describes the subtle structural changes of mucin in familial adenomatous polyposis as seen histochemically and in lectin binding. A discussion of the limitations of these techniques sets the right critical tone. The major and most consistent change in familial adenomatous polyposis, in both noncancerous and cancerous tissue, was a decrease in sialic acid content. Possibly related to this finding are the data of T. Muto that histochemical staining for sialomucins of flat colon (i.e., nonpolyps) biopsies of families of patients with familial adenomatous polyposis appeared to be associated with the carrier state. A. Quaroni's approach to plasma membrane glycoprotein changes that might define colon cancer was to study intestinal development and differentiation; differences associated with these states might re-emerge in cancer. Using monoclonal antibodies, he demonstrated intriguing relationships among rat small intestinal crypt cell surface glycoproteins, those of rat fetal cells, human colon cancer cells in tissue culture, and colon cancer tissue from biopsy material. Some of these monoclonal antibodies may be markers defining poorly differentiated cancer, a possible predictor of prognosis or responsiveness to therapy. Sakamoto and his colleagues describe a cytoplasmic-associated isoenzyme of thymidine kinase. This isoenzyme, in contrast to the mitochondrial-associated isoenzyme, was increased 12-fold in colon cancer. It also was found to be increased in DMH-treated rat normal mucosa. Somewhat disappointing, however, was the finding that random polyps from patients with familial adenomatous polyposis showed inconsistent and minimal elevation of this isoenzyme, possibly because of the heterogeneity of the polyps. The gene for this isoenzyme has been localized to chromosome 17, and Sakamoto et el. feel that their work lends support to a theory suggested by Dutrillaux and Muleris (ref. 40 of Sakamoto et al., chapter 38) that colorectal cancer "involves the deregulation of enzymes . . . of pyrimidine and purine synthesis via chromosomal imbalances involving 17q(thymidine kinase), 18(thymidylate synthetase), 5q(dihydrofolate reductase), and lp(cytidylate kinase)." Lastly, Guillem and Weinstein present their data demonstrating a consistent down-regulation of protein kinase C; all colon cancers appeared to have decreased protein kinase C activity. Although this activity was also shown to be decreased in ras-transfected cells, only 40% of human colon cancers showed increased ras-oncogene expression. This disparity, according to the authors, argues for the down-regulation of protein kinase C activity as the common pathway in the development of colon cancer.

The third group of chapters in this section is concerned with oncogenes, which Professor Kopelovich prefers to call *differentiation-related genes*. These chapters are difficult to summarize and must be carefully read; the relationship between oncogene expression and cancer has become blurred. The reader must be aware of what the author means by *amplification* and *increased expression* of a gene. The gene may be amplified without an increase in its RNA, its mRNA may be increased without an increase in product, or its product may be increased because of decreased destruction, and so forth. Forrester et al. emphasize mutations rather than differences in the level of expressions of the ras oncogene family. They point out that attempts to transform cells in tissue culture with ras oncogenes have been unsuccessful. Their data stress the high incidence of mutant c-K-ras oncogenes in villus adenomas and in carcinomas originating in villus adenomas, a possible indication of a precancerous event. These mutant genes can be found in primary colon cancers, but the incidence of the mutant genes appeared to be higher in metastatic lesions. The implication is that these mutants code for a product that is altered in a very slight manner but enough to effect tumor development.

Since there are no major differences in the expression of c-K-ras oncogenes between tumor and normal tissue, the association of tumor with mutant genes is hard to explain mechanistically. One proposal is that following c-K-ras mutations there are stepwise genetic alterations such as deletions at 5q, 18q, and 17q. It is the progressive accumulations of these genetic changes that leads to cancer, but which of these changes are important? Which alter growth control? For what functions or enzyme activities do these genes code? Michelassi presents some preliminary data that suggest that the product(p21) of the ras oncogene is increased in familial adenomatous polyposis. Herold and Rothberg describe their studies on the mechanisms of increased myc oncogene expression in most colon cancers. In many cases it is not due to an amplification of the gene itself. One colon cancer cell line appeared to be an exception in that there was a four- to eightfold increase in myc gene expression; the amount of myc RNA produced was the normal level per gene copy, but there were more gene copies. This was a relatively rare occurrence and does not account for the increased myc RNA expression found in 70% of colorectal cancers. Schwab et al. discuss the different changes in oncogene expression found in a number of tumor cell lines, including myc, myb, and her/neu. The fact that these are associated with different chromosomes and that Okamoto et al. (chapter 47, ref 13) found chromosomal deletions in familial adenomatous polyposis not only in 5q but also in chromosome 22, 6, 12q, 15, and other areas of 5, Schwab et al. suggest the possibility that more than one gene locus change is required for the development of colon cancer. They stress the importance of genetic instability as the important feature in the establishment of the cancer state.

The last group of chapters in this section are devoted to research on genetic markers in familial adenomatous polyposis. Wolman et al. give a fairly complete review of progress with genetic markers. They note that there have been multiple gene changes identified in the progression from polyp to colon cancer. The "most critical questions . . . are the identification and cloning of specific gene sequences and establishment of the exact order of alterations in multistep transformtion." Most readers of this book will be quite familiar with the fact that the editor, L. Herrera, was the first author of an article that appeared in the *American Journal of Medical Genetics* in 1986 describing a chromosome deletion in a man with Gardner's syndrome. Karyotype analysis of his blood lymphocytes as done by the Department of Genetics (Avery A. Sandberg) at Roswell Park Memorial Institute revealed a deletion in the long arm of chromosome 5 between either q13-q15 or q15-q22. A year later, work published in *Nature* from the Imperial Cancer Research Fund Laboratories (Walter Bodmer) in collaboration with other laboratories in England (University of Leicester) and Israel (Hadassah Medical School) used techniques of restriction fragment length polymorphism and cDNA probes to study 13 families (124 members) of patients with familial adenomatous polyposis. The results narrowed the chromosome location suggested by Herrera et al.; the gene responsible for this disease was in 5q21-5q22. Using an additional probe of this chromosome area (Pi227), Meera–Khan et al. (Chapter 46) present data that indicated that the gene was in band 5q22 close to 5q21. Thus, research gets closer and closer to the location of the gene responsible for familial adenomatous polyposis but it has not yet defined the gene. The cDNA probes do not identify the gene and the increased precision of its chromosome location will, at best, narrow it to the order of 10^2 genes. When the gene's product is functionally defined, will it be an "inhibitor" specific for colon epithelial growth of differentiation? Will the molecular biologist and the molecular pharmacologist be able to develop therapeutic agents to replace, enhance, or substitute for this gene product?

Dr. Herrera suggested other questions to be discussed in this introduction. His questions reflect the focus of the research described in most chapters of this section. Has a molecular pathway been demonstrated for the development of cancer from adenomatous polyps? Can one detect which polyps are committed to develop into cancer, i.e., is there a detectable premalignant change? Is there a panel of markers, histochemical, immunocytochemical, or serum, that can be used to predict increased risk or presence of cancer? The answer to all of Dr. Herrera's questions is maybe; progress is being made. These are questions that seek clinically useful results from basic research. Although much of basic science research is not oriented toward answering clinical questions specifically, it is basic research that has the greatest impact on how the more clinically oriented investigator tries to answer many clinical questions. Most of the authors listed in this section represent those clinical investigators who are able to synthesize basic science concepts and techniques and to apply them to clinical observations and research. The impact on each flows in both directions, as is evident particularly in genetics. We look forward to increasing interactions between basic and clinical investigators and a consequent logorithmic increase in progress against cancer.

Identification of Increased Susceptibility to Familial Polyposis and Other Diseases That Increase Susceptibility to Gastrointestinal Cancer: Proposed Application to Studies of Cancer Prevention in Human Subjects

Martin Lipkin, Eileen Friedman, Harold Newmark, and Sidney J. Winawer

Gastroenterology Service and Laboratory of Gastrointestinal Cancer Research, Department of Medicine, Memorial Sloan-Kettering Cancer Center (M.L., E.F., H.N., S.J.W.) and Department of Medicine, Cornell University Medical College, New York, New York (M.L., S.J.W.)

INTRODUCTION

Modified proliferation and differentiation of gastrointestinal epithelial cells have now been identified in familial polyposis and in other diseases that are associated with increased susceptibility to gastrointestinal cancer. In early stages of development of these disorders continued DNA synthesis occurs in maturing cells, with a delayed onset of normal terminal differentiation. In more advanced stages of precancerous disease, more extensive changes occur in gastrointestinal cells that exhibit progressively increasing degrees of abnormally delayed maturation.

In familial polyposis, and in rodents after treatment with chemical carcinogens, among the earliest modifications that develop in colonic epithelial cells is increased proliferative activity in the proliferative compartment. This expansion of the proliferative compartment develops in cancer-prone regions of the gastrointestinal tract that have been studied in humans with various precancerous diseases and in rodent models: the esophagus, stomach, and colon. Eventually excessive numbers of proliferating cells accumulate in the epithelium without undergoing normal maturation.

FAMILIAL ADENOMATOUS POLYPOSIS

An expanded proliferative compartment of epithelial cells in human subjects with increased susceptibility to colon cancer was originally found in studies carried out in familial polyposis. Familial polyposis is a disease with an autosomal dominant mode of inheritance that is characterized by the development of large numbers of adenomatous polyps throughout the entire colon and rectum. Carcinomas eventually develop in virtually all affected individuals. The cancers occur with highest frequency in the distal colon, a distribution that is similar to that of colorectal cancer in the general population.

While the existence of intestinal polyposis has been recorded for 250 years, it is only during the last century that researchers have further delineated the condition into subgroups [1]. In 1721, Menzel may have described the first case, one that was probably inflammatory in type. By 1881, Woodward had divided polyposis into two categories 1)primary or adenomatous, i.e., hyper-

Familial Adenomatous Polyposis, pages 227–244

plastic or neoplastic; and 2)inflammatory. At about the same time, researchers observed that primary polyposis had hereditary tendencies: "familial polyposis coli." Within 30 years, it became clear that this was a precancerous, hereditary condition in the large intestine. In 1882, Cripps observed two siblings with polyposis coli, and by 1900 the division was apparent: familial (adenomatosis) vs. nonfamilial (inflammatory polyposis).

Familial polyposis, an autosomal dominant genetic defect affecting each generation, is expressed phenotypically about 80% of the time. A typical pattern of inheritance in familial polyposis is shown in Figure 1. The probable genetic background of familial polyposis and its various associated syndromes has been debated by many investigators. There appears to be general agreement that classic familial polyposis is due to a single dominant gene. However, there is less agreement as to the genetics of sporadic cases and the various associated syndromes.

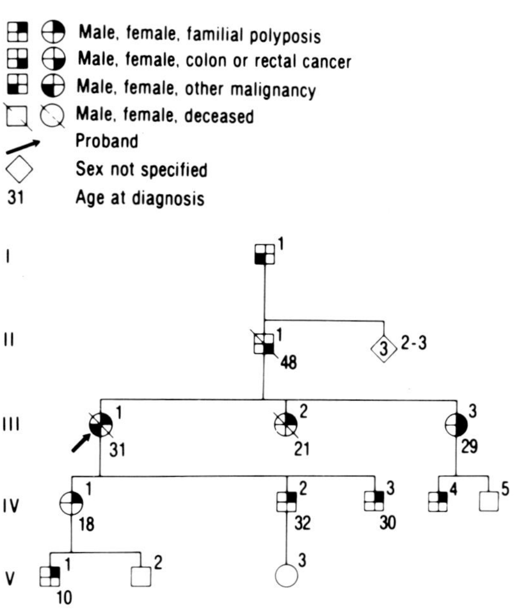

Fig. 1. Typical pattern of inheritance in familial polyposis, together with ages of onset in family members.

Some investigators believe that sporadic cases can be explained by new mutations. Others disagree, maintaining that a minor fraction of all sporadic cases would result from fresh mutation. It has also been suggested that environmental modification would render the expression of disease and inheritance virtually polygenic.

Records of the incidence of polyposis coli exist in Great Britain, the United States, and northern Europe, i.e., among Caucasians who have access to advanced medical services. The disease has also occurred, however, in Arabs, West Indians, African and African blacks, Orientals, and American Indians. Analysis of age at onset of disease is an important determinant in the identification of familial polyposis and other diseases in which familial predisposition increases the risk of colorectal cancer [2]. Figure 2 gives the cumulative age distributions of onset of familial polyposis and subsequent colon cancer, and comparisons are made with other population groups. From these data, the magnitude of increased risk at every age level can be estimated.

Environmental factors in polyposis coli have not been identified; however, it is possible that the known genetic predisposition could be modified by the environment. In our conceptual understanding of the development of cancer, the concept of a multistage evolution of neoplasms, with promotor or cocarcinogenic agents having a role, has become widely accepted [3–5]. Environmental or physiologic stimuli may contribute to the steps leading to neoplastic change, adenomas, and malignancy. In familial polyposis, although adenomas are scattered throughout the colon, carcinomas develop mainly in the distal colon. This is a pattern similar to that seen in the general population.

GARDNER'S SYNDROME

Gardner's syndrome, a variant of familial polyposis, is an autosomal dominant disorder showing a high degree of penetrance. Adenomatous polyps of the colon and occasionally of the small intestine are formed, and there is a propensity for development of adenocarcinoma in the adenomas. Recognized today on the basis of characteristic clinical findings, the incidence of the

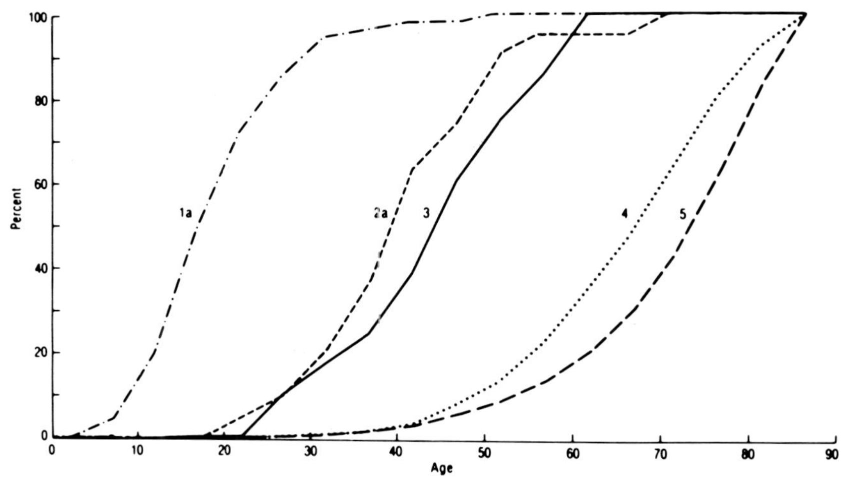

Fig. 2. Cumulative percentages of incident cases at various ages having familial polyposis compared with cumulative age incidence of colon cancer in other population groups. **1a:** The onset of nonmalignant polyposis. **2a:** The onset of familial polyposis derived from data on 38 cases seen at Memorial Hospital. **3:** Early age of onset of cancer in 28 affected individuals from a Memorial Hospital series who have familial colon cancer-prone disease without polyposis. **4:** The age of onset of colon and rectal cancer in the general population of the United States from the Third National Cancer Survey, NCI, and includes white and black males and females combined. **5:** The onset of colon and rectal cancer in males and females in Japan from data supplied by R.T. Hirayama.

syndrome is lower than familial polyposis and is estimated to be 1 in 14,000 births.

Adenomatosis of the large intestine, multiple osteomata of the skull and mandible, and multiple epidermoid cysts and soft tissue tumors of the skin were the symptoms reported by Gardner [6] in 1951. There had been previously studied cases in 1912 [7], 1935 [8], and 1943 [9]; Gardner and colleagues did follow-up work in 1952 [10] and 1953 and in 1962 and 1969, when the original case was reviewed. New observations showed impacted teeth, early dental caries, cysts and abnormal bone structure of the mandible and tibia, and desmoid tumors of the abdominal wall and small intestinal mesentery. It should be noted that an epidermoid cyst, uncommon before the age of puberty, may indicate polyposis.

Other possibly associated lesions include carcinoma of the thyroid, carcinomas of the ampulla of Vater, duodenum, and adrenal glands, adenomas of the small intestine, carcinoma in situ of the gallbladder, carcinomatous tumors of the small intestine, tumors of the brain and central nervous system, and lymphoid polyps of the ileum. Adenomas are distributed in the colon and rectum; they can, however, also occur in the small intestine, especially in the region of the ampulla of Vater, and in the stomach.

Gene expression is variable, with some persons having the various manifestations of the major triad of Gardner's syndrome and others with hereditary polyposis having only intestinal neoplasms. Periampullary carcinomas have been reported in the recent literature.

The desmoid tumors that arise following surgery present a particular problem. These can erupt between 1 and 3 years after an operation for polyposis, appearing in the abdominal wall or in the mesentery of the small intestine. They may be large and multiple, and, on occasion, they may precede the phenotypic expression of polyposis. At the Mayo Clinic, desmoid tumors developed in 3.5% of patients after surgery [11]. Similar observations have been made elsewhere. Clinically, desmoid tumors appear as carcinomatous recurrences, but they are considered benign or low-grade malignancies. Histologically, these intra-abdominal tumors often reach a stable size and afterward remain unchanged. They can obstruct the intestine or urinary tract.

The incidence of Gardner's syndrome among families in which more than one member has polyposis has been estimated at 14–18%. Only one or several family members may have obvious clinical manifestations of the disease. The expression of the disease is incomplete and, when made on the basis of clinical findings, is limited. As will be noted, abnormalities of epidermal cells and fibroblasts can be observed in family members lacking clinical manifestations of disease.

It is not yet clear whether features of the syndrome result from one dominant gene or from multiple genes. There are questions also as to the number, nature, and location of polyps in polyposis patients showing manifestations of Gardner's syndrome as compared with those with the typical non-Gardner familial polyposis. In terms of pathogenesis, the syndrome described by Gardner could represent the full manifestation of a spectrum of pathologic changes affecting all patients with multiple polyposis. It is possible that a single mutation may be responsible for most of the various associated syndromes. On that basis, Gardner's syndrome would include all adenomatous polyposis, with subsidiary lesions expressed in different degrees. There is, however, resistance from clinicians for a widespread use of this eponym.

EXPANSION OF THE PROLIFERATIVE COMPARTMENT OF EPITHELIAL CELLS IN THE COLONIC MUCOSA OF FAMILIAL POLYPOSIS AND IN OTHER DISEASES INCREASING SUSCEPTIBILITY TO GASTROINTESTINAL NEOPLASIA

Figure 3 shows examples of expansion of the proliferative compartment of colonic epithelial

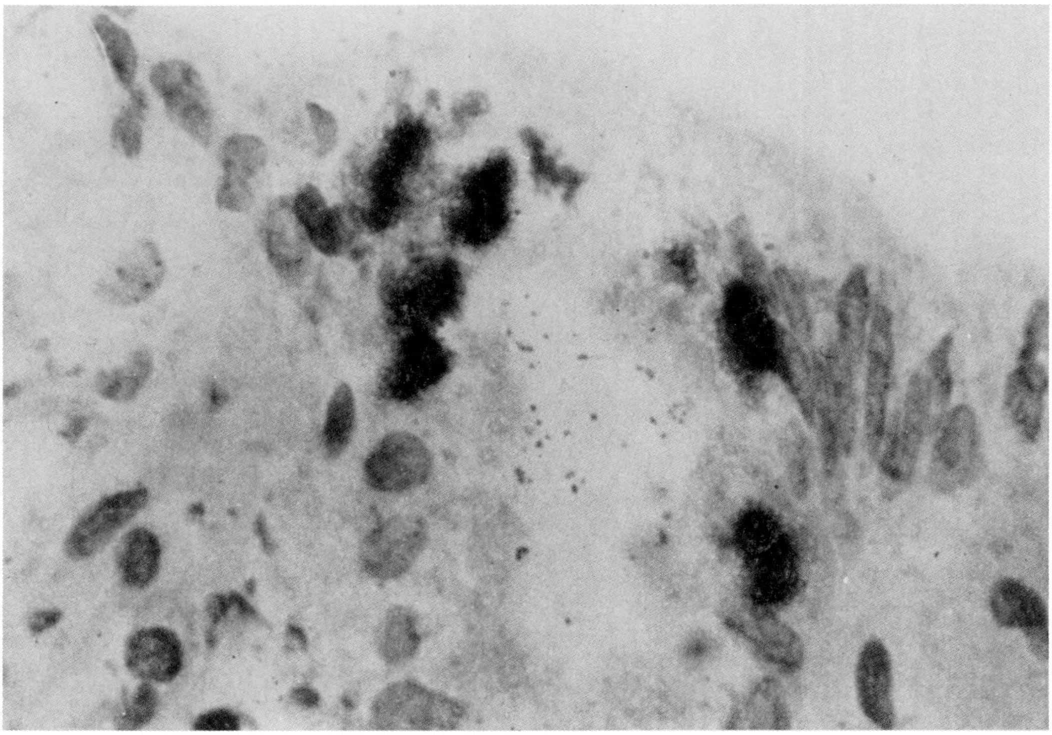

Fig. 3. Early net retention and accumulation of proliferative cells labeled with tritiated thymidine in an individual with familial polyposis.

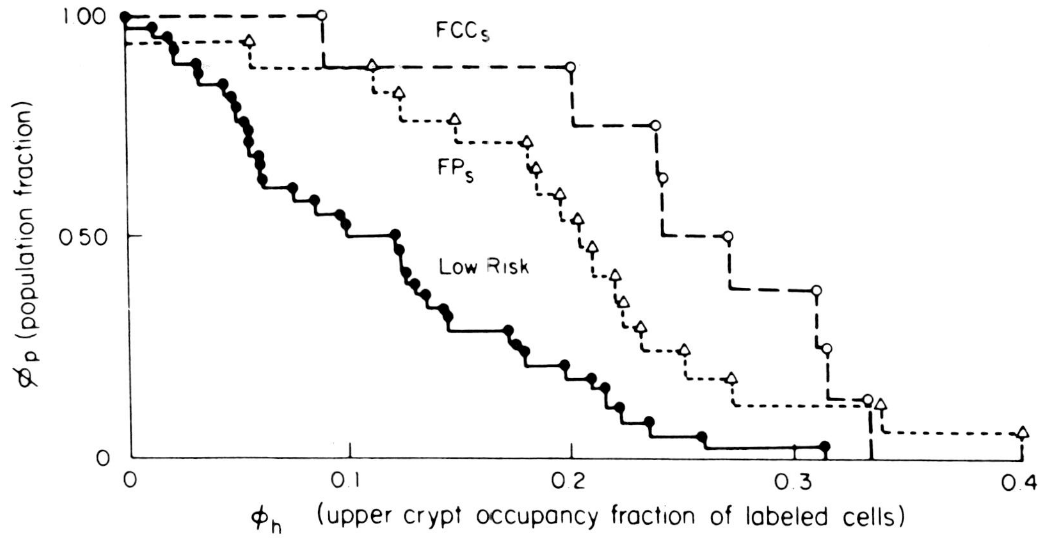

Fig. 4. Comparisons of the fractile distributions of ϕ_h between the high-risk populations FPs (symptomatic familial polyposis) and FCCs (symptomatic familial colon cancer) and low-risk subjects. Abscissa: The fraction of an individual's thymidine-labeled epithelial cells found in the upper 40% of the crypt. Ordinate: The fraction of all the individuals in a given population whose measured ϕ_h values equal or exceed the abscissa value. (Reproduced from Lipkin et al. [120]: Cancer Res 43:1899–1904, 1983.)

cells in individuals with familial polyposis. Figure 4 shows quantitation of this expansion of the proliferative compartment of epithelial cells, also in individuals with familial polyposis. Table 1 further summarizes similar information in various diseases of the esophagus, stomach, and colon of human subjects, all characterized by increasing susceptibility of affected individuals to gastrointestinal tract cancer. Figures 5 and 6 further illustrate expansions of the proliferative compartment of epithelial cells in multiple regions of the colon in diseases that predispose individuals to colonic cancer. Corresponding findings in the flat colonic mucosa of individuals having colonic carcinoma were recently noted, where DNA content in cells in the upper one-third of colonic crypts was increased, a finding not observed in the colonic mucosa of normal subjects [12]. In ulcerative colitis, it also was possible to identify subpopulations of hyperproliferating cells that expressed an antigen normally decreased in maturing cells [13].

ABNORMAL DIFFERENTIATION OF EPITHELIAL CELLS IN THE COLONIC MUCOSA IN FAMILIAL POLYPOSIS AND IN OTHER DISEASES INCREASING SUSCEPTIBILITY TO GASTROINTESTINAL NEOPLASIA

Further modifications occur in colonic epithelial cells as they undergo differentiation and migrate through the colonic crypts to be extended from the surface of the mucosa. Thus, benign colonic adenomas are believed to be an intermediate stage between normal colonic epithelial cells and carcinoma [1,14,15]; the probablity of carcinoma developing in benign colonic adenomas increases directly as adenomas increase in size. In the colonic adenomas of familial polyposis, in addition to an expansion of the proliferative compartment of epithelial cells, a marked shift of the entire proliferative region to the surface of the adenomas has been found [16].

TABLE 1.
Expansion of the Proliferative Compartment of Epithelial Cells: Studies of Human Subjects

Organ	Disease	References
Esophagus	Barretts esophagus	Herbst et al. [102]
		Pellish et al. [103]
	Esophagitis, reflux	Livstone et al. [104]
	Esophatitis, Linxian	Munoz et al. [105]
		Yang et al. [106]
Stomach	Pernicious anemia	Bell et al. [107]
		Willems et al. [108]
	Chronic gastritis	Winawer et al. [109]
		Deschner et al. [110]
		Sizikov et al. [111]
		Lipkin et al. [33]
	Partial gastrectomy	Assad et al. [112]
		Hansen et al. [113]
		Offerhaus et al. [114]
Large intestine	Familial polyposis	Deschner et al. [115]
		Bleiberg et al. [116]
		Lipkin et al. [117]
		Deschner et al. [118]
		Iwama [119]
		Lipkin et al. [120,121]
	Sporadic adenomas	Cole et al. [122]
		Maskens et al. [123]
		Lipkin et al. [131]
		Terpstra et al. [100]
		Lipkin et al. [99]
		Ponz de Leon et al. [101]
	Colon cancer	Maskens et al. [124]
		Romagnoli et al. [125]
		Lipkin et al. [120,121]
	Ulcerative colitis	Bleiberg et al. [126]
		Eastwood et al. [127]
		Serafini et al. [128]
		Deschner et al. [129]
		Lehy et al. [130]
		Biasco et al. [13]

Further abnormal properties also have been observed in colonic adenomas. These include the modulation of secretion of plasminogen activator by tumor promoters [17,18] and abnormal retrograde migration of adenomatous epithelial cells away from the surface of the mucosa deep into the crypts [16], as occurs with malignant cells; however, benign adenomatous epithelial cells did not invade through the basal layer.

During the abnormal development of colonic epithelial cells, blood group-related antigens of the ABH and Lewis systems also become modified, with neosynthesis of ABH specificities appearing in tumor cells together with accumulation of precursor antigens. Increased expression of Lewis antigens, especially Y and extended Y determinants, has been found, the latter not found in normal colonic mucosa and having a restricted pattern of distribution in normal tissues [19–22]. LeY expression in polyps was further correlated with histological type and degree of dysplasia [21,22]. Of particular importance, extended or trifucosyl LeY antigen expression was limited exclusively to premalignant adenomatous polyps and was invariably absent from nonpremalignant or hyperplastic polyps. Among

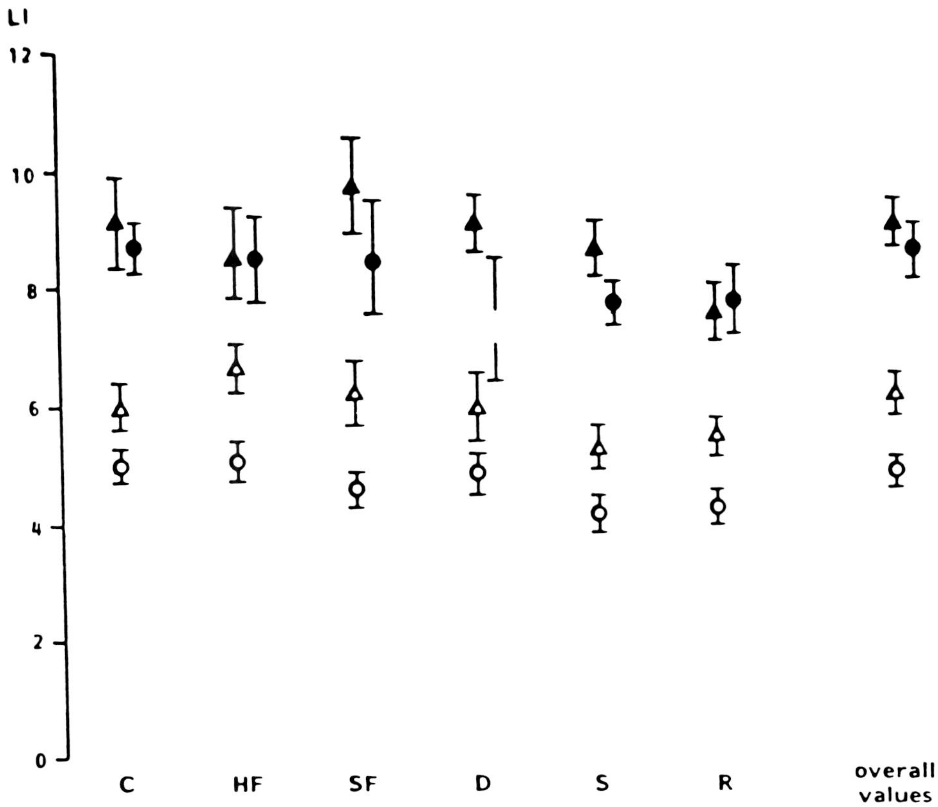

Fig. 5. Labeling index (LI, mean ± SE) at six sites in the colon: C, cecum; HF, hepatic flexure; SF, splenic flexure; D, descending colon; S, sigmoid; R, rectum. Open circles, control patients (N = 16); open triangles, patients with small adenomas (N = 21); closed triangles, patients with large adenomas (−1 cm diameter; N = 11); closed circles, patients with colon cancer (N = 13). Reprinted with permission from Terpstra et al. [100]: *Gastroenterology* 92:704–708. Copyright 1987 by The American Gastroenterology Association.)

adenomatous polyps extended LeY antigen expression tended to correlate with three known parameters of malignant potential: larger polyp size, villous histology, and severe dysplasia. Therefore, in human colon the LeY hapten appears to be an oncodevelopmental cancer-associated antigen, and extended LeY antigens may be highly specific markers for premalignancy and malignancy [22].

Further changes occur in colonic epithelial cells during abnormal differentiation and as neoplasms develop, including the expression of abnormal carbohydrate antigens and morphologic, immunologic, and biochemical modifications in the cells [23]. Alterations of gene expression also occur in the hereditary disease familial polyposis [24–26] and in carcinogen-induced and sporadic colonic cancer as colonic cells undergo abnormal differentiation and develop into adenomas and carcinomas [26–29]. In human studies, the structural changes seem to involve deletions of sequences as previously found in several other instances of inherited predisposition to cancer. Among the genes that change in expression during progression to colonic cancer, a subset has been identified in which changes of expression characterized induced differentiation of cells in culture [26].

p21 ras was expressed maximally in the normal midzone region of differentiating cells and in

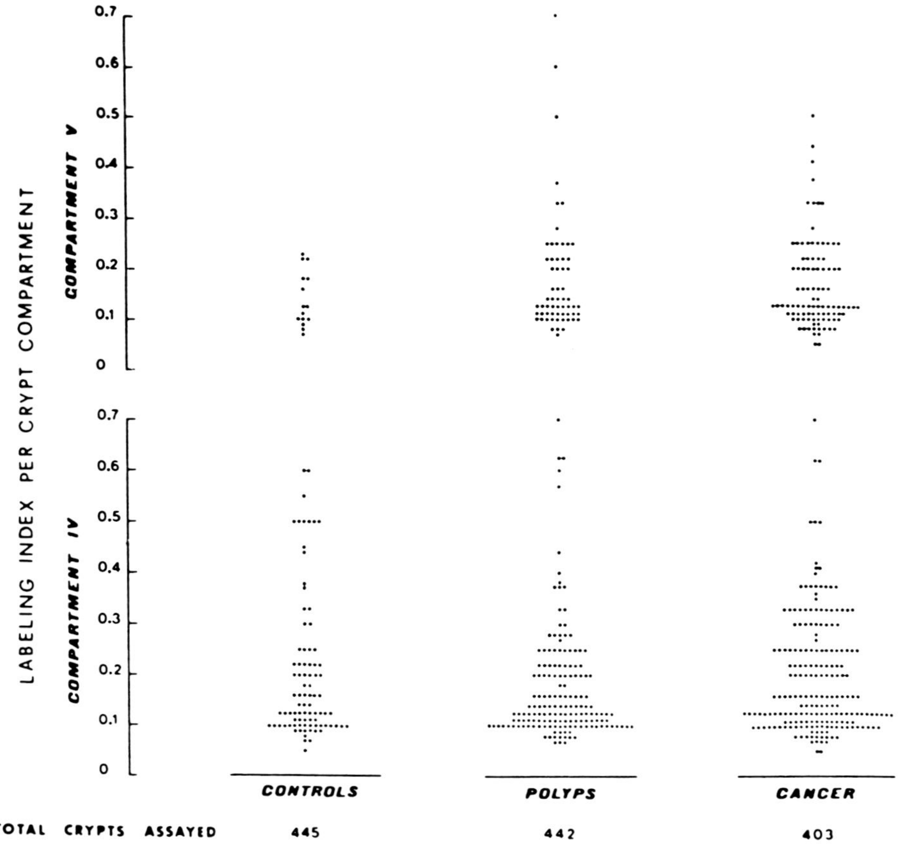

Fig. 6. Tritiated thymidine labeling index in the upper 40% of colonic crypts (compartments 4 and 5). Symbols indicate ratio between labeled and total cells. The number of crypt columns is given below each group. (Reproduced from Ponz de Leon et al. [101]: Cancer Res 48:4121–4126, 1988.)

dysplastic areas of adenomatous polyp cells [30]. ras gene expression was found highest in the most differentiated cells in the upper region of normal colonic crypts, and a high level of Ha-ras expression appeared to be a marker for a differentiated state of colonic carcinoma cells involving mucin production [31]. Colonic carcinoma cells also secrete TGFα and TGFβ [32]. As in keratinocytes, these may contribute to differentiation of the epithelial cells and an imbalance of these two endogenous growth modifiers to aberrant development of preneoplastic cells.

Thus, as noted above in humans, throughout the gastrointestinal tract, in diseases that lead to increased frequencies of cancer expanding populations of proliferating epithelial cells have been found before the development of observable tumors. Throughout the entire gastrointestinal tract, therefore, the normal mucosa is a comparatively *quiescent* mucosa in terms of cell proliferation, and fully mature cells are able to develop in order to function and to cover and protect the surface of the gastrointestinal tract. As cells progress through different stages of premalignancy, additional studies have begun to show a lack of terminal differentiation of epithelial cells [19–22,33], modifications of gene expression [23–31], and modified responses of the cells to growth factors and tumor promoters that may further contribute to abnormal cell development [17,18]. In various experimental models of tumor promotion increased cell proliferation also occurs [34,35]; that tumor promoters are capable of stimulating cell proliferation appears well established [35,36]. Properties of colonic epithelial cells, and also of other gastrointestinal epithelial cells that develop during abnormal differentiation, are summarized in Table 2. In precancerous diseases of the human cervix, an expansion of the proliferative compartment of epithelial cells and modifications of cell differentiation also occur [37–39].

APPLICATION OF THE BIOMARKERS OF INCREASED CANCER SUSCEPTIBILITY TO STUDIES OF CANCER PREVENTION

On the basis of these findings, it has been considered that biomarkers of abnormal gastrointestinal cell proliferation and differentiation might facilitate studies in the field of cancer prevention [40]. It has been well established that in human populations throughout the world [14,41 42], components of the ingested diet have a major influence on the incidence rates both of adenomas and of colon cancer, adding significantly to the influence of genetic predisposition [1,6,14 43,44]. This has stimulated many investigators to attempt to evaluate possible inhibitory effects of dietary elements on tumor formation. However, measurements of this type have generally been made in animal models in which the appearance of tumors can be studied over short time periods; findings have indicated that specific dietary factors can inhibit the induction and development of a wide variety of tumors in rodent models, including those arising in the gastrointestinal tract.

Table 3 summarizes many of the different classes of chemicals that lead to inhibition of tumor induction and development in animal models [45,46] and that have potential capability for chemoprevention in human populations; some of these are naturally occurring constituents of food. The chemopreventive agents have been classified into two broad categories [45,46]: inhibitors effective against the formation or activation of tumor-initiating agents (i.e., genotoxic agents) or against tumor promoters.

Within the first group are compounds that prevent the formation of carcinogens from precursor substances, i.e., ascorbic acid [47], α-tocopherol [48], and certain plant phenols (caffeic and ferulic acids) [49]; compounds that prevent carcinogenic substances from reaching or reacting with critical target sites in the tissues, i.e., phenols [45,50,51] and certain plant flavonoids, flavones, coumarins, and isothiocyanates [52–54]; and compounds that act after exposure to carcinogenic agents by inhibiting the expression of neoplasia, i.e., retinoids and carotenoids [55–57], selenium salts [58–60], protease inhibitors [61–63], inhibitors of arachadonic acid metabolism [64,65], sterols [66], and a steroid hormone [67].

Compounds that inhibit tumor promotion include retinoids [68,69], protease inhibitors [62,70,71], inhibitors of arachadonic acid metabolism [68,72], phenols [73], agents that increase intracellular cyclic adenosine monophosphate (AMP) [74], and modulators of calcium metabolism [75,76].

Thus new rationales for dietary intervention attempting to inhibit tumor development have emerged from epidemiological studies and from studies of animal models that might warrant evaluation in human populations. In human subjects, however, it is much more difficult to carry out studies attempting to inhibit tumor induction and development than in animal models or to determine whether dietary modifications or chemopreventive agents will actually inhibit the future appearance of tumors over many years. In studies of this type carried out in human populations, when neoplasia itself is used as an endpoint, large numbers of subjects tested for long durations are generally required. However, biomarkers that are directly associated with the evolution of neoplasia and that occur with much higher frequency in abnormal cells of susceptible individuals than do the actual tumors increase the possibility of carrying out studies of this type on fewer subjects for shorter durations. If biomarkers or intermediate endpoints were found to be modified in short-term studies by a particular intervention, leading to the regrowth of more normal and mature gastrointestinal cells, a rationale would

TABLE 2.
Abnormal Differentiation of Gastrointestinal Epithelial Cells

Organ	Biomarker	References
Esophagus	Histopathology of hyperplasia and dysplasia	Munoz et al. [135] Yang et al. [136]
	Ectopic and normal cytokeratins	Doran et al. [137] Tseng et al. [138] Scaramuzzino et al. [139]
	Tumor-associated antigens	Burg-Kurland [140]
	Modified response to growth factors	Banks-Schlegal [141]
Stomach	Histopathology of superficial, chronic, and atrophic gastritis	Correa [142]
	Metaplasia of gastric epithelial cells	Morson, [143] Stemmerman et al. [144] Matsukura et al. [145] Nardelli [146] Correa [142]
	Intestinal enzymes and mucin in metaplastic glands	Matsukura et al. [145] Jass et al. [147] Bara et al. [148] Nardelli et al. [146] Correa [142]
	Aneuploidy of epithelial cell nuclei	Capurso [149]
	Differential protein localization	Lipkin et al. [33]
	Modified gene expression	Noguchi et al. [150]
	Modified response to growth factors	Johnson [151,134]
Large intestine	Development of colonic adenomas	Gardner [6] Morson and Bussey [15] Bussey [1] Winawer et al. [98]
	Histopathology of inflammatory diseases	Morson and Bussey [15]
	Cytokeratin expression in polyposis	Garin Chesa et al. [132]
	Blood group antigens	Sakamato et al. [19] Cordon-Cardo et al. [20] Abe et al. [21] Kim et al. [22]
	Modified gene expression	Royston and Augenlicht [27] Garin Chesa et al. [30] Augenlicht et al. [31]
	Modified response to growth factors	Friedman [17] Friedman et al. [18] Coffey et al. [32]

be provided for carrying out longer-term studies to attempt to modify the later evolution of human tumors.

Since epithelial cell proliferation is increased in the colon, stomach, and esophagus of human subjects with increased susceptibility to gastrointestinal cancer before the appearance of tumors, the analysis of gastrointestinal cell proliferation patterns have been considered for possible application to this problem [40,77]. It is known that

TABLE 3.
Compounds With Potential Capability for Chemoprevention in Human Subjects[a]

Compounds	References
I. Inhibitors effective against the formation or activation of tumor-initiating agents	
A. Compounds that prevent formation of carcinogens from precursor substances	
Ascorbic acid	Mirvish [47]
α-Tocopherol	Newmark and Mergens [48]
Plant phenols (caffeic acid, ferulic acid, etc.)	Kuenzig et al. [49]
B. Compounds that prevent carcinogenic substance from reaching or reacting with target sites in tissues	
Plant phenols	Wattenberg [45,51]
	Tatsuta et al. [50]
	Newmark [152]
Plant flavonoids, flavones, coumarins, and isothiocyanates	Diamond et al. [52]
	Wattenberg [53,54]
C. Compounds that act after exposure to carcinogenic agents (inhibit expression of neoplasia)	
Retinoids and carotenoids	Seifter et al. [55]
	Sporn and Roberts [56]
	Moon et al. [57]
Selenium salts	Jacobs [58]
	Birt et al. [59]
	Medina et al. [60]
Protease inhibitors	Mozumi et al. [61]
	Nomura et al. [62]
	Yavelow et al. [63]
Inhibitors of arachadonic acid metabolism	Narisawa et al. [64]
	Murasaka et al. [65]
Sterols and steroid hormone	Cohen et al. [66]
	Schwartz et al. [67]
II. Compounds that inhibit tumor promotion	
Retinoids	Verma et al. [68,69]
Protease inhibitors	Troll [70], Troll et al. [71]
	Mozumi et al. [61]
Inhibitors of arachadonic acid metabolism	Viaje et al. [72]
	Verma et al. [68]
Plant phenols	Slaga et al. [73]
	Newmark [152]
Agents that increase intracellular cyclic AMP	Perchelet and Boutwell [74]
Modulators of calcium metabolism	Wood et al. [76]
	Newmark et al. [75]
	Lipkin et al. [77]

[a]From references [45,46]

human populations having increased incidences of colonic cancer consume greater amounts of dietary fat [14,41,42]. Studies in animal models have indicated that dietary fat acts as a tumor promoter [78]; in various animal models supplemental dietary calcium has now decreased the hyperproliferation of colonic epithelial cells induced by bile acids and fatty acids [79–81] or after partial resection of the small intestine [82]. The incidence of carcinogen-induced colonic tumors also decreased in several animal models after supplemental dietary calcium [83,84]. Further studies in rodents have indicated that supplementary dietary calcium decreased the hyperproliferation of mammary epithelial cells that was induced by increased dietary fat intake and the hyperproliferation and tumor yield induced by a carcinogen [85,86]. These findings are summarized in Table 4.

In human subjects at increased risk for familial colon cancer, the biomarker of increased colonic epithelial cell proliferation was recently studied before and after oral dietary supplementation with calcium. Following calcium supplementation epithelial cell proliferation was reduced in the group as a whole, yielding an altered colonic-crypt profile approaching that previously observed in subjects at low risk for colon cancer [77,87–90]. Reductions were greatest in individuals having pronounced hyperproliferation of colonic epithelial cells, while other inidividuals whose proliferation was close to normal remained unchanged [88,90]. Dietary supplementation with calcium also induced increased numbers of maturing cells in the crypts as is characteristic of low-risk populations [87,90].

Direct exposure of normal human colonic epithelial cells to physiological amounts of calcium in vitro has characteristically shown the cells capable of responding with decreased proliferation; however, when the neoplastic transformation of colonic cells progressed to adenomas and carcinomas, the cells become unresponsive to calcium [89]. Calcium also has induced a more quiescent proliferative state in normal epithelial cells of other tissues (Table 5), including keratinocytes, mammary epithelial cells, esophageal epithelium, bronchial epithelium, and urothelium and led to terminal differentiation together with growth inhibition in some of the cell systems [91–97]. Thus, in the various studies cited above, measurements of the proliferation and differentiation of epithelial cells have served as "intermediate biomarkers" with which to analyze early effects of nutritional intervention in the cells of both human subjects and animal models.

The application of intermediate biomarkers to human intervention studies in the field of cancer prevention can be considered in several stages, summarized in Table 6. It now appears possible to carry out initial pilot studies on small groups of human subjects using many nutritional and pharmacologic interventions, as conventionally carried out in animal models. Each study would evaluate the success of an intervention by deter-

TABLE 4.
Effects of Supplemental Dietary Calcium on Proliferation and Differentiation of Colonic and Mammary Cells of Rodents

Cell type	Calcium effect	References
Colon	Decreased hyperproliferation induced by deoxycholic acid	Wargovich et al. [79]
	Decreased hyperproliferation induced by fatty acids	Wargovich et al. [81]
	Decreased hyperproliferation induced by cholic acid	Bird et al. [80]
	Decreased hyperproliferation induced by partial enteric resection	Appleton et al. [82]
	Decreased tumor formation induced by partial enteric resection and carcinogen	Appleton et al. [83]
	Decreased proliferation and tumor formation induced by dietary fat and carcinogen	Pence and Buddingh [84]
	Decreased intestinal tumors after AOM	Skrypec et al. [133]
Mammary	Decreased proliferation induced by dietary fat	Zhang et al. [85]
	Decreased proliferation and tumor formation induced by dietary fat and carcinogen	Jacobson et al. [86]

TABLE 5.
Direct Effects of Calcium on Proliferation and Differentiation of Epithelial Cells in Vitro

Cell type	Calcium effect	References
Colonic	Decreased proliferation (2 mM)	Buset et al. [89]
	Decreased proliferation (2–4 mM)	Appleton et al. [82]
	Decreased proliferation (2 mM)	Arlow et al. [153]
	Decreased proliferation (2 mM)	Buset et al. [154]
Epidermal	Decreased proliferation (1.2 mM) induced terminal differentiation	Hennings et al. [92]
	Decreased proliferation (1 mM) induced terminal differentiation	Tsao et al. [94]
	Decreased proliferation (1 mM) induced terminal differentiation	Boyce et al. [134]
Esophageal	Decreased proliferation (1 mM) induced terminal differentiation	Babcock et al. [95]
Mammary	Decreased proliferation (>0.06 mM) induced terminal differentiation	McGrath and Soule [96]
	Decreased proliferation (>0.06 mM) induced terminal differentiation	Soule and McGrath [97]
Bronchial	Decreased proliferation (1 mM)	Lechner et al. [93]
Urothelial	Decreased proliferation (1 mM) induced terminal differentiation	Kirk et al. [91]

mining whether it modified a biomarker(s) in a direction characteristic of more normal cell development and lower risk for neoplasia.

If this was accomplished by an intervention in a pilot study, it then might be justified to consider larger expanded studies on more subjects for longer durations, measuring more advanced stages of neoplasia. In the case of colonic neoplasia, an appropriate second-stage biomarker is the colonic adenoma, which recurs at characteristic rates in individuals whose adenomas previously were removed [15,98]. Colonic adenomas are further believed to be the major precursors of colonic cancer [15]. However, reduced recurrence rates of adenomas in parallel with decreased hyperproliferation and increased maturation of gastrointestinal cells, would further validate the intervention as being of potential benefit in large-scale public health studies. To measure whether a specific dietary or pharmacologic intervention

TABLE 6.
Proposed Application of Intermediate Biomarkers to Studies of Human Cancer Prevention

I. Pilot studies
   A. Populations: Small test populations of individuals at increased risk for gastrointestinal cancer
      1. Preneoplastic biomarkers to be measured: Hyperproliferation of epithelial cells, aberrant cell differentiation and preneoplastic gene expression

II. Expanded studies
   A. Populations: Larger survey populations at increased risk for gastrointestinal neoplasia, including groups of individuals with sporadic colonic adenomas
      1. Preneoplastic biomarkers to be measured: Those enumerated in A.1, above, and further measurements of recurrence of colonic adenomas

III. Public health intervention studies
   A. Populations: Larger numbers of individuals in the general population studied for longer durations
      1. Endpoint: The incidence of gastrointestinal cancer

reduced the recurrence rate of adenomas, much larger numbers of subjects are needed for study for longer durations than are required for measuring whether more normal colonic cell proliferation and maturation are induced in the same subjects; in addition, much has been learned in recent years about the clinical and pathologic characteristic of adenomas [1,14,15,98].

Following expanded studies (Table 6), if results indicated inhibition of adenoma development, consideration could then be given to larger-scale public health intervention trials, which require much larger numbers of subjects for much longer durations, to measure the effect of the intervention on the actual evolution of cancer. In considering the possibility that increased calcium in diets consumed by Western populations might influence tumor incidence, if current studies continue to show efficacy, then large-scale public health intervention attempts to decrease colon cancer appear to be feasible [75].

References

1. Bussey HJR: Familial Polyposis Coli. Baltimore: The Johns Hopkins University Press, 1975.
2. Lipkin M, Scherf S, Schechter L, Braun D Jr: Memorial Hospital registry of population groups at high risk for cancer of the large intestine: Age of onset of neoplasms. Prev Med 9:335–345, 1980.
3. Lipkin M: Biology of large bowel cancer. Cancer 36:2319,1975.
4. Knudsen AG Jr: Genetic and environmental interactions in the origin of human cancer. In Mulvihill JJ, Miller RW, Fraumeni JF (eds): Genetics of Human Cancer. New York: Raven Press, 1977, pp 391–99.
5. Fraumeni JF: Clinical patterns of familial cancer. In Mulvihill JJ, Miller RW, Fraumeni JF (eds): Genetics of Human Cancer. New York: Raven Press, 1977, pp 223–233.
6. Gardner EJ: A genetic and clinical study of intestinal polyposis, a predisposing factor for carcinoma of the colon and rectum. Am J Hum Genet 3:167, 1951.
7. Devic A, Bussy M: Un cas de polypose adenomaoeuse generalisee a tout l'intestin. Arch Mal App Dig 6:278–289, 1912.
8. Cabot RC: Case records of the Massachusetts General Hospital: Case No. 21061, N Engl J Med 212:263, 1935.
9. Fitzgerald GM: Multiple composite odontomas coincidental with other tumorous conditions: Report of a case. J Am Dent Assoc 30:1408, 1943.
10. Gardner EJ, Plenk HP: Hereditary pattern for multiple osteomas in a family group, Am J Hum Genet 4:31, 1952.
11. Smith WG: Desmoid tumors in familial multiple polyposis, Mayo Clin Proc 34:31, 1959.
12. Suzuki H, Honda E, Matsumoto K, Iriyama K: Tissue CEA determination and cytophotometric DNA analysis of colorectal mucosa in patients with colorectal cancer. Jpn J Surg 15(6):449–454, 1985.
13. Biasco G, Lipkin M, Minarini A, Higgins P, Miglioli M, Luigi B: Proliferative and antigenic properties of the rectal cells in patients with chronic ulcerative colitis. Cancer Res 44:5450–5454, 1984.
14. Correa P, Haenszel W: The epidemiology of large bowel cancer. Adv Cancer Res 26:1, 1978.
15. Morson BC, Bussey JR: Predisposing causes of intestinal cancer. Curr Probl Surg, February, pp 1–46, 1970.
16. Lightdale C, Lipkin M, Deschner E: In vivo measurements in familial polyposis: Kinetics and location of proliferating cells in colonic adenomas. Cancer Res 42:4280–4283, 1982.
17. Friedman E: Differential response of premalignant epithelial cell classes to phorbol ester tumor promoters and to deoxycholic acid. Cancer Res 4:4588–4599, 1981.
18. Friedman E, Gillin S, Lipkin M: 12-O-tetradecanoylphorbol-13-acetate stimulation of DNA synthesis in cultured preneoplastic familial polyposis colonic epithelial cells but not in normal colonic epithelial cells. Cancer Res 44:4078–4086, 1984.
19. Sakamoto J, Furukawa K, Cordon-Cardo C, Yin BWT, Rettig WJ, Oettgen HF, Old LJ, Lloyd KO: Expression of Lewis^a, Lewis^b, X, and Y blood group antigens in human colonic tumors and normal tissue and in human tumor-derived cell lines. Cancer Res 46:1553–1561, 1986.
20. Cordon-Cardo C, Lloyd KO, Sakamoto J, McGroarty ME, Old LI, Melamed MR: Immunohistologic expression of blood group antigens in normal human gastrointestinal tract and colonic carcinoma. Int J Cancer 37(5):667–676, 1986.
21. Abe K, Hakomori S, Ohshiba S: Differential expression of difucosyl type 2 chain (LeY) defined by monoclonal antibody AH6 in different locations of colonic epithelia, various histological types of colonic polyps, and adenocarcinomas. Cancer Res 46(5):2639–2644, 1986.
22. Kim YS, Yuan M, Itzkowitz SH, Sun QB, Kaizu T, Palekar A, Trump BF, Hakomori S: Expression of LeY and extended LeY blood group-related antigens in human malignant, premalignant, and nonmalignant colonic tissues. Cancer Res 46(11):5985–5992, 1986.
23. Wolman SR, Mastromarino AJ: Markers of colonic cell differentiation: A summary. In Mastromarino AJ, Brattain MG (eds): Markers of Cell Differentiation. New York: Raven Press, 1984, pp 131–139.
24. Wolman SR: Genetic markers of colonic neoplasia Semin Surg Oncol 3:120–125, 1987.
25. Bodmer WF, Bailey CJ, Bodmer J, Bussey HJR, Ellis A, Gorman P, Lucibello VA, Murday VA, Rider SH, Scambler P, Sheer D, Solomon E, Spurr NK: Localization of the gene for familial adenomatous polyposis on chromosome 5. Nature 328:614–616, 1987.
26. Augenlicht LH, Wahrman MZ, Halsey H, Anderson L, Taylor J, Lipkin M: Expression of cloned sequences in biopsies of human colonic tissue and in colonic carcinoma cells induced to differentiate in vitro. Cancer Res 47:6017–6021, 1987.

27. Royston ME and Augenlicht LH: Biotinated probe containing a long-terminal repeat hybridized to a mouse colon tumor and normal tissue. Science 222:1339–1341, 1983.

28. Solomon E, Voss R, Hall V, Bodmer WF, Jass JR, Jeffreys AJ, Lucibello FC, Patel I, Rider SH: Chromosome 5 allele loss in human colorectal carcinomas. Nature 328:616–619, 1987.

29. Fearon ER, Hamilton SR, Vogelstein B: Clonal analysis of human colorectal tumors. Science 328:193–197, 1987.

30. Garin Chesa P, Rettig WJ, Melamed MR, Old LJ, Niman HL: Expression of p21 ras in normal and malignant tissues, lack of association with proliferation and malignancy. Proc Nat Acad Sci USA 84:3234–3238, 1987.

31. Augenlicht LH, Augeron C, Yander G, Laboisse C: Overexpression of ras in mucus-secreting colon carcinoma cells of low tumorigenicity. Cancer Res 47:3763–3765, 1987.

32. Coffey RJ, Shipley GD, Moses HL: Production of transforming growth factors by human colon cancer lines. Cancer Res 46:1164–1169, 1986.

33. Lipkin M, Correa P, Mikol YB, Higgins PJ, Cuello C, Zarama G, Fontham E, Zavala D: Proliferative and antigenic modifications in epithelial cells in chronic atrophic gastritis. J Natl Cancer Inst 75:613–619, 1985.

34. Slaga TJ: Antiinflammatory steroids: Potent inhibitors of tumor promotion. In Slaga TJ (ed): Carcinogenesis, Vol 5: Modifiers of Chemical Carcinogenesis, New York: Raven Press, 1980, pp 111–126.

35. Colburn NH: Tumor promotion and preneoplastic progression. In Slaga TJ (ed): Carcinogenesis, Vol 5: Modifiers of Chemical Carcinogenesis, New York: Raven Press, 1980, pp 33–56.

36. Boutwell RI: The function and mechanism of promoters of carcinogenesis. CRC Crit Rev Toxicol 2:419–443, 1974.

37. Wilbanks GD, Richart RM, Terner JY: DNA content of cervical intraepithelial neoplasia studied by two-wavelength Feulgen cytophotometry. Am J Obstet Gynecol 98:792–799, 1967.

38. Chi CH, Rubio CA, Lagerlof B: The frequency and distribution of mitotic figures in dysplasia and carcinoma in situ. Cancer 39:1218–1223, 1977.

39. Schubert B, Kunz J, Banaschak A: Labelling patterns of carcinomas of the cervix and their precancerous stages after ^{3}H-thymidine incorporation. Acta Histochem 27:111–115, 1983.

40. Lipkin M: Biomarkers of increased susceptibility to gastrointestinal cancer: New application to studies of cancer prevention in human subjects. Perspectives in Cancer Research. Cancer Research 48:235–245, 1988.

41. Doll R, Peto R: The causes of Cancer: Quantitative estimates of avoidable risks of cancer in the United States today. JNCI 66:1191–1308, 1981.

42. Weisburger JH, Reddy BS, Fiala ES, Barnes W, Wynder EL: Update on gastrointestinal carcinogenesis. In Jerzy Glass GB, Sherlock P (eds): Progress in Gastroenterology, Vol IV, New York: Grune & Stratton, 1983, pp 327–344.

43. Lipkin M, Sherlock P, de Cosse J: Risk factors and preventive measures in the control of cancer of the large intestine. Curr Probl Cancer 4:1–57, 1980.

44. Lynch HT, Lynch PM: In Lipkin M, Good RA (eds): Hereditary and Gastrointestinal Tract Cancer. In Gastrointestinal Tract Cancer. New York: Plenum Medical Book Co., pp 241–274, 1978.

45. Wattenberg LW: Inhibitors of chemical carcinogens. Adv Cancer Res 26:197–226, 1978.

46. Wattenberg LW: Chemoprevention of cancer. Cancer Res 45:1–8, 1985.

47. Mirvish SS: Ascorbic acid inhibition on *N*-nitrous compound formation in chemical food and biological systems. In: Zedeck MS and Lipkin M (eds): Inhibition of Tumor Induction and Development. New York: Plenum, pp 101–126, 1981.

48. Newmark H, Mergens W: α-Tocopherol (vitamin E) and its relationship to tumor induction. In Zedeck MS, Lipkin M (eds): Inhibition of Tumor Induction and Development, New York: Plenum Publishing Corp, 1981, pp 127–168.

49. Kuenzig W, Chau J, Norkus E, Holowaschenko H, Newmark H, Mergens W, Conney AN: Caffeic and ferulic acid as blockers of nitrosamine formation. Carcinogenesis (Lond) 5:309–314, 1984.

50. Tatsuta M, Mikuni T, Taniguchi H: Protective effect of butylated hydroxytoluene against induction of gastric cancer by N-methyl-N-nitro-N-nitrosoguanidine in Wistar rats. Int J Cancer 32:253–254, 1983.

51. Wattenberg L: Inhibitors of chemical carcinogens. In Burchenal JH (ed): Cancer: Achievements, Challenges and Prospects for the 1980's, New York: Grune & Stratton, 1981, pp. 517–539.

52. Diamond L, McFall R, Miller J, Gelboin HV: The effects of two isomeric benzoflavones on aryl hydrocarbon hydroxylase and the toxicity and carcinogenicity of polycyclic hydrocarbons. Cancer Res 32:731–736, 1972.

53. Wattenberg LW: Inhibition of carcinogenic effects of polycyclic hydrocarbons by benzyl isothiocyanate and related compounds. J Natl Cancer Inst 58:395–398, 1977.

54. Wattenberg LW: Inhibitors of chemical carcinogens. In Emmelot P, and Kriek E (eds): Environmental Carcinogenesis, Amsterdam: Elsevier/North-Holland Biomedical Press, 1979, pp 241–264.

55. Seifter E, Rettura G, Levenson SM: Dietary β-carotene is an effective tumor preventive agent. In Proceedings of the Thirteenth International Cancer Congress, Seattle, WA, September 8–15, 1982, p 30.

56. Sporn MB, Roberts AB: The role of retinoids in differentiation and carcinogenesis. Cancer Res 43:3034–3040, 1983.

57. Moon RC, McCormick DL, Mehta RG: Inhibition of carcinogenesis by retinoids. Cancer Res [Suppl] 43:2469–2475, 1983.

58. Jacobs MM: Inhibitory effects of selenium on 1,2-dimethylhydrazine and methytazoxymethanol colon carcinogenesis. Cancer (Phila) 40:2557–2564, 1977.

59. Birt DF, Lawson TA, Julius AD, Runice CE, Salmasi S: Inhibition by dietary selenium of colon cancer induced in the rat by bis-(2-oxopropyl)nitrosamine. Cancer Res 42:4455–4459, 1982.

60. Medina D, Lane HW, Shepherd F: Effect of dietary selenium levels on 7,12-dimethylbenzanthracene-

induced mouse mammary tumorigenesis. Carcinogenesis (Lond) 4:1159–1163, 1983.

61. Mozumi M, Ogawa M, Sugimura T, Takeuchi T, Umezawa H: Inhibition tumorigenesis in mouse skin by leupeptin, a protease inhibitor from actinomycetes. Cancer Res 32:1725–1728, 1972.

62. Nomura T, Hata S, Enomoto T, Tanaka H, Shibata K: Inhibiting effects of antipain on urethane-induced lung neoplasia in mice. Br J Cancer 42:624–626, 1980.

63. Yavelow J, Finlay TH, Kennedy AR, Troll W: Bowman-Birk soybean protease inhibitor as an anticarcinogen. Cancer Res [Suppl] 43:2454–2459, 1983.

64. Narisawa T, Sato M, Tani M, Kudo T, Takahashi T, Goto A: Inhibition of development of methylnitrosourea-induced rat colon tumors by indomethacin treatment. Cancer Res 41:1954–1957, 1981.

65. Murasaka G, Zenser TV, Davis BB, Cohen SM: Inhibition by aspirin of N-(4-[5-nitro-2-furyl]-2-thiazoly) -formamide–induced bladder carcinogenesis. Carcinogenesis (Lond) 5:53–55, 1984.

66. Cohen BI, Raicht RF: Plant sterols: Protective role in chemical carcinogenesis. In Zedeck MS, Lipkin M (eds): Inhibition of Tumor Induction and Development, New York: Plenum Publishing Corp, 1981, pp 189–201.

67. Schwartz AG, Tannen RH: Inhibition of 7,12-dimethylbenz(α)-anthracene- and urethan-induced lung tumor formation in A/J mice by long-term treatment with dehydroepiandrosterone. Carcinogenesis (Lond) 2:1335–1337, 1981.

68. Verma AK, Garcia CT, Ashendel CL, Boutwell RK: Inhibition of 7-bromoethylbenz[α]anthracene-promoted mouse skin tumor formation by retinoic acid and dexamethasone. Cancer Res 43:3045–3049, 1983.

69. Verma AK, Shapas BG, Rice HM, Boutwell RK: Correlation of the inhibition by retinoids of tumor promoter-induced mouse epidermal ornithine decarboxylase activity and of skin tumor promotion. Cancer Res 39:419–425, 1979.

70. Troll W: Blocking tumor promotion by protease inhibitors. In Magee PN et al. (eds): Fundamentals in Cancer Prevention, Baltimore: University Park Press, 1976, pp 41–55.

71. Troll W, Klassen A, Janoff A: Tumorigenesis in mouse skin: Inhibition by synthetic inhibitors of proteases, Science 169:1211–1213, 1970.

72. Viaje A, Slaga TJ, Wigler M, Weinstein B: Effects of antiinflammatory agents on mouse skin tumor promotion, epidermal DNA synthesis, phorbol ester-induced cellular proliferation, and production of plasminogen activator. Cancer Res 37:1530–1536, 1977.

73. Slaga TJ, Solanki W, Logani M: Studies on the mechanism of action of antitumor promoting agents: Suggestive evidence for the involvement of free radicals in promotion. In Nygaad OF, Simic MG (eds): Radioprotectors and Anticarcinogens, New York: Academic Press, Inc, 1983, pp417–485.

74. Perchellet JP, Boutwell RK: Comparison of the effects of 3-isobutyl-1-methylxanthine and adenosine cyclic 3′:5′-monophosphate on the induction of skin tumors by the initiation-promotion protocol and by the complete carcinogenesis process. Carcinogenesis (Lond) 3:53–60, 1982.

75. Newmark HL, Wargovich MJ, Bruce WR: Colon cancer and dietary fat, phosphate and calcium: A hypothesis. J Natl Cancer Inst 72:1323–1325, 1981.

76. Wood AW, Chang RL, Huang MT, Uskokovic M, Conney AH: 1,-25-Dihydroxyvitamin D_3 inhibits phorbol ester-dependent chemical carcinogenesis in mouse skin. Biochem Biophys Res Commun 116:605–611, 1983.

77. Lipkin M, Newmark H: Effect of added dietary calcium on colonic epithelial cell proliferation in subjects at high-risk for familial colon cancer. N Eng J Med 313:1381–1384, 1985.

78. Bull AW, Soullier BK, Wilson PS, Hayden MT, Nigro ND: Promotion of azoxymethane-induced intestinal cancer by high fat in rats. Cancer Res 39:4956–4959, 1979.

79. Wargovich MJ, Eng VWS, Newmark HL, Bruce WR: Calcium ameliorates the toxic effect of deoxycholic acid on colonic epithelium. Carcinogenesis 4:1205–1207, 1983.

80. Bird RP, Schneider R, Stamp D, Bruce WR: Effect of dietary calcium and cholic acid on the proliferative indices of murine colonic epithelium. Carcinogenesis 7:1657–1661, 1986.

81. Wargovich MJ, Eng VWS, Newmark HL, Bruce WR: Calcium inhibits the damaging and compensating proliferative effects of fatty acids on mouse colon epithelium. Cancer Lett 23:253–258, 1984.

82. Appleton GVN, Bristol JB, Williamson RCN: Increased dietary calcium and small bowel resection have opposite effects on colonic cell turnover. Br J Surg 73:1018–1021, 1986.

83. Appleton GVN, Davies PW, Bristol JB, Williamson RCN: Inhibition of intestinal carcinogenesis by dietary supplementation with calcium. Br J Surg 74:523–525, 1987.

84. Pence BC, Buddingh F: Inhibition of dietary fat promotion of colon carcinogenesis by supplemental calcium or vitamin D. Proc Assoc Cancer Res 28:154, 1957.

85. Zhang L, Bruce WR, Bird RP: Influence of dietary fat and calcium on the proliferative indices of mouse mammary glands. Cancer Res 47:4905–4508, 1987.

86. Jacobson EA, Russell R, Newmark HL, Amer MA, Carroll KK: Fat calcium and tumor development in dimethylbenz(α)anthracene (DMBA)-treated rats. Proc Can Fed Biol Soc [Abstr], 1987.

87. Lipkin M, Newmark M: Application of intermediate biomarkers and prevention of cancer of the large intestine In Basic and Clinical Perspectives of Colorectal Polyps and Cancer Steele G, et al (eds): Alan R. Liss, Inc., New York, pp 135–150, 1988.

88. Lipkin M, Friedman E, Winawer S, Newmark H: Colonic epithelial cell proliferation in responders and nonresponders to supplemental dietary calcium. Cancer Research 49:248–254, 1989.

89. Buset M, Lipkin M, Winawer S, Swaroop S, Friedman E: Inhibition of human colonic epithelial cell proliferation in vivo and in vitro by calcium. Cancer Res 46:5426–5430, 1986.

90. Rozen P, Fireman Z, Wax Y, Ron E: Oral calcium suppresses increased colonic mucosal proliferation of persons at risk for colorectal neoplasia. Gastroenterology [Part 2] 92:1603, 1987; Gut, in press.

91. Kirk D, Kagawa S, Vener G, Narayan KS, Ohnuki Y, Jones LW: Selective growth of normal adult human urothelial cells in serum-free medium. In Vitro 22:165–171, 1985.

92. Hennings H, Michael D, Cheng N, Steinert P, Holbrook K, Yuspa SH: Calcium regulation of growth and differentiation of mouse epidermal cells in culture. Cell 19:245–254, 1980.

93. Lechner JK, Haugen A, McClendon IA, Pettis EW: Clonal growth of normal adult human bronchial epithelial cells in a serum-free medium. In Vitro 18:633–642, 1982.

94. Tsao MC, Walthall BJ, Ham RC: Clonal growth of normal human epidermal keratinocytes in a defined medium. J Cell Physiol 110:219–229, 1982.

95. Babcock MS, Marino MR, Gunning WT III, and Stoner GD: Clonal growth and serial propagation of rat esophageal epithelial cells. In Vitro 19:403–415, 1983.

96. McGrath CM, Soule HD: Calcium regulation of normal mammary epithelial cell growth in culture. In Vitro 20:652–662, 1984.

97. Soule HD, McGrath CM: A simplified method for passage and long-term growth of human mammary epithelial cells. In Vitro 22:6–12, 1986.

98. Winawer SJ, Ritchie MT, Diaz BJ, Gottlieb LS, Stewart ET, Zauber A, John EH: The National Polyp Study. Front Gastrointest Res 10:216–225, 1986.

99. Lipkin M, Uehara K, Winawer S, et al.: Seventh Day Adventist vegetarians have quiescent proliferative activity in colonic mucosa. Cancer Lett 26:139–144, 1985.

100. Terpstra OT, Van Blankenstein M, Dees J, Eilers GAM: Abnormal pattern of cell proliferation in the entire colonic mucosa of patients with colon adenoma or cancer. Gastroenterology 92:704–708, 1987.

101. Ponz de Leon M, Roncucci L, Donato PD, Tassi L, et al.: Patterns of epithelial cell proliferation in colorectal mucosa subjects and of patients with adenomatous polyps or cancer of the large bowel. Cancer Res 48:4121–4126, 1988.

102. Herbst JJ, Berenson MM, McCloskey DW, Wiser WC: Cell proliferation in esophageal columnar epithelium (Barrett's esophagus). Gastroent 75:683–687, 1978.

103. Pellish LJ, Hermos JA, Eastwood GL: Cell proliferation in three types of Barrett's epithelium. Gut 21:26–31, 1980.

104. Livstone EM, Sheahan DG, Behar J: Studies of esophageal epithelial cell proliferation in patients with reflux esophagitis. Gastroent 73:1315–1319, 1977.

105. Munoz N, Lipkin M, Crespi M, Wahrendorf J, Grassi A, Lu S: Proliferative abnormalities of the oesophageal epithelium of Chinese populations at high and low risk for oesophageal cancer. Int; J ;Cancer 36:187–189, 1985.

106. Yang G-C, Lipkin M, Yang K, Wang G-Q, Li J-Y, Yang CS, Winawer S, Newmark H, Blot W, Fraumeni JF, Jr: Proliferation of esophageal epithelial cells in individuals in Linxian, China. J Natl Cancer Inst 79:1241–1246, 1987.

107. Bell B, Almy TP, Lipkin M: Cell proliferation kinetics in the gastrointestinal tract of man. III Cell renewal in esophagus, stomach, and jejunum of a patient with treated pernicious anemia. J Natl Cancer Inst 38:615–628, 1967.

108. Willems G, Bleiberg H: Proliferative changes in the gastric mucosa of patients with pernicious anemia. In A. Gerard (ed): Gastrointestinal Tumors: A Clinical and Experimental Approach. New York: Pergamon Press, 1978, p. 39.

109. Winawer SJ, Lipkin M: Cell proliferation kinetics in the gastrointestinal tract of man. IV. Cell renewal in the intestinalized gastric mucosa. J Natl Cancer Inst 42:9, 1969.

110. Deschner EE, Winawer SJ, Lipkin M: Patterns of nucleic acid and protein synthesis in normal human gastric mucosa and atrophic gastritis. J Natl Cancer Inst 48:1567–1574, 1972.

111. Sizikov AI, Azykbekov R: Histoautoradiographic study of gastric epithelial DNA synthesis in precancerous lesions of the stomach. Vopr Onkol 27:19–22, 1981.

112. Assad RT, Eastwood GL: Epithelial proliferation in human fundic mucosa after antrectomy and vagotomy. Gastroent 79:807–811, 1980.

113. Hansen OH, Larsen JK, Svendsen LB: Changes in gastric mucosal cell proliferation after antrectomy or vagotomy in man. Scand J Gastroenterol 13:947–952, 1978.

114. Offerhaus GJA, van de Stadt J, Samson G, Tytgat GNJ: Cell proliferation kinetics in the gastric remnant. Eur J Cancer Clin Oncol 21(1):73–79, 1985.

115. Deschner E, Lewis CM, Lipkin M: In vitro study of human rectal epithelial cells. I. Atypical zone of H^3 thymidine incorporation in mucosa of multiple polyposis. J Clin Invest 42:1922–1928, 1963.

116. Bleiberg H, Mainguet P, Galand P: Cell renewal in familial polyposis: comparision between polyps and adjacent healthy mucosa. Gastroent 63:240–245, 1972.

117. Lipkin M: Phase 1 and phase 2 proliferative lesions of colonic epithelial cells in diseases leading to colonic cancer. Cancer 34:878–888, 1974.

118. Deschner EE, Lipkin M: Proliferative patterns in colonic mucosa in familial polyposis. Cancer 35: 413–418, 1975.

119. Iwama T, Utsunomiya J, Sasaki J: Epithelial cell kinetics in the crypts of familial polyposis of colon. Jpn J Surg 7:230–234, 1977.

120. Lipkin M, Blattner WE, Fraumeni JF Jr, Lynch HT, Deschner EE, Winawer S: Tritiated thymidine (øp, øh) labeling distribution as a marker for hereditary predisposition to colon cancer. Cancer Res 43:1899–1904, 1983.

121. Lipkin M, Blattner WA, Gardner EJ, Burt RW, Lynch H, Deschner E, Winawer S, Fraumeni JF, Jr: Classification and risk assessment of individuals with familial polyposis, Gardner Syndrome, and familial nonpolyposis colon cancer from [^{3}H]dThd-labeling patterns in colonic epithelial cells. Cancer Res 44:4201–4207, 1984.

122. Cole JW, McKalen A: Studies on the morphogenesis of adenomatous polyps in the human colon. Cancer 16:998–1002, 1963.

123. Maskens AP, Meersseman F, Beckers C: In vitro radioautographic study of adenomatous polyp and hyperplasia of the rectocolic mucosa in man. Scand J Gastroent 7:43, 1982.

124. Maskens AP, Deschner EE: Tritiated thymidine incorporation into epithelial cells of normal-appearing

colorectal mucosa of cancer patients. J Natl Cancer Inst 58:1221–1224, 1977.

125. Romagnoli P, Filipponi F, Bandettini L, Brugnola D: Increase of mitotic activity in the colonic mucosa of patients with colorectal cancer. Dis Colon Rectum 27:305–308, 1984.

126. Bleiberg H, Mainguet P, Galand P, Chretien J, Dupont-Mairesse N: Cell renewal in the human rectum: In vitro autoradiographic study on active ulcerative colitis. Gastroent 58:851–855, 1970.

127. Eastwood GL, Trier JS: Epithelial cell renewal in cultured rectal biopsies in ulcerative colitis. Gastroent 64:383–390, 1973.

128. Serafini EP, Kirk AP, Chambers TJ: Rate and pattern of epithelial cell proliferation in ulcerative colitis. Gut 22:648–652, 1981.

129. Deschner EE, Winawer SJ, Katz S, Kahn E: Proliferative defects in ulcerative colitis patients. Cancer Invest 1:41–47, 1983.

130. Lehy T, Mignon M, Abitbol JL: Epithelial cell proliferation in the rectal stump of patients with ileorectal anastomosis for ulcerative colitis. Gut 24:1048–1056, 1983.

131. Lipkin M, Enker WF, Winawer SJ: Tritiated thymidine labeling of rectal epithelial cells in "non-prep" biopsies of individuals at increased risk for colonic neoplasea. Cancer Lett 37:153–161, 1987.

132. Garin Chesa P, Rettig WJ, Melamed MR: Expression of cytokeratins in normal and neoplastic colonic epithelial cells—implications for cellular differentiation and carcinogenesis. Am J Surg Path 10:829–835, 1986.

133. Skrypec DJ, Bursey RG: Effect of dietary calcium azoxymethane-induced intestinal carcinogenesis in male F344 rats fed high fat diets. FASEB Journal 2:A857, 1988.

134. Boyce ST, Hann RG: Calcium-regulated differentiation of normal human epidermal keratinocytes in chemically defined clonal culture and serum-free serial culture. J Invest Dermatol 81:33s–40s, 1983.

135. Munoz N, Crespi M, Grassi A et al.: Precursor lesions of oesophageal cancer in high-risk populations in Iran and China: Lancet i, 876–879, 1972.

136. Yang GC, Lipkin M, Yang K, Wang G-Q, Li J-Y, Yang CS, Winawer S, Newmark H, Blot WJ, Fraumeni JF, Jr: Proliferation of esophageal epithelial cells among residents of Linxian, China. J Natl Cancer Inst 79:1241–1246, 1987.

137. Doran TI, Vidrich A, Sun T: Intrinsic and extrinsic regulation of the differentiation of skin, corneal and esophageal epithelial cells. Cell 22:17–25, 1980.

138. Tseng SCG, Hatchell D, Tierney N, Huang AJW, Sun T: Expression of specific keratin markers by rabbit corneal, conjunctival, and esophageal epithelia during Vitamin A deficiency. J Cell Biol 99:2279–2286, 1984.

139. Scaramuzzino D, Stoner GD, Goldblatt PJ: Keratin protein expression in nontumorigenic and tumorigenic rat esophageal epithelial cells (meeting abstract). Proc Annu Meet Am Assoc Cancer Res 27:69, 1986.

140. Burg-Kurland CL, Purnell DM, Combs JW, Hillman EA, Harris CC, Trump BF: Immunocytochemical evaluation of human esophageal neoplasms and preneoplastic lesions for beta-chorionic gonadotropin, placental lactogen, alphafetoprotein, carcinoembryonic antigen, and nonspecific cross-reacting antigen. Cancer Res 46(6):2936–2943, 1986.

141. Banks-Schlegel SP, Quintero J: Human esophageal carcinoma cells have fewer, but higher affinity epidermal growth factor receptors. J Biol Chem 261(10): 4359–4962, 1986.

142. Correa P: Chronic gastritis as a cancer precursor. Scand J Gastroenter 19:131–136, 1984.

143. Morson B: Carcinoma arising from areas of intestinal metaplasia in the gastric mucosa. Br J Cancer 9:377–385, 1955.

144. Stemmermann, GN, Hayashi T: Intestinal metaplasia of the gastric mucosa: A gross and microscopic study of its distribution in various disease state. J Natl Cancer Inst 4:627–634, 1968.

145. Matsukura N, Susuki K, Kawachi T, Aoyagi M, Sugimura T, Kitaoka H, Numajiri H, Itahashi M, Hirota T: Distribution of marker enzymes and mucin in intestinal metaplasia in human stomach and incomplete types of intestinal metaplasia in minute gastric carcinomas. J Natl Cancer Inst 65:231–240, 1980.

146. Nardelli J, Bara J, Rosa B, Burtin PJ: Intestinal metaplasia and carcinomas of the human stomach: An immunohistologic study. Histochem Cytochem 31: 366–375, 1983.

147. Jass JR, Filipe MI: Sultamucins and precancerous lesions of the human stomach. Histopathology 4:271–279, 1980.

148. Bara J, Loisillier F, Burtin P: Antigen gastric and intestinal mucous cells in human colonic tumors. Br J Cancer 41:209–221, 1980.

149. Capurso L, Teodori L, DeVita R, Galloni L, Tarquini M et al.: DNA content as a marker of precancerous lesions of the digestive tract. Gastroenterology 82(5):1029, 1982.

150. Noguchi M, Hirohashi S, Shimosato Y, Thor A, Schlom J, Tsunokawa Y, Terada M, Sugimura T: Histologic demonstration of antigens reactive with anti-p21 ras monoclonal antibody (RAP-5) in human stomach cancers. J Natl Cancer Inst 77(2):379–385, 1986.

151. Johnson LR: Regulation of Gastrointestinal growth. In: Physiology for the Gastrointestinal tract, Second Edition, eds. Johnson LR, Raven Press, New York, 1987, pp 301–333.

152. Newmark HL: Plant phenolics as inhibitors of mutational and precarcinogenic events. Canad J Physiol & Pharmcol 65:461–466, 1987.

153. Arlow FL, Walczak SM, Majumdar APN: The role of calcium in deoxycholic acid-induced hyperproliferation of colonic mucosal explants. Gastroenterology 94:A12, 1988.

154. Buset M, Lipkin M, Winawer S, Friedman E: Direct and indirect protection of human colonic epithelial cells by calcium. Gastroenterology 92 (Part 2):1334, 1987.

29

Inhibition of Intestinal Carcinogenesis by Dietary Supplementation with Calcium

G.V.N. Appleton and R.C.N. Williamson

Department of Surgery, Royal Postgraduate Medical School, Hammersmith Hospital, London, England

INTRODUCTION

Therapeutic advances in large bowel cancer over the past 40 years have been unsuccessful in improving the overall prognosis of the disease: large bowel cancer causes almost as many deaths now as it did in 1945 [1,2]. The slight benefit provided by innovations in surgical, anesthetic, and oncological techniques has been balanced by a slow rise in incidence [2,3]. It is becoming increasingly clear that research efforts must be directed toward prevention (and very early detection) of the disease rather than treatment of the established cancer.

A propensity to colorectal cancer is carried within certain high-risk families [4], yet environmental factors dominate the etiology of this disease. Haenszel's classic studies on migrants in the 1960s [5,6] together with subsequent population studies [7,8] suggest that diet is the main risk factor in the majority of cases. Interest in calcium as a chemopreventative agent began when the IARC Working Party in Scandinavia showed that the incidence of colorectal cancer was lower in areas where the inhabitants consumed more dairy products, despite a high-fat diet [9]. Since then, many different aspects of the effect of calcium on the gastrointestinal epithelium have been investigated, including changes in adaptive potential and carcinogenesis.

An intake of approximately 1 g/day calcium is required for normal health [10]. About 230 mg are absorbed from the gut, specifically in the duodenum and upper jejunum; 130 mg is secreted into the distal small bowel, and 100 mg appears in the urine. Almost no calcium transport occurs in the colon: fecal calcium is unchanged after total colectomy, and an isolated colonic loop secretes no calcium into its lumen [11]. Milk, cheese, and flour provide 75% of the normal intake of calcium, the rest coming from small amounts in several other foodstuffs[10]. The Western diet of the 1980s, increasingly dominated by "fast food" and sweet-tasting products, may be deficient in calcium. In the United Kingdom a study of 375 11–14 year olds indicated that many children require additional dietary calcium for normal growth and development [10]. Drinking water usually provides 5% of the total daily calcium input, although there is considerable regional and annual variation.

Cytokinetic techniques have been extensively used to study the action of calcium on epithelial surfaces. A large body of data collected in our laboratory [12] and from others [4] indicates that the rate of epithelial cell turnover in the colonic crypts determines an individual's susceptibility to colorectal carcinoma. Accelerated rates of DNA synthesis (measured by autoradiography) and crypt cell production (measured by a stathmokinetic technique) are associated with increased numbers of experimentally induced neoplasms [4,12]. Colonoscopic biopsies at multiple sites in patients with adenomas or carcinomas show increased labeling indices [13,14]; patients with such a "field change" are, therefore, particu-

Familial Adenomatous Polyposis, pages 245–251

larly prone to adenoma formation and consequent malignant change. Evaluating cytokinetic data in the gastrointestinal epithelium is a useful biomarker of a subject's cancer risk [4].

Current research on the inhibition of tumor formation by intraluminal calcium centers around population studies, the effect on colonic adaptation and carcinogenesis, and possible mechanisms of action.

POPULATION STUDIES

During the 1960s, Garland noted that the death rate from colorectal cancer was highest in American cities receiving the least exposure to sunlight, and he postulated that vitamin D and calcium might be intermediaries in this effect [15]. He thus initiated a 19 year prospective dietary study on 1,954 men from Chicago, which showed that a high calcium intake (>1,500 mg/day) was associated with a 65% reduction in cancer incidence [16]. Diets rich in vitamin D were similarly protective.

Conversely, low calcium diets (<500 mg/day) lead to a greater cancer risk [17]. A study of 110 Hawaiian-Japanese subjects carried out by Heilbrun and colleagues [18] failed to confirm these data, but total calcium intake was particularly low and numbers were small. Despite the uncertainty surrounding the conclusions drawn from the study of Heilbrun et al., it seems that populations consuming high-calcium diets enjoy a relative freedom from colon cancer [19].

ACTION OF CALCIUM IN VIVO

Adaptation

Clinical trials and animal models have both shown that dietary supplementation with calcium causes striking adaptation in the large bowel [20–24]. Patients who are at high risk for developing colorectal carcinoma, e.g., first-degree relatives of colon cancer patients, have raised proliferative indices in their colonic crypts [22]. If high-risk patients are given 1.25 g calcium carbonate daily, their labeling indices fall to those seen in the normal population [22]. In rodents, the promoting effects of intrarectally administered bile acids and fatty acids on cell division in the colon are negated by concomitant oral gavage with either calcium lactate or gluconate [23,24].

Massive small bowel resection in rats normally causes a 50–100% increment in crypt cell production rate (CCPR) within the left colon. Doubling the rats' daily intake of calcium from 0.5% to 1.0% (by adding 24 g/liter calcium lactate to the drinking water) prevents the adaptive response; it also causes a fall in colonic CCPR among control animals without resection (Table 1) [20].

Carcinogenesis

If dietary manipulation with calcium is combined with exposure to a specific colorectal carcinogen (azoxymethane), the yield of large bowel tumors obtained in rats closely parallels the data on adaptation (see above) [21]. Animals receiving added calcium develop about one-half the number of colorectal neoplasms compared with controls given ordinary tap water [21] (Table 1). As before, merely doubling the intake of calcium abolishes the expected effect of small bowel resection, namely, promotion of colorectal carcinogenesis. Tumor inhibition by calcium is also seen in rats fed high-fat diets [25]. Using the classification of colorectal tumors of Sunter et al. [26], we have shown that the main effect of calcium is to reduce the yield of adenomas and type 1 carcinomas; no significant differences in type 2 or type 3 carcinomas were observed between treated and nontreated groups (Table 2).

Laboratory rats are particularly susceptible to carcinogens such as azoxymethane and dimethylhydiazine. Newmark [27] argues that commercially available rat chow contains a 10-fold excess of calcium (on a relative scale) over that found in human diets. A recent study in rats using calcium concentrations approximating to "human nutrient density" indicates that when overall dietary calcium concentrations are very low (0.03%), calcium still offers protection against colorectal tumor development; however, the effect is limited to malignant neoplasms (M.J. Wargovich, personal communication). Within the small intestine calcium also inhibits the formation of azoxymethane-induced tumors in Sprague-Dawley rats [21]: 46–51% fewer duodenal tumors

TABLE 1.
Effect of Calcium on Colorectal Adaptation and Carcinogenesis in Sprague-Dawley Rats†

Group	Colonic CCPR (cells/crypt/hour)	Colonic tumor yield (mean No. tumors/rat)
Jejunal trans, tap water	4.49 ± 0.33	4.34 ± 0.62
Jejunal trans, added calcium	3.32 ± 0.40	1.83 ± 0.44
80% SBR, tap water	7.23 ± 0.44*	6.74 ± 1.87*
80% SBR	4.98 ± 0.70*	3.69 ± 1.35*

†Jejunal trans, transection of jejunum 10% along length of small bowel (acting as control for the resection groups); 80% SBR, resection of the middle 80% of the small bowel; added calcium, = 24 g/liter calcium lactate added to drinking water. Data are based on those of Appleton et al. [20,21].
*$P < 0.01$ vs. equivalent group with jejunal transection.

were seen in animals given supplemental calcium lactate.

ACTION OF CALCIUM IN VITRO

In addition to its intraluminal effect, calcium modifies the behavior of cell lines and small explants in vitro. An extensive study of cultured epidermal cells by Hennings et al. [28] has shown that the extracellular concentration of calcium is critical in the regulation of proliferation and differentiation. Keratinocytes divide rapidly in 0.05–0.1 mM calcium and form a monolayer with a high growth fraction; the cells do not stratify and they continue to produce keratin. After raising calcium concentrations, epidermal cells undergo terminal differentiation, cell-to-cell contact occurs rapidly, and desmosomes form within 2 hours. Cells then stratify, become cornified, and detach from the dish [28]. Calcium has also been shown to induce a quiescent proliferative state in mammary, esophageal, bronchial, and urothelial cells [4]. CCPR in organ-cultured rat colonic explants falls by 33% when the extracellular calcium concentration is raised from 2 to 4 mM, and a further fall of 26% is seen when levels reach 6 mM [29]. A similar response is seen in colonic biopsies from high-risk patients, and calcium reverses deoxycholate-induced hyperproliferation (and raised ODC levels) in human and rodent colonic explants [30].

TABLE 2.
Classification of Colorectal Tumors*

Type of neoplasm	Control	Added calcium	P
Adenoma	1.09 ± 0.23	0.50 ± 0.21	<0.05
Type 1 carcinoma	1.68 ± 0.37	0.41 ± 0.40	<0.01
Types 2+3 carcinomas	1.39 ± 0.41	1.01 ± 0.22	NS

*According to Sunter et al. [26]. Data are based on those of Appleton et al. [21].

The effect of calcium on cultured neoplastic colonic tissue is less clear. In a limited study in man by Buset et al. [31], no restraint of proliferation was seen in either polyps or carcinomas. Transformed mouse 3T3 cells and neoplastic rat liver cells are also unresponsive [32,33]. By contrast, LoVo, a human adenocarcinoma cultured cell line, undergoes restricted proliferation when calcium is added to serum-free media, and a spindle-like pattern of growth ensues [34].

CIRCULATING LEVELS OF CALCIUM AND PHOSPHATE

Serum concentrations of calcium alter little with dietary variation. This phenomenon was first recognized in the 1920s [35], and it has subsequently been confirmed in both man and the rat [20,21] (Table 3). It is therefore unlikely that the observed effect of calcium supplementation is mediated systemically. By contrast, calcium binds phosphate intraluminally, with a resultant decrease in phosphate absorption and corresponding hypophosphatemia (Table 3) [20,35]. Volunteers taking oral calcium salts excreted 49% more phosphate in their feces [36]. Although calcium could conceivably exert a systemic effect on cell proliferation by altering serum phosphate levels,

TABLE 3.
Serum Levels of Calcium and Phosphate (mmol/liter)†

Group	Calcium	Phosphate
Transection	2.73 ± 0.08	2.43 ± 0.24*
Transection + calcium	2.68 ± 0.08	1.93 ± 0.14
SBR	2.73 ± 0.09	2.57 ± 0.34*
SBR + calcium	2.93 ± 0.16	2.19 ± 0.23

†SBR, 80% mid-small bowel resection; transection, jejunal transection; calcium, 24 g/liter calcium lactate added to drinking water.
*$P < 0.05$ vs. equivalent group with added calcium.
Data are based on those of Appleton et al. [20,21].

therefore, a direct luminal effect on the colonic epithelium seems a more plausible mechanism.

MECHANISM OF ACTION OF INTRALUMINAL CALCIUM

Direct Effects

As already stated, a local increase in calcium concentrations has a ''direct'' antitropic effect on colonic mucosa in culture, i.e., it inhibits cell proliferation. Exact physiological concentrations relevant in vivo are unknown. Calcium stabilizes cellular membranes [28]: higher concentrations may thus prevent loss of cell-to-cell contact by preserving tight junctions, thus reducing a tendency toward proliferation [37]. Alternatively, the action of the ubiquitous calcium-binding protein calmodulin may be modulated by local fluctuations in calcium concentration [38]. Protein kinases, which are involved in the initiation of DNA synthesis, are activated when calcium forms bonds with calmodulin [39]. At present, the exact processes involved in calcium transport across the intestinal wall are poorly understood.

Indirect Effects

In 1984 Newmark and colleagues [40] put forward an intuitive hypothesis that the effect of dietary calcium was mediated by an ''indirect'' mechanism. Calcium is known to be a powerful chelator of fats; it binds to them even more strongly than it does to the powerful calcium-binding agent EDTA [40], especially in a basic pH environment. Both fats and bile acids are implicated as potent promoters of colorectal carcinogenesis. By binding fatty acids and bile acids intraluminally to form insoluble, nonirritant calcium soaps, their potentially harmful effect could be negated [40]. Sparse, mainly historical evidence is available to support this attractive theory. In 1967, LeVeen et al. [41] found that large doses of calcium given to volunteers prevented castor oil-induced diarrhea. Studying a 17-year-old man with only 18 cm small bowel remaining, Winawer et al. [42] showed that calcium balance was negative unless either dietary fat was severely restricted or 3 g calcium carbonate was given daily. Patients after jejunoileal bypass (for morbid obesity) usually have diarrhea, possibly because of large amounts of unabsorbed bile acids entering the colon; calcium supplementation helps to control this unpleasant side effect [43].

Fecal Studies

Fecal analysis in rats fed high-calcium diets demonstrates that bile acid levels are reduced, while excretion of both saturated and unsaturated fats is increased [29] (Table 4). After extracting fatty acids and bile acids from fecal residues, careful examination has found presumptive evidence of soaps with fats, but no calcium-bile acid complexes can be detected (unpublished data). In another study, twice as many calcium soaps were found in rats fed 1% calcium diets compared with 0.5% calcium diets, and the effect was especially pronounced in animals on fiber-free diets [44]. In man, treatment with 1,500 mg calcium (as calcium carbonate) for 1 week is sufficient nearly to double the fecal output of bile acids, which are found as calcium–phosphate–bile

TABLE 4.
Levels of Fecal Bile Acids, Calcium, Fats, and Sterols†

	Control	Added calcium	Percent change
Total FBA	1.66 ± 0.23	1.14 ± 0.13	31
Bound BA	0.16 ± 0.19	0.09 ± 0.06	44
Total BA	1.82	1.23	33
Sat FA	3.09 ± 1.45	6.50 ± 2.47	110
Unsat FA	2.63 ± 0.93	6.07 ± 2.38	131
Other FA	1.04 ± 0.34	2.09 ± 0.88	
Total FFA	6.76	14.68	117
Cholesterol	1.09 ± 0.35	1.08 ± 0.36	
Sterols	4.89 ± 1.32	5.29 ± 1.04	

†FBA, free bile acids; BA, bile acids; Sat, Unsat, saturated, unsaturated; FA, fatty acids; FFA, free fatty acids.
Data are based on those of Appleton et al. [29].

acid complexes [36]. More work along this interesting line of approach is required.

CONCLUSIONS

Deprivation of calcium within the gastrointestinal tract has profound consequences on mucosal morphology, cellular kinetics, and carcinogenesis. Available data suggest that both direct and indirect mechanisms of action are important. Further research must consider the roles of vitamin D3 and pH. Vitamin D3 has already been shown to protect independently against the development of colorectal cancer [16,25], and it reduces the proliferation of LoVo cells [45]. This vitamin has a pivotal role in the regulation of calcium transport across the mucosal barrier. Oral calcium compounds may alter luminal pH. 7-α-Dehydroxylase, an inducible bacterial enzyme that converts primary bile acids into secondary bile acids, is inhibited when cecal pH is low [46]. It may thus be possible to eat a high-fat diet with impunity if the colon is sufficiently acidified. Nevertheless, data thus far suggest that calcium lactate and calcium carbonate have an equivalent therapeutic effect despite their different pH values.

The weight of evidence, both clinical and experimental, supports the premise that doubling the dose of calcium in the diet offers significant protection against the development of colorectal cancer. Thus far it would seem that calcium's action is more likely to be preventative than therapeutic. Large bowel cancer is so common in affluent countries that long-term dietary trials are surely justified. If hyperproliferative mucosa is the forebear of malignant epithelial change in the colon, it could take 20–25 years to observe any significant effect of oral calcium (as with ulcerative colitis and Crohn's disease). More rapid results are likely to be obtained by studying the effect of oral calcium on adenoma formation, especially in patients with familial adenomatous polyposis. A combined trial along these lines is currently under way in London and New York.

Lastly, there is no indication that taking supplemental calcium is harmful. Indeed calcium may convey the added benefit of a reduced tendency toward atherosclerosis and coronary heart disease [47].

References

1. Gill PG, Morris PJ: The survival of patients with colorectal cancer treated in a regional hospital. Br J Surg 65:17–20, 1978.
2. Reasbeck PG: Colorectal cancer: The case for endoscopic screening. Br J Surg 74:12–17, 1987.
3. Krakoff I: Cancer chemotherapeutic agents. CA 37:93–105, 1987.
4. Lipkin M: Biomarkers of increased susceptibility to gastrointestinal cancer: New application to studies of cancer prevention in human subjects. Cancer Res 48:235–245, 1988.
5. Haenszel W: Cancer mortality among the foreign-born in the U.S. J Natl Cancer Inst 26:37–132, 1961.
6. Haenszel W, Dawson EA: A note on mortality from cancer of the colon and rectum from the United States. Cancer 18:265–272, 1965.

7. Jain M, Cook GM, Davis FG, Grace MG, Howe GR, Miller AB: A case-control study of diet and colo-rectal cancer. Int J Cancer 26:757–768, 1980.

8. Potter JD, McMichael AJ, Bonnett AZ: Diet, alcohol and large bowel cancer: A case-control study. Proc Nutr Soc Aust 7:123–126, 1982.

9. IARC Working Party: Diet, bowel function, fecal characteristics and large bowel cancer in Denmark and Finland. Nutr Cancer 4:5–17, 1982.

10. Hackett AF, Rugg-Gunn AJ, Allinson M, Robinson CJ, Appleton DR, Eastoe JE: The importance of fortification of flour with calcium and the sources of Ca in the diet of 375 English adolescents. Br J Clin Nutr 51:193–197, 1984.

11. Nicolaysen R, Eeg-Larsen N, Malm OJ: Physiology of calcium metabolism. Physiol Rev 33:424–444, 1953.

12. Williamson RCN, Rainey JB: The relationship between intestinal hyyperplasia and carcinogenesis. Scand J Gastroenterol [Suppl 104] 19:57–76, 1984.

13. Terpstra OT, van Blankenstein M, Dees J, Eilers GAM: Abnormal pattern of cell proliferation in the entire colonic mucosa of patients with colon adenoma or cancer. Gastroenterology 92:704–708, 1987.

14. Fozard JBJ, Watkins A, Dixon MF, Giles GR: Abnormal crypt kinetics: A means of identifying subjects at risk of colon cancer. Br J Surg 74:1155, 1987.

15. Garland C, Garland F: The Calcium Connection. New York: Putnam, 1988.

16. Garland C, Barrett-Connor E, Rossof AH, Shekelle RB, Crique MH, Paul O: Dietary vitamin D and calcium and risk of colorectal cancer: A 19-year prospective study in men. Lancet i:307–309, 1985.

17. Garland CF, Garland FC: Calcium and colon cancer. Clin Nutr 5:161–166, 1985.

18. Heilbrun LK, Hankin JH, Nomura AMY, Stemmermann GN: Colon cancer and dietary fat, phosphorus and calcium in Hawaiian-Japanese men. Am J Clin Nutr 43:306–309, 1986.

19. Newmark HL, Wargovich MJ: Letter to the editor. Am J Clin Nutr 4:998–1000, 1986.

20. Appleton GVN, Bristol JB, Williamson RCN: Increased dietary calcium and small bowel resection have opposite effects on colonic cell turnover. Br J Surg 73:1018–1021, 1986.

21. Appleton GVN, Davies PW, Bristol JB, Williamson RCN: Inhibition of intestinal carcinogenesis by dietary supplementation with calcium. Br J Surg 74:523–552, 1987.

22. Lipkin M, Newmark H: Effect of added dietary calcium on colonic epithelial cell proliferation in subjects at high risk for familial colonic cancer. N Engl J Med 313:1381–1384, 1985.

23. Wargovich MJ, Eng VW, Newmark HL, Bruce WR: Calcium ameliorates the toxic effect of deoxycholate on colonic epithelium. Carcinogenesis 4:1205–1207, 1983.

24. Wargovich MJ, Eng VWS, Newmark HL: Calcium inhibits the damaging and compensatory proliferative effects of fatty acids on mouse colon epithelium. Cancer Lett 23:253–258, 1984.

25. Pence BC, Buddingh F: Inhibition of dietary fat promotion of colon carcinogenesis by supplemental calcium or vitamin D. Proc Am Assoc Cancer Res 28:154, 1987.

26. Sunter JP, Appleton DR, Wright NA, Watson AJ: Pathological features of colonic tumors induced in rats by the administration of 1,2-dimethylhydrazine. Virchows Arch [B] 29:211–223, 1979.

27. Newmark HL: Nutrient density: An important and useful tool for laboratory animal studies. Carcinogenesis 8:871–875, 1987.

28. Hennings H, Holbrook K, Yuspa SH: Factors influencing calcium-induced terminal differentiation in cultured mouse epidermal cells. J Cell Physiol 116:265–281, 1983.

29. Appleton GVN, Wheeler EE, Challacombe DN, Williamson RCN: Intraluminal calcium and colonic cancer: Possible mechanisms of action. Gastroenterology 94:A10, 1988.

30. Rafter JJ, Eng VWS, Furrer R, Medline R, Bruce WR: Effects of calcium and pH on the mucosal damage produced by deoxycholic acid in the rat colon. Gut 27:1320–1329, 1986.

31. Buset M, Lipkin M, Winawer S, Swaroop S, Friedman E: Inhibition of human colonic epithelial cell proliferation in vivo and in vitro by calcium. Cancer Res 46:5426–5430, 1986.

32. Swoerenga SHH, Whitfield JH, Morris HP: The reduced extracellular requirement for proliferation by neoplastic hepatocytes. In vitro 14:527–535, 1978.

33. Boyton AL, Whitfield JF, Issacs RT, Martin HJ: Control of 3T3 cell proliferation by calcium. In Vitro 10:12–17, 1974.

34. Wargovich MJ, Lointer PH: Calcium and vitamin D modulate mouse colon epithelial proliferation and growth characteristics of a human colon tumor cell line. Can J Physiol Pharmacol 65:472–477, 1987.

35. Telfer SV: Studies in calcium and phosphorus metabolism (IV). The influence of free fatty acids in the intestine on the absorption and excretion of the mineral elements. Q J Med XX:1–6, 1926.

36. Welberg JWM, Meer Rvd, Kleibeuker JH, et al.: Short-term effects of dietary calcium supplementation on fecal excretion of minerals and bile acids. Gastroenterology 94:A492, 1988.

37. Wargovich MJ: Calcium and colon cancer. J Am Coll Nutr 7 (in press), 1988.

38. Hait WN, Lazo JS: Calmodulin: A potential target for cancer therapeutic agents. J Clin Oncol 4:994–1012, 1986.

39. Cheung WY: Calmodulin plays a pivotal role on cellular regulation. Science 207:19–26, 1980.

40. Newmark HL, Wargovich MJ, Bruce WR: Colon cancer and dietary fat, phosphate and calcium: A hypothesis. J Natl Cancer Inst 72:1323–1325, 1984.

41. LeVeen HH, Borek B, Axelrod DR, Johnson A: Cause and treatment of diarrhea following resection of small intestine. Surg Gynecol Obstet 95:766–770, 1967.

42. Winawer SJ, Broitman SA, Wolochow DA, Osborne MP, Zamcheck N: Successful management of massive small bowel resection based on assessment of absorption defects and nutritional needs. N Engl J Med 274:72–78, 1966.

43. Joffe SN: Surgical management of morbid obesity. Gut 22:252–254, 1981.

44. Radulovich D, Lupton JR: In vivo calcium soap formation with two levels of calcium and fat and three fibers. Faseb 2:A430, 1988.

45. Lointier P, Wargovich MJ, Saez S, et al.: The role of vitamin D3 in the proliferation of a human colon cancer cell line in vitro. Anticancer Res 7:817–822, 1987.

46. Hill MJ: Microbes and Human Carcinogenesis. London: Edward Arnold, 1986.

47. Carlson LA, Olsson AG, Rossner S: Effects of oral calcium upon serum cholesterol and triglycerides in patients with hyperlipidaemia. Atherosclerosis 14:391–400, 1971.

30

Prospects for the Chemoprevention of Cancer in Humans

John S. Bertram

Director, Basic Science Program, Cancer Research Center of Hawaii, University of Hawaii, Honolulu, Hawaii

INTRODUCTION

It is the goal of this chapter to review prospects for the chemoprevention of cancer in general, with specific reference to colon carcinogenesis when appropriate. The justification for this general approach stems from a growing understanding of the process of carcinogenesis and the realization that common events occur in different organs. In this view of carcinogenesis the disparate nature of diverse malignancies owes more to the differentiated state of the cell to be transformed than to the nature of the causative agent. In support of this approach, recent advances in the molecular biology of cancer have identified dominantly acting cancer genes (oncogenes) that become activated by identical mechanisms in different human tumors. Furthermore, these genes become activated in rodent model systems used in laboratory research into cancer causation and its prevention [1]. Additionally, chemicals that are known carcinogens in animal models and that induce DNA adducts strongly implicated in subsequent genetic changes leading to neoplasia have been demonstrated to induce the identical DNA adducts in human DNA [2]. Thus events occurring during the neoplastic conversion of colonic polyps, for example, may be viewed with reasonable confidence in a wider picture of carcinogenesis in general.

The term *chemoprevention* refers to the use of defined pharmacological agents to prevent or reverse the process of carcinogenesis [for review, see 3]. Thus, by definition, chemoprevention does not deal with the treatment of existing malignancy; indeed, chemopreventive agents are in general without direct effect on established cancer cells. To understand the requirements for a chemopreventive agent and to discuss the prospects for chemoprevention, it is first necessary to review briefly what is known of the carcinogenic process. The scientific rationale for the concept of chemoprevention of cancer in humans will then be reviewed, with reference to specific agents. Finally, special problems concerning the design and conduct of clinical chemoprevention trials will be discussed.

ETIOLOGY OF HUMAN CANCER AND THE CARCINOGENIC PROCESS

Epidemiologic studies, principally conducted in migrant populations, have led to the realization that the majority of human cancer in the most commonly involved organs is induced by exogenous agents rather than being of genetic origin [4]. In concept, at least, these tumors are preventable. The major exogenous factors identified are, of course, tobacco and diet; together they are believed to contribute to about 70% of excess cancer mortality in the United States [4]. Only a small proportion of cancers appear genetically linked, of which bilateral retinoblastoma [5] and familial adenomatous polyposis are two important examples. In these diseases, it appears that cells progress spontaneously to an early stage in the carcinogenic process, and then subsequent events required for the production of a neoplastic

Familial Adenomatous Polyposis, pages 253–262

cell may occur spontaneously. While these secondary events may be rare on a per cell basis, the target cell population may be sufficiently large (in multiple polyps, for example) to make these events frequent at the level of the organ.

Steps in the Carcinogenic Process

Evidence for multiple steps in the carcinogenic process comes from animal studies, from studies of cultured mammalian cells, and from studies in humans exposed to industrial carcinogens or nuclear radiation. The prolonged latency between exposure and clinical tumors in humans is entirely consistent with the data obtained in rodent models.

To illustrate the potential sites for active intervention, an overview of the carcinogenic process is presented diagramatically in Figure 1. As shown, the steps may be separated mechanistically and temporally. The processes of metabolic activation, DNA adduct formation, and repair all occur rapidly, the first two within a few hours of exposure (virtually instantaneously for physical carcinogens). Rates of repair of potentially carcinogenic lesions vary extensively from organ to organ and species to species. In experimental systems utilizing rodent fibroblasts, repair appears essentially complete within 48 hours. Cell replication must occur before the DNA lesion is repaired if an initiated cell is to result from this chemical damage. Thus any protocol aimed at reducing the formation of initiated cells (Steps 1,2,3,4) must be instituted rapidly after exposure or continuously if exposure is continuous. In contrast, the conversion of an initiated cell to a premalignant or fully malignant cell, either spontaneously or induced by tumor promoters, is a prolonged process taking decades in humans. Inhibition of this process at any time prior to the onset of frank malignancy can be expected to delay the onset

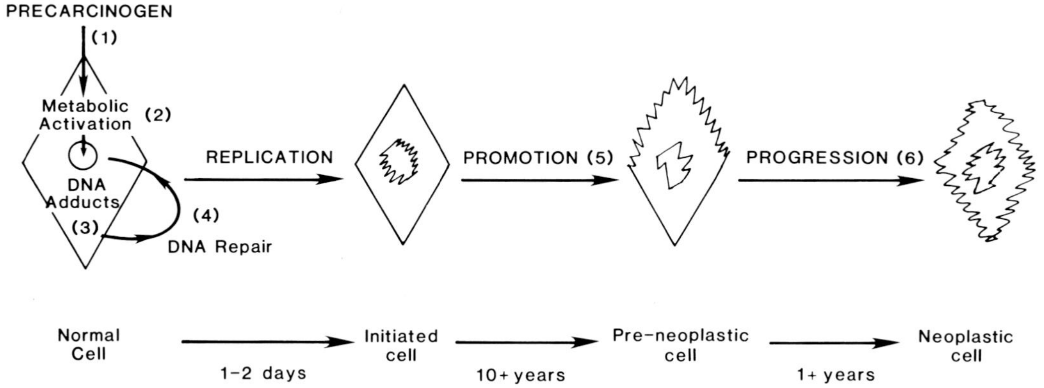

Fig. 1. Steps in the chemical induction of neoplasia: Loci for intervention. **Step 1:** Avoidance of exposure is clearly the most desirable form of cancer prevention, but is outside the scope if this chapter. In the special case of endogenous formation of nitrosamines and of fecal mutagens, chemopreventive agents can block formation and presumably alter exposure. **Step 2:** Most chemical carcinogens require metabolic activation; chemoprevention can be achieved by blocking or diverting this metabolism toward less genotoxic products. **Step 3:** The proximate or ultimate carcinogenic form of a carcinogen may be intercepted prior to its reaction with DNA. **Step 4:** DNA replication past carcinogen-induced DNA lesions appears to be an important step converting chemical damage to genetic alteration. Stimulation of DNA repair or inhibition of cell proliferation do not seem viable prospects for clinical intervention at this time. **Step 5:** The conversion of initiated cells to preneoplastic cells is a lengthy process and appears currently to offer the best prospects for clinical intervention. Even a small delay in this process would result in a significant decrease in incidence. **Step 6:** The phenotypic reversion of preneoplastic cells to normality, thus preventing the progression to frank neoplasia, is feasible and offers the advantage of rapid assessment of drug efficiency. (Reprinted from Bertram et al. [3], with permission of *Cancer Research*.)

of disease. Thus intervention can be started after exposure or during continuous exposure.

The final site for intervention is the progression of premalignant cells to malignant cells of increasing virulence (Fig.1, step 5). For many epithelial tissues, early pathological changes (preneoplasia) appear to be reversed by agents such as the retinoids; however, there is no evidence yet that this reversal is permanent. The ability to block the progression of malignant cells to cells wih increasing invasive or metastatic properties has to our knowledge not yet been demonstrated.

In patients with familial adenomatous polyposis there is evidence that genetic abnormalities exist in lymphocytes and skin fibroblasts [6,7], and in these patients other tumors occur with high frequency [8], indicating a widespread predisposition of somatic cells to abnormal growth. It seems likely that one or more secondary events are then required for the conversion of these abnormal cells to malignancy. Multistep origination of neoplasia is currently being dissected at the molecular level [9], and, while a detailed discussion of this field is beyond the scope of this chapter, in most cases examined at least two discreet genetic alterations in oncogene structure and/or expression have been found necessary for oncogenic transformation [10]. It appears likely that the inherited predisposition to polyposis provides the first event in multistep carcinogenesis. While the nature of these required secondary events leading to adenocarcinoma of the colon are unknown, it is likely that both DNA damage caused by initiating agents and the multiple effects caused by the tumor promoters influence this process.

Potential Sites for Chemoprevention: Prevention of Initiation

While the relevance of prevention of initiating events may not at first glance be obvious in a discussion of familial adenomatous polyposis, in which polyps may be considered as clones of initiated cells, there is evidence from studies in mouse skin that the subsequent events leading to carcinoma may be accelerated by genotoxic initiating agents [11]. As outlined in Figure 1, initiation involves the chemical reaction of an activated carcinogen with a relevant DNA base and the subsequent attempt by the cell to replicate this damaged DNA during normal mitogenesis. However, because of the presence of the carcinogen adduct, normal base-pairing cannot occur and a mutation is introduced into the daughter DNA. The simplest example of carcinogen activation and DNA adduct formation is the formation of a methylcarbonium ion from the widely distributed carcinogen dimethynitrosamine and its subsequent reaction to form a 0-6-methyl adduct on guanine. The presence of this adduct prevents normal base-pairing with cytosine and makes likely the erroneous incorporation of thymidine [for review, see 12]. It is of interest that activated oncogenes of the ras family, which have been isolated from human bladder, and colon carcinomas have apparently been activated by a cytosine → thymidine point mutation consistent with the mechanism outlined above [13].

Nitrosamines such as dimethylnitrosamine can be formed in foodstuffs by the reaction of nitrite with secondary amines or may be formed in the stomach driven by the low pH of the stomach contents. Ascorbate is an effective scavenger of nitrite ions and will reduce nitrosamine formation in experimental animals [14] and will reduce the mutagenicity of human gastric juice [15]. There is persuasive epidemiologic evidence that ascorbic acid protects against esophageal and stomach cancer [16–18], and the declining stomach cancer rates over the past 50 years parallel the increased availability of fresh fruits. Mutagens are also found in human feces, but epidemiologic data have not identified colon cancer as being responsive to dietary ascorbate. However, levels of fecal mutagens can be reduced by supplemental vitamins C and E [19]. Mutagenicity appears to be primarily caused by the presence of fecapentaenes [20], compounds that also cause DNA breakage in colonic cells [21]. Because of the correlation between high levels of fecal mutagens and diets associatd with high risks for colon cancer [22], several interventional trials of high-dose ascorbate have been conducted in familial adenomatous polyposis. In both trials, the polyps decreased in number and/or size

[23,24]. These studies suggest that polyp formation as well as their ultimate conversion to adenocarcinomas requires the interplay of environmental factors (i.e., diet, fecal flora) as well as a genetic predisposition.

Inhibition of the Promotional Phase of Carcinogenesis: Promotion and Promoters

The promotional phase is the longest, the least understood, and yet is the phase with the greatest potential for clinical intervention. This potential stems from several separate lines of evidence: 1) Consequences of exposure to chemicals and radiation demonstrate that this phase is of many years duration in humans. It is possible, therefore, unlike anti-initiation therapy, to begin treatment long after commencement of carcinogen exposure. 2) Since late stages of carcinogenesis are affected, it should be possible to detect results in a few years rather than the decades required to demonstrate the effectiveness of anti-initiation therapy. 3) From the results of animal studies, and from epidemiologic evidence, drugs are available that demonstrate activity without appreciable side effects. 4) Experience in both humans and animals has shown that early preneoplastic lesions can be reversed. A potential disadvantage of drugs active in this phase is that studies in both animals and in cell culture show that inhibition of promotion by retinoids is reversible, requiring continuous treatment for continuous effect. Thus, should clinical efficacy be unequivocally demonstrated, the ethics of discontinuing therapy in clinical trial volunteers will require careful consideration.

As originally defined [25], *promotion* is an operational term referring to the ability of compounds or procedures to facilitate the production of mouse skin tumors resulting from a single subcarcinogenic exposure to the skin carcinogen dimethylbenzanthracene (DMBA). Thus promotion in this experimental system is defined in terms of promoters. Promoters, classically those derived from croton oil, have properties quite distinct from carcinogens: 1) They are themselves nontumorigenic; 2) they require repeated applications in order to promote tumor formation; 3) their effects are reversible, leading to the observation that promoter treatment prior to carcinogen exposure is ineffective; and 4) a minimum frequency of promoter treatment is required to effect promotion. Although exposure to croton oil is not a major public health factor, lessons learned from experimental studies using this model are considered highly relevant to the human carcinogenic process. For example, studies of tobacco carcinogenesis have led to the conclusion that tobacco smoke contains both potent promoters and initiators [25]. Furthermore bile salts, whose output is stimulated by a high-fat diet, have promoting activities in experimental systems [27], suggesting a mechanistic link between diet and colon cancer.

In spite of much investigation, the biochemical mode of action of tumor promoters is poorly understood. The active principal of croton oil, tetradecanoylphorbol acetate (TPA), has been studied most. A major recent finding has been the identification of what appears to be its receptor as a calcium-dependent protein kinase (C kinase) [28,29], which it activates upon binding. Future research must now identify the crucial protein substrates for the phosphate group transferred by this kinase. This finding has important ramifications that may help to integrate laboratory studies of TPA promotion with the general phenomenon of the conversion of initiated cells to neoplastic cells, a process I have operationally called *promotion* without regard to the identification of a known promoter. This integration may be possible because of the realization that the endogenous activator of C kinase is a membrane degradation product called *diacylglycerol* (DG). The production of this endogenous activator may be enhanced by growth factors implicated in human and experimental tumor induction [30]. Thus ''spontaneous'' promotion in humans may be very similar mechanistically to experimental promotion in mouse skin induced by the phorbol ester tumor promoters. In a model currently being developed, growth factors activate kinases that phosphorylate phosphatidylinositol (P1), a component of the plasma membrane, to phosphatidylinositol 4,5-bisphosphate (PIP_2). This intermediate can then be hydrolyzed to DG and inositol 1,4,5-trisphosphate (IP_3). The former compound has been discussed above. IP_3 acts to mobilize Ca^{2+}, an ion with multiple intracellular regulatory activities [31]. DG can be metabolized by a lipase to arachidonic acid, the precursor of prostaglandin synthesis. Prostaglandins in turn are major mediators of inflammation and are strongly implicated as mediators in experimental tumor promotion, since both steroidal and nonsteroidal anti-inflammatory agents, such as aspirin and indomethacin, block prostaglandin synthesis from arachidonic acid and inhibit two-stage carcinogenesis in mouse skin [32]. The final links in the sequence between activation of protein kinase C and/or release of prostaglandins, and the conversion of initiated cells to progressively growing tumors, have yet to be clarified. It is to be hoped that this search will reveal other sites for intervention.

Intervention in the Promotional Process: Experimental Studies

Retinoids and carotenoids. The most widely studied chemopreventive agents are the retinoids, natural and synthetic analogs of vitamin A. It is unfortunate in the present context that while these compounds are potent preventive agents against a wide range of chemically induced carcinomas, they have thus far not demonstrated activity in the colon. Furthermore, epidemiologic evidence does not provide much support for a potential role of retinoids in this organ [3]. In two experimental studies, retinoids either failed to modify the carcinogenic response to nitrosomethylurea [33] or actually resulted in an increase in tumors induced by methylnitrosoguanidine [34]. In this latter study, however, the retinoid-treated group weighed and ate more than the retinoid-free controls, which may have influenced the results. This lack of activity of retinoids against colon carcinoma is disappointing in view of their impressive effects against mammary [35,36], bladder [37,38], skin [34], oral cavity [40], and esophageal and forestomach carcinomas [41]. Retinoids furthermore are highly active inhibitors of the in vitro neoplastic transformation of mouse fibroblasts [42]. It should be noted in passing that in certain situations retinoids have deleterious effects on carcinogenesis and possess additional significant toxicity, indicating that their use is not without hazard [for review, see 3].

The other component to epidemiologic studies involving vitamin A is β-carotene and the carotenoids. β-Carotene is both converted in the ilium to vitamin A and at higher levels of intake is absorbed intact and stored throughout the body [43]. Much of the epidemiologic data suggest it is the carotenoid content of the diet rather than the preformed retinoid content that is protective for cancer [44]. It is clear that carotenoids themselves will inhibit UV-induced skin cancer in the mouse [45], and we have recently demonstrated that carotenoids can inhibit the in vitro neoplastic conversion of mouse fibroblasts [46] in the absence of their conversion to retinoids [47]. In both in vivo and in vitro studies, inhibition occurred during the promotional phase of carcinogenesis. To my knowledge, no studies have yet examined carotenoid effects on colon carcinogenesis.

Selenium. The trace element selenium is a component of the enzyme glutathione peroxidase and as such might be expected to enhance the repair of oxidatively damaged membranes [48]. The epidemiologic evidence for a protective effect of selenium against cancers in general is conflicting; studies both demonstrating and failing to demonstrate an association between dietary Se and decreased risk for cancer have been reported [for review, see 3]. One study of colorectal cancer failed to show an association [49]. In contrast, animal studies have consistently shown Se to be protective against carcinomas at a number of sites, including the colon [50]. Interpretation of these studies is hampered by the fact that, in most cases examined, protective levels of Se were also associated with body weight reduction in treated versus control animals. This in itself could contribute to the observed effect.

α-Tocopherol. As previously mentioned, α-tocopherol in combination with ascorbic acid will cause a major reduction in fecal mutagenicity [19], suggesting it should reduce initiating events in the colon. The postulated role of peroxidation reactions in the process of tumor promotion [51] implies that the antioxidant properties of α-tocopherol and of other antioxidants should protect against promoting events. Epidemiologic evidence in humans for a protective effect of α-tocopherol on cancer rates are conflicting [3]. Part of the problem is the difficulty of accurately assessing intake for this widely distributed vitamin; furthermore, potential interactions with other antioxidants may well influence the overall response. Studies in experimental animals have likewise yielded equivocal results.

Early reports of inhibitory actions of this compound on polycyclic aromatic carcinogen-induced tumors [52,53] have not in general been substantiated by later studies [for review, see 54], although a recent report has shown that topical application to DMBA-treated hamster buccal mucosa can lead to a reduction in tumor yield [55]. In the DMBA rat mammary carcinoma model, while α-tocopherol was not active alone, it was shown to potentiate the antitumor effects of selenium. Treatment was accompanied by a decrease in the lipid-peroxidation state of the target mammary tissue and liver [56]. A study of dimethylhydrazine-induced colon carcinomas in rats concluded that a diet high in α-tocopherol reduced the number, but not the incidence, of tumors [57]. The role of α-tocopherol in association with ascorbic acid in reducing fecal mutagens and polyp area in humans [58] suggests its potential protective role in colon cancer. Accordingly, a number of clinical trails are currently underway to examine this relationship [for review, see 3].

Miscellaneous Compounds Active Against Experimental Colon Cancer

Antiflammatory agents. As described above, one effect of TPA-type tumor promoters is to increase the production of arachidonic acid metabolites, principally prostaglandins. Inhibition of prostaglandin synthesis by anti-inflammatory agents such as indomethacin, or of arachidonic acid release by the anti-inflammatory steroids, causes a reduction in mouse skin carcinogenesis. When tested in a rat colon carcinogenesis model, indomethacin was shown to reduce the incidence of carcinoma [59]. To my knowledge, no human studies have examined this potential relationship.

Bile acids, calcium, and fiber. There is persuasive evidence that bile acids, whose output is stimulated by a high-fat diet, have properties that parallel in many respects those of the potent phorbol ester tumor promoter TPA [60] and in addition may directly cause gentoxicity [61]. Furthermore, skin fibroblast cells from individuals with familial adenomatous polyposis can be neoplastically transformed by exposure to TPA, suggesting that these cells exist in an initiated state and that promoter alone is capable of inducing some second event required for transformation [6]. Strategies designed to reduce the exposure of the colonic epithelium to bile acids such as deoxycholate may be predicted to reduce cancer risk, especially in genetically predisposed individuals.

Exposure of normal colonic epithelium to bile acids induces cell proliferation and this action can be attenuated by concurrent treatment with Ca^{2+}, probably because of the formation of insoluble salts. Calcium supplementation will reduce the incidence of experimentally induced colorectal carcinomas [62]. Preliminary epidemiologic evidence also supports the concept of a preventive role of calcium in human colon cancer [63], although these findings have not been confirmed by others [64]. A preliminary intervention trial of calcium in familial adenomatous polyposis demonstrated that supplementation was associated with a decreased proliferation rate of colonic epithelium [65], further substantiating the concept of a negative association between calcium and colon cancer. Because of the proposed interaction between dietary calcium and bile acids, this provides further indirect evidence for the role of these acids in the carcinogenic process. An interventional clinical trial of supplemented calcium is currently underway in patients with familial adenomatous polyposis.

A second means of reducing exposure of colonic epithelium to bile acids is by dietary supplementation with fiber, and there is much suggestive evidence from epidemiologic studies [65] and studies in experimental animals [66] that high-fiber diets are protective against colon cancer. Fiber can have multiple effects on colon contents, increasing their bulk, reducing transit time, complexing with bile salts, etc, and it is at present unclear as to the precise role played by this material in modulating colon carcinogenesis. The interpretation of these studies is further complicated by the realization that the term fiber encompasses a very heterogenous group of molecules with diverse properties [67]. While the use of dietary fiber to reduce colon cancer risk cannot, strictly speaking, be defined as chemoprevention, since it involves the use of ill-defined chemicals that may simply act physically to reduce exposure, the relevance of dietary fiber to colon cancer risk is undoubtably significant. On the basis of this evidence, at least one interventional trial with fiber (wheat bran) in familial adenomatous polyposis is currently underway.

CLINICAL TRIALS AND TRIBULATIONS

A detailed discussion of ethical and logistical problems confronting the planning and execution of a major chemoprevention clinical trial is outside the scope of this chapter. However, it should be notd that many difference exist between clinical trials of chemopreventive agents and chemotherapeutive agents. For example, because the latter involves patients with existing malignancy, appreciable toxicity is acceptable; in contrast, chemoprevention trials involve healthy individuals, or those with minimal disease, and expected risks must be carefully weighed against possible benefits. Because of the protracted nature of most chemoprevention trials and, in most cases, the low frequency of expected malignancies among the study population, logistical problems of recruitment, compliance, and long-term follow-up differ dramatically from those encountered in chemotherapy trials. For example, to measure low-frequency events within a reasonable (5–10 year) time period, many thousands of individuals need to be involved; maintaining compliance among these low-risk individuals over a protracted time period presents severe problems. This should be less of a problem with familial adenomatous polyposis, in which the risks of malignancy are evident, than with a group at risk for skin cancer, for example [for a more detailed discussion of these issues, see 3,68].

In the cervix [69–71], lung [72], oral cavity [73–81], and skin [82–85] topical, or in some cases systemic, administration of retinoids has resulted in a significant induction of complete or partial remissions of preneoplasia in these organs. In the colon, ascorbic acid was shown to reduce the polyp area and/or size in patients with familial adenomatous polyposis [86,87], while in the bladder, systemic retinoid treatment reduced the recurrence rate of bladder carcinomas at anatomically new sites [88]. Finally, retinoids have been shown to have chemotherapeutic activity against basal cell carcinomas [82–85, 89,90], probably because of their actions on the differentiated state of cells rather than a consequence of any cytotoxic properties.

At the present time in the United States, approximately 20 phase III clinical intervention trials are underway. Of these, five target the colon and involve the use of ascorbic acid, α-tocopherol, wheat bran, calcium, and β-carotene singly or in combination. For most of these studies, it will be several years before effects on intermediate endpoints are available and still longer before effects on cancer incidence are known. This delay is a consequence of the protracted nature of the carcinogenic process in humans, as discussed previously. An additional consequence of the slow progression of many human cancers is that the outgrowth of a malignant cell to form a clinically detectable tumor may also take many months to several years; such latent tumor cells in most cases cannot be expected to respond to chemopreventive agents. Therefore, cancer incidence rates in treated and control groups may be identical during the early phases of the study because of the outgrowth of these pre-existing, initially latent malignancies. For example, the first study of retinoids in patients at high risk for recurrent (at new sites) bladder carcinoma did not recognize this problem and was abandoned after 4–8 months because of an identical outcome in treated and control groups [91]. A second study recognized this problem and found highly significant differences in recurrence rates when treatment with retinoids had continued longer than 8 months [88].

In summary, there appear to be many opportunities for the chemoprevention of cancer, including colon cancer, and, as our knowledge of the molecular defects associated with this disease becomes more complete, it is predicted that new strategies will be possible. The protracted nature of clinical intervention trials will demand much patience from the public and physicians and, it is also hoped, from funding agencies.

ACKNOWLEDGMENTS

This work was supported by USPHS grant CA 39947.

References

1. Varmus H: The molecular genetics of cellular oncogenes. Annu Rev Genet 18:553–612, 1984.
2. Autrup H, Harris CC: Metabolism of chemical carcinogens by human tissues. In Harris CC, Autrup H (eds): Human Carcinogenesis. New York: Academic Press, 1983, pp 169–194.
3. Bertram JS, Kolonel LN, Meyskens FL Jr: Rationale and strategies for chemoprevention of cancer in humans. Cancer Res 47:3012–3031, 1987.
4. Doll R, Peto R: The causes of cancer: Quantitative estimates of avoidable risks of cancer in the United States today. J Natl Cancer Inst 66:1192–1308, 1981.
5. Cavenee WK, Dryja TP, Phillips RA, Benedict WF, Godbout R, Gallie BC, Murphree AL, Strong LC, White RL: Expression of recessive alleles by chromosomal mehanisms in retinoblastoma. Nature 305:779–784, 1983.
6. Gardner EJ, Rogers SW, Woodward S: Numerical and structural chromosome aberrations in cultured lymphocytes and cutaneous fibroblasts of patients with multiple adenomas of the colorectum. Cancer 49:1413–1419, 1982.
7. Kopelovich L, Bias NE, Helson L: Tumour promoter alone induces neoplastic transformation of fibroblasts from humans genetically predisposed to cancer. Nature 282:619–621, 1979.
8. Utsonomiya J, Nakamura T: The occult osteomatous changes in the mandible in patients with familial polyposis coli. Br J Surg 62:45–51, 1975.
9. Land H, Parada LF, Weinberg RA: Cellular oncogenes and multistep carcinogenesis. Science 222:771–778, 1983.
10. Thomassen DG, Gilmer TM, Annab LA, Barrett JC: Evidence for multiple steps in neoplastic transformation of normal and preneoplastic Syrian hamster embryo cells following transfection with Harvey murine sarcoma virus oncogenes (v-Ha-ras). Cancer Res 45:726–732, 1985.
11. Hennings H, Shores R, Weak ML, Spangler EF, Tarone R, Yuspa SH: Malignant conversion of mouse skin tumors is increased by tumor initiators and unaffected by tumor promoters. Nature 304:67–69, 1983.
12. Margison GP, O'Connor PJ: Nucleic acid modification by N-nitroso compounds. In Grover PL (ed): Chemical Carcinogenesis and DNA. Boca Raton, FL: CRC Press, 1979, pp 111–158.
13. Tabin CJ, Bradley SM, Bargmann CI, Weinberg RA, Papageorge, AG, Scolnick EM, Dhar R, Lowy DR, Chang EH: Mechanism of activation of a human oncogene. Nature 300:143–152, 1982.
14. Ohshima H, Bereziat JC, Bartsch H: Monitoring N-nitrosoamino acids excreted in the urine and faeces of rats as an index of N-nitrosation. Carcinogenesis 3:115–120, 1982.
15. O'Connor HJ, Habibzedah N, Schorah CJ, Axon ATR, Riley SE, Garner RC: Effect of increased intake of vitamin C on the mutagenic activity of gastric juice and intragastric concentrations of ascorbic acid. Carcinogenesis 6:1675–1676, 1985.
16. Cook-Mozaffari PJ, Azordegan F, Day NE, Ressicaud A, Sabai C, Aramesh B: Oesophageal cancer studies in the Caspian Littoral of Iran: Results of a case-control study. Br J Cancer 39:293–309, 1979.
17. Meinsma L: Nutrition and cancer [in Dutch, English summary]. Voeding [The Hague] 25:357–365, 1964.
18. Bjelke E: Dietary factors and the epidemiology of cancer of the stomach and large bowel. Aktuel Ernaehrungsmed Klin Prax [Suppl] 2:10–17, 1978.
19. Dion PW, Bright-See EB, Smith CC, Bruce WR: The effect of dietary ascorbic acid and α-tocopherol on fecal mutagenicity. Mutat Res 102:27–37, 1982.
20. Gingerich JS, Gupta I, Krepinsky JJ: General structure of "fecapentanes," the mutagenic substances in human faeces. Naturwissenschaften 69:557–558, 1982.
21. Hinzman MJ, Novotny C, Ullah A, Shamsuddin AM: Fecal mutagen fecapentaene-12 damages mammalian colon epithelial DNA. Carcinogenesis 8:1475–1479, 1987.
22. Reddy BS, Sharma C, Darby L, Laakso T, Wynder EL: Metabolic epidemiology of large bowel cancer. Mutat Res 72:511–522, 1980.
23. DeCosse JJ, Adams MB, Kuzma JF, Logerfo P, Codon RE: Effect of ascorbic acid on rectal polyps of patients with familial polyposis. Surgery 78:608–612, 1975.
24. Bussey HJR, DeCosse JJ, Deschner EE, Eyers AA, Lesser ML, Morson BC, Ritchie SM, Thomson JPS, Wadsworth J: A randomized trial of ascorbic acid in polyposis coli. Cancer 50:1434–1439, 1982.
25. Boutwell RK: Some biological aspects of skin carcinogenesis. Prog Exp Tumor Res 4:207–250, 1964.
26. Doll R: An epidemiological perspective on the biology of cancer. Cancer Res 38:3573–3583, 1978.
27. Kaibara N, Yurugi E, Koga S: Promoting effects of bile acids on the chemical transformation of C3H/10T1/2 fibroblasts in vitro. Cancer Res 44:5482–5485, 1984.
28. Nishizuka Y: The role of protein kinase C in cell surface signal transduction and tumor promotion. Nature 308:693–698, 1984.
29. Niedel JE, Kuhn LJ, Vandenbark GR: Phorbol diester receptor copurifies with protein kinase C. Proc Natl Acad Sci USA 80:36–40, 1983.
30. Berridge MJ: Inositol trisphosphate and diacylglycerol as second messengers. Biochem J 220:345–360, 1984.
31. Whitfield JE, Boynton AL, Rixon RH, Youdale T: The control of cell proliferation by calcium, Ca^{2+}-calmodulin, and cyclic AMP. In Boynton AL, Leffert HL (eds): Control of Animal Cell Proliferation, New York: Academic Press, 1985, pp 331–365.
32. Schwarz JA, Viaje A, Slaga TJ, Yuspa SH, Hennings

H, Lichi U: Fluocinolone acetonide—A potent inhibitor of mouse skin tumor promotion and epidermal DNA synthesis. Chem Biol Interact 17:331–347, 1977.

33. Silverman J, Katayama S, Zelenakas K, Lauber J, Musser TK, Reddy M, Levenstein MJ, Weisberger JH: Effect of retinoids on the induction of colon cancer in F344 rats by N-methyl-N-nitrourea or by 1,2-dimethylhydrazine. Carcinogenesis 2:1167–1172, 1981.

34. Narisawa T, Reddy BS, Wong C, Weisberger JH: Effect of vitamin A deficiency on rat colon carcinogenesis by N-methyl-N-nitro-N-nitrosoguanidine. Cancer Res 36:1376–1382, 1976.

35. Moon RC, Grubbs CJ, Sporn MB: Inhibition of 7, 12-dimethyl-benz[a]anthracene-induced mammary carcinogenesis by retinyl acetate. Cancer Res 36:2626–2630, 1976.

36. Thompson HJ, Becci PJ, Brown CC, Moon RC: Effect of the duration of retinyl acetate feeding on inhibition of 1-methyl-1-nitrosourea-induced mammary carcinogenesis in the rat. Cancer Res 39:3977–3980, 1979.

37. Sporn MB, Squire RA, Brown CC, Smith JM, Wenk ML, Springer S: 13-cis-Retinoic acid: Inhibition of bladder carcinogenesis in the rat. Science 195:487–489, 1977.

38. Becci PJ, Thompson HJ, Grubbs CJ, Squire RA, Brown CC, Sporn MB, Moon RC: Inhibitory effect of 13-cis-retinoic acid on urinary bladder carcinogenesis induced in C57BL/6 mice by N-butyl-N-(4-hydroxybutyl)nitrosamine. Cancer Res 38:4463–4466, 1978.

39. Verma AK, Shapas BG, Rice HM, Boutwell RK: Correlation of the inhibition by retinoids of tumor promoter-induced mouse epidermal ornithine decarboxylase activity and of skin tumor promotion. Cancer Res 39:419–425, 1979.

40. Shklar G, Schwartz J, Gran D, Trickler DP, Wallace KD: Inhibition of hamster buccal pouch carcinogenesis by 13-cis-retinoic acid. Oral Surg 50:45–52, 1980.

41. Smith DM, Rogers AE, Herndon BJ, Newberne PM: Vitamin A (retinyl acetate) and benzo[a]pyrene-induced respiratory tract carcinogenesis in hamsters fed a commercial diet. Cancer Res 35:11–16, 1975.

42. Merriman RL, Bertram JS: Reversible inhibition by retinoids of 3-methylcholanthrene-induced neoplastic transformation in C3H/10T1/2 clone 8 cells. Cancer Res 39:1661–1666, 1979.

43. Underwood BA: Vitamin A in animal and human nutrition. In Sporn MB, Roberts AB, Goodman DS (eds): The Retinoids. New York: Academic Press, Vol 1, 1984, pp 281–392.

44. Peto R, Doll R, Buckley JD, Sporn MB: Can dietary β-carotene materially reduce human cancer rates? Nature 290:201–208, 1981.

45. Mathews-Roth MM, Krinsky NI: Carotenoids affect development of UV-β-induced skin cancer. Photochem Photobiol 46:507–509, 1987.

46. Pung A, Rundhaug JE, Yoshizawa CN, Bertram JS: β-Carotene and canthaxanthin inhibit chemically- and physically-induced neoplastic transformation in 10T1/2 cells. Carcinogenesis 9:1533–1539, 1988.

47. Rundhaug JE, Pung A, Read CM, Bertram JS: Uptake and metabolism of β-carotene and retinal by C3H/10T1/2 cells. Carcinogenesis 9:1541–1545, 1988.

48. Griffin AC: Role of selenium in the chemoprevention of cancer. Adv Cancer Res 29:419–442, 1979.

49. Jansson B, Jacobs MM, Griffin AC: Gastrointestinal cancer: Epidemiology and experimental studies. In Schrauzer GN (ed): Inorganic and Nutritional Aspects of Cancer, New York: Plenum Publishing Corp, 1978, pp 305–322.

50. Birt DF, Lawson TA, Julius AD, Runice CE, Salmasi S: Inhibition by dietary selenium of colon cancer induced in the rat by bis(2-oxopropyl)nitrosamine. Cancer Res 42:4455–4459, 1982.

51. Cerutti PA: Prooxidant states and tumor promotion. Science 227:375–381, 1985.

52. Jaffe WG: The influence of wheat germ oil on the production of tumors in rats by methylcholanthrene. Exp Med Surg 4:278–282, 1946.

53. Haber SL, Wissler RW: Effect of vitamin E on carcinogenicity of methylcholanthrene. Proc Soc Exp Biol Med 111:774–775, 1962.

54. Wattenberg LW: Inhibition of carcinogenic and toxic effects of polycyclic hydrocarbons by phenolic antioxidants and ethoxyquin. J Natl Cancer Inst 48:1425–1430, 1972.

55. Odukoya O, Hawah F, Shklar G: Retardation of experimental oral cancer by topical vitamin E. Nutr Cancer 6:98–104, 1984.

56. Horvath PM, Ip C: Synergistic effect of vitamin E and selenium in the chemoprevention of mammary carcinogenesis in rats. Cancer Res 43:5335–5341, 1983.

57. Cook MG, McNamara P: Effect of dietary vitamin E on dimethylhydrazine-induced colonic tumors in mice. Cancer Res 40:1329–1331, 1980.

58. Bruce WR, McKeown-Eyssen G, Ciampi A, Dion PW, Boyd N: Strategies for dietary intervention studies on colon cancer. Cancer 47:1121–1125, 1981.

59. Narisawa T, Hermanek P, Habs M, Schmahl D: Reduction in carcinogenicity of N-nitroso methylurea by indomethacin and failure of resuming effect of prostaglandin E_2 (PGE_2) against indomethacin. J Cancer Clin Oncol 108: 239–242, 1984.

60. Fitzer CJ, O'Brian CA, Guillem JG, Weinstein IB: The regulation of protein kinase C by chenodeoxycholate, deoxycholate and several structurally related bile acids. Carcinogenesis 8:217–220, 1987.

61. Watanabe J, Bernstein H: The mutagenicity of bile acids using a fluctuation test. Mutat Res 158:45–51, 1985.

62. Appleton GU, Davies PW, Bristol JB, Williamson RC: Inhibition of intestinal carcinogenesis by dietary supplementation with calcium. Br J Surg 74:523–525, 1987.

63. Garland C, Shekelle R, Barrett-Connor M, Criqui MH, Rossof AH, Paul O: Dietary vitamin D and calcium and risk of colorectal cancer: A 19-yr prospective study in men. Lancet 1:307–309, 1985.

64. Heibrun LK, Nomura A, Hankin JH, Stemmermann GN: Dietary vitamin D and calcium and risk of colorectal cancer. Lancet 1:925, 1985.

65. Krichevsky D: Diet, nutrition and cancer. The role of fiber. Cancer 58:1830–1836, 1986.

66. Galloway DJ, Owen RW, Jarrett F, Boyle P, Hill MJ, George WD: Experimental colorectal cancer: The relationship of diet and faecal bile acid content concentration to tumor induction. Br J Surg 73:233–237, 1986.

67. Jacobs LR: Effect of dietary fiber on colonic cell prolif-

eration and its relationship to colon carcinogenesis. Prev Med 16:566–571, 1987.

68. Sestili MA (ed): Chemoprevention Clinial Trials: Problems and Solutions. Washington, DC: NIH Publication No. 85-2715, 1984.

69. Surwit EA, Graham V, Droegemueller W, Chvapil M, Dorr RT, Davis JR, Meyskens FL Jr: Evaluation of topically applied trans-retinoic acid in the treatment of cervical intraepithelial lesions. Am J Obstet Gynecol 143:821–823, 1982.

70. Meyskens FL Jr, Grahanam V, Chvapil M, Dorr RT, Alberts DS, Surwit EA: A phase I trial of β-all-trans-retinoic acid for mild or moderate intraepithelial cervical neoplasia delivered via a collagen sponge and cervical cap. J Natl Cancer Inst 71:921–925, 1983.

71. Graham V, Surwit ES, Weiner S, Meyskens FL: Phase II trial of β-all-trans-retinoic acid for cervical intraepithelial neoplasia delivered via a collagen sponge and cervical cap. West J Med 145:192–195, 1986.

72. Misset JL, Mathe G, Santelli G, Gouveia J, Homasson JP, Sudve NC, Gaget H: Regression of bronchial epidermoid metaplasia in heavy smokers with etretinate treatment. Cancer Detect Prevent 9:167–170, 1986.

73. Shah JP, Strong EW, DeCosse JJ, Itri L, Sellers P: Effect of retinoids on oral leukoplakia. Am J Surg 146:466–469, 1983.

74. Pindborg JJ, Jolst O, Renstrup G, Roed-Peterson B: Studies in oral leukoplakia. J Am Dent Assoc 76:767–771, 1968.

75. Koch HF: Biochemical treatment of precancerous oral lesions: The effectiveness of various analogs of retinoic acid. J Max Fac Surg 6:59–63, 1978.

76. Koch HF: Effect of retinoids on precancerous lesions in oral mucosa. In Orfanos CE, et al. (eds): Retinoids: Advances in Basic Research and Therapy. Berlin: Springer-Verlag, 1981, pp307–312.

77. Hong WJ, Itri L, Endicott J, Bell R, Vaughan C, Doos W, Gunter P, Strong S: The effectiveness of 13-cis-retinoic acid in the treatment of premalignant lesions in oral cavity. Proc Am Soc Clin Oncol 4:906, 1985.

78. Alberts DS, Coulthard SW, Meyskens FL Jr: Regression of aggressive laryngeal papillomatosis with 13-cis-retinoic acid. J Biol Respir Mod 5:124–128, 1984.

79. Bichler E: The role of aromatic retinoid in treatment of laryngeal keratinizing disorders and dysplasias. In Spitzy KH, Karrer K (eds): Proceedings of the 13th International Congress of Chemotherapy. Symposium Retinoids, A New Approach to Prevention and Therapy of Cancer. Vienna, 1983.

80. Stich HF, Rosin MP, Vallejera MO: Reduction with vitamin A and beta-carotene administration of proportion of micronucleated buccal mucosal cells in Asian betel nut and tobacco chewers. Lancet 1:1204–1206, 1984.

81. Stich HF, Stich W, Rosin M, Vallejera MO: Use of the micronucleus test to monitor the effect of vitamin A, beta-carotene and canthaxanthin on the buccal mucosa of betel nut/tobacco chewers. Int J Cancer 34:745–750, 1984.

82. Bollag W, Ott F: Vitamin A acid in benign and malignant epithelial tumors of the skin. Acta Dermatovener (Stockh) [Suppl] 74:163–166, 1975.

83. Belisario JC: Recent advances in topical cytotoxic therapy of skin cancer and pre-cancer. In Melanoma and Skin Cancer. Proc Int. Canc. Conf. (Sydney), 1972, pp 349–365.

84. Grupper Ch, Beretti B: Cutaneous neoplasia and etretinate. In Spitzy KH, Karrer K (eds): Proc 13th International Congress of Chemotherapy. Symposium Retinoids: A New Approach to Prevention and Therapy of Cancer. Vienna, 1983.

85. Moriarty M, Dunn J, Derregh A, Lambe R, Brick I: Etretinate in treatment of actinic keratosis: A double-blind crossover study. Lancet i:364–365, 1982.

86. DeCosse JJ, Adams MB, Kuzma JF, Logerfo P, Codon RE: Effect of ascorbic acid on rectal polyps of patients with familial polyposis. Surgery 78:608–612, 1975.

87. Bussey HJR, DeCosse JJ, Deschner EE, Eyers AA, Lesser ML, Morson BC, Ritchie SM, Thompson JPS, Wadsworth J: A randomized trial of ascorbic acid in polyposis coli. Cancer 50:1434–1439, 1982.

88. Alfthan O, Tarkkanen J, Grohn P, Heinonen E, Pyrhonen S, Saila K, Tigason (etretinate) in prevention of recurrence of superficial bladder tumors: A double-blind study. Eur Urol 9:6–9, 1983.

89. Peck GL, Olson TG, Butkus D, Pandya M, Arnaud-Battandier J, Yoder F, Lezif WR: Treatment of basal cell carcinomas with 13-cis-retinoic acid. Proc Am Assoc Cancer Res 20:56, 1979.

90. Lippman S, Kessler J, Meyskens FL Jr: Retinoids as preventive and therapeutic anti-cancer agents. Cancer Treatment Rep 71:493–515, 1987.

91. Pedersen H, Wolf H, Jensen SK, Lund F, Hansen E, Olsen PR, Sorenson BL: Administration of a retinoid as prophylaxis of recurrent non-invasive bladder tumors. Scand J Urol Nephol 18:121–123, 1984.

31

Role of Fecal Bile Acids and Bacteria in Patients With Genetic Predisposition to Cancer of the Large Bowel

Michael Hill

Public Health Laboratory Service Centre for Applied Metabolism and Research, Porton Down, Salisbury, England

BACKGROUND

Bile acids are produced by the human liver as the end products of cholesterol metabolism. The two bile acids synthesized are cholic acid (3,7, 12-trihydroxy-5-cholan-24-oic acid) and chenodeoxycholic acid (3-7-dihydroxy-5-cholan-24-oic acid), and these are secreted in bile as the conjugates with glycine or taurine via a C-24 amide bond. The function of the bile acids is fat digestion; the conjugates are poorly absorbed from the intestine by a passive absorption mechanism but are efficiently recovered from the terminal ileum by an active transport process and returned via the portal vein to the liver. The efficiency is such that less than 5% of the bile acids escape recovery and enter the colon each cycle, but since they are cycled 6–10 times per day 300–600 mg enters the large bowel. The enterohepatic circulation of bile aids has been reviewed in more detail elsewhere [1,2].

The large intestine contains a rich bacterial flora (Table 1) dominated by the nonsporing, strictly anaerobic, rod-shaped organisms (*Bacteroides* spp., *Bifidobacterium* spp., *Eubacterium* spp., *Propionibacterium* spp.). This flora is able to metabolize extensively the bile conjugates entering the colon, the principal reactions being 1) deconjugation, 2) dehydroxylation, and 3) hydroxyloxidoreduction. The deconjugation reaction releases free bile acids from the conjugates by hydrolyzing the amide bond; the enzyme is at very high activity in the normal colon to the extent that virtually all of the bile acids are deconjugated within 1–4 hours of entering the colon. The free bile acids are much more readily recovered from the colon by passive diffusion, and approximately 30% of the bile acids entering the colon are recovered in this way and returned to the liver. The 7-dehydroxylase yields the principal fecal bile acids lithocholic and deoxycholic acids from chenodeoxycholic and cholic acids, respectively; in most persons more than 90% of the fecal bile acids have undergone this dehydroxylation reaction. The enzyme is only produced under highly anaerobic conditions and requires similarly anaerobic conditions for its action. The hydroxyl oxidoreductase yields oxo bile acids and hydroxyl groups with the β-configuration from the α-hydroxyl groups produced by the liver. In vitro these oxidoreductases tend to be the dominant enzymic products of the gut flora, but the anaerobic conditions in the gut are unfavorable to both the production and the action of the enzymes. As a consequence, the oxo bile acids and those with β-hydroxyl groups are minor fecal bile acids, accounting for only 1–20% of the total. The normal fecal bile acids are summarized in Table 2 [for detailed review of the bacterial metabolism of bile acids, see 3,4].

In addition to bile acids, feces also contain neutral steroids produced by bacterial action on cholesterol and plant steroids. Cholesterol is syn-

Familial Adenomatous Polyposis, pages 263–266

TABLE 1.
Bacterial Flora in the Feces of Healthy Adult Humans

Organisms	No. per gram of feces
Anaerobes	
Bacteroides spp.	10^{11}
Bifidobacterium spp.	10^{10}–10^{11}
Eubacterium spp.	10^{9}–10^{11}
Propionibacterium spp.	10^{9}–10^{11}
Clostridium spp.	10^{6}–10^{8}
Veillonella spp.	10^{4}–10^{6}
Microaerophilic	
Lactobacillus spp.	10^{7}–10^{8}
Streptococcus spp.	10^{6}–10^{8}
Facultative and others	
Escherichia coli	10^{6}–10^{8}
Micrococci/staphylococci	10^{3}–10^{6}
Bacillus spp.	ND to 10^{4}
Yeasts and fungi	10^{3}–10^{5}

ND, not determined.

thesized in the liver and secreted in bile and is also present in large amounts in the diet. Only a small proportion of the cholesterol entering the small bowel (from whatever source) is absorbed, and a high proportion enters the colon where it is 1) reduced to coprostanol (3-hydroxy-5β-cholestane), coprostanone (3-oxo-5β-cholestane), and cholestenone (3-oxo-cholest-4-ene). In most reports, in normal healthy persons 60–70% of the fecal cholesterol metabolites are in the form of coprostanol, 5–15% are coprostanone, 0–5% are cholestenone, and 10–25% are undegraded cholesterol (Table 3).

It has been hypothesized that colorectal cancer is caused at least in part by bacterial metabolites of the bile acids [5–7] the role of which is the promotion of carcinogenesis probably by stimulating adenoma growth [8] and dysplasia [9,10]. Since the risk of colorectal carcinogenesis is very high in patients with familial adenomatous polyposis (FAP) and in the so-called cancer families, it was natural to expect the fecal bile acids (FBA) and other fecal steroids of such persons to be very extensively metabolized and for the gut bacterial flora to show a high level of metabolic activity in general.

TABLE 2.
Fecal Steroids of Normal Adult Humans

Bile acid	Proportion of fecal bile acids (% of total)
Deoxycholic acid	Important (45–55)
Lithocholic acid	Important (30–40)
Cholic acid	Minor (3–5)
Chenodeoxycholic acid	Minor (3–5)
Conjugated bile acids	Minor (less than 5)
Oxo-bile acids	Minor (1–20)
Unsaturated bile acids	Minor (much less than 1)

FECAL ANALYSES IN FAP PATIENTS

The first report of fecal steroids in patients with FAP was by Core and Watne [11], who assayed fecal cholesterol and metabolites. In contrast to the result that might have been expected, they found a very low extent of metabolism of cholesterol to coprostanol in a small number of patients with FAP. This observation was confirmed and extended by Bone et al. [12], who found that in six patients with FAP less than 25% of the cholesterol had undergone metabolism to coprostanol during colonic transit. Further, in a

TABLE 3.
Fecal Neutral Steroids in Various Populations*

Country of origin	No. analyzed	Percent normal type[a]
United States	53	93
Scotland	15	100
Denmark	21	100
England	198	97
South Africa, white	13	100
South Africa, black	23	74
Finland	23	100
India	11	100
Uganda	11	91
Japan	36	56
Hong Kong	64	84
English Vegans	15	100

*For details, see Hill [3].
[a]More than 50% of cholesterol reduced to coprostanol.

group of 13 as yet unaffected children six had low cholesterol metabolism while in the other seven more than 70% of the cholesterol had been reduced to coprostanol (i.e., had normal cholesterol metabolism). In addition, two patients with Peutz-Jegher's syndrome had normal metabolism of cholesterol while one patient with juvenile polyposis had test results similar to those seen in FAP patients. Finally, in all 24 patients a low extent of metabolism of cholesterol appeared qualitatively to be accompanied by a low extent of degradation of fecal bile acids.

These observations were quickly confirmed and extended by other investigators [13,15]. In our studies we developed the work along two lines; the first was to investigate the causes of the lack of metabolism, and the second was to test the predictive value of the fecal analyses in identifying which of the children of FAP patients would actually develop the disease.

FAP patients have an intestinal flora that fails to metabolize completely not only cholesterol but also, for example, bile acids and some amino acids. Cholesterol and bile acids and their metabolites are excreted in feces; in contrast, the metabolites of tyrosine (urinary volatile phenols [UVPs]) and of the basic amino acids lysine, arginine, and ornithine (piperidine and pyrrolidine) are absorbed from the colon and excreted in the urine. Table 4 summarizes the results obtained when these metabolites were assayed in FAP patients compared with control persons. In normal healthy persons the fecal bile acids are almost completely deconjugated and dehydroxylated; in FAP patients a proportion of the bile acids remain conjugated and a high proportion remains undehydroxylated [13,14]. Similarly, in normal healthy persons the urine contains 50–100 mg per day of UVP (from tyrosine metabolism), 500–1000 μg per day of piperidine (from lysine), and 100–500 μg per day of pyrrolidine (from arginine and ornithine); in FAP patients the urine contained only 10–15 mg per day of UVP and no detectable piperidine or pyrrolidine. Thus the intestinal bacterial flora in FAP patients metabolizes a range of substrates very poorly.

The factors controlling the metabolic activity of the intestinal flora include rate of intestinal transit, intestinal pH and Eh, and the composition of the bacterial flora. All of these wer examined by Drasar et al. [13]; in six FAP patients the transit time (as measured using radio-opaque markers) was not unusually rapid, and most FAP patients produced well-formed stools; the fecal pH was in the range 6.5 to 7.5 (as in normal, healthy persons); the redox potential in feces was similar to that in the feces of normal, healthy persons, and the composition of the fecal bacterial flora in FAP patients was indistinguishable from that in normal, healthy control persons. Further, when feces from FAP patients were incubated with cholesterol or bile acids in vitro their meta-

TABLE 4.
Metabolic Activity of the Gut Bacterial Flora Toward Four Substrates in FAP Patients Compared With Disease-Free Control Persons

Substrate	Reaction	Route of excretion of the product	Extent of the reaction: FAP	Extent of the reaction: Normal
Bile acids	Deconjugation	Feces	50% (150–250 mg/day)	95% (300–500 mg/day)
	7-Dehydroxylation	Feces	20% (50–100 mg/day)	80–90% (250–450 mg/day)
Cholesterol	4–5-Reduction	Feces	10–30% (50–100 mg/day)	60–90% (500–800)
Tyrosine	Catabolism to phenol and cresol	Urine	10–20 mg/day (mainly phenol)	60–100 mg/day (mainly p-cresol)
Basic amino acids	Formation of cyclic secondary amines	Urine	Not detected	1,000–1,500 μg/day

bolic activity was normal. Thus in FAP patients the fecal bacterial flora is not unusual, the physicochemical conditions are normal, there is ample time during transit for metabolism to take place, and the flora is fully active in vitro. Nevertheless, the bacterial flora fails to metabolize a range of substrates in vivo.

PREDICTIVE VALUE OF FECAL ANALYSES

Initially it was hoped that there would be predictive value in fecal analysis, since in the initial study all of the FAP patients failed to metabolize any of the four substrates studied. When almost 100 of the teenaged children of such patients were investigated, they segregated into two types: They had either a very low (FAP type) or a high (normal type) metabolism. Almost all of those with FAP-type results progressed to develop FAP, while those with normal results in general remained free of polyposis; there was, however, a number of families in which all members had normal results, including those who developed FAP, while a few patients who consistently had FAP-type results have remained disease free. The predictive value of the fecal analyses is not sufficiently good to be of clinical value (and in one batch of patients was not sufficient even to be notable). Nevertheless, the lack of metabolism by the gut flora in a high proportion of FAP patients remains an enigma and should contain clues to the biochemical abnormalities that are the phenotypic expression of the FAP genetic abnormality.

References

1. Hoffmann AF: The enterohepatic circulation of bile acids in man. Clin Gastroenterol 6:3–24, 1977.
2. Hill MJ: Conservation of bile aids. In Fumagalli R, Kritchevsky D, Paoletti R (eds): Drugs Affecting Lipid Metabolism. Amsterdam: Elsevier, 1980, pp 89–96.
3. Hill MJ: The role of unsaturated bile acids in the etiology of large bowel cancer. In Hiatt H, Watson J, Winsten J (eds): Origins of Human Cancer. New York: Cold Spring Harbor Lab Press, 1977, 1627–1640.
4. Hill MJ: Microbes and Human Carcinogenesis. London: Edward Arnold, 1986.
5. Aries VIC, Crowther JS, Drasar BS, Hill MJ: Degradation of bile salts by human intestinal bacteria. Gut 10:575–577, 1969.
6. Hill MJ, Drasar BS, Williams REO: Faecal bile acids and *Clostridia* in patients with cancer of the large bowel. Lancet, i:535–538, 1975.
7. Hill MJ: Mechanisms of colorectal carcinogenesis. In Joossens J, Hill M, Geboers J (eds): Diet and Human Carcinogenesis. Amsterdam: Excerpta Medica, 1985, pp 149–164.
8. Hill MJ: Bacteria and colorectal adenomas. Top Gastroenterol 13: 237–252, 1985.
9. Hill MJ: Biochemical approaches to the intervention in large bowel cancer. In Ingall JRF, Mastromarino AJ (eds): Carcinoma of the Large Bowel and Its Precursors. New York: Alan R. Liss, 1985, pp 263–276.
10. Hill MJ, Melville D, Lennard-Jones J, Neale K, Ritchie J: Faecal bile acids, dysplasia in carcinoma in ulcerative colitis. Lancet 2: 185–186, 1987.
11. Core SK, Watne AL: Fecal steroids and colon cancer [abstr]. Fed Proc 33:260, 1974.
12. Bone E, Drasar BS, Hill MJ: Gut bacteria and their metabolic activities in familial polyposis. Lancet i:1117–1120, 1975.
13. Drasar BS, Bone ES, Hill MJ, Marks CG: Colon cancer and bacterial metabolism in familial polyposis. Gut 16:824, 1975.
14. Watne A, Lai H-Y, Mance T, Core S: Fecal steroids and bacterial flora in patients with polyposis coli. Am J Surg 131:42–46, 1976.
15. Reddy BS, Mastromarino A, Gastafson C, Lipkin M, Wynder EL: Fecal bile acids and neutral sterols in patients with familial polyposis. Cancer 38:1694–1698, 1976.

32

Tissue Culture Studies in Familial Adenomatous Polyposis: Biomarkers, Genetics, and Cancer[1]

Levy Kopelovich

Laboratory of Cancer Genetics and Cancer Prevention, VA Medical Center, Bay Pines and Departments of Pathology and Cellular and Molecular Biology, University of South Florida College of Medicine, Tampa, Florida

INTRODUCTION

Here is a dilemma: Although specific chromosomes have been assigned to each of several distinct autosomal dominant forms of inherited cancer [1–3], experiments show the systemic expression of abnormal biomarkers that are commonly shared by these syndromes, viz., hereditary adenomatosis of the colon and rectum (ACR), Von Recklinghausen's neurofibromatosis (VRNF), retinoblastoma (RB), and lung and breast cancer [for review, see 4]. The occurrence of abnormal biomarkers in clinically unaffected skin cells from patients who are predisposed to different forms of cancer led to the concept of a global expression of the cancer trait [4]. Accordingly, distinct forms of cancer may each represent a *single* and *specific* gene defect, but additional gene(s) can pleiotropically control the expression of these cancer-predisposing genes.

Even in the case of RB, the RB1 locus, presumed to be RB specific, is apparently also a target of somatic mutations in mesenchymal tumors among patients having no obvious predisposition to RB and no previous evidence of RB [5]. Thus the cloned RB1 sequence is representative of a gene that is a frequent target of mutation during cancer development [5–7]. The product of the RB gene was identified as a nuclear phosphoprotein that is associated with DNA binding activity [8]. Whether these results can also be used in support of the role of a higher hierarchy of control in cancer development has yet to be established.

EXPERIMENTAL SYSTEM

As part of a study on genetic mechanisms that predispose to cancer, we investigated cultured skin fibroblasts from ACR and VRNF patients. An autosomal dominant pattern of inheritance in both ACR and VRNF is manifested by a tendency toward tumor formation, including those arising from skin [9,10]. This knowledge led us to consider the use of skin fibroblasts to study genetic determinants of cancer predisposition in these two precancer syndromes. Clearly, it is an easier task to scan cultured fibroblasts than it is to obtain cells from most tissues at high risk for a variety of cancers.

By using only cultured skin fibroblasts from patients (including those with preneoplastic skin lesions) and from healthy individuals, we were able to examine a single cell type under comparable conditions in vitro. Phenotypic expressions occurring in vitro in early-passage fibroblastic cell strains apparently reflect biologic properties occurring in vivo. Only adult (6–70 year) human fibroblasts were investigated. Human embryo

[1]In this chapter, familial adenomatous polyposis is referred to as *hereditary adenomatosis of the colon and rectum* (ACR).

Familial Adenomatous Polyposis, pages 267–274

and foreskin fibroblasts are readily distinguished from adult fibroblasts [11].

Fibroblasts are ubiquitous and provide the stromal elements of all organs. The embryologic derivation of the fibroblast lends itself to a variety of proliferative expressions. The fibroblast itself also has a remarkable range of oncogenic potentials [12]. Defects in fibroblast growth control and organization may possibly be related to the development of a tumor that is different histologically, as well as to induction of metastasis in some experimental systems [4,13].

From our observations, the following terminology of basic concepts has developed [4,14, 15]. *Transformed cell* describes cells with an abnormal phenotype in vitro. The term *cancer initiation,* or *cancer predisposition,* describes the transformed cell phenotype in conjunction with genetic susceptibility in vivo. *Cancer-specific expressions,* or *global expression of the cancer trait,* as distinct from *cancer-specific genes,* refers to the occurrence of similar biomarkers in cells from patients who are predisposed to different dominantly inherited forms of cancer.

INITIATED CELL PHENOTYPE

To date, many abnormal phenotypic expressions have been identified in fibroblastic cells from ACR and VRNF patients. The abnormalities include altered nutrient requirements; loss of growth control, including anchorage independence; deformed cytoarchitecture; alterations of membrane-associated parameters; loss of sensitivity to hydrocortisone; augmented expression of host–cell coded antigens; and differential susceptibility to a variety of physical, chemical, and viral agents [4] (Table 1). Extension of these experiments in a number of laboratories confirmed the occurrence of these alterations not only in cells from ACR patients but also in VRNF, RB, and lung and breast cancer patients [4,14,15].

The studies also showed that not all cells from patients genetically at risk of cancer express the transformed phenotype to the same extent. The magnitude of change of all experimental parameters reported by the different laboratories was variable. This variation ranged from 1.3-fold to about threefold for unperturbed cells and from about fivefold to 1000-fold for virus-treated cells. Thus, despite high gene penetrance, phenotypic heterogeneity at the cellular level, like clinical signs, shows considerable variability. Experimental conditions would have also contributed to this variation. Nevertheless, skin fibroblasts from ACR, VRNF, RB, and lung and breast cancer patients were consistently identified at a $P < 0.05$ level of significance by the various laboratories [for review, see 4].

The abnormal expressions observed in fibroblasts from ACR and VRNF patients describe the changing phenotype of cells undergoing neoplastic transformation (Table 1). Such cells presumably represent an inititated state that, for the first time, provides a means of characterizing cancer initiation in humans. Our presumption of the initiated cell is based on the identification of biomarkers that, collectively, are usually found during neoplastic transformation. These abnormal biomarkers are intrinsically linked to cancer, since all affected individuals eventually develop cancer. However, additional mutations are apparently necessary, with certain promoters acting to increase the probability for expression of the malignant phenotype. The probability of such a transition occurring spontaneously is extremely rare, since, for example, very few initiated cells become tumorigenic even in the target organs of ACR or NF patients. This observation is consistent with in vitro studies, as well [4]. Thus clinical manifestations, like phenotypic expressions at the cellular level, show considerable heterogeneity.

ONCOGENES AND THE INITIATED CELL PHENOTYPE

The role of oncogenes in cancer predisposition has yet to be determined [3,4,16,17]. The study of dominant forms of cancer shows that changes in structure or level of expression of oncogenes during cancer development may be secondary to an effect by the cancer gene itself [4,15]. For example, the association between increased transformation by the Kirsten murine sarcoma virus (KiMSV)/Harvey murine sarcoma virus (HaMSV) and colorectal cancer was first

TABLE 1.
Phenotypic Profile of an Inititiated ACR Cell*

A. Growth parameters
   1. Growth in nutrient-deprived environment
   2. Loss of contact inhibition
   3. Inceased cloning efficiency
   4. A partial loss of anchorage sensitivity
   5. Decreased sensitivity to hydrocortisone-induced cell proliferation in monolayers and in agar
B. Cytoskeletal structures
   1. Defective actin-containing cables
   2. Normal organization of microtubules
   3. Normal organization of intermediate filaments
C. Membrane-associated parameters
   1. Increased 2-deoxyglucose uptake
   2. Increased Con A agglutination (in suspension and onto derivatized matrices)
   3. Increased intra- and extracellular levels of plasminogen activator
   4. Defective polymerization of collagen (tertiary structure)
   5. Normal expression of fibronectin
   6. Lack of restoration of deformed cytoskeletal actin by fibronectin
D. Expression of cellular oncogenes
   1. No apparent change in c-ras oncogenes
   2. Increased expression of the transformation-association host–cell coded p53 protein that is further amplified during cancer progression
E. Cytotoxic effects of chemical and physical agents
   1. Apparently normal sensitivity to γ-rays and UV-irradiation. Increased tolerance to γ-rays and UV irradiation during cancer progression
   2. Decreased cytotoxic response to retinoic acid
   3. Decreased cytotoxic response to 5-azacytidine that is further amplified during cancer progression
   4. Decreased cytotoxic response to TPA that is bimodally expressed and becoming progressively hyperbolic during cancer development
F. Increased sensitivity to further transformation by oncogenic viruses
   1. Kirsten murine sarcoma virus (associated with an expression of a human fetal-like antigen)
   2. SV40 (associated with an expression of a human placenta-like antigen)
G. Increased sensitivity to further transformation by chemical and physical agents
   1. TPA (also characterized by a marked increase in cell ploidy and by expression of a human fetal-like antigen)
   2. MNNG (also characterized by a marked increase in cell ploidy)
   3. γ-rays (associated with a progressive increase in radiotolerance during cancer development)
H. Metabolic parameters
   1. Normal cholesterol feedback regulation (HMG CoA reductase)
   2. Normal methionine requirement
   3. Increased lactate production[a]
   4. Decreased prostaglandins production[a]

*These results (updated from 1982) have been recently summarized in great detail [4]. In general, the pattern of abnormal biomarkers found in initiated ACR cells becomes progressively amplified during cancer development (for additional information, see Tumor Progression).
[a]Preliminary observations.

seen in skin fibroblasts from ACR patients [4,18]. In this instance, however, no differences were found between normal and ACR cells at the level of DNA, RNA transcripts, or gene products of the ras gene family (R. Ellis and L. Kopelovich, unpublished observation, 1982). DNA from ACR cells also lacked transforming activity in the NIH/3T3 DNA transfection assay [19]. It was concluded that the increased sensitivity of ACR cells to transformation by the ras family of oncogenes is dissociated, at least in part, from the ability of such cells to express an altered c-ras proto-oncogene. How the increased sensitivity of ACR cells to transformation by KiMSV and HaMSV might be related to an altered c-ras gene expression in colon adenomas [20] and colon and lung adenocarcinomas [20,21] has yet to be established.

We also found increased expression of the tranformation-associated p53 antigen in ACR and NF cells [22]. The increased expression of p53 antigen prior to any alterations in expression, or to transforming potential of the c-ras family of oncogenes, indicates that it is an early event associated with cancer initiation. Moreover, fibroblasts from clinically identifiable precursor states in NF showed increasingly greater amounts of the p53 antigen, suggesting a correlation with cancer progression as well [22,23].

Based on our experience, certain viral oncogenes appear to induce transformation/neodifferentiation of human skin fibroblasts in the presence of glucocorticosteroids [24–27]. We have recently demonstrated conversion of skin fibroblasts histiocytes through the use of a feline-derived oncogene [27]. These studies suggest that oncogenes may be instrumental during reprogramming as constitutive genes whose role is to facilitate differentiation in both normal and cancer cells. This interpretation may also be true with respect to spontaneous changes involving oncogenes in clinical forms of human cancer [20,21]. Differentiation-related genes and/or growth-regulatory genes may be more appropriate labels for oncogenes [4,14,15].

TUMOR PROGRESSION

Promotion is apparently the single most important step in the genesis of human cancer. Intervention at the level of promotion may, in reality, be the most effective phase of cancer control [4]. Study of cells from clinically identifiable preneoplastic lesions in ACR and NF has provided insight into cancer progression vis à vis the initiated human cell phenotype (Table 1).

For example, we determined the sensitivity to γ-rays of cultured fibroblasts derived from normal skin and from clinically identifiable preneoplastic lesions on the skin of ACR and VRNF patients. Fibroblasts from skin of normal appearance in these patients were normally sensitive to γ-irradiation [28,29]. However, an ACR cell clone with a 45X(-Y) karyotype [29] and fibroblasts from café-au-lait lesions and from neurofibromas were abnormally radiotolerant (about twofold) to treatment with γ-rays [28]. Virus-transformed human skin fibroblasts and human tumor cells (fibrosarcoma, colon adenocarcinoma, malignant melanoma), in that order, were found to be increasingly more radiotolerant (D_os 195–300 rad) than were fibroblasts from clinically identifiable preneoplastic lesions [28]. Significantly, ACR cells were apparently also more sensitive to transformation by γ-irradiation [4].

Taken together, the results suggest that increased propensity to cancer in the human cell system is associated with increased radiotolerance and increased transformation by low-level ionizing radiation. Similar conclusions were subsequently made through the cancer family syndrome originally described by Chang et al. [30]. A corollary finding is the observation that the c-RAF-1 proto-oncogene regulates both tumorigenic and radiation-resistant phenotypes of human squamous cell carcinoma [31]. The clinical significance of these observations with regard to radiation therapy of certain types of cancer should be noted [4,28]. For example, the use of radiotherapy in treating tumors on ACR, VRNF, or RB patients has caused some controversy because secondary malignancies have developed in the field of radiation [4,10,32].

The tumor-promoting effects of 12-O-tetradecanoyl phorbol-13-acetate (TPA) on human cells are highly complex [33]. These effects presumably consist of both short- and long-term alterations [4]. For example, we observed both low- and high-affinity receptors for TPA. The high-affinity receptors for TPA can apparently be modulated by cell density in a transient fashion (down-regulation), or they can be completely inactivated through a sequence of constitutive changes leading to neoplastic transformation. While the significance of this transition has yet to be understood, it does appear to be diagnostic of neoplastic progression in vitro [4]. Although induction of hyperploidy apparently occurs to a comparable degree in normal and ACR cells it may, in reality, represent the most important effect by TPA as a tumor promoter [for review, see 4].

The reduced sensitivity of ACR cells to hydrocortisone-induced cell proliferation in vitro may possibly be linked to mechanisms associated with progression of colorectal cancer [34]. For example, colon adenocarcinoma is refractory to glucocorticosteroid therapy in such patients. Recent experiments showed that steroid-insensitive cells contain functional receptors and that the defect occurs at the level of transcriptional control during cancer progression [35].

Fibroblasts from normal-appearing skin and from cancer-prone tissues of ACR and NF patients were also increasingly more resistant to 5-azacytidine–induced cytotoxicity [36]. Although cytotoxicity induced by 5-azacytidine is presumably a complex phenomenon [37], our data suggest that it is associated with the expression of an autosomal dominant gene in cancer-predisposed persons and with preneoplastic lesions in such patients. Determination of overall 5-methylcytosine patterns and of specific methylation domains in the DNA of such cells is in progress.

These studies represent only a few of many that illustrate the relevance of biomarkers to the understanding of cancer initiation and cancer progression in man. In general, the abnormal biomarkers found in unperturbed initiated cells became progressively more amplified during cancer development.

GENETIC PREDISPOSITION TO CANCER IS AN AUTOSOMAL DOMINANT TRAIT

We believe that autosomal dominant traits that predispose individuals to cancer truly provide genetic information directly related to this disease. Genetic predisposition to cancer in the autosomal dominant syndromes at the cellular level is associated with cancer initiation [4,14,15]. Remarkably, in a recent study [38], a patient with both ACR and NF was identified through information from his family and by his clinical features, suggesting that these two dominant genes can be coexpressed in a single cell of such persons.

An autosomal dominant pattern has been recognized in a large number of familial aggregates predisposed to a specific form(s) of cancer. These families comprise a large segment of all cancer reported in the United States and elsewhere [39]. It has been our belief that a strong genetic component exists in the sporadic forms of cancer, in which such expression would be consistent with a variably penetrant dominant trait [14,40]. More recently, inheritance of susceptibility to colonic adenomatous polyps and associated colorectal cancers was demonstrated [41].

It is conceivable that the basic genetic mechanisms underlying a predisposition to cancer are essentially similar qualitatively in the autosomal dominant cancer syndromes, the familial cancer syndromes, and the sporadic forms of cancer. A fundamental assumption is that the site of mutation in nonhereditary cancers is similar to that of hereditary cancers for the same tumor type(s) [14]. This is in line with recent experiments suggesting that chromosome 5 is apparently involved in both ACR and sporadic forms of colon adenocarcinoma [42–44]. However, quantitative differences could occur because of gene-dosage at the primary locus and/or at ancillary loci that modulate the expression of malignancy [4,14]. In our view, the question of whether homozygosity is obligatory during cancer development [45], including examples of RFLP probes [20, 42,43,46–49], has yet to be determined.

CLINICAL AND GENETIC CONSIDERATIONS

It is our belief that, at present, predisposition to cancer as a global syndrome can best be detected at the phenotypic cellular level. Much of diagnostic medicine is based on the identification of secondary effects that occur systemically. A systemic expression of the cancer-predisposed phenotype is also consistent with an autosomal dominant mode of inheritance. This conclusion is supported by experimental results to date [4,14].

The present studies further indicate that genotypic distinctions previously attributed to Gardner's syndrome and ACR [50], central VRNF, peripheral VRNF, and mixed peripheral/ central VRNF [12] are not substantiated by the use of biological or biochemical markers. These genotypic distinctions should, therefore, be considered clinical subsets that are manifestations of the heterogeneity found in genetic traits. The possibility that DNA polymorphism may yet distinguish these clinical subsets as discrete disease entities has been raised [44].

Gene penetrance in the autosomal dominant syndromes, both ACR and VRNF, is assumed to be in the range of about 85–100% [9,10]. This range is derived from pedigree analysis, in which the probability of trait expression through several generations appears to support this contention. To date, approximations of gene penetrance were based on clinical expression. Considering the variability of clinical signs, particularly in VRNF, accurate diagnosis may be difficult [10]. Biologic characterization of cells from cancer-predisposed patients, together with clinical signs, should be used to ascertain gene expression more accurately than clinical signs alone. RFLPs emerge as powerful probes for linkage analysis in cancer-predisposed syndromes [2].

These considerations make the ethical issue with respect to treatment more complex and suggest that we should act conservatively with regard to prophylactic measures in the case of individuals identified as gene carriers. A proportion of such individuals may never develop the clinical signs. However, genetic counseling that uses biological markers, including DNA polymorphism, is prudent. Records of membership in high-cancer-risk families, in which organ(s) specificity is indicated, is very important in interpreting potential clinical symptoms and clinical sites of cancer. Extension of studies on biomarkers may permit early detection of cancer in the general poplation, including ''cancer-cured'' individuals [4].

ACKNOWLEDGMENTS

I thank Drs. Lee Weber and Eric Wickstrom for discussions and Mrs. Ana Mackino for typing the manuscript. This work was supported, in part, by grants from the Veterans Administration, VAMC, Bay Pines, Florida.

References

1. Sandberg AA: The chromosomes in human cancer and leukemia. New York: Elsevier, 1980.
2. White R, Caskey CT: The human as an experimental system in molecular genetics. Science 240:1483–1488, 1988.
3. Friend SH, Dryja TP, Weinberg RA: Oncogenes and tumor suppressing genes. N Engl J Med 318:618–622, 1988.
4. Kopelovich L: The transformed (initiated) human cell phenotype: Study of cultured skin fibroblasts from individuals predisposed to cancer. Mutat Res 199:369–385, 1988.
5. Friend SH, Horowitz JM, Gerber MR, Wang XF, Bogenmann E, Li PF, Weinberg RA: Deletions of a DNA sequence in retinoblastomas and mesenchymal tumors: Organization of the sequence and its encoded protein. Proc Natl Sci USA 84:9059–9063, 1987.
6. Lee EY-HP, To H, Shew JY, Bookstein R, Scully P, Lee WH: Inactivation of the retinoblastoma susceptibility gene in human breast cancer. Science 241:218–221, 1988.
7. Harbour JW, Lai SL, Whang-Peng J, Gazdar AF, Minna JD, Kaye FJ: Abnormalities in structure and expression of the human retinoblastoma gene in SCLC. Science 241:353–356, 1988.
8. Lee WH, Shew JY, Hong FD, Sery TW, Domoso LA, Young L-J, Bookstein R, Lee Y-HP: The retinoblastoma susceptibility gene encodes a nuclear phophoprotein associated with DNA binding activity. Nature 329:642–645, 1987.
9. Morson BC, Bussey JR: Predisposing causes of intestinal cancer. Curr Probl Surg: 1–46, 1970.
10. Rubenstein AE, Bunge RP, Housman DE (eds): Neurofibromatosis. Ann NY Acad Sci 486:1–414, 1986.
11. Kopelovich L: Are all normal diploid human cells strains alike: Relevance to carcinogenic mechanisms in vitro. Exp Cell Biol 50:266–270, 1982.
12. Hardy JD: The ubiquitous fibroblast: Multiple oncogenic potentials with illustrative cases. Ann Surg 205:445–455, 1987.
13. Picard O, Rolland Y, Poupon MF: Fibroblast-dependent tumorigenicity of cells in nude mice: Implication for implantation of metastases. Cancer Res 46:3290–3295, 1986.
14. Kopelovich L: Hereditary adenomatosis of the colon and rectum: Relevance to cancer promotion and cancer control in humans. Cancer Genet Cytogenet 5:333–336, 1982.

15. Kopelovich L: Tissue culture assays in familial polyposis coli: Observations and considerations. Semin Surg Oncol 3:159–164, 1987.

16. Weinberg RA: The action of oncogenes in the cytoplasm and nucleus. Science 230:770–776, 1985.

17. Duesberg PH: Retroviruses as carcinogens and pathogens: Expectations and reality. Cancer Res 47:1199–1220, 1987.

18. Pfeffer L, Kopelovich L: Differential genetic susceptibility of cultured human skin fibroblasts to transformation by Kirsten murine sarcoma virus. Cell 10:313–320, 1977.

19. Needleman SE, Yuasa Y Srivastava S, Aaronson SA: Normal cells of patients with high cancer risk syndromes lack transforming activity in the NIH/3T3 transfection assay. Science 222:173–174, 1983.

20. Vogelstein B, Fearon ER, Hamilton SR, Kern SE, Preisinger AC, Leppert M, Nakamura Y, White R, Smits AMM, Bos JL: Genetic alterations during colorectal tumor development. N Engl J Med 319:525–532, 1988.

21. Rodenhuis S, van de Wetering ML, Mooi WJ, Evers SG, van Zandwijk N, Bos JL: Mutational activation of the K-ras oncogene. N Engl J Med 317:929–935, 1987.

22. Kopelovich L, DeLeo AB: Elevated levels of p53 antigen in cultured skin fibroblasts from patients with hereditary adenocarcinoma of the colon and rectum and its relevance to oncogenic mechanisms. J Natl Cancer Inst 77:1241–1246, 1986.

23. Kopelovich L, DeLeo AB: Increased levels of p53 antigen in cultured fibroblasts from preneoplastic lesion in neurofibromatosis patients. Cancer Genet Cytogenet (in press), 1989.

24. Kopelovich L, Rich R, Wallace A: Hydrocortisone promotes the neodifferentiation of Kirsten murine sarcoma virus transformed human skin fibroblasts to adipose cells. Relevance to oncogenic mechanisms. Exp Cell Biol 54:25–33, 1986.

25. Kopelovich L, Wallace A, Rich RF: The kinetics of neodifferentiation of Kirsten murine sarcoma virus transformed human skin fibroblasts to adipose cells by hydrocortisone. Cancer Invest 5:567–581, 1987.

26. Kopelovich L: 5-Azacytidine inhibits adipocytic conversion of human skin fibroblasts by Kirsten murine sarcoma virus and dexamethasone. Exp Cell Biol 55:276–280, 1987.

27. Kopelovich L, Fenyk J: Transformation/neodifferentiation of human skin fibroblasts by acute oncornaviruses and dexamethasone. Exp Cell Biol 56:311–320, 1988.

28. Kopelovich L, Rich RF: Enhanced radiotolerance to ionizing radiation is correlated with increased cancer proneness of cultured fibroblasts from precursor states in neurofibromatosis patients. Cancer Genet Cytogenet 22:203–210, 1986.

29. Kopelovich L, Chapman T: An imbalance in sex chromosomes alters cell survival of human skin fibroblasts exposed to ionizing irradiation. Cancer Genet Cytogenet 20:115–120, 1986.

30. Chang EH, Pirollo DF, Zou ZQ, Cheung HY, Lawler EL, Garner R, White E, Bernstein WB, Fraumeni JW Jr, Blattener WA: Oncogenes in radioresistant, noncancerous skin fibroblasts from a cancer-prone family. Science 237:1036–1039, 1987.

31. Kasid U, Pfeifer A, Brennan T, Beckett M, Weichselbaum RR, Dritschilo A, Mark GE: Antisense human c-RAF-1 cDNA transfection and expression modulates tumorigenic and radiation-resistant phenotypes of a human squamous cell carcinoma. Am Assoc Cancer Res 29:471, 1988.

32. Winawer SJ, Schottenfeld D, Sherlock P: Colorectal cancer: Prevention, epidemiology and screening. In Winawer SJ, Schottenfeld D, Sherlock P (eds): Progress, Cancer Research and Therapy, New York: Raven Press, 1980, Vol 13.

33. Rozengurt E: Early signals in the mitogenic response. Science 234:161–167, 1986.

34. Kopelovich L: Effect of hydrocortisone on the proliferation of cultured skin fibroblasts from normal individuals and individuals at high risk of colon cancer. Exp Cell Biol 51:308–314, 1983.

35. Darbre PD, King JB: Progression to steroid insensitivity can occur irrespective of the presence of functional steroid receptors. Cell 51:521–528, 1987.

36. Kopelovich L, Fenyk J: Fibroblasts from persons predisposed to cancer are abnormally resistant to 5-azacytidine-induced cytotoxicity. Exp Cell Biol 55:281–284, 1987.

37. Jones PA: DNA methylation and cancer. Cancer Res 46:461–466, 1986.

38. Lynch HT, Fitzgibbons RJ Jr, Lanspa SJ, Marcus JN, Lynch JF, Kopelovich L: Familial polyposis coli and neurofibromatosis in the same patient: A family study. Cancer Genet Cytogenet 28:245–251, 1987.

39. Guirgis HA, Lynch HT (eds): Biomarkers, Genetics, and Cancer. New York: Van Nostrand, Reinhold, Inc., 1985, 204 pp.

40. Schneider NR, Chaganti SR, German J, Chaganti RSK: Familial predisposition to cancer and age at onset of disease in randomly selected cancer patients. Am J Hum Genet 35:454–467, 1983.

41. Cannon-Albright LA, Skolnick MH, Bishop T, Lee RG, Burt RW: Common inheritance of susceptibility to colonic adenomatous polyps and associated colorectal cancers. N Enl J Med 319:533–537, 1988.

42. Bodmer WF, Bailey CJ, Bodmer J, Bussey HJR, Ellis A, Gorman P, Lucibelo FC, Murday VA, Rider SH, Scambler P, Sheer D, Solomon E, Spurr NK: Localization of the gene for familial adenomatous polyposis on chromosome 5. Nature 328:614–616, 1987.

43. Solomon E, Voss R, Hall V, Bodmer WF, Jass JR, Jeffreys AJ, Lucibelo FC, Patel I, Rider SH: Chromosome 5 allele loss in human colorectal carcinomas. Nature 328:616–619, 1987.

44. Leppert M, Dobbs, M, Scambler P, O'Connell P, Nakamura Y, Stauffer D, Woodward S, Burt R, Hughes J, Gardner E, Lathrop M, Wasmuth J, Lalouel J-M, White R: The gene for familial polyposis coli maps to the long arm of chromosome 5. Science 238:1411–1413, 1987.

45. Knudson AG: Genetics and etiology of human cancer. In: Harris H, Hirchhorn K (eds): Advances in Human Genetics. New York: Raven Press, 1977, pp 1–66.

46. Cavenee WK, Dryja TP, Phillips RA, Benedict WF,

Godbout R, Gallie BL, Murphree AL, Strong LC, White RL: Expressions of recessive alleles by chromosomal mechanisms in retinoblastoma. Nature 305:779–784, 1983.

47. Okamoto M, Saski M, Sugio K, Sato C, Iwama T, Ikeuchi T, Tonomura A, Sasazuki T, Miyaki M: Loss of constitutional heterozygosity in colon carcinoma from patients with familial polyposis coli. Nature 331:273–277, 1988.

48. Law DJ, Olschwang S, Monpezat J-P, Lefrancois D, Jagelman D, Petrelli NJ, Thomas G, Feinberg AP: Concerted nonsyntenic allelic loss in human colorectal carcinoma. Science 241:961–965, 1988.

49. James CD, Carlbom E, Dumanski JP, Hansen M, Nordenskjold M, Collins VP, Cavenee WK: Clonal genomic alterations in glioma malignancy stages. Cancer Res 48:5546–5551, 1988.

50. Gardner E, Richards R: Multiple cutaneous and subcutaneous lesions occurring simultaneously with hereditary polyposis and osteomatosis. Am J Genet 5:139–148, 1953.

33

Familial Polyposis Colonic Epithelial Cells Respond Inappropriately to Endogeneous Modulators of Colonic Cell Growth

Eileen A. Friedman

Department of Medicine, Memorial Sloan-Kettering Cancer Center, New York, New York

INTRODUCTION

Response to inappropriate growth stimuli and lack of response to normal growth modulators characterize tumors. Colonic epithelial cells from normal-appearing "flat mucosa," biopsied from patients with familial adenomatous polyposis (FAP), display some of these inappropriate, tumor-like responses. Thus mutation or deletion of one of the alleles of the FAP gene [1] makes colonic epithelial cells respond to their environment in a different manner than do normal cells. Since the product of the FAP gene is not known at this writing, its molecular mechanism has yet to be elucidated. Yet we believe, based on the data summarized in this chapter, that loss of one allele of the FAP gene, either directly or indirectly, induces loss of normal cellular response to the calcium differentiation signal. Loss of this normal cellular response is also tightly linked to the acquisition of an inappropriate mitogenic response to tumor promoters of the class that activate protein kinase C.

Epithelial cells from colonic biopsies were primary-cultured either in the presence or absence of the phorbol ester tumor promoter TPA. The epithelial nature of these cultured cells was proven by the presence of characteristic epithelial cell substructures as revealed by electron microscopy [2] and by the presence of cytokeratins as defined by three different monoclonal antibodies [3]. As summarized in Table 1, normal cells from seven patients with a family history of colon cancer and normal cells from eight patients with colonic adenomas or carcinoma displayed no mitogenic response to TPA. However, cells from five familial polyposis patients displayed a strong mitogenic response to TPA, a fivefold increase in the growth fraction [2]. Cells from one FAP patient displayed no mitogenic response to TPA. Since the FAP syndrome develops during adolescence and early adulthood, it is possible that less than 100% of the flat mucosal cells in this individual's colon were expressing the FAP phenotype. If the FAP phenotype (abnormal differentiation pattern, slower DNA replication but expanded zone of proliferation, mitogenic response to tumor promoters) is expressed in cell patches throughout the colon, the biopsy specimen we analyzed might well have been taken from one of the non-FAP phenotype patches.

The TPA response was measured by tubular adenomas: the histologically simplest adenoma class, the earliest class to arise in a colon cleaned of pre-existing adenomas, and the adenoma class with the least malignant potential. Each of six tubular adenomas responded to TPA by a small, but significant, increase in the tumor growth fraction (Table 1). Since the colons of patients symptomatic for FAP are filled with hundreds to thousands of adenomas, the majority of which are tubular, these data show that a protein kinase C-activating tumor promoter can stimulate the growth of FAP preneoplastic cells and premalig-

Familial Adenomatous Polyposis, pages 275–277

TABLE 1.
Mitogenic Effects of TPA Limited to Flat Mucosa From Familial Polyposis Symptomatic Patients and to Tubular Adenomas

	Cumulative ^{3}H-thymidine labeling index (%) growth fraction (mean ± SE)	
	No TPA	+TPA
Normal-appearing cells from seven patients with family history of colon cancer	16.8 ± 2.5	19.8 ± 2.7
Normal-appearing cells from eight patients with tumors	14.7 ± 2.4	11.8 ± 3.9
Preneoplastic cells from five patients symptomatic with familial polyposis	4.7 ± 1.4	24.6 ± 6.1
Preneoplastic cells from one FP patient	3.7 ± 0.8	1.8 ± 1.2
Premalignant cells from six tubular adenomas	24.1 ± 2.5	40.3 ± 5.6

nant tubular adenoma cells, relative to the normal cells, leading to a relative increase in the number of preneoplastic, and then premalignant, cells. Recent data from our laboratory [4] have shown that 10 of 10 adenomas respond to the diglyceride dimyristin with a twofold mitogenic stimulation, while none of the normal cells from seven biopsy specimens were stimulated. These long-chain diglycerides can be derived from partial breakdown of fecal fats and can serve as endogeneous tumor promoters that activate protein kinase C.

FAP cells have lost the capacity to respond to the differentiation signal of elevated external Ca^{2+} levels [5,6]. Normal colonic epithelial cells, cultured from colonic biopsy specimens of nine patients, exhibited a typical dose-response curve when cultured with $CaCl_2$ concentrations of 0.001 to 2.2 mM [5]. The optimum for proliferation was observed at 0.1 mM, while $CaCl_2$ of ≥1 mM inhibited growth. This was quantitated by averaging the growth fractions of these biopsy specimens at 0.1 and 2.2 mM $CaCl_2$ (Table 2). The mean growth fraction decreased from 16.7 ± 1.5% to 10.7 ± 1.2%, a statistically significant decrease, $P < 0.005$. This response to Ca^{2+} was not observed with two adenomas and two carcinomas (Table 2). Ten patients symptomatic with FAP were biopsied and the response of their cells to exogeneous Ca^{2+} concentrations assayed. Eight of the biopsy specimens exhibited no response to Ca^{2+}, while two responded like normal cells. Thus the majority of FAP biopsies were composed of Ca^{2+}-insensitive cells.

The observation that a majority of FAP cells had lost the normal cell response to Ca^{2+} and had gained the tumor cell response to tumor promoters led us to test FAP cells with both agents. One patient, over a period of several months, underwent a biopsy three times, yielding five biopsy specimens. Cells from each of these specimens exhibited the normal cell response to Ca^{2+} of growth inhibition (patient 1, Table 3).

TABLE 2.
Response of Primary-Cultured Colonic Epithelial Cells (Normal, Preneoplastic, and Neoplastic) to Growth in the Presence of Different $CaCl_2$ Concentrations

	Growth fraction (%, mean ± SE)		
Tissue	In 0.1 mM $CaCl_2$	In 2.2 mM $CaCl_2$	*P* value
Normal (9)[a]	16.7 ± 1.5	10.7 ± 1.2	<0.005
Tumors (4)	12.2 ± 0.9	17.9 ± 5.2	>0.1
FP (8)	9.5 ± 1.8	9.1 ± 2.1	>0.1
FP (2)	10.6 ± 1.4	6.0 ± 1.0	>0.01

[a]Number of patients assayed.

TABLE 3.
Colonic Epithelial Cells From Familial Polyposis Symptomatic Patients Respond Either to Calcium or to TPA

Patient	Response to calcium	Response to TPA	No. of Biopsies
1	Growth inhibition	None	5
2	None	Growth stimulation	3
3	None	Growth stimulation	3

TABLE 4.
Summary

	Response to Ca[a]	Response to protein kinase C-activating tumor promoters
Normal cells	+	−
↓		
Familial polyposis cells	−	+
↓		
Neoplastic tubular adenoma cells	−	+

+, Present; −, absent.

Two other patients, from the larger FAP subgroup, underwent a biopsy three times. Cells from each of these specimens exhibited no response to Ca^{2+} but had gained a mitogenic response to the tumor promoter TPA (patients 2 and 3, Table 3).

We conclude that mutation or deletion in one allele of the FAP gene, leading to the phenotypic expression of the FAP gene in colonic epithelial cells, leads directly or indirectly to loss of the normal cell response to Ca^{2+} (Table 4). Concomitant with this loss of normal growth regulation is the acquisition by the FAP cell of an abnormal mitogenic response to tumor promoters of the class that activates protein kinase C. This loss of response to a normal cell regulator, and gain in response to another compound that elicits no mitogenic response in normal cells, is maintained when cells become overtly neoplastic and form adenomas. Since ionized calcium is present in the colonic lumen and diglycerides are also present from partial digestion of dietary fats, both of these regulators are endogenous agents. Thus the FAP cell has two ways to circumvent normal colonic growth controls. The FAP cell can be stimulated to divide and overgrow its normal cell neighbors by diglycerides, while the normal regulation of cell growth by Ca^{2+} is disregarded.

References

1. Bodmer WF, Bailey CJ, Bodmer J, Bussey HJR, Ellis A, Gorman P, Lucibello FC, Murday VA, Rider SH, Scambler P, Sheer D, Solomon E, Spurr NK: Localization of the gene for familial adenomatous polyposis on chromosome 5. Nature 328:614–616, 1987.
2. Friedman E, Gillin S, Lipkin M: TPA stimulation of DNA synthesis in cultured preneoplastic familial polyposis colonic epithelial cells but not in normal colonic epithelial cells. Cancer Res 44:4078–4086, 1984.
3. Buset M, Winawer S, Friedman E: Defining conditions to promote attachment of colon epithelial cells. In Vitro 23:403–412, 1987.
4. Friedman E, Isaksson P, Rafter J, Marian B, Winawer S, Newmark H: Fecal diglycerides as selective endogenous mitogens for premalignant and malignant human colonic epithelial cells. Cancer Res 49:544–548, 1989.
5. Buset M, Lipkin M, Winawer S, Swaroop S, Friedman E: Inhibition of human colonic epithelial cell proliferation *in vivo* and *in vitro* by calcium. Cancer Res 46:5426–5430, 1986.
6. Friedman E, Lipkin M, Newmark H, Winawer S: Heterogeneity in the response of familial polyposis epithelial cells and adenomas to increasing levels of calcium *in vitro*. Cancer, 1989 (in press).

34

Gap Junctional Intercellular Communication in Neoplasia: Implications for the Cause and Treatment of Cancer

James E. Trosko and Chia-Cheng Chang

Department of Pediatrics/Human Development, Michigan State University, East Lansing, Michigan

> It appears that modern cancer research has taken a position contrary to that outlined in the present account—theories are to be avoided and it is assumed that masses of descriptive data will make the solution obvious.
>
> V.R. Potter [1988]

INTRODUCTION: BANKRUPTCY OF THE CURRENT CHEMOTHERAPEUTIC STRATEGIES

Today, the general feeling is that the underlying basis for the current strategies of cancer therapy is bankrupt in that, while scores of different modes of therapy against many types of cancers have been tried, few have produced the kinds of results expected from the success of medical intervention seen with other kinds of diseases. While newer approaches are now being considered, even here major theoretical and practical barriers will prevent the development of the so-called magic bullet therapy.

The objective in this brief overview is to suggest that a completely different approach to cancer prevention and treatment might be possible based on newer concepts of carcinogenesis [Trosko, 1987]. It is based on the assumption that, unlike many diseases that have been prevented or cured without their underlying mechanisms fully known, effective control of this disease will only result from detailed understanding of the mechanisms of carcinogenesis. Concepts of the multistage nature of carcinogenesis, oncogenes, anti-oncogenes, intercellular communication, and cancer as a "stem-cell disease" or "disease of differentiation" should be considered when cancer intervention strategies are being designed [Trosko et al., 1988a].

MULTISTAGE NATURE OF CARCINOGENESIS: MULTIPLE MECHANISMS AFFORD MULTIPLE POINTS OF INTERVENTION

From experimental animal studies and from epidemiological/clinical studies of human cancer, the emerging picture of carcinogenesis is that it is a multistep process [Cairns, 1975; Pitot et al., 1981]. Operationally, the process has been conceptualized to consist of an *"initiation"* phase, whereby a normal stem cell has a critical gene (possibly an "oncogene") *irreversibly* altered to form a single premalignant or "initiated" cell by a single low dose of a "carcinogen." Next, until and unless the initiated cell is released from some "suppressing" factors from surrounding cells, this initiated cell will not be able to develop into a malignant cell. The *promotion* phase of carcinogenesis is viewed as the

Familial Adenomatous Polyposis, pages 279–288

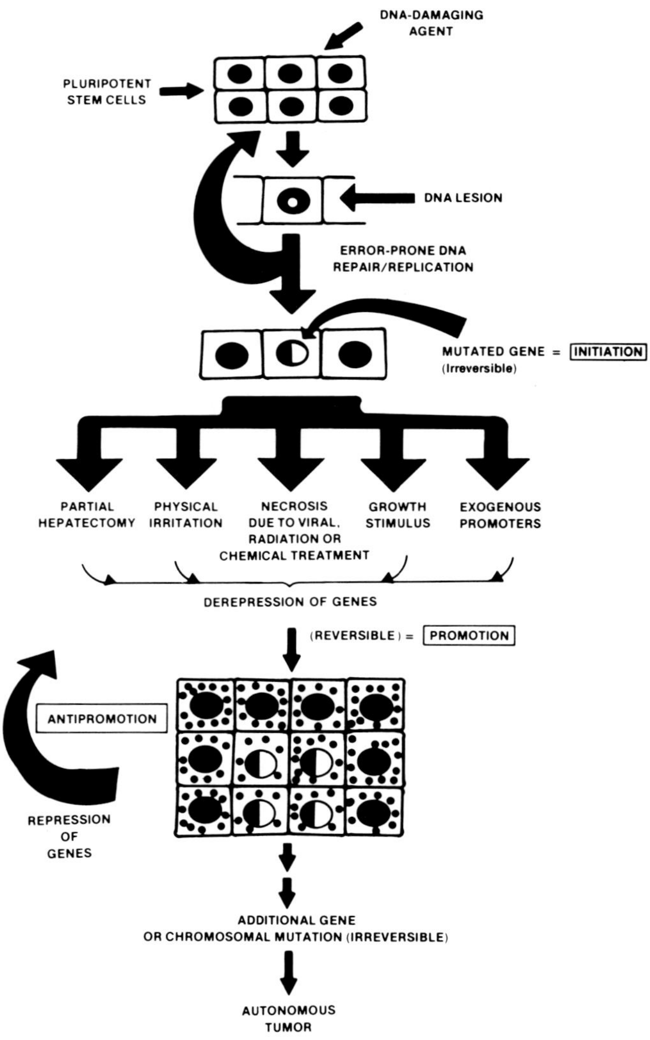

Fig. 1. Multiple modes by which initiated cells can be promoted. Promotion is conceptualized as a process allowing cells with a specific carcinogen-induced mutation to multiply, enabling them to reach either a "critical mass" in order to become resistant to the antiproliferative influences of normal cells or to increase the chance that one of these mutated cells would accumulate a second mutation (Reproduced from Trosko and Chang, 1980, with permission of Churchill Livingstone.)

result of those processes by which the single initiated cell is clonally multiplied, thereby helping to facilitate the conversion of the premalignant cell to a malignant one (the *progression* phase) [Trosko et al., 1988b] (Fig. 1).

Although the molecular mechanisms for the initiation, promotion, or progression phases are still unknown, the mechanisms underlying the initiation and promotion phases are different. Because the initiating event is an irreversible event, mutagenesis has been implicated as the basis for initiation [Trosko and Chang, 1981; Yuspa and Morgan, 1981].

To help explain the clonal nature of cancer

[Fialkow, 1979] and the stem cell [Steel and Stephens, 1983] or disease of differentiation [Markert, 1968; Pierce, 1980; Potter, 1978] theories of cancer, as well as to be consistent with the operational definition of promotion, the single initiated cell must be increased. Therefore, among other things that might happen during the promotion phase, *mitogenesis* must occur to allow the selective increase of the initiated cell (Fig. 2).

Within this hypothesis, initiation is viewed as a process that induces an irreversible lesion (i.e., mutation) in a gene that is needed for the terminal differentiation of a stem cell. Recent evidence seems to support this idea that initiation blocks the ability of a cell to differentiate [Yuspa and Morgan, 1981; Kawamura et al., 1985; Scott and Maercklein, 1985]. Although the prevailing view of cancer is that carcinogenesis is the process that induces a "mortal" cell to become "immortal," this hypothesis assumes the stem cell to be naturally "immortal" and the initiation event prevents the "mortalization" of the stem cell.

CANCER AS A DISEASE OF GROWTH CONTROL AND OF DIFFERENTIATION

While the empirical evidence suggests that cancer cells have problems related to growth regulation and to terminal differentiation, it would seem that understanding the mechanisms for mitogenesis and differentiation would lead to understanding cancer. Although the molecular mechanisms for mitogenesis and differentiation are not known, the control of cell division and differentiation of potential proliferable cells (i.e., stem cells) seems to be linked to the phenomenon of "contact inhibition." In general, normal cells seem to "contact–inhibit" while cancer cells do not [Borek and Sachs, 1966; Corsaro and Migeon, 1977]. It is here that a possible connection between the concept of intercellular communication can be linked to the concept of tumor promotion, to cancer as a disease of differentiation, and to oncogenes [Trosko et al, 1988b].

Two major forms of intercellular communication exist: transfer of molecules (e.g., growth

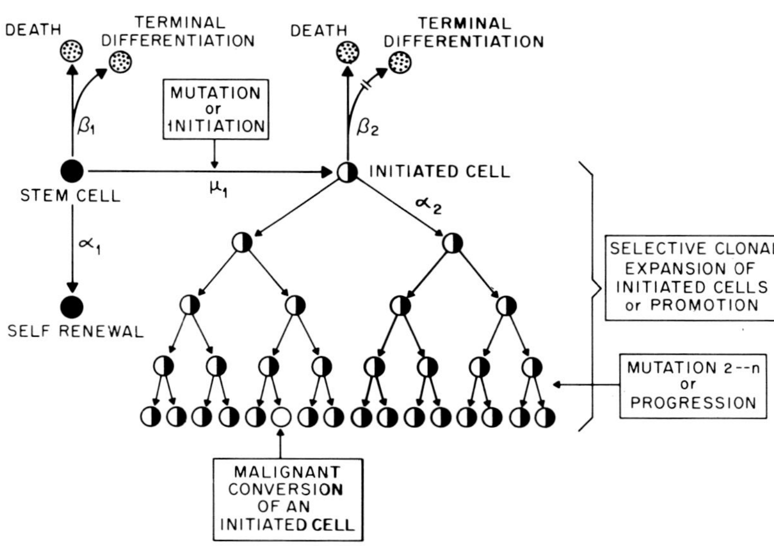

Fig. 2. The initiation/promotion/progression model of carcinogenesis. β_1, rate of terminal differentiation and death of stem cell; β_2, rate of death, but not of terminal differentiation of the initiated cell —||→ α_1, rate of cell division of stem cells; α_2, rate of cell division of initiated cells; μ_1, rate of the molecular event leading to initiation (i.e., possibly mutation); μ_2, rate at which second event occurs within an initiated cell. (Reproduced from Trosko et al., 1988, with permission of the publisher.)

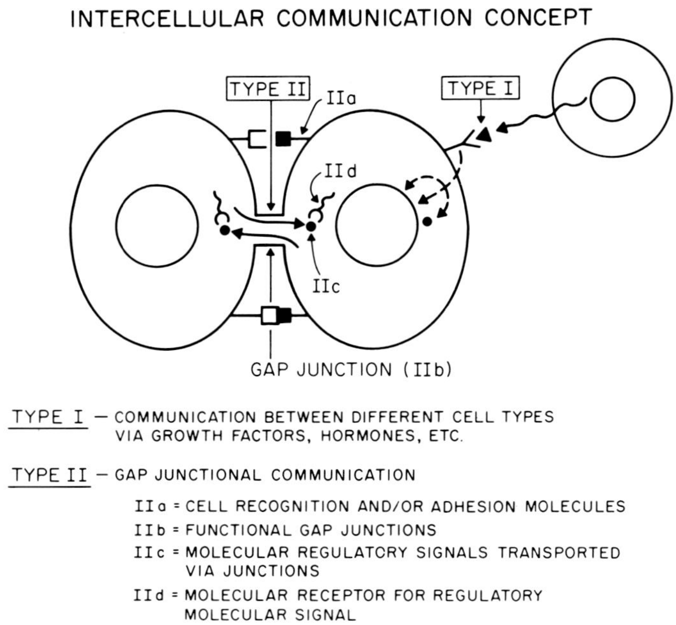

Fig. 3. Heuristic diagram illustrating two general forms of intercellular communication. One involves the production and transmission of "signal" molecules over a distance through extracellular space to a target tissue. The other involves the transfer of signal molecules via permeable intercellular junctions between coupled cells. Clearly, the one form could influence the other form of intercellular communication if the transmitted signal stimulates molecules of the target cell that modulate the function of gap junctions. (From Trosko and Chang, 1986, with permission of Plenum Press.)

factors, neurotransmitters, hormones) from one cell type, extracellularly, to another cell type; and the transfer of ions and small molecular weight molecules, via the membrane-bound protein channel—the gap junction [Pitts and Finbow, 1986]. Both have been implicated in the regulation of proliferation and differentiation [Loewenstein, 1979; Schultz, 1985] (Fig. 3). In fact, there is evidence that the two can influence each other [Larsen and Risinger, 1985; Neyton and Trautman, 1986].

Many cells derived from tumors have been shown to have some dysfunction in their ability to perform gap junctional intercellular communication in vitro, as well as in vivo [Kanno, 1985]. More recently, many tumor-promoting chemicals have been shown to inhibit gap junctional intercellular communication in vitro [Trosko and Chang, 1988, 1989] and that altered gap junctional communication is found during in vitro transformation [Enomoto and Yamasaki, 1984]. The tumor promoter phorbol ester has been shown to reduce the frequency of gap junctions in mouse skin [Kalimi and Sirsat, 1984]. Partial hepatectomy, a tumor-promoting stimulus triggering regenerative hyperplasia in the rat, has also been shown to reduce gap junctions during the regenerative growth phase [Meyer et al., 1980]. Reduced numbers of gap junctions in rat hepatocarcinomas have been noted using monoclonal antibodies to a gap junction protein [Dermietzel et al., 1987].

At this point, the connection between oncogenes, intercellular communication, and the concept of cancer as a disease of differentiation can be made. In the last few years, the expression of various cellular proto-oncogenes has been correlated with a cell's commitment to either proliferate or differentiate [Weinberg, 1985; Adamson, 1987; Ohlsson and Pfeifer-Ohlsson, 1987]. Recently several oncogenes, such as the src, ras, and mos, as well as the polyomavirus and the SV40 T antigen genes, were shown to be associated with a decrease in gap junction communication [Atkinson and Sheridan, 1984; Azarnia and Loewenstein, 1984, 1987; Chang et al., 1985; Atkinson et al, 1986; El-Fouly et al., 1986; Azarnia et al., 1988).

Several growth factors, transforming growth factor-β (TGF-B) and epidermal growth factor have also been shown to modulate gap junction function [Madhukar et al., 1989]. These observations allow us to postulate a mechanism by which "extracellular" communication via growth factors can modulate gap junctional communication. In addition, the idea that oncogenes, which code for growth factors, growth factor receptors, or transmembrane signaling elements, can modulate gap junctions allows for the integration of chemical tumor promoters, oncogenes, and growth factors by their common cellular consequence, namely, the inhibition of intercellular communication.

MECHANISMS OF THE MODULATION OF GAP JUNCTIONAL INTERCELLULAR COMMUNICATION

The idea now emerges that a structure, the gap junction, can be modulated, transiently with exogenous or endogenous chemicals, or stably with altered oncogene products, and therefore lead to transient or stable alteration of the control of differentiation and growth. On the molecular biochemical level, one would surmise that the mechanisms by which chemical tumor promoters, various oncogenes, and growth factors modulate gap junctions would be quite different.

For example, the tumor promoter 12-O-tetradecanoylphorbol-13-acetate (TPA) seems to mediate its tumor-promoting activity through the activation of protein kinase C [Nishizuka, 1986]. However, DDT and dieldrin, pesticides and tumor promoters, can inhibit intercellular communication in cells down-regulated or insensitive to TPA (our unpublished results). This indicates these two chemical tumor promoters act through different mechanisms [Warngard et al., 1987].

In a more general sense, conditions that modulate intracellular levels of Ca^{2+}, intracellular pH, or cAMP, or generate oxygen radicals, have been correlated with the modulation of gap junction function [Spray and Bennett, 1985]. This provides a unifying explanation for a wide variety of structurally unrelated chemicals that are known to influence tumor promotion (Fig. 4).

The different oncogene products and the growth factors have been associated with various receptor-linked protein kinases and transmembrane signaling elements needed for the mitogenesis process. However, in each case, whether the cell is induced to enter the mitogenic process by chemical promoters, oncogenes, or growth factors, the cell has to alter its physiological state from a quiescent cell to a cell that must prepare for mitogenesis. The inhibition of gap junctional communication is seen to play a major role for this mitogenesis event [Trosko and Chang, 1984].

EXTRACELLULAR, INTRACELLULAR, AND INTERCELLULAR COMMUNICATION: MECHANISM FOR THE HOMEOSTATIC CONTROL OF GROWTH AND DIFFERENTIATION

Starting with the hypothesis that cell proliferation and replacement in a tissue must start from stem cells and that cancer is derived from a stem cell that is "blocked or partially blocked" in its ability to differentiate [Potter, 1978], one has to account, first, for how a stem cell is normally regulated, particularly in internal organs, which must maintain a constant volume in adult animals. A clue comes from the observation that presumptive human kidney epithelial stem cells do not have gap junctional intercellular communication [Chang et al., 1987]. Since these cells must be under some negative growth control, it is assumed that they must be suppressed from growth by negative growth regulators derived from their differentiated daughter cells or from the end-stage differentiation of other cells in the immediate environment (Fig. 5). This form of extracellular communication by diffusible factors has been documented in several systems, including tumor necrosis factor [Yarden and Kimchi,

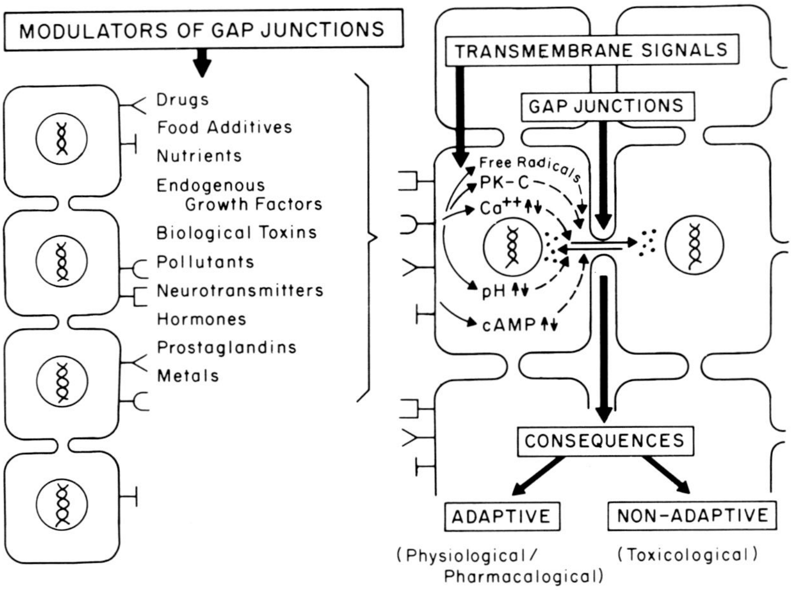

Fig. 4. Diagram summarizing how a variety of chemicals might modulate gap junction function by receptor- or nonreceptor-mediated second messengers or by other mechanisms. The consequences of either decreasing or inducing gap junctional communication will depend on the circumstances (e.g., compensatory hyperplasia leading either to wound healing or to tumor promotion).

1986], tumor growth factor [Takehara et al., 1987], β-interferon [Resnitzky et al., 1986], and a factor from differentiating spermatogonia that acts on undifferentiated spermatogonia [de Rooij et al., 1985]. Clearly, a reduction in the extracellular factor, a reduction in the receptors for the extracellular factor, and an interference of the transmembrane signaling elements will cause the stem cell to proliferate, giving rise to a stem cell progeny and to a cell destined to differentiate. If the cell is able to differentiate, it can now produce the negative growth factor and suppress the stem cell proliferation. However, if a stem-like cell loses its ability to respond to negative growth regulators because of the carcinogenic process, it will continue to grow and not differentiate. Recently, Kimchi et al. [1988] demonstrated that retinoblastoma cells did not have TGF-β receptors, as did the normal retinal cells, and these retinoblastoma cells were not responsive to the antimitogenic effects of the TGF-β.

This now raises the question of the observation that many, if not all, malignant cancer cells have dysfunctional gap junctional intercellular communication [Kanno, 1985]. If normal stem cells have no gap junctional intercellular communication, but are suppressed by extracellular communication via diffusible negative growth regulators, and if malignant cancer cells have no gap junctional intercellular communication but are not suppressed, then this implies a link between extracellular communication and gap junctional intercellular communication. Several observations have demonstrated that diffusible, extracellular communicating molecules can modulate gap junctional intercellular communication. For example, hormones [Larsen and Risinger, 1985], neurotransmitters [Neyton and Trautman, 1986], and growth factors [Madhukar et al., 1989] can alter gap junctional intercellular communication. In these cases, several intracellular transmembrane signaling systems can link the extracellular communication system to the gap junctional intercellular communication system, possibly via protein kinases, G protein, adenyl cyclase, intracellular free Ca^{2+}, cytoplasmic pH changes, and second-message systems [Rozengurt, 1986; Hollenberg, 1986; Moolenaar et al.,

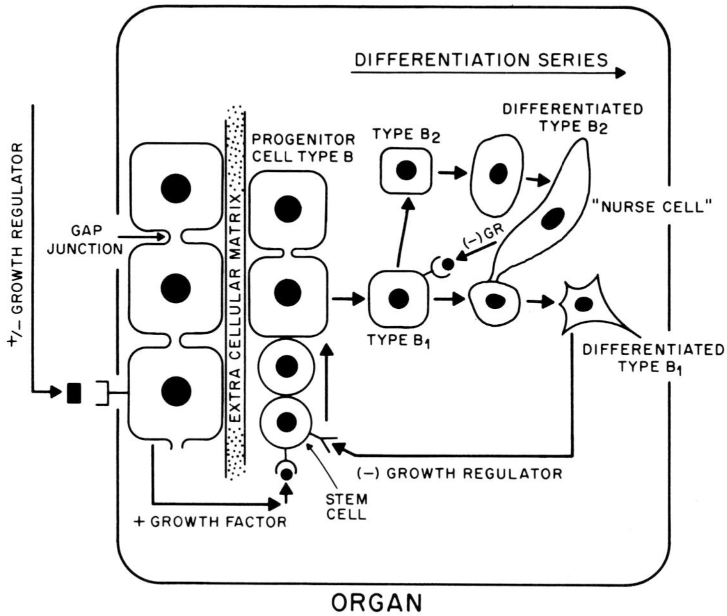

Fig. 5. Diagram illlustrating the inter-relationship of intercellular communication by positive and negative growth regulators on stem cell growth and differentiation and intercellular communication via gap junctions in a closed organ system. (Reproduced from Trosko and Chang, 1988b, with permission of Lewis Publishers.)

1986; Sekar and Hokin, 1986; Castagna, 1987].

Within this framework, if a stem cell is initiated (i.e., it can self-renew but cannot terminally differentiate), then, from in vivo observations these initiated cells can be suppressed by surrounding normal cells. From in vitro studies, tumor promoters can release these initiated cells from the suppressing effects of the normal cells. Since many, if not most, tumor promoters (extracellular-like communicating molecules) can down-regulate gap junctional communication, these initiated cells can proliferate into a clone of dysfunctional cells that apparently can communicate with normal cells via extracellular communication and with themselves via gap junctional communication. Yamasaki et al. [1987] have shown that, in their in vitro transformation system, the early transformed cells can communicate with themselves but not with their normal neighbors ("selective communication"). If this represents the universal sequence of events, the demonstration that metastasizing cells seem to lack all gap junctional communication (Iijima et al., 1969; Nicolson et al., 1988] suggests a correlation with the loss of growth control and the ability to differentiate with gap junctional communication.

If the persistent reduction of gap junctional communication is correlated with the loss of growth control and the ability to differentiate terminally, then, in principle, if one could circumvent this block and up-regulate gap junctional communication in malignant cells that are in contact with surrounding normal cells, terminal differentiation might ensue. Several chemicals have been shown to up-regulate or increase gap junctional communication (e.g., retinoic acid [Maden, 1982] and those chemicals increasing cAMP [Flagg-Newton et al., 1981; Azarnia and Russell, 1985; DeMaziere and Scheuermann, 1985; In't Veld et al., 1985; Saez et al., 1986]. Reversal of the transformed phenotype in several in vitro systems seems to have been correlated with increased gap junctional communication induced by increased intracellular cAMP [Mehta et al., 1986; Matsukawa and Bertram, 1988].

In conclusion, if the homeostatic regulation of growth and differentiation of cells in a multicellular organism dependends on the coordinated linkage of extra-, inter-, and intracellular communication by specific messages that trigger a limited number of second messages that regulate gap junctional communication, it seems that persistent or stable disruption of communication by altered endogenous (mutations, amplified expression, and so forth) and exogenous (tumor promoter) factors would contribute to the carcinogenesis process. Consequently, a new strategy would be to restore intercellular communication in cancer cells [Vitkauskas and Canellakis, 1985; Trosko, 1987]. Since one would predict that the breakdown in the extra-, intra-, and intercellular communication linkage could occur in any phase, restoration of this complex homeostatic system will probably not occur via a universal ''golden bullet.'' On the other hand, if the ultimate consequence of the disruption during carcinogenesis is the lack of gap junctional intercellular communication, then, at least, a new specific and testable hypothesis for future chemotherapeutic drug development is now possible.

ACKNOWLEDGMENTS

We acknowledge present and former students and coworkers for their contributions to the development of the ideas expressed in this chapter. In particular, our on going dialogue with Dr. Van R. Potter has been an inspiration for our work. We also thank Mrs. Darla Conley for her excellent wordprocessing skills. The research, on which this chapter is based was supported in part by grants from the National Cancer Institute (CA-21104), the U.S.Air Force Office of Scientific Research (AFOSR-86-0084), and a gift from the R.J. Reynolds Company.

References

Adamson ED (1987): Oncogenes in development. Development 99:449–471.

Atkinson MM, Anderson SK, Sheridan JD (1986): Modification of gap junctions in cells transformed by a temperature-sensitive mutant of Rous sarcoma virus. J Membr Biol 9:53–64.

Atkinson M, Sheridan J (1984): Decreased junctional permeability in cells transformed by 3 different viral oncogenes: A quantitative video analysis. J Cell Biol 99:401A.

Azarnia R, Loewenstein WR (1984): Intercellular communication and the control of growth: Alteration of junctional permeability by the src gene: A study with temperature-sensitive mutant Rous sarcoma virus. J Membr Biol 82:191–205.

Azarnia R, Loewenstein WR (1987): Polyomavirus middle T antigen down regulates junctional cell to cell communication. Mol Cell Biol 7:946–950.

Azarnia R, Reddy S, Kmiecki TE, Shalloway D, Loewenstein WR (1988): The cellular src gene product regulates junctional cell to cell communication. Science 239:398–401.

Azarnia R, Russell TR (1985): Cyclic AMP effects on cell to cell junctional membrane permeability during adipocyte differentiation of 3T3-L1 fibroblasts. J Cell Biol 100:265–269.

Borek C, Sachs L (1966): The difference in contact inhibition of cell replication between normal cells and cells transformed by different carcinogens. Proc Natl Acad Sci USA 56:1705–1711.

Cairns J (1975): Mutation, selection and the natural history of cancer. Nature 225:197–200.

Castagna M (1987): Phorbol esters as signal transducers and tumor promoters. Biol Cell 59:3–14.

Chang CC, Trosko JE, El-Fouly MH, Gibson-D'Ambrosio RE, D'Ambrosio SM (1987): Contact insensitivity of a subpopulation of normal human fetal kidney epithelial cells and of human carcinoma cell lines. Cancer Res 47:1634–1645.

Chang CC, Trosko JE, Kung HJ, Bombick D, Matsumura F (1985): Potential role of the src gene product in inhibition of gap junctional communication in NIH 3T3 cells. Proc Natl Acad Sci USA 82:5360–5364

Corsaro CM, Migeon BR (1977): Comparison of contact-mediated communication in normal and transformed human cells in culture. Proc Natl Acad Sci USA 74:4476–4480.

DeMaziere AMG, Scheuermann DW (1985): Increased gap junctional area in the rat liver after administration of dibutyryl cAMP. Cell Tissue Res 239:651–655.

Dermietzel R, Yancey SB, Traub O, Willecke K, Revel J-P (1987): Major loss of the 28-KD protein of gap junction in proliferating hepatocytes. J Cell Biol 105:1925–1934.

de Rooij DK, Lok D, Weenk D (1985): Feedback regulation of the proliferation of the undifferentiated spermatogonia in the Chinese hamster by the differentiating spermatogonia. Cell Tissue Kinet 18:71–81.

El-Fouly MH, Warren ST, Trosko JE, Chang CC (1986): Inhibition of gap junction-mediated intercellular communication in cells transfected with the human H-ras oncogene. Am J Human Genet 39:A30.

Enomoto T, Yamasaki H (1984): Lack of intercellular communication between chemically transformed and surrounding non-transformed BALB/c 3T3 cells. Cancer Res 44:5200–5203.

Fialkow PJ (1979): Clonal origin of human tumors. Annu Rev Med 30:135–176.

Flagg-Newton JL, Dahl G, Loewenstein WR (1981): Cell junction and cyclic AMP: I. Upregulation of junctional membrane permeability and junctional membrane particles by administration of cyclic nucleotide or phosphodiesterase inhibitor. J Membr Biol 63:105–121.

Hollenberg MD (1986): Mechanisms of receptor-mediated transmembrane signalling. Experientia 42:718–727.

Iijima N, Yamamoto T, Inoue K, Soo S, Matsuzawa A, Kanno Y, Matsui Y (1969): Experimental studies on dynamic behavior of cells in subcutaneous solid tumor (MH 134–C3H/HE). Jpn J Exp Med 39:205–221.

In't Veld P, Schuit F, Pipeleers D (1985): Gap junctions between pancreatic β-cells are modulated by cyclic AMP. Eur J Cell Biol 36:269–276.

Kalimi GH, Sirsat SM (1984): The relevance of gap junctions to stage I tumor promotion in mouse epidermis. Carcinogenesis 5:1671–1677.

Kanno Y (1985): Modulation of cell communication and carcinogenesis. Jpn J Physiol 35:693–707.

Kawamura H, Strickland SE, Yuspa SH (1985): Association of resistance to terminal differentiation with initiation of carcinogenesis in adult mouse epidermal cells. Cancer Res 45:2748–2752.

Kimchi A, Wang X-F, Weinberg RA, Cheifetz S, Massague J (1988): Absence of TGF-β receptors and growth inhibitory responses in retinoblastoma cells. Science 240: 196–199.

Larsen WJ, Risinger MA (1985): The dynamic life histories of intercellular membrane junctions. Mod Cell Biol 4:151–216.

Loewenstein WR (1979): Junctional intercellular communication and the control of growth. Biochim Biophys Acta 605:33–91.

Maden M (1982): Vitamin A and pattern formation in the regenerating limb. Nature 295:672–675.

Madhukar BV, Trosko JE, Chang CC (1988): Chemical, oncogene and growth factor modulation of gap junctional communication in carcinogenesis. In Sperelakis NS, Cole WC (eds): "Cell Interactions and Gap Junctions." Boca Raton, FL: CRC Press (in press).

Madhukar BV, Oh SY, Chang CC, Wade M, Trosco JE (1989): Altered regulation of intercellular communication by epidermal growth factor, transforming growth factor-β and peptide hormones in normal human keratinocytes. Carcinogenesis 10:13–20.

Markert C (1968): Neoplasia: A disease of cell differentiation. Cancer Res 28:1908–1914.

Matsukawa T, Bertram JS (1988): Augmentation of post-confluence growth arrest of 10T1/2 fibroblasts by endogenous cyclic adenosine 3′:5′-monophosphate. Cancer Res 48:1874–1881.

Mehta PP, Bertram JS, Loewenstein WR (1986): Growth inhibition of transformed cells correlates with their junctional communication with normal cells. Cell 44:187–196.

Meyer DJ, Yancey SB, Revel JP (1980): Intercellular communication in normal and regenerating rat liver. A quantitative analysis. J Cell Biol 91:505–523.

Moolenaar WH, Defize LHK, deLaat SW (1986): Ionic signalling by growth factor receptors. J Exp Biol 124:359–373.

Neyton J, Trautman A (1986): Acetylcholine modulation of the conductance of intercellular junctions between rat lacrimal cells. J Physiol 377:283–295.

Nicolson GL, Dulski KM, Trosko JE (1988): Loss of intercellular junctional communication correlates with metastatic potential in mammary adenocarcinoma cells. Proc Natl Acad Sci USA 85:473–476.

Nishizuka Y (1986): Studies and perspectives of protein kinase C. Science 233:305–312.

Ohlsson RI, Pfeifer-Ohlsson SB (1987): Cancer genes, proto-oncogenes and development. Exp Cell Res 173:1–16.

Pierce GB (1980): Neoplasms, differentiation and mutations. Am J Pathol 77:103–118.

Pitot HC, Goldsworthy T, Moran S (1981): The natural history of carcinogenesis: Implications of experimental carcinogenesis in the genesis of human cancer. J Supramol Cell Biochem 17:133–146.

Pitts JD, Finbow ME (1986): The gap junction. J Cell Sci 4:239–266.

Potter VR (1978): Phenotypic diversity in experimental hepatomas: The concept of partially blocked ontogeny. Br J Cancer 38:1–23.

Potter VR (1988): On the road to the blocked ontogeny theory. Adv Oncol 4:2–8.

Resnitzky D, Yarden A, Zipori D, Kimchi A (1986): Autocrine B-related interferon controls c-myc suppression and growth arrest during hematopoietic cell differentiation. Cell 46:31–40.

Rozengurt E (1986): Early signals in the mitogenic response. Science 234:161–166.

Saez JC, Spray DC, Nairn AC, Hertzberg E, Greengard P, Bennett MVL (1986): C-AMP increases junctional conductance and stimulates phosphorylation of the 27-KDa principal gap junction polypeptide. Proc Natl Acad Sci USA 83:2473–2477.

Schultz RM (1985): Roles of cell to cell communication in development. Biol Reprod 32:27–42.

Scott RE, Maercklein PB (1985): An initiation of carcinogenesis selectively and stably inhibits stem cell differentiation: A concept that initiation of carcinogenesis involves multiple phases. Proc Natl Acad Sci USA 82:2995–2999.

Sekar MC, Hokin LE (1986): The role of phosphoinositides in signal transduction. J Membr Biol 89:193–210.

Spray DC, Bennett MVL (1985): Physiology and pharmacology of gap junctions. Annu Rev Physiol 47:281–303.

Steel GG, Stephens TC (1983): Stem cells in tumours. In Potten CS (ed): "Stem Cells: Their Identification and Characterization," New York: Churchill Livingstone, pp 271–293.

Takehara K, LeRoy EC, Grotendorst GR (1987): TGF-β inhibition of endothelial cell proliferation: Alteration of EGF binding and EGF-induced growth-regulatory gene expression. Cell 49:415–422.

Trosko JE (1987): Mechanisms of tumor promotion: Possible role of inhibited intercellular communication. Eur J Cancer Clin Oncol 23:599–601.

Trosko JE, Chang CC (1980): An integrative hypothesis linking cancer, diabetes and atherosclerosis: The role of mutations and epigenetic changes. Med Hypotheses 6:455–468.

Trosko JE, Chang CC (1981): The role of radiation and chemicals in the induction of mutations and epigenetic changes during carcinogenesis. In Lett JT, Adler A (eds): "Advances in Radiation Biology," Vol 9, New York: Academic Press, pp 1–36.

Trosko JE, Chang CC (1984): Adaptive and nonadaptive consequences of chemical inhibition of intercellular communication. Pharmacol Rev 36:137–144.

Trosko JE, Chang CC (1986): Role of intercellular communication in modifying the consequences of mutations in somatic cells. In Shankel DM, Hartman PE, Kada T, Hollaender A (eds): "Antimutagenesis and Anticarcinogenesis Mechanisms." New York: Plenum Press, pp 439–456.

Trosko JE, Chang CC (1988): Nongenotoxic mechanisms in carcinogenesis: Role of inhibited intercellular communication. In Hart RW, Hoerger FD (eds): "Banbury Report 31: Carcinogen Risk Assessment: New Directions in the Qualitative and Quantitative Aspects." New York: Cold Spring Harbor Laboratory Press, pp 139–171.

Trosko JE, Chang CC (1989): The role of inhibited intercellular communication in carcinogenesis: Implications for risk assessment from exposure to chemicals. In Gehrs CJ (ed): "Bioindicators: Exposure and Effects." Chelsea, MI: Lewis Press (in press).

Trosko JE, Chang CC, Madhukar BV, (1988a): Chemical and oncogene modulation of intercellular communication in tumor promotion. In Milman HA, Elmore E (eds): "Biochemical Mechanisms and Regulation of Intercellular Communication," Vol XIV. Princeton, NJ: Princeton Scientific Publ, pp 209–236.

Trosko JE, Chang CC, Madhukar BV, Oh Sy, Bombick D, El-Fouley MH (1988b): Modulation of gap junction intercellular communication by tumor promoting chemicals, oncogenes and growth factors during carcinogenesis. In Johnson R, Hertzberg E (eds): "Gap Junctions," New York: Alan R. Liss, Inc., pp 435–448.

Vitkauskas GV, Canellakis ES (1985): Intercellular communication and cancer chemotherapy. Biochim Biophys Acta 823:19–34.

Warngard L, Flodstrom S, Ljungquist S, Ahlborg UG (1987): Interaction between quercetin, TPA and DDT in the V79 metabolic cooperation assay. Carcinogenesis 8:1201–1205.

Weinberg RA (1985): The action of oncogenes in the cytoplasm and nucleus. Science 230:770–776.

Yamasaki H, Hollstein M, Mesnil M, Martel N, Aguelon A-M (1987): Selective lack of intercellular communication between transformed and nontransformed cells as a common property of chemical and oncogene transformation of BALB/3T3 cells. Cancer Res 47:5658–5664.

Yarden A, Kimchi A (1986): Tumor necrosis factor reduces c-myc expression and cooperates with interferon-γ in HeLa cells. Science 234:1419–1421.

Yuspa SH, Morgan DL (1981): Mouse skin cells resistant to terminal differentiation associated with initiation of carcinogenesis. Nature 293:72–74.

35

Biochemical Markers in Colonic Polyposis Syndromes

Ann L. Silverman, Tusar K. Desai, and Gordon D. Luk

Division of Gastroenterology, Department of Medicine, Wayne State University School of Medicine and Harper-Grace Hospitals, Detroit, Michigan

INTRODUCTION

Colorectal cancer is second only to lung cancer in prevalence in men and women in the United States. In 1988, it was estimated that approximately 147,000 new cases would be diagnosed and that 62,000 deaths were expected [1]. Despite active and ongoing research into the chemotherapy of this illness, little success has been achieved. Currently the only potential cure available for this tumor is definitive surgery of localized disease [2]. Therefore, it is appropriate to focus attention on potential methods of early cancer detection.

Early diagnosis of colorectal cancer depends on identifying markers in the serum or colonic mucosa present in neoplastic tissues in early stages but not present in normal mucosa [3]. Early diagnosis is the key issue, since this is a stage at which the tumor is potentially curable. Currently, considerable attention is being devoted to developing biochemical and genetic markers to diagnose patients at risk of developing colorectal cancer as well as to diagnosis curable disease early. This clearly implicates the adenomatous polyp.

GENOTYPIC AND PHENOTYPIC MARKERS

Familial adenomatous polyposis is atypical of dominantly inherited cancers, like Wilm's tumor or retinoblastoma, in that it expresses many phenotypic markers that identify it early [4–10]. These clinical features are discussed in some detail in the chapters by Drs. Watne, Bulow, Carl, Herrera, and Trabousli (this volume). Common to all of these clinical syndromes is the development of multiple adenomatous polyps in the colon that, if left untreated (by removal of the colon), lead to colorectal cancer in virtually every patient by the end of the third decade [5]. These polyps therefore are an important phenotypic marker of eventual malignancy. Understanding the evolution of this precursor lesion will help to identify factors important in the progression of transformation.

Earlier diagnosis of affected patients will become possible as we learn more about the region of deletion on chromosome 5 originally described by Herrera et al. [11]. Certainly, familial adenomatous polyposis appears to be one of the cancers described by Knudson [12] in which the patient is born with one gene deletion or mutation in the germ cell and a second event occurs at the somatic level that results in cancer expression. A marker on the long arm of chromosome 5 close to the gene for familial adenomatous polyposis was uncovered by examining lymphocyte DNA from kindreds of patients with this syndrome [13,14]. This chromosomal segmental defect appears to be involved in at least 20% of sporadic colorectal cancers [15,16]. Of particular interest, the loss of heterozygosity of genetic alleles observed in carcinomas is not seen in adenomas [15,16]. This latter finding suggests that the deleted gene on chromosome 5 is important

Familial Adenomatous Polyposis, pages 289–297

specifically in the progression to cancer. The loss of one chromosomal allele to heterozygosity has been described in other chromosomes in colon cancer as well as the point mutation of specific oncogenes [16–19]. These genotypic events in the evolution of AFP and colon cancer are discussed in greater detail in the chapter by Drs. Wolman, Okamoto, and Khan (this volume).

MARKERS SPECIFIC FOR FAP

Before the identification of a marker close to the gene responsible for familial adenomatous polyposis, many investigators sought to find markers specific for this syndrome. HLA antigens were examined in the hopes that a particular locus would segregate with the gene responsible for this disorder. Two independent studies failed to show a linkage between familial adenomatous polyposis and HLA haplotype [20,21].

Differences in cellular carbohydrate immunodeterminants have been described in colon cancer and normal colonic mucosa [for review, see 22]. These carbohydrate moieties are attached to lipids and proteins by specific enzymes called *glycosyltransferases* [22]. It is thought that the difference in carbohydrate moieties results from either blocked synthesis of a precursor or enhanced synthesis of a new precursor [22]. Therefore, studying the level of activity of the glycosyltransferase in normal mucosa and neoplasm might help to determine the mechanism of this difference. Slomski et al. [23] compared glycosyltransferase levels in normal mucosa, mucosa from patients with sporadic colorectal cancer, and mucosa from the polyps of patients with familial adenomatous polyposis. Of the eight enzymes studied, three were significantly decreased in activity in the carcinomas and the adenomatous polyps from patients with familial adenomatous polyposis compared with normal mucosa. One enzyme was significantly increased in activity in both cancers and adenomas compared with normal mucosa [23]. These findings confirm the observation of altered carbohydrate side chains in neoplastic mucosa.

Antigenic determinants of immunoglobulin chains have been correlated with many disorders. A Danish group attempted to correlate the antigenic determinants of IgG heavy chains and κ light chains in patients with familial adenomatous polyposis compared with controls. They observed that individuals with the Gm3;5,13 phenotype had a twofold increase in risk for familial adenomatous polyposis, although they noted that there is a 5% chance that this correlation may occur by chance [24]. Other populations need to be examined before any conclusions can be drawn.

Lipkin [25] has shown an increase in the proliferation index in the mucosa of patients with familial adenomatous polyposis and colorectal cancer by measuring incorporation of [^{3}H]thymidine into the mucosa. Lipkin specifically looked at regional crypt compartment labeling and was able to identify patients with familial cancer predisposition from patients with sporadic tumors with a sensitivity and specificity ranging from 70 to 90% [26,27]. These studies are described in greater detail in the chapter by Dr. Lipkin (Chapter 28, this volume).

Danes et al. [27] have used dermal fibroblast monolayers from patients with a familial predisposition to colorectal cancer compared with normals as a model of an abnormal chromosomal complement predisposing to cancer by evaluating in vitro tetroploidy. They examined tetraploidy by three criteria: 1) metaphase chromosome preparations, 2) [^{3}H]thymidine incorporation, and 3) flow cytometry to measure DNA content. They found that this technique had a high sensitivity (81–96%) and a high specificity (81–96%) for identifying those without a family cancer history and for some patients with a family history, Gardner's syndrome, or Lynch's syndrome. However, the sensitivity for familial adenomatous polyposis was quite low.

In an attempt to use familial adenomatous polyposis as a model of lesions that ultimately progress to malignancy, Garin Chesa et al. [28] examined the differences in cytokeratins (proteins that form the cell's structural backbone) by monoclonal antibody histocytochemical staining in flat ("normal") and adenomatous mucosa from patients with familial adenomatous polyposis compared with normal mucosa and neoplastic mucosa from patients with sporadic colorectal cancer. Of interest, they observed that the flat ("normal") mucosa of patients with familial adenomatous polyposis had the same keratin expression as malignant tumors and villous adenomas from patients with sporadic tumors. Tubular adenomas and cells of the proliferative compartment of normal mucosa did not express these keratins, suggesting that cells destined to become malignant may derive from the maturational compartment of the colonic epithelium.

BIOCHEMICAL MARKERS IN COLON CANCER

CARCINOEMBRYONIC ANTIGEN

Carcinoembryonic antigen (CEA), initially described in 1965 [29], was the first protein available for use in a blood test to diagnose colon cancer. It belongs to a class of proteins referred to as *oncofetal proteins,* which are normally expressed in the fetus but only in very small amounts in normal adults. CEA is a group of related glycoproteins whose immunoreactivity resides on the protein moities. It has been and still is the standard that other oncofetal antigens are measured against. Unfortunately its sensitivity and specificity for diagnosing early colon cancer is not high. It may have a role in the postoperative monitoring of patients with known colorectal cancer both to determine if surgery has been successful in removing all malignant tissue and in following the patient for recurrent disease [30,31].

Its lack of sensitivity derives from a very low detection rate for early resectable lesions and no sensitivity for colonic polyps, which are the ultimate premalignant lesion [31]. Although it was first demonstrated to be elevated abnormally in gastrointestinal malignancies, it is also elevated in other epithelial tumors. In addition, it is abnormally high in many nonmalignant conditions, including liver disease, renal failure, and fibrocystic breast disease, and in smokers [31–33]. Therefore CEA is not useful as a screening test in asymptomatic patients.

CEA may have a role in evaluating for the presence of residual tumor after surgery for definitive resection, as well as following tumor burden after chemotherapy [31,34]. Unfortunately, in poorly differentiated tumors CEA is not produced and therefore may not be useful [33]. Many investigators have sought to use CEA as a tool for early diagnosis of tumor recurrence after initial surgery. The results have been disappointing in most studies because of the inability of CEA to detect early resectable disease. A recent study examined whether frequent determinations of CEA may allow for earlier detection of recurrence and increase resectability in "second look" operations. When CEA was measured every 4–6 weeks for the first 2 years, and small rises in serum levels were calculated based on a nomogram, "second look" surgery resulted in a resectability rate of 55% with a 5 year survival of 31% [34]. This study needs to be confirmed, but it suggests that monitoring of CEA may need to be more frequent than every 3 months and that more sensitive criteria for evaluating elevations may need to be developed to enhance its value as a marker for recurrence.

Other investigators have attempted to use CEA in combination with other markers of malignant proliferation with little success. Mercer and Talamo [35] used CEA with 10 other biochemical markers in malignant and benign colonic epithelial disease. CEA in combination with four of the most sensitive markers increased the sensitivity in detecting early disease; however, the specificity was decreased by 30% [35]. More investigation into the combined use of multiple biochemical markers needs to be done.

The use of CEA as a diagnostic tool for familial adenomatous polyposis has been investigated. Patients with multiple polyps have higher levels than controls. However, the overlap is sizable and the differences are small [36]. In patients with familial adenomatous polyposis, CEA levels do decrease after colectomy [36]. No longitudinal studies have yet been done correlating CEA levels with progression of disease.

CEA is still the best serum marker available for diagnosing colon cancer; however, because of its low sensitivity for early disease, its usefulness is limited. Additional clinical trials are needed to evaluate its sensivity and specificity for following curative surgery.

ABNORMAL GLYCOSYLATION IN CANCER CELL MEMBRANES

The presence of abnormal carbohydrates on epithelial cell surface lipids and proteins was briefly mentioned in an earlier section in this chapter. This topic will also be covered in some detail in the chapters by Drs. Boland and Muto (this volume). Many cell surface lipids and proteins undergo post-translational modifications that consist of glycosylations and phosphorylation. Many of these modifications are known to alter protein function and are important in cell transport, cell receptors, and intercellular interactions [22,37]. Of interest in colon cancer is the identification of changes in the glycosylation patterns of premalignant and malignant colonic cells. Many of the aberrant carbohydrate structures seen on tumor cells are also seen in fetal tissue. Because of their enhanced specificity over CEA, these abnormal carbohydrate moieties have implications not only in studying colonic tissue directly but also as a potential diagnostic test for detecting early disease in the blood.

CA-19 is a monoclonal antibody to a glycolipid in tissues but recognizes a mucin-type glycoprotein in serum [38]. It was developed by using the human carcinoma cell line SW1116 as an immunogen, and it recognizes the carbohydrate moiety (a monosialoganglioside) [39,40]. This antibody, although originally developed against colon cancer to aid in its diagnosis, is more sensitive for gastric, pancreatic, and hepatobiliary tumors as a serum test and has a very high specificity for these tumors in some studies [41–43]. Its usefulness in immunocytochemical studies is limited by its lack of specificity. Many benign tissues, such as pancreas, gallbladder, and gastric epithelial cells, also stain [41,44]. Improved serological diagnosis of colon cancer may be obtained by a combination of antibodies that recognize different abnormal carbohydrate determinants. The combination of CSLEA1 (a carbohydrate antigen that recognizes a monosialoganlioside similar to CA-19) and CSLEX1 (an antibody to a sialylated Lewis^x antigen) was more sensitive than either alone in the serologic diagnosis of colorectal cancer [45]. For serological detection of colon cancer, CEA was found to be more sensitive than CA-19, although CA-19 was more sensitive in pancreatic cancer [42].

Many of the carbohydrate cancer markers that are now recognized are similar to carbohydrates seen on human blood group antigens. CA-19 is a sialylated Lewis^a antigen and, as mentioned previously, CSLEX1 is a sialylated Lewis^x antigen. The Lewis antigen, like other blood group antigens, is not expressed on cells other than erythrocytes in a small percentage of persons designated as nonsecreters. Of interest, some nonsecretors express blood group antigens in malignant tissue [46]. Many of these blood group antigens are abnormally expressed in colon malignancy as will be discussed below. Their usefulness in the serological diagnosis of colon cancer is currently being explored.

Normal expression of blood group antigens is limited to the proximal half of the colon in patients with a blood group secretor status [46,47]. The only exception is the Lewis^a, which is expressed throughout the entire colon and is independent of secretor status [46]. In fetal colonic epithelial tissue, all antigens are expressed throughout the colon [46,47]. In colorectal cancer and some adenomatous polyps, the expression of blood group antigens in the tumor tissue and surrounding normal mucosa is altered in several ways. These alterations in blood group antigen expression include 1) in distal colon, lesions expressing fetal blood group antigens; 2) loss of blood group antigen expression in normal colon; 3) appearance of blood group antigens in nonsecretors; and 4) expression of blood group antigens incompatible with the host. The significance of the alteration in blood group antigen expression is unclear at present. Many explanations have been offered, including increased glycosyltransferase activity and increased glycosidase activity, either intrinsic to the tumor or from anaerobic bacteria in the colon.

The advent of monoclonal antibody technology has allowed us to understand and characterize further abnormal blood group antigen expression in colorectal cancer. Colorectal neoplasms express not only normal blood group antigens in an altered manner but also they express altered blood group antigens [48–51]. These altered blood group antigens include polymeric Le^x and its sialylated derivatives and Le^y, a fucosylated derivative of Le^x [48–51]. These antigens are considered "oncofetal antigens" because they are expressed in fetal colonic epithelium but not normally expressed in adult tissue. Of interest, their expression in adenomatous polyps closely correlates with malignant potential, i.e., the larger the polyp and the more villous the component present, the more likely are these antigens expressed [49,51]. The T antigen (Thomsen-Friedenreich antigen), a precursor carbohydrate for the blood group system M and N antigens, has also been used to study colon tissue by immunohistochemical methods to localize its expression [52]. Currently these are only research tools but may serve as potential diagnostic markers in the future in high-risk populations.

ORNITHINE DECARBOXYLASE

Ornithine decarboxylase (ODC) is a key enzyme in the synthesis of polyamines from arginine and ornithine. The precise function of the polyamines in vivo is unknown; however, much experimental data suggest that they are very important in cellular functions. Some of their functions include cell differentiation, membrane stabilization, free radical scavenging, and promotion of RNA, DNA, and protein synthesis [for review, see 53–55]. Both polyamines and ODC have been shown to be important in cell proliferation in intestinal mucosa 1) during recovery after cytotoxic injury [56], 2) during lactation [57], 3) during postintestinal resection adaptation [58,59], and 4) during newborn maturation [56] in a rat model. Of particular importance, both ODC and polyamines have been demonstrated to be elevated in many malignant tissues, including colorectal cancer [60,61]. Data from our laboratory and others suggest that ODC and polyamines are elevated in tissues that progress to malignancy, and they may serve as a marker of tissues predisposed to malignant transformation [62]. Finally, there is much experimental evidence in animal models to suggest that lowering ODC and polyamines may be an effective adjunct in cancer chemotherapy [63] and potentially in chemoprevention in high-risk groups such as familial adenomatous polyposis (patients' family members).

Studies in our laboratory suggest that measuring ODC in the colonic mucosa of persons at risk for developing familial adenomatous polyposis may serve as a marker to identify those who will later express manifestations of multiple colonic polyposis and cancer [62]. ODC activity was measured in the colonic mucosa of patients with familial adenomatous polyposis and stratified according to gross and histologic criteria from normal-appearing flat mucosa to dysplastic polyps and compared with normal controls. There was a statistically significant increase in ODC activity from flat mucosa to polyp to dysplastic polyp. We have now found that ODC activity in colorectal cancers from patients with familial adenomatous polyposis is another threefold higher than seen in the dysplastic polyps.

Furthermore, in colonic mucosa from clinically unaffected first-degree relatives of patients with FAP, who have a 50% chance of inheriting the gene, there was a bimodal distribution of ODC activity. One peak occurred at the mean for normal controls and the other was near the mean for the normal-appearing mucosa from patients with familial adenomatous polyposis [62]. Since that study was published, one person with high ODC was noted to express the phenotype with multiple polyps. None of the 17 patients with low ODC have expressed the phenotype. Although further follow-up is necessary, the data suggest that measuring ODC activity in colonic mucosa may identify persons at risk for FAP who will express the phenotype.

Other studies have shown elevations in ODC in adenomatous polyps and cancers from patients with sporadic colon cancer as well as in carcinogen-induced rat colorectal cancers. Rozhin et al. [64] showed a significant increase in the ODC activity of polyps and colorectal cancers from humans as well as an increase in ODC activity in tumors from rats induced with azoxymethane compared with normal control mucosa. Of interest, the normal-appearing control mucosa from rats treated with azoxymethane showed a trend toward higher ODC activity compared with normal mucosa from untreated rats. LaMuraglia et al. [65] found the ODC activity in 34 colorectal carcinomas and six polyps to be elevated compared with ODC activity in the uninvolved mucosa in the same patient. They also found the ODC activitiy in the normal mucosa of patients with cancer to be elevated compared with normals without cancer or polyps. Porter et al. [66] again documented a trend in increasing ODC activity from normal-appearing mucosa to polyp and ultimately to colon cancer. They also showed a trend in the increase of another enzyme in the biosythesis of polyamines, S-adenosylmethionine [66]. While ODC is not specific for colorectal cancer, it may serve as a marker for mucosa at risk for malignant change.

POLYAMINES

Like ODC activity, polyamines have been investigated as a potentional diagnostic tumor marker in colorectal cancer. An early study documented that up to two-thirds of patients with colorectal carcinomas had elevated serum polyamine levels compared with persons with adenomatous polyps, normal colon, and nonmalignant colon disorders [67]. Other investigators have measured polyamines in colonic mucosa as a marker of malignant proliferation. Kingsnorth et al. [68] measured polyamine levels in the mucosa of colorectal cancer and compared them with levels in the mucosa of patients that was removed for diverticular diseases. All polyamines individually as well as total polyamine levels were elevated compared with normal tissue. However, the polyamine levels were independent of histological grade of tumor, stage, or metastatic involvement. LaMuraglia et al. [65] also confirmed that polyamines were elevated in adenomatous polyps and cancers compared with normal mucosa. Further investigations are necessary to varify this as a diagnostic marker of colonic neoplasia.

THERAPEUTIC IMPLICATIONS

Ornithine decarboxylase and polyamines may serve not only as potential diagnostic markers for colorectal cancer, but, because they are involved in cell proliferation, they may provide potential targets for the treatment and/or prevention of colorectal neoplasia. Currently inhibitors of polyamine synthesis at all levels of the pathway are available [for review, see 63]. Difluoromethyl ornithine (DFMO), a specific inhibitor of ornithine decarboxylase that has been shown to be well tolerated with few side effects, has been used to suppress tumor growth in vitro and in vivo [63]. DFMO has been used in our laboratory and in others to suppress mucosal growth processes in rats [56–58] and to suppress both carcinogen-induced colonic tumors in mice and rats [64,69] and the growth of implants of human colon carcinoma cells in athymic mice [70]. DFMO has also been documented to inhibit tumor metastases [71].

DFMO is limited in the treatment of established cancers because of an incomplete inhibition of the polyamine pathway [63]. Other polyamine synthesis inhibitors and antagonists are currently being tested for use in malignancy. Because of its low toxicity and side effects, DFMO may still be useful in the chemoprophylaxis of persons at high risk of developing colon cancer. DFMO may be useful in patients who have undergone colectomy with ileal-rectal anastomosis for FAP, because of their continued risk of developing cancer in the retained rectum.

SUMMARY

There has been much progress in the identification of the gene involved in FAP. For molecular biological techniques to be useful in the early and prenatal diagnosis of FAP, much work is still needed to identify the gene locus and to characterize the gene product. Markers that are now in use are not specific or sensitive enough to detect early colon cancer. Newer tumor markers such as polyamines, ornithine decarboxylase, and altered blood group antigen carbohydrates may have a potential as future tumor markers. Additional studies into these markers as well as developing new biochemical markers are warranted in the future to enhance the sensitivity and specificity of diagnosis of early colon cancer, and those at risk for developing cancer. Finally, understanding events involved in abnormal cell proliferation (i.e., elevated polyamines and ODC in colorectal cancer) may help to direct future chemotherapy and possibly chemoprevention in high risk groups such as familial adenomatous polyposis.

References

1. Silverberg E, Lubera J: Cancer Statistics, 1988. CA 38(1):16–17, 1988.
2. Sugarbaker PH, Gunderson LL, Wittes RE: Colorectal Cancer. In DeVita VT, Hellman S, Rosenberg SA (eds): Cancer Principles and Practice of Oncology. Philadelphia: J.B. Lippincott, 1985, pp 795–884.
3. Sherlock P, Lipkin M, Winawer SJ: The prevention of colon cancer. Am J Med 68:917–930, 1980.
4. Gardner EJ, Richards RC: Multiple cutaneous and subcutaneous lesions occurring simultaneously with hereditary polyposis and osteomatosis. Am J Hum Genet 5:139–147, 1953.
5. Bussey HJR: Familial Polyposis Coli: Family Studies, Histopathology, Differential Diagnosis, and Results of Treatment. Baltimore: John Hopkins University Press, 1975, pp 1–104.
6. Burt RW, Bishop DT, Cannon LA, Dowdle MA, Lee RG, Skolnick MH: Dominant inheritance of adenomatous colonic polyps and colorectal cancer. N Engl J Med 312:1540–1544, 1985.
7. Offerhaus GJA, Giardiello FM, Levin LS, Krush AJ, Hasler JF, Booker SV, Welsh SB, Hamilton SR, Yardley JH, Luk GD: Jaw lesions as predictors for colonic adenomatous polyposis in Gardner's Syndrome (GS): A follow-up study [Abstr]. Gstroenterology 90:1570, 1986.
8. Lewis RA, Crowder WE, Eiderman LA, Nessbaum RL, Ferrell RE: The Gardner's syndrome. Significance of ocular features. Ophthalmology 9:916–925, 1984.
9. Gardner EJ: Follow-up study of a family group exhibiting dominant inheritance for a syndrome including intestinal polyps, osteomas, fibromas, and epidermal cysts. Am J Hum Genet 14:376–390, 1962.
10. Traboulsi EI, Krush AJ, Gardner EJ, Booker SV, Offerhaus GJA, Yardley JH, Hamilton SR, Luk GD, Giardiello FM, Welsh SB, Hughes JP, Maumenee IH: Prevalence and importance of pigmented ocular fundus lesions in Gardner's syndrome. N Engl J Med 316:661–667, 1987.
11. Herrera L, Kakati S, Gibas L, Pietrzak E, Sandberg AA: Gardner's Syndrome in a man with an interstitial deletion of 5q. Am J Med Genet 25:473–476, 1986.
12. Knudson AG Jr: Hereditary cancer, oncogenes and antioncogenes. Cancer Res 45:1437–1443, 1985.
13. Bodmer WF, Bailey CJ, Bodmer J, Bussey HJR, Ellis A, Gorman P, Lucibello FC, Murday VA, Rider SH, Scambler P, Sheer D, Solomon E, Spurr NK: Localization of the gene for familial adenomatous polyposis on chromosome 5. Nature 328:614–616, 1987.
14. Leppert M, Dobbs M, Scambler P, O'Connell P, Nakamura Y, Stauffer D, Woodward S, Burt R, Hughes J, Gardner E, Lathrop M, Wasmuth J, Lalouel JM, White R: The gene for familial polyposis coli maps to the long arm of chromosome 5. Science 238:1411–1413, 1987.
15. Solomon E, Voss R, Hall V, Bodmer WF, Jass JR, Jeffreys AJ, Lucibello FC, Patel I, Rider SH: Chromosome 5 loss in human colorectal carcinomas. Nature 328:616–619, 1987.
16. Okamoto M, Sasaki M, Sugio K, Sato C, Iwama T, Ikeuchi T, Tonomura A, Susazuki T, Miyaki M: Loss of constitutional heterozygosity in colon carcinoma from patients with familial polyposis coli. Nature 331:273–277, 1988.
17. Fearon ER, Hamilton SR, Vogelstein B: Clonal analysis of human colorectal tumors. Science 238:193–197, 1987.
18. Bos JL, Fearon ER, Hamilton SR, Verlaan-de Vries M, van Boom JH, van der Eb AJ, Vogelstein B: Prevalence of ras gene mutations in human colorectal cancers. Nature 327:293–297, 1987.
19. Forrester K, Almoguera C, Han K, Grizzle WE, Perucho M: Detection of high incidence of K-ras oncogenes during humor colon tumorigenesis. Nature 327:298–303, 1987.
20. Sasaki M, Sugio K, Soejima JI, Ikeuchi T, Tonomura A, Iwama T, Utsunomiya J, Sasazuki T: Lack of association and linkage between HLA and familial polyposis coli. Hum Genet 77:36–39, 1987.
21. Bodmer J, Kennedy L, Brennan J, Bodmer W: HLA and genetic marker studies in adenomatous polyposis. Br J Surg [Suppl] 72:S32–S35, 1985.
22. Hakomori S: Aberrant glycosylation in cancer cell membranes as focused on glycolipids: Overview and perspectives. Cancer Res 45:2405–2414, 1985.
23. Slomski CA, Durham JP, Watne AL: Glycosyltransferase levels in familial polyposis coli. J Surg Res 40:406–410, 1986
24. Pandey JP, Ebbesen P, Bülow S, Svendsen LB, Fudenberg HH: IgG heavy-chain (Gm) allotypes in familial polyposis coli. Am J Hum Genet 39:133–136, 1986.
25. Lipkin M: Phase 1 and phase 2 proliferative lesions of colonic epithelial cells in diseases leading to colonic cancer. Cancer 34:878–888, 1974.
26. Lipkin M, Blattner WE, Fraumeni JF, Lynch HT, Deschner E, Winawer SJ: Tritiated thymidine labeling distribution as a marker for hereditary predisposition to colon cancer. Cancer Res 43:1899–1904, 1983.
27. Danes BS, Garder EJ, Lipkin M: Studies on the identification of genetic risk for heritable colon cancer. Cancer Detect Prevent 8:349–365, 1985.
28. Garin Chesa P, Rettig WJ, Melamed MR: Expression of cytokeratins in normal and neoplastic colonic epithelial cells. Am J Surg Pathol 10:829–835, 1986.
29. Gold P, Freeman SO: Demonstration of tumor-specific antigens in human colonic carcinomata by immunological tolerance and absorption techniques. J Exp Med 121:439–462, 1965.
30. Green JB III, Trowbridge AA: The use of carcinoembryonic antigen in the clinical management of colorectal cancer. Surg Clin North Am 59:831–839, 1979.
31. Fletcher RH: Carcinoembryonic antigen. Ann Intern Med 104:66–73, 1986.
32. Zamcheck N, Kupchik HZ: Summary of clinical use and limitations of the carcinoembryonic antigen assay and some methodological considerations. In Rose NR, Friedman H, (eds): Manual of Clinical Immunology ed 2. Washington, DC: American Society of Microbiology, 1980.

33. Go VLW, Zamcheck N: The role of tumor markers in the management of colorectal cancer. Cancer 50:2618–2623, 1982.

34. Martin EW Jr, Minton JP, Carey LC: CEA-directed second-look surgery in the asymptomatic patient after primary resection of colorectal carcinoma. Ann Surg 202:310–317, 1985.

35. Mercer DW, Talamo TS: Multiple markers of malignancy in sera of patients with colorectal carcinoma: Preliminary clinical studies. Clin Chem 31:1824–1828, 1985.

36. Krush AJ, Zamcheck N, Lynch HT: CEA and genetics: Gardner's syndrome. Dis Colon Rectum 26:404–408, 1983.

37. Feizi T: Demonstration by monoclonal antibodies that carbohydrate structures of glycoproteins and glycolipids are onco-developmental antigens. Nature 314:53–57, 1985.

38. Magnani JL, Steplewski Z, Koprowski H, Ginsburg V: Identification of the gastrointestinal and pancreatic cancer-associated antigen detected by monoclonal antibody 19-9 in the sera of patients as a mucin. Cancer Res 43:5489–5492, 1983.

39. Koprowski H, Herlyn M, Steplewski Z, Sears HF: Specific antigen in serum of patients with colon carcinoma. Science 212:53–55, 1981.

40. Magnam JL, Borckhaus M, Smith DF, Ginsburg V, Blaszczyk M, Mitchell KE, Steplewski Z, Koprowski H: A monosialoganglioside is a monoclonal antibody-defined antigen of colon carcinoma. Science 212:55–56, 1981.

41. Itzkowitz SH, Kim YS: New carbohydrate tumor markers. Gastroenterology 90:491–494, 1986.

42. Steinberg WM, Gelfand R, Anderson KK, Glenn J, Kurtzman SH, Sindelar WF, Toskes PP: Comparison of the sensitivity and specificity of the CA 19-9 and carcinoembryonic antigen assays in detecting cancer of the pancreas. Gastroenterology 90:343–349, 1986.

43. Gupta MK, Arciaga R, Bocci L, Tubbs R, Bukowski R, Deodhar SD: Measurement of a monoclonal-antibody-defined antigen (CA 19-9) in the sera of patients with malignant and nonmalignant diseases. Cancer 56:277–283, 1985.

44. Atkinson BF, Ernst CS, Herlyn M, Steplewski Z, Sears HF, Koprowski H: Gastrointestinal cancer-associated antigen in immunoperoxidase assay. Cancer Res 5:957–972, 1979.

45. Chia D, Terasaki PI, Suyama N, Galton J, Hirota M, Katz D: Use of monoclonal antibodies to sialyated Lewis^x and sialyated Lewis^a for serological tests of cancer. Cancer Res 45:435–437, 1985.

46. Schoentag R, Primus FJ, Kuhns W: ABH and Lewis blood group expression in colorectal carcinoma. Cancer Res 47:1695–1700, 1987.

47. Yuan M, Itzkowitz SH, Palekar A, Shamsuddin AM, Phelps PC, Trump BF, Kim YS: Distribution of blood group antigens A,B,H, Lewis^a, and Lewis^b in human normal, fetal and malignant colonic tissue. Cancer Res 45:4499–4511, 1985.

48. Kim YS, Yuan M, Itzkowitz SH, Sun Q, Kaizu T, Palekar A, Trump BF, Hakomori S: Expression of Le^y and extended Le^y blood group-related antigens in human malignant, premalignant, and nonmalignant colonic tissues. Cancer Res 46:5985–5992, 1986.

49. Abe K, Hakomori S, Ohshiba S: Differential expression of difucosyl type 2 chain (Le^y) defined by monoclonal antibody AH6 in different locations of colonic epithelia, various histological types of colonic polyps and adenocarcinomas. Cancer Res 46:2639–2644, 1986.

50. Itzkowitz SH, Yuan M, Fukushi Y, Palekar A, Phelps PC, Shamsuddin AM, Trump BF, Hakomori S, Kim YS: Lewis^x and sialylated Lewis^x-related antigen expression in human malignant and non-malignant colonic tissues. Cancer Res 46:2627–2632, 1986.

51. Yuan M, Itzkowitz SH, Ferrell LD, Fukushi Y, Palekar A, Hakomori S, Kim YS: Expression of Lewis^x and sialylated Lewis^x antigens in human colorectal polyps. JNCI 78:479–488, 1987.

52. Boland CR, Montgomery CK, Kim YS: Alterations in human colonic mucin occurring with cellular differentiation and malignant transformation. Proc Natl Acad Sci USA 79:2051–2055, 1982.

53. Pegg AE, McCann PP: Polyamine metabolism and function. Am J Physiol 243:C212–C221, 1982.

54. Tabor CW, Tabor H: Polyamines. Annu Rev Biochem 53:749–790, 1984.

55. Pegg AE: Recent advances in the biochemistry of polyamines in eukaryotes. Biochem J 234:249–262, 1986.

56. Luk GD, Marton LJ, Baylin SB: Ornithine decarboxylase is important in intestinal mucosal maturation and recovery from injury in rats. Science 210:195–198, 1980.

57. Yang P, Baylin SB, Luk GD: Polyamines and intestinal growth: Absolute requirement for ODC activity in adaptation during lactation. Am J Physiol 247:G553–G557, 1984.

58. Luk GD, Baylin SB: Inhibition of intestinal epithelial DNA synthesis and adaptive hyperplasia after jejunectomy in the rat by suppression of polyamine biosynthesis. J Clin Invest 74:698–704, 1984.

59. Luk GD, Baylin SB: Polyamine and intestinal growth-increased polyamine biosynthesis after jejunectomy. Am J Physiol 245:G656–660, 1983.

60. O'Brien TG: The induction of ornithine decarboxylase as an early, possibly obligatory, event in mouse skin carcinogenesis. Cancer Res 36:2644–2653, 1976.

61. Luk GD, Hamilton SR, Yang P, Smith JA, O'Cellaigh D, McAvinchey D, Hyland J: Kinetic changes in mucosal ornithine decarboxylase activity during azyoxymethane-induced colonic carcinogenesis in the rat. Cancer Res 46:4449–4452, 1986.

62. Luk GD, Baylin SB: Ornithine decarboxylase as a biologic marker in familial colonic polyposis. N Engl J Med 311:80–83, 1984.

63. Pegg AE: Polyamine metabolism and its importance in neoplastic growth and as a target for chemotherapy. Cancer Res 48:759–774, 1988.

64. Rozhin J, Wilson PS, Bull AW, Nigro ND: Ornithine decarboxylase activity in the rat and human colon. Cancer Res 44:3226–3230, 1984.

65. LaMuraglia GM, Lacaine F, Malt RA: High ornithine decarboxylase activity and polyamine levels in human colorectal neoplasia. Ann Surg 204:89–93, 1986.

66. Porter CW, Herrera-Ornelas L, Clark L, Pera P, Petrelli NJ, Mittleman A: Polyamine biosynthetic enzyme activities correlate with neoplastic progression in human colorectal tissues [Abstr]. Proc Am Assoc Cancer Res 27:159, 1986.

67. Nishioka K, Romsdahl MM, McMurtrey MJ: Serum polyamine alterations in surgical patients with colorectal carcinoma. J Surg Oncol 9:555–562, 1977.

68. Kingsnorth AN, Lumdsen AB, Wallace HM: Polyamines in colorectal cancer. Br J Surg 71:791–794, 1984.

69. Kingsnorth AN, King WW-K, Diekema K, McCann PP, Ross JS, Malt RA: Inhibition of ornithine decarboxylase with 2-difluoromethylornithine: Reduced incidence of dimethylthydrazine-induced colon tumors in mice. Cancer Res 43:2545–2549, 1983.

70. Zhang S, Luk GD, Hamilton SR: Difluoromethyl ornithine induced inhibition of growth of autochthonous experimental colonic tumors produced by azoxymethane in male F344 rats. Cancer Res 48:6498–6503, 1988.

71. Sunkara PS, Baylin SB, Luk GD: Inhibitors of polyamine biosynthesis: Cellular and in vivo effects of tumor proliferation. In McCann PP, Pegg AE, Sjoerdsma A (eds): Inhibition of Polyamine Metabolism: Biological Significance and Basis for New Therapies. Orlando, FL: Academic Press, 1987, pp 121–140.

36

Mucin Abnormalities in Colonic Mucosa in Patients With Familial Adenomatous Polyposis

T. Muto, K. Sugihara, and M. Ooya

Department of Surgery 1, University of Tokyo, Tokyo, Japan

INTRODUCTION

It has been well-documented with several well-known histochemical techniques [1] that patterns of mucus secretion are altered in colonic carcinomas, adenomas, and inflammatory bowel diseases. Not only overt lesions but also flat, normal-appearing mucosa adjacent to carcinoma or adenoma was found to show similar mucin changes [2]. It would be interesting and moreover clinically useful if such mucin changes were also present in the flat mucosa between adenomas in familial adenomatous polyposis (FAP). Although there are several reports regarding the abnormality of the skin fibroblasts or colonic epithelium in patients with FAP, none of the investigative methods, because of technical difficulties [3–7], seems to be reliable or clinically available for the early detection of the genetic carrier in a FAP family. However, the presence of a mucin abnormality in the background mucosa of FAP family members detected with rather simple technique may shed light on the early detection of the genetic carrier.

Colonic mucus is a mixture of neutral, sialo- and sulfomucins, and the latter two types are important constituents of the colonic mucins [1]. Neutral mucins and sialomucins contribute to the periodic acid-Schiff (PAS) reaction, whereas the high-iron diamine-Alcian blue (HID-AB) technique stains sialo- and sulfomucins in blue and brown, respectively [8]. The periodic acid-thionin Schiff/potassium hydroxide/periodic acid-Schiff (PAT/KOH/PAS) reaction distinguishes the composition of side-chain acylation in sialomucin [9], whereas the mild sodium periodate oxidation/Schiff (mPAS) staining demonstrates non-O-acylated sialomucin (NANA) more accurately [10] (Table 1). These staining techniques have been used to determine the presence or absence of mucin abnormalities in the background mucosa of FAP patients.

HIGH-IRON DIAMINE-ALCIAN BLUE (HID-AB)

The sulfate radicals are specifically identified with the high-iron diamine to give a brown-black color, while the sialomucins are colored blue when the HID staining is followed by Alcian blue at pH 2.5. The detailed staining technique has been described elsewhere [8].

In the normal colonic mucosa of the left colon sulfomucins predominate in the lower half of the crypt, while in the right colon sulfomucins occupy the upper two-thirds [1]. Filipe [11] proposed the term *transitional* mucosa to describe mucosa adjacent to the edge of colonic carcinoma where altered mucus secretion was found in the absence of morphological atypia, being characterized by increased sialomucins and decreased or absent sulfomucins in contrast to normal colonic mucosa. She confirmed that similar changes of mucus secretion are also found in isolated patches

Familial Adenomatous Polyposis, pages 299–303

TABLE 1.
Classification of Mucosubstance According to Histochemical Methods

		Acid mucin		
			Sialomucin	
	Neutral mucin	Sulfomucin	NANA	O-acylated sialomucin
AB-PAS	Red	Blue	Blue	Blue
HID-AB		Brown	Blue	Blue
PKP	Blue		Blue	Red
Mild-PAS	(−)	(−)	Pink (+)	(−)

AB-PAS, Alcian blue (pH 2.5)-PAS; HID-AB, high-iron diamine-Alcian blue (pH 2.5); PKP, PAT/KOH/PAS.

distant from frank tumors, and the increase in sialomucins was directly related to the extent of invasion by carcinoma [2]. She suggested that the mucin changes may be a primary rather than secondary affect of tumor growth and reflect a transformation to a fatal type of epithelium indicating an early stage in carcinogenesis.

Filipe et al. [12] used HID-AB staining in 24 colectomy specimens resected for FAP to see patterns of mucus secretion. Numerous fragments were taken from the various regions, and the percentage of the length of mucosa with a predominance of sialomucins was calculated (Table 2). The flat mucosa between polyps showed an abnormal mucus secretion pattern characterized by increased sialomucins. These changes were patchy and widespread but more pronounced adjacent to carcinomas and larger adenomas. These mucin changes were more extensive in the left colon than in the right and more marked in the noninvolved mucosa from patients with carcinoma than in the noncancer group. They concluded that abnormal glycoprotein synthesis characterized by changes of mucous secretory pattern in the colonic flat mucosa in FAP could antedate morphological changes and prove useful as an additional biological marker to detect high-risk family members in the FAP family.

PERIODIC ACID-THIONIN SCHIFF/POTASSIUM HYDROXIDE/PERIODIC ACID-SCHIFF (PAT/KOH/PAS)

This staining technique, originated by Culling et al. [9], stains non-O-acylated sialomucin (N-acetyl neuraminic acid [NANA]) blue and

TABLE 2.
Familial Adenomatous Polyposis: Distribution of Sialomucins in the Colonic Mucosa*

		Patients with carcinoma	
Regions	Patients without carcinoma	Noninvolved mucosa	Tumor-adjacent mucosa
Cecum	6.8 (14)	2.5 (4)	84.8 (1)
Ascending colon	3.8 (18)	14.7 (5)	—
Hepatic flexure	1.8 (8)	12 (1)	—
Transverse colon	4.8 (19)	32.5 (5)	—
Splenic flexure	5.7 (2)	—	82 (1)
Descending colon	24.7 (15)	31.5 (4)	—
Sigmoid colon	37.7 (17)	70 (4)	77 (4)

*Results are shown as percentages of sialomucins/length of mucosa. Values in parentheses are numbers of cases examined. (Reproduced from Filipe et al. [12], with permission of the publisher.)

TABLE 3.
PAT/KOH/PAS Staining Procedure

1. Mix the solution (cold thionin Schiff's reagent[a]; distilled water, 100 ml; thionin, 1.0 g; sodium metabisulfite, 2.5 g; concentrated HCl 4 ml) using magnetic stirrer overnight; after dissolving, add 1 g fresh activated charcoal and shake 1–2 minutes.
2. 1% periodic acid, 1% KOH in 70% alcohol, 0.1% $NaBH_4$ in 1% Na_2HPO_4, 1% Schiff's reagent

Staining procedure

1. Deparaffinize sections and bring to running water
2. Rinse with distilled water
3. 1% Periodic acid; 60 min[b]
4. Running water, 10 min
5. Rinse with distilled water
6. Cold thionin Schiff's reagent, 60 min[b]
7. Running water, 10 min
8. Rinse with distilled water
9. Sodium borohydride solution; 0.1% $NaBH_4$ in 1% Na_2HPO_4
10. Running water, 10 min
11. Rinse with distilled water
12. Rinse with 70% alcohol
13. 1% KOH in 70% alcohol, 60 min[b]
14. Running water, 10 min
15. Rinse with distilled water
16. 1% Periodic acid; 10 min
17. Running water, 10 min
18. Rinse with distilled water
19. 1% Schiff's reagent
20. Running water, 10 min
21. Rinse with distilled water
22. Dehydrate up graded alcohol to xylol and mount

[a]Standard thionin Schiff's reagent in Culling's original method.
[b]Thirty minutes in Culling's original method.

O-acylated sialomucin red. According to Culling et al. [9,13] and Reid et al. [14], sialomucins of the normal colonic mucosa have acylated side chain at the C_8 and stain red, while colonic carcinomas stain blue-purple, indicating the altered position of the acylated side chain in sialomucins. Muto et al. [15] adopted this staining technique with some minor modification to the colonic flat mucosa in patients with FAP (Table 3). As the right colon mucosa predominantly stains blue-purple, only the flat mucosa specimens from the left colon or the rectum with various pathology were selected for the study (Table 4). There were 41 FAPs, 155 carcinomas, 107 adenomas, and 121 normal controls. The flat mucosa specimens were collected either from the surgically resected specimens or from colonoscopic biopsy specimens. Colonoscopic consecutive biopsy specimens from the left colon, including the rectum, in 121 persons proved to be normal by total colonoscopy were used as control. It is interesting to note that the flat mucosa between adenomas of the left colon in FAP stained blue-purple in 82.9% (significantly different), whereas the background flat mucosa of carcinoma and adenoma stained the same color in 34.8% and 40.2%, respectively (no significant difference) compared with normal controls (Table 5).

Although the PAT/KOH/PAS technique distinguishes sialomucins by the different position of the O-acylated side chain, it also stains PAS-positive substances such as neutral mucin. Sugihara and Jass [16] suggested that the different staining property of the right and left colonic mucin obtained with this technique is due to the presence of neutral mucin in the right colon. They also interpret the blue-purple staining patterns in normal control to indicate goblet cell mucin heterogeneity in the general population and do not apparently associate it with neoplastic dis-

TABLE 4.
PAT/KOH/PAS Staining Properties of Right and Left Colonic Mucin in Normal Colon†

	Blue/purple (%)	Red	Total
Right colon	73 (73.0)	27	100
Left colon	46 (38.0)	75	121*

†Reproduced from Muto et al. [15], with permission of the publisher.
*Statistically significant ($P < 0.01$).

TABLE 5.
PAT/KOH/PAS Staining Properties of Left Colonic Mucin in Various Colonic Pathology†

	Blue/purple (%)	Red	Total
Background mucosa of			
Carcinoma	54 (34.8)	101	155
Adenoma	43 (40.2)	64	107
FAP	34 (82.9)	7	41*
Normal control	43 (35.5)	78	121*

†Reproduced from Muto et al. [15], with permission of the publisher.
*Statistically significant ($P < 0.01$).

ease. Therefore, it is assumed that the staining properties of sialomucin obtained by this technique cannot be properly compared without taking account of the sampling site.

Although it is not clear yet whether the differences in the mucin properties are genetic or acquired, the results obtained here seem to be valuable from a clinical point of view, because members of FAP family having abnormal mucin, stained blue or purple by this particular technique, may well be regarded as at high risk for being the disease carrier and should be carefully followed until adenomas actually develop. There are several reports on the early detection of the genetic carrier in a FAP family, but none of the methods seems to be reliable or clinically applicable because of technical difficulties [3,7]. Compared with other methods, the PAT/KOH/PAS technique has a great advantage in its simplicity. It is not clear yet whether the mucin abnormality in FAP is the same as that in carcinoma, and further detailed analyses are needed.

MILD PERIODIC ACID-SCHIFF (mPAS)

This modified PAS technique, introduced by Veh et al. [10], stains neither O-acylated sialomucins (except, possibly, 7-O-acylated sialomucin) nor neutral mucins; if stains N-acylated sialomucin exclusively. As compared with other staining technique such as HID-AB and PAT/KOH/PAS, this technique seems to be most specific in terms of identifying N-acylated sialomucin (NANA). Sugihara and Jass [17] adopted this technique to determine the presence or absence of the sialomucin abnormality in FAP and malignant disease of the colon. They collected 92 tissue blocks from the left colon and 52 from the right colon in 112 patients with FAP, and the pattern of mucin secretion of the flat mucosa between adenomas was examined. Tissues from 137 patients with other conditions served as controls.

Mild PAS shows two staining patterns: diffuse and focal. Diffuse staining was graded according to the intensity as negative (−), weak (+), and intense (+ +). Focal staining was recorded when isolated crypts stained intensely. They found no difference between FAP and controls in both the left and right colon in terms of either diffuse or focal staining (Table 6). They also confirmed that all forms of sialomucins stained by saponification/periodic acid/phenylhydrazine/Schiff (KOH/PAPS) showed no noticeable difference between FAP and controls. They also examined staining properties with HID-AB in the left colon of 25 patients with FAP and in controls, and they found no significant difference between those conditions. They postulated that blue reaction product might not necessarily indicate an abundance of sialomucin but that it could be due to decreased sulfomucin. The only difference between patients with FAP and controls was the indirect demonstration of less neutral mucins in the right colon in FAP as assessed by the reduction in PAS staining after phenylhydrazine blockade, which blocked neutral mucin. Although they used a more specific technique for identifying non-O-acylated sialomucin, they

TABLE 6.
Diffuse Staining With Mild PAS in Patients With FAP and in Controls*

	Left colon (%)		Right colon (%)	
	FAP	Control	FAP	Control
−	36 (39.1)	47 (52.8)	28 (53.8)	34 (70.8)
+	46 (50.0)	34 (38.2)	15 (28.9)	11 (22.9)
+ +	10 (10.9)	8 (9.0)	9 (17.3)	3 (6.3)
	92	89	52	48

*Reproduced from Sugihara and Jass [17], with permission of the British Medical Journal.

failed to detect mucin changes in the normal-appearing mucosa in patients with FAP.

CONCLUSIONS

The data described here are based on the histochemical study of the mucin secretion pattern of the flat mucosa in patients with FAP. Various techniques have been used for detecting mucin changes: HID-AB for sialomucin/sulfomucin, PAT/KOH/PAS for altered O-acylated side chains in sialomucin, and mPAS for non-O-acylated sialomucin. They have thus far yielded varying results. Although the PAT/KOH/PAS technique seems to be helpful for the early detection of high-risk family members in the FAP family, the observed mucin abnormalities are contradictory to those found with the mPAS technique. The proof of the usefulness of the PAT/KOH/PAS technique in the early detection of genetic carriers in FAP family members remains to be determined. The mucin study of the colonic goblet cells requires further progress to identify the metabolic changes that precede morphological atypia and may be an early expression of cell transformation from the normal to neoplastic state.

References

1. Filipe ML: Mucins in the human gastrointestinal epithelium: A review. Invest Cell Pathol 2:195–216, 1979.
2. Filipe ML, Branfoot AC: Abnormal patterns of mucus secretion in apparently normal mucosa of large intestine with carcinoma. Cancer 34:282–290, 1974.
3. Pfeffer L, Lipkin M, Stutman O, Kopelovich L: Growth abnormalities of cultured human skin fibroblasts derived from individuals with hereditary adenomatosis of the colon and rectum. J Cell Physiol 89:29–38, 1976.
4. Kopelovich L, Colons S, Pollack R: Defective organization of actin in cultured skin fibroblasts from patients with inherited adenocarcinoma. Proc Natl Acad Sci USA 74:3019–3022, 1977.
5. Barfknecht TR, Little JB: Abnormal sensitivity of skin fibroblasts from familial polyposis patients to DNA alkylating agents. Cancer Res 42:1249–1254, 1982.
6. Lipkin M, Blattner WA, Gardner EJ, Burt RW, Lynch H, Deschner E, Winawer S, Fraumeni JF Jr: Classification and risk assessment of individuals with familial polyposis, Gardner's syndrome, and familial non-polyposis colon cancer from [^{3}H]thymidine labeling patterns in colonic epithelial cells. Cancer Res 44:4201–4207, 1984.
7. Luk GD, Baylin SB: Ornithine decarboxylase as a biologic marker in familial colonic polyposis. N Engl J Med 311:80–83, 1984.
8. Spicer SS: Diamine methods for differentiating mucosubstances histochemically. J Histochem Cytochem 13:211–234, 1965.
9. Culling CF, Reid PE, Dunn WL: A new histochemical method for the identification and visualization of both side chain acylated and nonacylated sialic acid. J Histochem Cytochem 24:1225–1230, 1976.
10. Veh RW, Moessen D, Kuntz D, May B: Histochemical demonstration of side-chain substituted sialic acids. In Malt RA, Williamson RCN (eds): Colonic Carcinogenesis. Lancaster: MTP Press, Ltd, 1981, pp 355–365.
11. Filipe ML: Value of histochemical reactions for mucosubstances in the diagnosis of certain pathological conditions of the colon and rectum. Gut 10:577–586, 1969.
12. Filipe ML, Mughal S, Bussey HJ: Patterns of mucus secretion in the colonic epithelium in familial polyposis. Invest Cell Pathol 3:329–343, 1980.
13. Culling CF, Reid PE, Worth AJ, Dunn WL: A new histochemical technique of use in the interpretation and diagnosis of adenocarcinoma and villous lesions in the large intestine. J Clin Pathol 30:1056–1062, 1977.
14. Reid PE, Culling CF, Ramey CW, Dunn WL, Clay MG: A simple method for the determination of the O-acetyl substitution pattern of the sialic acids of colonic epithelial glycoprotein. Can J Biochem 55:493–503, 1977.
15. Muto T, Agawa S, Ooya M, Morioka Y: Mucin abnormality in colonic mucosa in patients with familial polyposis coli. Semin Surg Oncol 3:179–182, 1987.
16. Sugihara K, Jass JR: Colorectal goblet cell mucin heterogeneity and its relation to malignant disease. Clin J Pathol 39:1088–1095, 1986.
17. Sugihara K, Jass JR: Colorectal goblet cell mucins in familial adenomatous polyposis. J Clin Pathol 40:608–611, 1987.

Glycoconjugate Abnormalities of Colonic Epithelium in Familial Adenomatous Polyposis

C. Richard Boland

Department of Internal Medicine, University of Michigan Medical School, and Veterans Administration Medical Center, Ann Arbor, Michigan

BACKGROUND

Glycoconjugates are complex substances in which carbohydrates are covalently linked to other molecules such as lipids or proteins. Most membrane-bound and secreted proteins are glycoproteins; many important determinants of cell identity and behavior on the cell surface membrane are glycoconjugates [1]. The carbohydrate portion of a glycoconjugate molecule consists of a relatively short chain of sugar residues, usually less than 20 in number; however, there may be several identical chains or different chains per molecule. Of interest, only six different sugar residues are found in mammalian glycoproteins (these being galactose, n-acetylgalactosamine, n-acetylglucosamine, fucose, sialic acids, and mannose). However, because of the large number of possibilities for sequence and anomeric linkage between these sugar residues, an enormous degree of diversity is possible for oligosaccharide structure [2,3]. Certain patterns of oligosaccharide modification have been identified for normal cellular processes in the colon, such as cell differentiation [4,5], and for certain diseases, such as ulcerative colitis [6]. Because of the assumed importance of glycoconjugate structure in cellular behavior, many laboratories have attempted to identify characteristic cancer-associated patterns of glycoconjugate structure in humans [7,8].

Mucins are the principal secreted glycoconjugates of colonic, as well as other, epithelia. Changes in the normally expressed antigenic and biochemical structures of colonic mucins have been appreciated in colonic cancer [4,9–12]. The structural basis of "cancer-associated mucins" in the colon is poorly understood at this time; however, at least part of the difference appears to be attributable to modifications in the glycosylation of the molecule [2–4,10,11].

Several experimental approaches have been used to identify mucins associated with gastrointestinal cancer in an attempt to characterize the biochemical or metabolic mechanisms associated with the neoplastic process and to develop potential diagnostic approaches for the identification of premalignant epithelium. Although mucins are thought primarily to play a protective role in the colon, their easy identification on histological sections and the growing availability of tools to measure differences in their structure have made them the focus of attention in the histochemist's search for tumor-specific glycoprotein determinants. However, it is not certain what structural relationship exists between mucins, which are secreted, and those glycoproteins destined for the cell surface membrane.

Some glycoconjugate structures initially identified in colonic cancers have also been identified in adenomatous polyps of the colon [13–18].

Familial Adenomatous Polyposis, pages 305–314

Thus, it has become apparent that glycoconjugates found in malignancy may be expressed in the premalignant phase of neoplasia. Furthermore, it has been demonstrated that certain cancer-associated antigenic structures are quantitatively expressed in direct proportion to the likelihood of cancer developing in the premalignant lesion [14,15].

Other chapters in this volume discuss in greater detail the biological abnormalities seen in familial adenomatous polyposis (FAP). This disease is an autosomal dominantly inherited disease in which countless benign adenomatous polyps develop within the colon [19]. Several laboratories have demonstrated that abnormalities exist throughout the body in this disorder, even in tissues that may not appear to be affected [19,20]. Although a genetic locus associated with this disorder has recently been identified [21], the gene product of the locus and the pathophysiology of this disease remain completely unknown at the time of this writing. The remainder of this chapter will review attempts made at identifying abnormalities of glycoconjugate synthesis in the colonic mucosa of patients with FAP.

TRADITIONAL HISTOCHEMICAL TECHNIQUES

A traditional method for staining carbohydrate-containing structures on tissue sections involves the use of the periodic acid-Schiff (PAS) technique. The histochemical principle is that periodic acid oxidizes available hydroxyl residues to aldehydes (and there may be as many as five in a hexose), and the pigmented Schiff reagent reduces and covalently binds to adjacent pairs of aldehyde groups. Therefore, the PAS technique will stain red any area that contains vicinal diol groups. An abundant (but not exclusive) source of these groups resides in unsubstituted sialic acid residues, which are richly represented in mucins. The source of the vicinal hydroxyl groups in sialic acid is found on the seventh, eighth, and ninth carbon atoms of this nine-member carbon chain [1]. Sometimes, carbons 7, 8, or 9 may contain a covalently linked acyl group, i.e., an esterified carbon chain derived from an organic acid. If the sialic acid is O-acylated at carbon 8 or at both carbons 7 and 9, this portion of the residue will not bind PAS. This is the basis for one of the manipulations of mucin histochemistry. If a site on a histological slide is not stained by the standard PAS technique, but stains red after removing the acyl side chains and restaining with PAS, this suggests the presence of O-acylated sialic acids [22].

A second method for identifying differences in mucins utilizes two other stains: Alcian blue (AB) and high-iron diamine (HID) [23]. Alcian blue is a histochemical stain that binds to anionic residues such as sialic acid and sulfate on mucins by an unidentified chemical reaction. AB stains sialic residues best at pH 2.5 and sulfate groups best at pH 1.0. HID stains sulfate groups black and does not stain sialic acid residues. By combining these two techniques (HID-AB) at pH 2.5, sulfated mucins tend to stain black or brown, and sulfomucins tend to stain blue. The interpretation of the staining reaction is somewhat complicated, since the more intense brown-black stain of sulfomucins will obscure the weaker blue stain of sialomucins.

In 1980, Filipe et al. [24] studied a group of 24 colectomy specimens resected for FAP. Her prior work had revealed that sulfomucins predominated in the normal colon; however, there were some regional differences between the proximal and distal colon, in which sialomucins were seen at the base of the crypt in the right colon. Transitional mucosa, the minimally abnormal but apparently non-neoplastic epithelium immediately adjacent to a cancer, had a predominance of sialomucins. Her study on FAP revealed an increased proportion of sialomucins in FAP colons compared with normals. These changes were more extensive in the distal colon, were consistently present immediately adjacent to cancers and large polyps, but were also seen in flat mucosa not involved by obvious neoplasia. Thus changes previously seen in association with cancer were found in the flat, apparently non-neoplastic colonic tissues in FAP. For the reasons stated above, it is difficult to conclude whether there has been a decrease in sulfation or an increase in sialylation using histochemical techniques.

In 1985, Muto et al. used a modification of

the PAS technique in which they removed the O-acylated side chains from sialomucins by saponification with potassium hydroxide [25]. They reported that 100% of 41 adenocarcinomas of the colon contained unacylated mucins, which was also seen in 82% of villous or tubulovillous adenomas, 33% "of adenomas" (presumably tubular adenomas), 64% of transitional mucosa, and 82% of flat mucosa from patients with FAP. Unfortunately, 39% of normal control colons stained in a similar manner. Conversely, acylated mucins (ie., those that stained with PAS only after saponification) were seen in none of the cancers, 18% of flat FAP tissues, and 61% of normal control colons. Thus, it would appear that there is a decrease in the acylation of sialic acid residues in neoplastic tissues and that this characteristic is also present in flat FAP tissues, as well as in a proportion of controls.

Sugihara and Jass [26] pursued this issue in greater detail in 1986. They utilized additional manipulations of the PAS technique, such as mild periodic acid Schiff staining (which they believe selectively stains "N-acetyl sialic acid" lacking in O-acetyl groups) and phenylhydrazine interpositioning (which does not stain O-acylated sialic acids and also blocks PAS staining of neutral mucins). They reported heterogeneity in goblet cell sialomucins within the general patient population, but were unable to confirm a specific association between the different forms of sialomucins and colon cancer.

In 1987, these investigators studied FAP colons with modified PAS stains [27]. Although there appeared to be perhaps less neutral mucin in the proximal colon of patients with FAP compared with controls, there were no important differences in O-acylated sialic acids in the FAP patients. It was again concluded that there is underlying heterogeneity in colonic sialic acid structure, but that these differences are not related to neoplastic events in the colon. Thus there is currently some controversy regarding the value of traditional histochemical stains in identifying cancer-associated glycoconjugate structures in the human colon.

In 1984, Nishiura et al. [28] reported their histochemical study of gastric polyps of FAP. When they compared fundic gland polyps in FAP to those occurring in patients without this genetic disease, they found an increase in O-acylated sialic acids in the FAP cases. This small but provocative study requires confirmation and amplification.

LECTIN HISTOCHEMISTRY IN FAP

Lectins are naturally occurring proteins and glycoproteins extracted from plants and other sources that can be used as probes of glycoconjugate structure [29]. Lectins bind to exposed carbohydrate residues and are used histochemically to determine patterns of glycosylation that occur in tissue glycoconjugates. A large number of lectins is currently available that possess relative degrees of specificity for different carbohydrate structures. For example, one lectin, *Ricinis communis* agglutinin$_1$ (RCA$_1$), will bind to terminal, β-linked galactose residues, whereas peanut agglutinin (PNA) selectively labels galactose residues that are bound through a β-1,3 linkage to N-acetylgalactosamine (i.e., the Thomsen-Friedenreich antigen) [29]. Some lectins are relatively specific for certain blood group structures; for example, *Dolichos biflorus* agglutinin (DBA) recognizes blood group A, and *Ulex europeus* agglutinin$_1$ (UEA$_1$) will agglutinate blood group O (or H) erythrocytes. Although most lectins bind terminal, nonreducing carbohydrate residues (such as those mentioned above), other lectins can bind "internal" carbohydrate structures, such as wheat germ agglutinin, which binds N-acetylglucosamine residues, or *Lens culinaris* agglutinin, which binds best to a mannose-containing N-linked pentasaccharide core structure containing an internally placed fucose residue. In fact, many lectins have more complex structural requirements for binding than just the terminal sugar residue [29]. Although lectins can bind any carbohydrate present on tissue sections, the dense carbohydrate content of mucins made them prime targets for study using these probes. The variety of lectins available for histochemical studies permitted an additional perspective on glycoconjugate structure by the histochemist.

In 1982, Yonezawa et al. [16] used the lectin UEA$_1$ to study normal and neoplastic human colons. They reported a marked site-specific binding with this lectin, in which labeling was uniformly seen in the normal proximal colon, but was not seen in the distal colon. Moreover, UEA_1 bound to 78% of all colorectal cancers and to 12 of 18 adenomatous polyps, all of which came from the rectum. Yonezawa et al. [30] then studied UEA_1 binding in FAP. The study focused on the distal colon, since the initial study showed the lectin to be most informative in this region. In the four specimens of rectosigmoid mucosa from FAP patients, UEA_1 staining was observed not only in the adenomatous epithelium but also in the non-neoplastic epithelium intervening between the polyps. Although UEA_1 binds a blood group-related structure, the labeling was independent of the patient's blood type.

Sugihara and Jass [27] attempted to confirm this observation; they also used PNA and the lectin *Helix pomatia* agglutinin (HPA), which binds N-acetylgalactosamine residues, making it similar in specificity to DBA [4,29]. A total of 22 patients with FAP were studied, including specimens from both the proximal and distal colon. Staining results for each tissue were classified as: none, up to 50%, or more than 50% (however, it was not clear how these estimates were derived from the slides). They confirmed the finding of Yonezawa et al. that most specimens of proximal colon were stained by UEA_1, but found somewhat greater staining in the distal colon than did the prior group. However, no differences were found between FAP and control colons. No goblet cell mucin was stained using PNA in either group; however, in some instances, portions of the epithelial cell were stained with this lectin. Again, no differences were found between FAP and control colons [27]. Thus, the results of Yonezawa et al. were only partially confirmed, and no differential staining was found in FAP colons with the other two lectins.

Our laboratory has been interested in the use of lectin histochemistry to study colonic neoplasia. Because of the avid labeling of secreted glycoconjugates in the colon, this became the focus of our investigations. It was initially noted in 1982 that goblet cell mucins in the lower portion of the crypt (the locus of less mature epithelial cells) tended to bind the lectins RCA_1 and *Bauhinia purpurea* agglutinin (BPA), and the binding of these lectins was selectively inhibited in the presence of the hapten sugar galactose [4]. Contrariwise, goblet cell mucin in the upper half of the colonic crypt bound RCA_1 and BPA less well, but bound DBA and soybean agglutinin (SBA), which were selectively inhibited by the presence of the hapten sugar N-acetylgalactosamine. To date, these characteristics of goblet cell mucin are the best markers of colonic cell differentiation, and they suggest a relationship between the glycosylation of mucin and the state of cellular differentiation.

The lectin PNA (which selectively binds the galactose β-1,3-N-acetylgalactosamine disaccharide) does not bind goblet cell mucin in the normal colon, but will bind secreted glycoconjugates in most colon cancers [4,5,13]. This observation has been confirmed by other laboratories [31,32]; however, it has become apparent that some variations in PNA binding in the normal and neoplastic colon may be observed because of differences in the lectin binding technique [15,32]. PNA labeling of secreted glycoconjugates in the colon appears to be an oncofetal characteristic [33,34]. Although one cannot tell what molecular species is being labeled in a histochemical study, we have shown that PNA binds to mucins secreted in xenografts derived from cultured human colon cancer cells [35].

We have found that PNA binds to glycoconjugates in neoplastic polyps of the colon as well [13–15], and that a larger proportion of each polyp is labeled as a function of size, the presence of villous architecture, and the presence of carcinoma in the polyp. This has been recently reviewed in greater detail elsewhere [13].

We have recently studied FAP colons with five lectins, as listed in Table 1 [36]. Many of the problems previously encountered by histochemists have revolved around the difficulty one has in achieving an objective assessment of histochemical staining. Our study involved the staining of 22 colectomy specimens from patients with familial adenomatous polyposis and comparing them with rectal biopsies from 27 sex-matched controls who had no personal or family history of colorectal neoplasia. For the purpose of the

TABLE 1.
Lectins Used to Study FAP Colons

Lectin (abbreviation)	Inhibitory Binding Specificity [29]
Ulex europeus agglutinin-1 (UEA)	α-Fucose
Peanut agglutinin (PNA)	β-Gal 1,3αGalNAc
Succinylated WGA (s-WGA)	β-GlcNAc
Dolichos biflorus agglutinin (DBA)	α-GalNAc
Wheat germ agglutinin (WGA)	β-GlcNAc or sialic acid

Gal, galactose; GalNAc, N-acetylgalactosamine; GlcNAc, N-acetylglucosamine.

study, 100–200 colonic crypts were independently scored on a scale of 0 to 4 for intensity of fluorescence, ranging from absent (0) to intense or maximal (4). Then a weighted average was calculated for each slide by summing the individual scores of all the crypts and expressing the sum per 100 crypts, producing a score that ranged from 0 (all 100 crypts negative) to 400 (all 100 crypts intensely stained). We had previously shown that a histochemical estimate of the labeling on a slide with a fluorescent lectin correlated well with lectin bound to mucin isolated biochemically from paired tissue specimens [37]. However, this study [37] demonstrated that the histochemical estimate of lectin binding was most accurate in confirming zero binding or intense degrees of binding, but had difficulty discriminating among intermediate and more intense degrees of staining. The biometric technique developed for the histochemical scoring of the FAP slides provided a means for quantitating crypt-to-crypt heterogeneity within a tissue section.

The labeling of control colonic tissues is depicted in Figure 1, in which the five lectins are listed on the x axis, and the lectin binding score (0–400) is listed on the y axis. It is apparent that PNA and UEA_1 have very low binding scores in the normal colon. The weighted average ± SD for PNA was 19 ± 36; the score for UEA_1 was 1 ± 1. The very low binding scores for these rectal biopsies using UEA_1 confirmed the findings of Yonezawa et al. [16], and it is interesting to note that although the score for PNA was low, it was not zero. The scores for DBA and WGA were 361 ± 31 and 375 ± 18, much as expected. The score for sWGA was 133 ± 79, suggesting that the very high score for WGA represented a large component of binding to sialic acid residues, since binding by sWGA indicates the presence of N-acetylglucosamine residues, which are not expressed as abundantly.

FAP colons contained polypoid lesions, flat adenomatous areas, and flat but morphologically normal areas. The apparently normal areas were scored as "FAP normal," and the polypoid or flat adenomatous areas were scored together as "FAP abnormal." Figure 2 depicts the lectin scores in FAP normal tissue. The binding score using PNA was 9 ± 36, which was not significantly different from controls. The score using UEA_1 was 30 ± 59, which was significantly higher than that seen in controls ($p < 0.05$). Thus, the observations of Yonezawa et al. were confirmed with UEA_1; however, the change in lectin binding was quite subtle. The binding score for sWGA on FAP normal tissues was 188 ± 38 (which was significantly greater than control, $p < 0.05$). Contrariwise, the WGA binding score was 259 ± 68, which was significantly less than that seen in control ($p < 0.001$). One interpretation of these findings is that there was a diminution of terminal sialylation of glycoconjugate residues in FAP normal tissues. Moreover, the increase in sWGA binding suggests an increased "exposure" of N-acetylglucosamine residues, and it is possible that this has occurred as a result of a failure of terminal sialylation. The binding score for DBA on FAP normal tissues was 339 ± 69, which was no different from controls.

The lectin labeling in FAP abnormal tissues is depicted in Figure 3. The score for PNA on FAP abnormal tissues was 18 ± 40, which was no different from controls or FAP normal tissues. The labeling score for UEA_1 on FAP abnormal tissues was 24 ± 72, which was not significantly different from FAP normal (or control) tissues. However, the score for DBA was 219 ± 105,

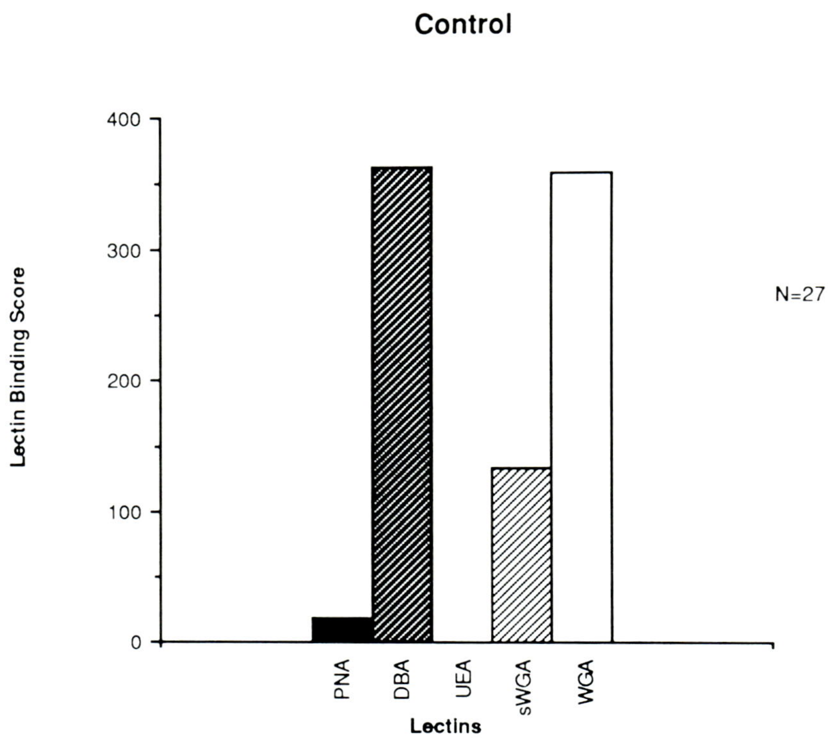

Fig. 1. Lectin binding scores in control colons. Twenty-seven rectal biopsies were studied from patients with no personal or family history of colonic neoplasia. The lectins are listed on the x axis (PNA, peanut agglutinin; DBA, *Dolichus biflorus* agglutinin; UEA, *Ulex europeus* agglutinin$_1$; sWGA, succinylated wheat germ agglutinin; WGA, wheat germ agglutinin). The lectin binding score, ranging from 0 to 400, is listed on the y axis (see text for description of scoring biometry). This figure indicates that most of the crypts stained intensely with DBA and WGA, very few stained with PNA or UEA, and sWGA had an intermediate score.

which was significantly less than that seen in either FAP normal or control tissues ($p < 0.005$). This was compatible with our prior observation that DBA binding tended to be diminished in adenomatous polyps [14]. The binding score in FAP abnormal tissues was 61 ± 63 for sWGA, which was significantly less than that in control tissues ($p < 0.03$) or FAP normal tissues ($p < 0.0001$). The binding score for WGA in FAP abnormal tissues was 265 ± 84, which was significantly less than controls ($p = 0.0001$), but was not significantly different from FAP normal tissues.

Thus we were able to document changes in glycoconjugate expression in FAP normal tissues, in which two lectins stained more intensely (UEA and sWGA) and one lectin stained less intensely (WGA) than controls. FAP abnormal tissues showed reduced binding by DBA, sWGA, and WGA compared with control tissues. FAP abnormal tissues showed significantly less binding by DBA and sWGA when compared with normal-appearing tissues from FAP. All of these findings were relatively subtle, but could be used to identify FAP tissues if careful scoring biometry were employed.

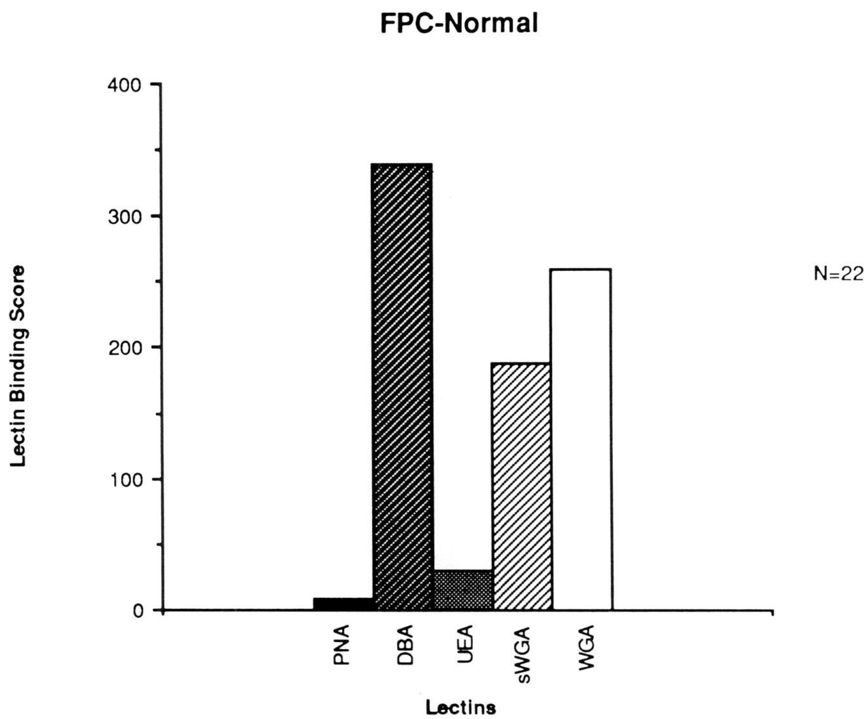

Fig. 2. Lectin binding scores in FAP normal tissues. The lectins are listed on the x axis, and the lectin binding scores on the y axis (see Fig. 1). Twenty-two specimens of normal-appearing colonic epithelium from resected specimens of FAP were used in the study. Compared with control colons, the binding scores for UEA and sWGA were significantly greater, and that for WGA was significantly less. There were no significant differences in binding scores for PNA or DBA.

OTHER APPROACHES

Glycosyltransferase Activity

A number of additional approaches are on the horizon that may aid in the interpretation of routine histochemical studies and lectin histochemistry in FAP. Oligosaccharide chains are synthesized by the stepwise addition of sugars, a reaction that is catalyzed by a group of enzymes known as *glycosyltransferases*. The appearance of a novel transferase or the disappearance of a critical transferase would result in the synthesis of modified carbohydrate antigens. One group has studied glycosyltransferase levels in FAP [39]. Although appropriate controls were selected, the investigators were only able to analyze neoplastic tissues from FAP, but not the uninvolved mucosa (i.e., FAP normal).

The results were interesting with regard to the sialyltransferases and one of the galactosyltransferases, the activities of which were reduced in colon cancer tissue (obtained from nonpolyposis patients), and FAP tissues. A reduction in sialyltransferase activity is compatible with the data we obtained with the lectin WGA, which binds terminal sialic acid residues. Our studies did not use a lectin that could be used to correlate with their galactosyltransferase studies. This work also suggested that a change in the anomeric linkage of fucose residues was produced by the fucosyltransferases in cancers and FAP tissues when compared with controls, but there were no appar-

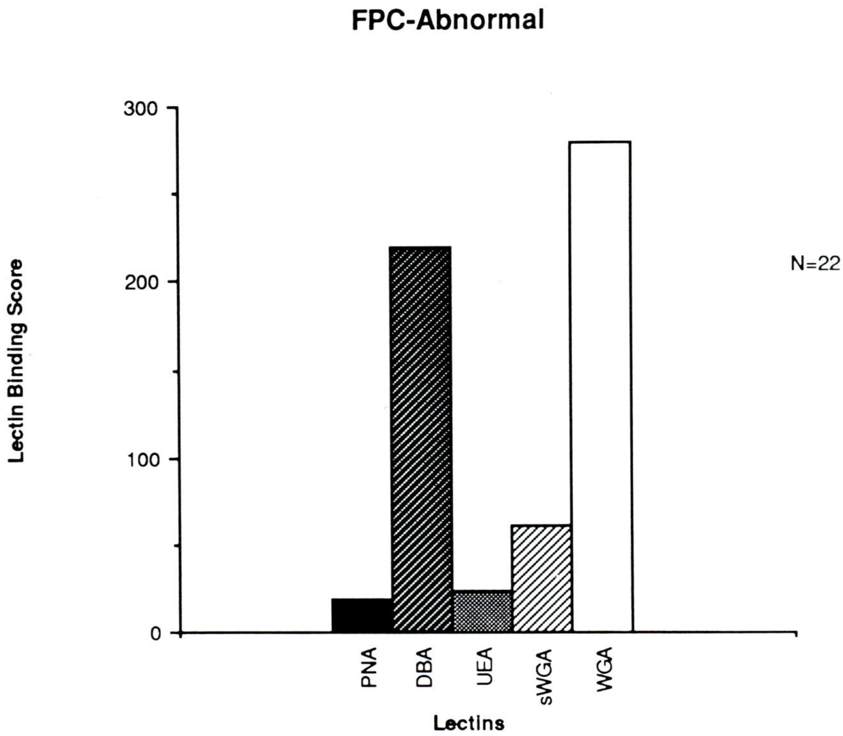

Fig. 3. Lectin binding scores in FAP abnormal tissues. The lectins are listed on the x axis and the lectin binding scores on the y axis as described in the legend for Figure 1. Compared with control colons, the lectin binding scores were significantly less for DBA, sWGA, and WGA. Compared with FAP normal tissues (Fig. 2), the lectin binding scores were significantly less for DBA and sWGA.

ent differences between the FAP tissues and cancers. This type of work may help to clarify the mechanisms responsible for changes in lectin binding and traditional histochemistry seen in this disease.

Monoclonal Antibodies

Many monoclonal antibodies have recently been developed against putative tumor antigens in the colon [40]. The monoclonal antibody B72.3 [41] has been used in radioimmunoassays and immunohistochemistry and found to be valuable in distinguishing between normal and neoplastic tissues. The epitope recognized by this monoclonal antibody has not been fully characterized, although it is known to recognize a high molecular weight glycoprotein (TAG-72) that may be a mucin. Other monoclonal antibodies, such as those directed against Lewis^x and sialylated Lewis^x antigen have been found to bind preferentially to neoplastic lesions in the colon, including adenomatous polyps [42]. Similarly, a monoclonal antibody has been raised to the Lewis^y determinant (a difucosyl type 2 chain), and the binding of this antibody to tissues using immunohistochemistry correlates with the degree of neoplasia present in the tissue (i.e., the labeling is strongest in cancer, intermediate in adenomatous polyps, and least in nonneoplastic lesions) [43]. To date, none of these probes has been used to study the polyposis syndromes. It would be of greatest interest to determine the temporal sequence by which tumor-associated carbohydrate structures appear in the colon, particularly if they should appear in FAP tissue that is histologically normal or in presymptomatic patients carrying the FAP gene. Additional work into the glycoconjugate structures expressed in preneoplastic epithelium or in normal-appearing FAP tissues will surely involve the use of probes that are more specific and informative than those that have been used to date.

References

1. Lance P, Boland CR, Kim YS: Glycoconjugates of the small intestine and colon. In Glass GBJ, Sherlock P (eds): Progress in Gastroenterology, Vol IV. Grune and Stratton, New York, 1983, pp 31–56.
2. Podolsky DK: Oligosaccharide structures of human colonic mucins. J Biol Chem 260:8262–8271, 1985.
3. Podolsky DK: Oligosaccharide structures of isolated human colonic mucin species. J Biol Chem 260:15510–15515, 1985.
4. Boland CR, Montgomery CK, Kim YS: Alterations in human colonic mucin occurring with cellular differentiation and malignant transformation. Proc Natl Acad Sci USA 79:2051–2055, 1982.
5. Boland CR, Kim YS: Lectin markers of differentiation and malignancy. In Wohlman SR, Mastromarino AJ (eds): Progress in Cancer Research and Therapy, Vol 29. New York: Raven Press, 1984, pp 253–266.
6. Podolsky DK, Isselbacher KJ: Composition of human colonic mucin: Selective alteration inflammatory bowel disease. J Clin Invest 72:142–153, 1983.
7. Smets LA, Van Beek WP: Carbohydrates of the tumor cell surface. Biochem Biophys Acta 738:237–249, 1984.
8. Richman PI, Bodmer WF: Monoclonal antibodies to human colorectal epithelium: Markers for differentiation and tumour characterization. Int J Cancer 39:317–328, 1987.
9. Nairn RC, Fothergill JE, McEntegart MG, Richmond HG: Loss of gastrointestinal-specific antigen in neoplasia. Br Med J 1:1791–1993, 1986.
10. Gold D, Miller F: Chemical and immunological differences between normal and tumoral colonic immunoprotein antigen. Nature 255:85–87, 1975.
11. Gold DV, Miller F: Comparison of human colonic mucoprotein antigen from normal and neoplastic mucosa. Cancer Res 38:3204–3211, 1978.
12. Kurosaka A, Nakajima H, Funakoshi I, Matsuyama M, Nagayo T, Yamashima I: Structures of the major oligosaccharides from a human rectal adenocarcinoma glycoprotein. J Biol Chem 258:11594–11598, 1983.
13. Boland CR: Mucin histochemistry in colonic polyps and cancer. Semin Surg Oncol 3:183–189, 1987.
14. Boland CR, Montgomery CK, Kim YS: A cancer-associated mucin alteration in benign colonic polyps. Gastroenterology 82:664–672, 1982.
15. Yuan M, Itzkowitz SH, Boland CR, Kim YD, Tomita JT, Palekar A, Bennington JL, Trump BF, Kim YS: Comparison of T-antigen expression in normal, premalignant and malignant human colonic tissue using lectin and antibody immunohistochemistry. Cancer Res 46:4841–4847, 1986.
16. Yonezawa S, Nakamura T, Tanaka S, Sato E: Glycoconjugate with *Ulex europaeus* agglutinin-1-binding sites in normal mucosa, adenoma, and carcinoma of the human large bowel. JNCI 69:777–785, 1982.
17. Stramignoni D, Bowen R, Atkinson BF, Schlom J: Differential reactivity of monoclonal antibodies with human colon adenocarcinomas and adenomas. Int J Cancer 31:543–552, 1983.
18. Culling CF, Reid PE, Worth AJ, Dunn WL: A new histochemical technique of use in the interpretation and diagnosis of adenocarcinomas and villous lesions in the large intestine. J Clin Pathol 30:1056–1062, 1977.
19. Boland CR, Itzkowitz SI, Kim YS: Colonic polyps and the gastrointestinal polyposis syndromes. In Sleisenger MH, Fordtran JS (eds): Gastrointestinal Diseases, ed 4. Philadelphia: W.B.Saunders Company, 1988, Chapter 80:1483–1518.
20. Kopelovich L, Bias NE, Helson L: Tumour promoter alone induces neoplastic transformation of fibroblasts from humans genetically predisposed to cancer. Nature 282:619–621, 1979.
21. Bodmer WF, Bailey CJ, Bodmer J, Bussey HJR, Ellis A, Gorman Y, Lucibello FC, Murday VA, Rider SH, Scambler P, Sheer D, Solomon E, Spurr NH: Localization of the gene for familial adenomatous polyposis on chromosome 5. Nature 328:614–616, 1987.
22. Culling CFA, Reid PE: Specific techniques for the identification of O-acylated sialic acids in the colon. J Microsc 119:415–425, 1980.
23. Filipe MI: Mucins in the human gastrointestinal epithelium. Invest Cell Pathol 2:195–216, 1979.
24. Filipe MI, Mughal S, Bussey HJ: Patterns of mucus secretion in the colonic epithelium in familial polyposis. Invest Cell Pathol 3:329–343, 1980.
25. Muto T, Kamiya J, Sawada T, Agawa S, Morioka Y, Utsunomiya J: Mucin abnormality of colonic mucosa in patients with familial polyposis coli. Dis Colon Rectum 28:147–148, 1985.
26. Sugihara K, Jass JR: Colorectal goblet cell sialomucin heterogeneity: Its relationship to malignant disease. J Clin Pathol 39:1088–1095, 1986.
27. Sugihara K, Jass JR: Colorectal goblet cell mucins in familial adenomatous polyposis. J Clin Pathol 40:608–611, 1987.
28. Nishiura M, Hirota T, Itabashi M, Ushio K, Yamada T, Oguro U: A clinical and histopathological study of gastric polyps in familial polyposis coli. Am J Gastroenterol 79:98–103, 1984.
29. Goldstein IJ, Poretz RD: Isolation, physiochemical characterization, and carbohydrate-binding specificity of lectins. In Leiner IE, Sharon N, Goldstein IJ (eds): The Lectins: Properties, Functions, and Applications in Biology and Medicine, Orlando FL: Academic Press, Inc, 1986, pp 35–247.
30. Yonezawa S, Nakamura T, Tanaka S, Maruta K, Nishi M, Sato E: Binding of *Ulex europaeus* agglutinin-1 in polyposis coli: Comparative study with solitary adenomas in the sigmoid colon and rectum. JNCI 71:19–24, 1983.
31. Cooper HS: Peanut lectin-binding sites in large bowel carcinoma. Lab Invest 47:383–390, 1982.
32. Orntoft TF, Mors NPO, Eriksen G, Jacobsen NO, Poulsen HS: Comparative immunoperoxidase demonstration of T-antigens in human colorectal carcinomas and morphologically abnormal mucosa. Cancer Res 45:447–452, 1985.

33. Boland CR, Kim YS: Peanut lectin binding identifies human colonic onco-fetal mucin [Abstr]. Clin Res 30:34A, 1982.

34. Coapman RA, Cooper HS: Peanut lectin binding sites in human fetal colon. Arch Pathol Lab Med 110:124–127, 1986.

35. Boland CR, Roberts JA, Siddiqui B, Byrd JC, Kim YS: Cancer-associated colonic mucins in cultured tumor cells and nude mouse xenografts. Cancer Res 46:5724–5729, 1986.

36. Sams JS, Lynch HT, Burt RW, Boland CR: Abnormalities in lectin binding profiles in familial colon cancer in familial polyposis coli [Abstr]. Gastroenterology 88:1568, 1985.

37. Boland CR, Bresalier RS, Roberts JA: Assay of lectin binding sites in colonic cancer-associated mucins: Comparison of fluorescence microscopy with a quantitative chromatographic technique. J Histochem Cytochem 1988 36:1329–1334, 1988.

38. Hounsell EF, Feizi T: Gastrointestinal mucins. Structures and antigenicities of their carbohydrate chains in health and disease. Med. Biol. 60:227–236, 1982.

39. Slomski CA, Durham JP, Watne AL: Glycosyltransferase levels in familial polyposis coli. J Surg Res 40:406–410, 1986.

40. Schlom J: Basic principles and applications of monoclonal antibodies in the management of carcinomas. Cancer Res 46:3225–3228, 1986.

41. Johnson VG, Schlom J, Paterson AJ, Bennett J, Magnani JL, Colcher D: Analysis of a human tumor-associated glycoprotein (TAG-72) identified by monoclonal antibody B72.3. Cancer Res 46:850–857, 1986.

42. Yuan M, Itzkowitz SH, Ferrell LD, Fukushi Y, Palekar A, Hakomori S-I, Kim YS: Expression of Lewis^x and sialylated Lewis^x antigens in human colorectal polyps. JNCI 78:479–488, 1988.

43. Abe K, Hakomori S-I, Ohshiba S: Differential expression of difucosyl type 2 chain (Le^y) defined by monoclonal antibody AH6 in different locations of colonic epithelia, various histological types of colonic polyps, and adenocarcinomas. Cancer Res 46:2639–2644, 1986.

38

Thymidine Kinase Activities in Familial Adenomatous Polyposis, Adenomatous Polyps, and Carcinoma of the Colon

Shinobu Sakamoto, Noriyuki Kasahara, and Takeo Iwama

Medical Research Institute, Tokyo Medical and Dental University, Tokyo, Japan (S.S.); Department of Physiology, University of California, San Francisco, California (N.K.); Second Department of Surgery, Tokyo Medical and Dental University, Tokyo, Japan (T.I.)

INTRODUCTION

Familial adenomatous polyposis (FAP), a genetic disorder characterized by the development of numerous adenomatous polyps in the colon and rectum, is associated with a high incidence of colorectal carcinoma; thus this disease represents a case of heritable predisposition to the development of cancer and is a useful model for the study of biochemical mechanisms underlying carcinogenesis. We have long been using isozymes of thymidine kinase to examine such issues in general and, using this tool, have recently focused our attention on FAP in particular.

THYMIDINE KINASE AND THE SALVAGE PATHWAY OF TMP SYNTHESIS

The rapid replication of DNA, which is commonly found to occur in malignant neoplasms, requires an adequate supply of deoxyribonucleotides to serve as the substrates for the DNA polymerase reaction. One such essential substrate, thymidine monophosphate (TMP), is a pyrimidine deoxyribonucleotide that may be synthesized via two pathways: 1) the de novo pathway, which involves the direct modification of the uridine base of the precursor nucleotide deoxyuridine monophosphate (dUMP) in a methylation reaction catalyzed by the enzyme thymidylate synthetase (TS) and requiring N^5,N^{10}-methylenetetrahydrofolate as the methyl donor; and 2) the salvage pathway, which involves only the phosphorylation and reutilization of pre-existing thymidine deoxyribonucleosides (Fig. 1a).

Thymidine kinase (TK; EC 2.7.1.21) is the key enzyme that catalyzes the phosphorylation of deoxythymidine to form TMP via the pyrimidine salvage pathyway (Fig. 1a) [1]. The activity of this enzyme has been shown to be regulated in response to alterations in DNA replicative activity. Bollum and Potter [2] originally demonstrated that initiation of DNA synthesis in regenerating rat liver is preceded by a dramatic increase in the level of TK activity. High TK activity has also been consistently observed in rapidly proliferating normal and neoplastic tissues, including fetal tissue [3,4], hepatomas [5,6], pulmonary tumors [7,8], lymphomas [9,10], leukemias [11,12], mammary tumors [13–15], and colon tumors [4,16–25].

ISOZYMES OF THYMIDINE KINASE

Two distinct forms of TK have been shown to exist that differ in molecular weight, electrophoretic mobility, intracellular localization, and biochemical properties (Table 1) [1,3,26–30]. One of these isozymes is the predominant form seen in terminally differentiated adult tissues and is associated with the mitochondrial cell fraction;

Familial Adenomatous Polyposis, pages 315–324

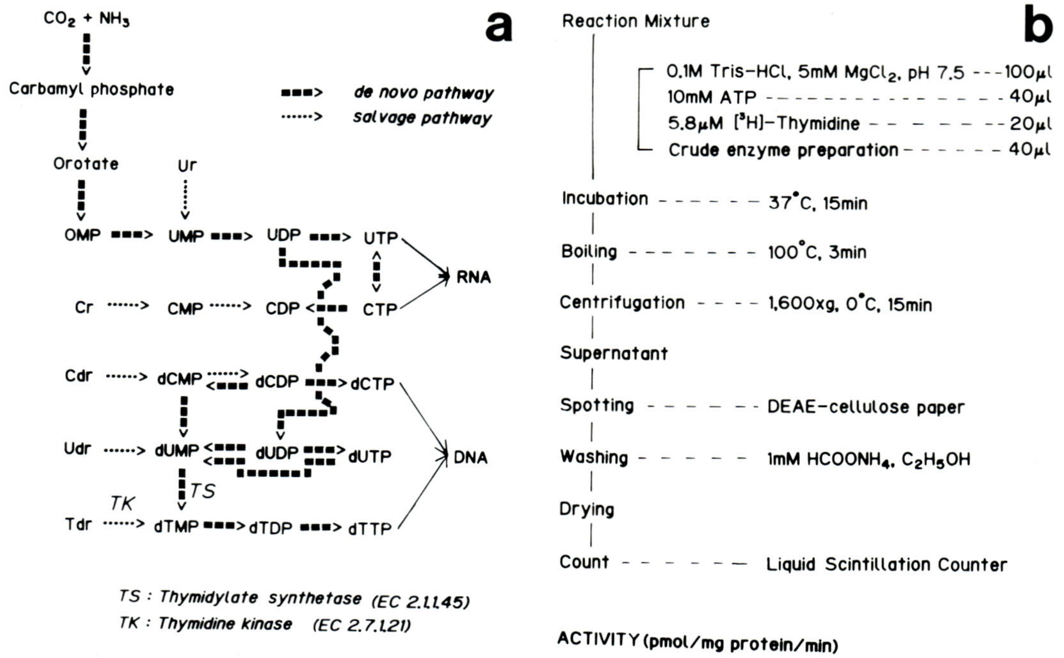

Fig. 1. **a:** Metabolic pathways of pyrimidine nucleotide synthesis: The de novo and salvage pathways are shown by, respectively, the dashed and dotted arrows. OMP, orotidine monophosphate; Ur, uridine ribonucleoside; UMP, UDP, and UTP, uridine mono-, di-, and triphosphate; Cr, cytidine ribonucleoside; CMP, CDP, and CTP, cytidine mono-, di-, and triphosphate; Cdr, cytidine deoxyribonucleoside; dCMP, dCDP, and dCTP, deoxycytidine mono-, di-, and triphosphate; Udr, uridine deoxyribonucleoside; dUMP, dUDP, and dUTP, deoxyridine mono-, di-, and triphosphate; Tdr, thymidine deoxyribonucleoside; dTMP, dTDP, and dTTP, deoxythymidine mono-, di-, and triphosphate; TS, thymidylate synthetase; TK, thymidine kinase. TS and TK catalyze, respectively, the de novo and salvage pathways of dTMP synthesis. **b:** Protocol for assay of thymidine kinase activity. This protocol is based on the method of Taylor et al. [3]. See text for details.

it is often therefore referrred to as "TK-A" or "TK-M." The molecular weight of this isozyme is about 50,000–70,000, and it migrates rapidly during polyacrylamide gel electrophoresis. Its K_m for (ATP) adenosine triphosphate is 0.65×10^{-6} M; however, it can also utilize nucleotides other than ATP as phosphate donors. It is active over a broad range of pH optima, ranging from 7 to 9, is relatively heat-stable up to 45°C, and its activity is almost totally inhibited by thymidine triphosphate (TTP). In addition, the activity of this mitochondrial isozyme is also significantly inhibited by low concentrations of deoxycytidine triphosphate (dCTP), which, like TTP, is also an end-product of pyrimidine nucleotide biosynthesis. The gene that encodes this isozyme has been localized to human chromosome 16 and has been designated TK-2.

The other TK isozyme is associated with the cytosolic cell fraction and is usually seen in significant quantity only in cells undergoing rapid proliferation, such as fetal or neoplastic cells; accordingly, it is often referred to as "TK-F" or "TK-C." It has a molecular weight of about 90,000–100,000, and it migrates slowly during polyacrylamide electrophoreses. Its K_m for ATP is 2.3×10^{-6} M, and it specifically utilizes ATP most efficiently as its phosphate donor. Its pH optimum is in a narrower range than the mitochondrial isozyme, and it seems to have less ther-

TABLE 1.
Summary of the Biochemical Properties of the Two TK Isozymes

Gene	TK-1	TK-2
Chromosomal location	17 q21–22	16
Subcellular localization	Cytosol	Mitochondria
Cell cycle-specific activity	Low during G1 phase, increases just prior to S	Relatively constant throughout cycle
Predominanat form in	Fetal, neoplastic tissues	Adult tissues
Molecular weight	90,000–100,000	50,000–70,000
Phosphate donors	ATP only	ATP, CTP, GTP, UTP
K_m for ATP	2.3×20^{-6}	0.65×10^{-6}
Range of pH optima	Narrow	Broad (pH 7–9)
Thermal stability	Loss of >50% activity at 45°C	90% active at 45°C
Inhibition by TTP	+	+
Inhibition by dCTP	–	+
PAGE migration	Slow	Rapid
DEAE-cellulose column chromatography	Eluted at 0 M NaCl (peak A)	Eluted at 0.1 M NaCl (peak B)

mal stability, losing more than 50% of its activity at 45°C. The activity of this cytosolic TK isozyme is inhibited by TTP; however, it is not subject to negative regulation by low concentrations of dCTP. The gene encoding this isozyme has been localized to q21-22 of human chromosome 17 and has been designated TK-1.

These two isozymes of TK have been separated and purified by various methods, including polyacrylamide gel electrophoresis [3,28], subcellular fractionation [28,29], affinity column chromatography [6,9,13,24,30], and DEAE-cellulose column chromatography [14,15,19, 20,22,27].

For DEAE-cellulose column chromatography, which is the procedure we commonly use, a crude enzyme extract is first prepared by pulverizing the tissue specimens under liquid nitrogen, followed by homogenization at 0°C with buffer containing 5mM Tris-HCl (pH 7.5)/0.1 mM EDTA/1 mM mercaptoethanol/0.25 M sucrose and then colllecting the supernatant after centrifugation at 105,000g for 1 hour at 4°C. The crude extract is then fractionated by adding saturated ammonium sulfate to 50% saturation and stirring for 1 hour, followed by centrifugation at 10,000g for 20 minutes, overnight dialysis of the precipitate resuspended in buffer containing 5 mM Tris-HCl (pH 7.5)/20% glycerol/1 mM $MgCl_2$, and centrifugation again at 10,000g for 30 minutes. The resultant supernatant is loaded onto a DEAE-cellulose column and eluted with the same buffer containing increasing concentrations of NaCl (0,0.1,0.2, and 0.3 M). The activities of the cytosolic and mitochondrial TK isozymes are typically eluted at NaCl concentrations of 0 and 0.1 M, and we have designated these as peaks "A" and "B," respectively.

MEASUREMENT OF THYMIDINE KINASE ACTIVITIES

We can measure either total TK activity in a given tissue sample, or, as described above, we can separate the isozymes by DEAE-cellulose column chromatography and measure their activities individually. TK activity is measured by the method of Taylor et al. [3]. An assay mixture consisting of 5 mM $MgCl_2$, 10 mM ATP, 2 μl [6-^{3}H]thymidine, and 0.1 M Tris-HCl buffer (pH 7.5) in a total volume of 200 μl is incubated with the enzyme preparation for 15 minutes at 30°C. A 100 μl aliquot of the mixture is spotted onto DEAE-cellulose paper, which is then washed extensively with 1 mM ammonium formate and methanol to remove all unphosphorylated substrate, dried, and the radioactivity remaining on the paper is measured in a liquid scintillation counter (Fig. 1b). In addition, the differential inhibitory effect of pyrimidine nucleotides on these two isozymes may be demonstrated by including TTP or dCTP in the reaction mixture at final concentrations of 0.5 mM, 1.0 mM, and 5.0 mM to confirm biochemically the identities of the two peaks eluted from the DEAE-cellulose column.

THYMIDINE KINASE ACTIVITIES IN CARCINOMA OF THE COLON

We [19,20] and others [4,16,17,18] have previously determined that total TK activity in human colon carcinoma tissue was significantly higher than that seen in normal human colon mucosa. Weber et al. [16] have reported that TK activity rose to 331% that of normal mucosa in colonic adenocarcinoma samples obtained from nine patients and that TK activities in rapidly growing xenografts of human colon carcinoma in nude (athymic) mice were markedly higher than those in slowly growing xenografts [17]. Furthermore, Herzfeld et al. [4,18] have also suggested that progressive elevations in TK activity seem to correlate with increasing histological dedifferentiation of the tumor.

These results were confirmed by our own findings [19], which demonstrated an increase in total TK activity of 328% in 13 samples of human colon carcinoma as compared with normal colon mucosa. We then further extended these studies to examine specific changes in the activities of the two TK isozymes; our results indicate that the rise in total TK activity associated with colorectal carcinogenesis may be attributable, at least partially, to a great increase in the activity of the cytosolic TK isozyme, which elutes as peak A on DEAE-cellulose column chromatography (Fig. 2). Peak A activity, which was greatly reduced in normal mucosa, rose to 12-fold that of normal in colon carcinoma tissue, whereas peak B, the mitochondrial or "adult" isozyme, increased only 1.8-fold [19]. These findings are therefore indeed in accord with studies of TK isozyme activity in other neoplastic tissues; thus, in human colorectal carcinoma, as is true in general, total TK activity has been observed to be increased in concert with a specific rise in cytosolic TK isozyme activity in tissues undergoing malignant transformation.

THYMIDINE KINASE ACTIVITIES IN DMH-INDUCED COLON CARCINOMA

It has been shown that a high incidence of adenocarcinoma in the distal colon can be induced by subcutaneous injections of 1,2-dimethylhydrazine (DMH) into rats at weekly intervals and that such tumors are analogous to human colon carcinoma in their mode of growth and metastasis [23,31]. Weber et al. [25] and Balis et al. [32] have reproted that TK activity is increased in DMH-induced colon carcinoma, approaching levels such as are seen in fetal intestine. We have also found that total TK activity in DMH-induced colon carcinoma rises to as high as 594% compared wih normal mucosa in rats 7 weeks after completion of DMH treatment [21]. Such increases were found to be associated with a great increase in cytosolic (peak A) TK isozyme activity of up to 23.6-fold that of normal, whereas mitochondrial (peak B) activity was increased only 1.6-fold [22].

Of further interest was the fact that increases in TK activity have also been noted in morphologically normal-appearing colon mucosa after treatment with DMH [23]. Though we were not able to detect any significant increase in total TK activity, we noted that peak A TK isozyme activity was indeed moderately increased (to 368% of normal) in DMH-treated "normal" mucosa [22]. This may suggest that DMH-induced changes in DNA synthesis occur in otherwise apparently normal mucosa prior to the onset of overt malignancy. These biochemical studies complement previous observations concerning the morphology and dynamics of crypt cell populations after DMH treatment. On the basis of these observations, it has been suggested [33,34] that DMH-induced colon carcinogenesis may involve a two step process: 1) an initial increase in the population of mitotically active cells followed by 2) eventual transformation of some of these cells.

THYMIDINE KINASE ACTIVITIES IN ADENOMATOUS POLYPS OF THE COLON

Polyps developing in the gastrointestinal tract have long been regarded by many as "premalig-

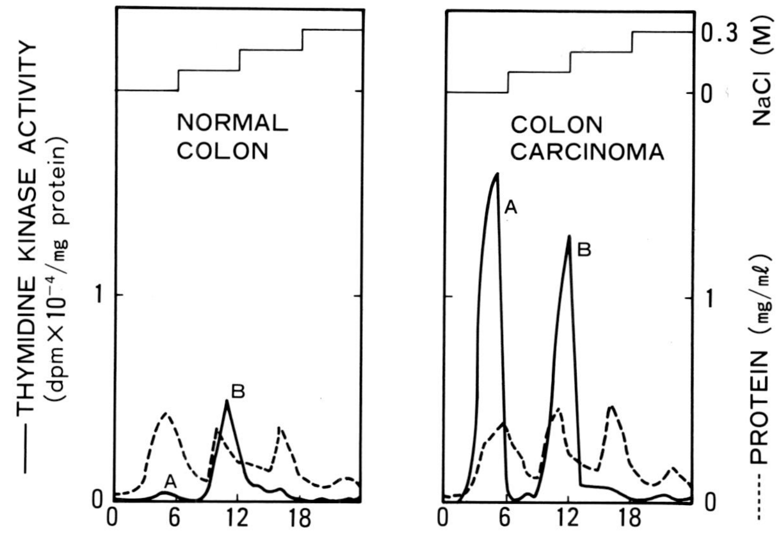

Fig. 2. Typical elution profiles of thymidine kinase activity (solid lines, dpm × 10^{-4}/mg protein) and protein content (dashed lines, mg/ml) after DEAE-cellulose column chromatography of normal human colon mucosa and human colon carcinoma tissues. The column was eluted with 5 mM Tris-HCl (pH 7.5)/20% glycerol/1 mM $MgCl_2$ buffer containing increasing concentrations of NaCl (0,0.1,0.2, and 0.3 M). Fractions of 1.0 ml were collected to a total of 6.0 ml for each NaCl concentration. Thymidine kinase activities eluted at NaCl concentrations of 0 and 0.1 M were designated peaks A and B, and their biochemical properties were found to correspond to the cytosolic and mitochondrial TK isozymes, respectively.

nant'' lesions. However, much debate has centered on whether carcinoma actually does arise from polyps that are predisposed to subsequent malignant change (the so-called polyp-cancer sequence) or whether both arise de novo from previously normal mucosa via independent (though perhaps related) processes. Thus we were interested in determining whether benign and well-differentiated neoplastic tissue, i.e., adenomatous polyps of the colon, would exhibit the same enzymatic characteristics as malignant adenocarcinoma or whether some differences, quantitative or qualitative, would be apparent. Previously, Balis et al. [32] had reported that skin fibroblasts from patients with Gardner's syndrome reacted by indirect immunofluorescence with antibodies generated against TK purified from placental extacts and that TK from these fibroblasts seemed to have fetal or tumor-like properties in terms of thermal stability and activation by various effectors. However, quantitative data on the differential activities of specific TK isozymes inherent in polypoid lesions had yet to be determined.

Accordingly, we examined total TK and TK isozyme activities in 14 samples of sporadic polyps taken from human colon and compared these with the corresponding values in both normal and carcinomatous human colon tissues. Histologically, all of the polyps were identified as adenomas and all of the carcinoma specimens as moderately well-differentiated adenocarcinomas. Total TK activity in colon carcinoma was found to be, on average, 2.9-fold that of normal, a value consistent with previous studies. However, in tissue samples obtained from sporadic adenomatous polyps of the colon, total TK activity was found to be only 1.9-fold that of normal, i.e., a value slightly higher than that seen in normal colon mucosa but that did not reach levels such as those seen in malignant disease. Furthermore, we found that, in contrast to the situation in colon carcinoma, this moderate increase in TK activity in colon polyps seems to be attributable mainly to an increase in mitochondrial (peakB) TK isozyme activity, i.e., mitochondrial TK isozyme activities were elevated in both colon polyp and colon carcinoma tissue to, respectively, 158% and 151% of normal, whereas cytosolic (peak A) TK isozyme activity was increased to 510% only in colon carcinoma and was not significantly elevated in colon polyps [20]. These results suggest that increased activity of the mitochondrial TK isozyme alone is sufficient to support the relatively slow growth of benign neoplasms such as adenomatous polyps; in contrast, increased activity of the cytosolic TK isozyme seems to be specifically associated with the development of colon carcinoma, perhaps indicating a specific induction of this enzyme that is necessitated by and that contributes to the faster growth rates observed in malignant neoplasms.

THYMIDINE KINASE ACTIVITIES IN FAMILIAL ADENOMATOUS POLYPOSIS

Recently, we obtained sufficient material from FAP patients to enable us to make preliminary comparisons of TK activities in FAP polyp tissue with those in normal or cancerous colon tissue (manuscript in preparation). In terms of total TK activity, colon carcinoma tissue was increased to about threefold (consistent with previous studies), whereas FAP polyp samples from 15 patients showed an average elevation of only 1.8-fold over normal colon tissue (Fig. 3). Interestingly, only 5 of the 15 FAP samples showed significant elevations in total TK activity. Furthermore, TK isozyme analysis revealed variable patterns of peak A activity, with the cytosolic isozyme being elevated in some cases (8 of 15) and remaining low in others (Fig. 4). Thus the polypoid lesions in FAP seem to be a heterogeneous population with respect to TK activities and, accordingly, DNA replicative activity. It remains to be determined, although it seems likely, that this biochemical heterogeneity in fact reflects the heterogeneity of the individual polyps in their potential for malignant change. The precise pathogenesis of colon carcinoma in FAP remains unclear; whether carcinoma arises in situ via a polyp-cancer sequence or whether it arises de novo from adjacent tissue is still a topic of controversy. However, the present observations seem to suggest that some polyps are more active in DNA synthesis than others, as manifested by increased total TK activity and/or increased activity of the cytosolic (peakA) TK isozyme and therefore may either be more advanced along the biochemical

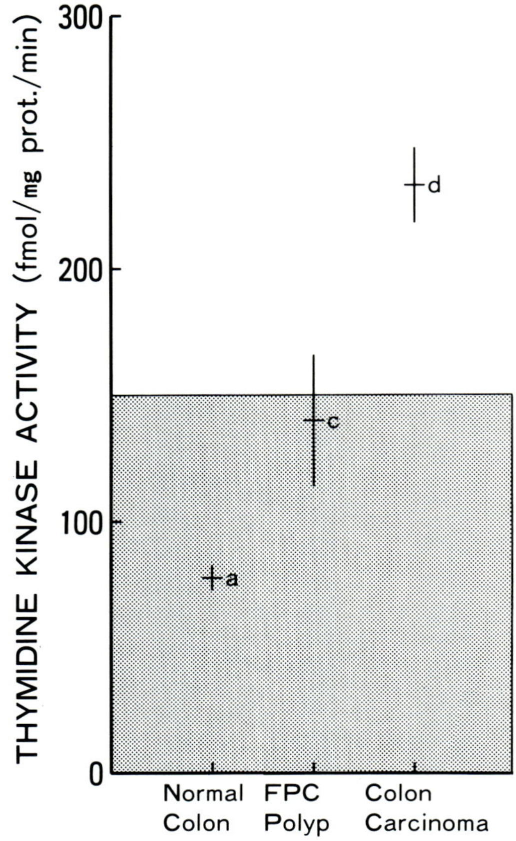

Fig. 3. Total thymidine kinase activity in normal human colon mucosa, polyps resected from familial polyposis coli patients, and human colon carcinoma tissues. TK activity is expressed as fmol/mg protein/min. The actual values obtained (mean ± S.E.M.) were, for normal colon (N = 60), 78.44 ± 4.67; for FPC polyps (N = 15), 139.97 ± 26.50; and for colon carcinoma (N = 60), 232.81 ± 14.92. Each value was found to be significantly different from either of the other values ($P < 0.05$) by the Student's t test; ^{a}vs^{c,d} and ^{c}vs^{d}.

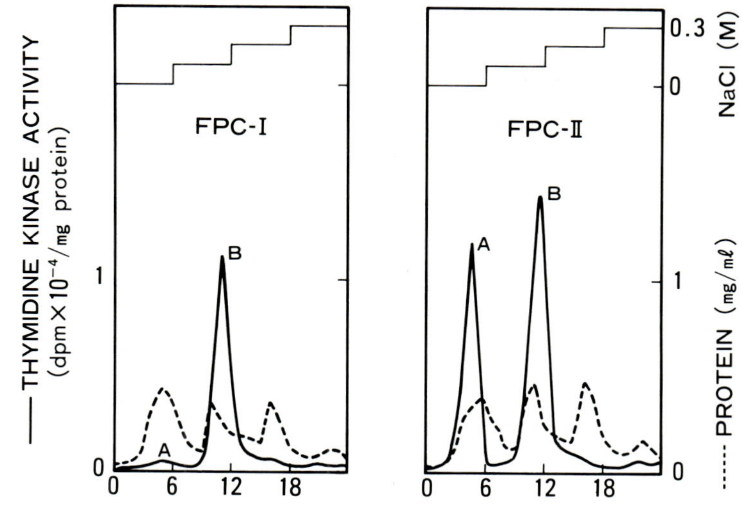

Fig. 4. Typical elution profiles of thymidine kinase activity (solid lines, dpm $\times 10^{-4}$/mg protein) and protein content (dashed lines. mg/ml) from DEAE-cellulose column chromatography of FPC polyp samples. Elution procedures were the same as described in Figure 2 and in the text. TK isozyme activities in polyp samples from 15 patients with familial polyposis coli were examined in this manner. Of these, 7 of 15 showed elution profiles similar to the pattern on the left panel (designated FPC-l), with cytosolic TK (peak A) isozyme activity remaining low. In contrast, 8 of 15 showed elution profiles similar to the pattern on the right panel (designated FPC-ll), with marked elevations of peak A activity.

path to overt malignant transformation or more susceptible to other factors that subsequently induce carcinogenesis.

FUTURE DIRECTIONS IN THYMIDINE KINASE RESEARCH

The ultimate goal of studies aimed at the elucidation of biochemical and enzymatic changes that accompany neoplasia in the colon is the understanding of the causes and processes involved in malignant transformation and thereby the development of improved strategies for detection, treatment, monitoring, and perhaps even prevention of carcinogenesis. At present, we are reasonably certain that the activation of the cytosolic TK isozyme is specifically associated wih the development of colon carcinoma. We first hope to apply this observation to the early detection of initial carcinogenesis of the colon as well as recurrent or metastatic disease. To this end, we are presently investigating the diagnostic value of serum TK measurements as a means for such detection. Serum TK measurements have previously been shown to be of prognostic use in lung cancer [8], lymphoma [10], and leukemia [11,12]. The sensitivity and specificity of such measurements would be further enhanced if a radioimmunoassay that utilized an antibody specific for the cytosolic isozyme could be developed. Accordingly, we are also presently trying to generate just this type of monoclonal antibody.

The efficacy of various anticancer treatments may also be tested by monitoring their effects on various parameters such as DNA synthesis and TK activities. We [21] have previously examined the effects of UFT (a combination of tegafur and uracil) on TK and thymidylate synthetase (TS) activities in DMH-induced colon carcinoma in rats and found that low doses of UFT, which contains fluoropyrimidines that inhibit TS activity and the de novo pathway of pyrimidine synthesis, actually enhance the activity of TK and the salvage pathway, thus offsetting any therapeutic gain; this suggests that adequate consideration of the dosage is a vitally important factor in obtaining maximum benefit from anticancer drugs and that optimum dosages may possibly in the future be determined by monitoring TK activities in individual patients.

Finally, now that the genetic locus for FAP has been localized [35] to bands q21-q22 on chromosome 5, one may anticipate that the gene itself will soon be identified and the sequence of its gene product elucidated. At the same time, the cytosolic TK gene, located on chromosome 17 [26], has already been cloned an sequenced [36], and the regulatory mechanisms governing its expression, at both transcriptional and post-transcriptional levels, have been studied [37–39]. Such advances may perhaps shed some light on the molecular events that lead to malignant transformation. A possible sequence of chromosomal modifications that may result in a series of defined metabolic perturbations leading to colorectal carcinogenesis has already been proposed [40] from the standpoint of classic cytogenetics. Interestingly, this scenario involves the deregulation of enzymes that catalyze the salvage and de novo pathways of pyrimidine and purine synthesis via chromosomal imbalances involving 17q (thymidine kinase), 18 (thymidylate synthetase), 5q (dihydrofolate reductase), and 1p (cytidylate kinase). In the future, it may be possible to test directly such hypotheses by utilizing the techniques of reverse genetics and molecular biology to examine, for example, the interactions that might be taking place between the FAP gene product and the 5′-flanking region of the cytosolic TK gene. Such studies will hopefully add to our understanding of the precise molecular mechanisms underlying carcinogenesis in the colon and open the way to the formulation of better strategies for its prevention and treatment.

CONCLUSIONS

In summary, it seems that increased activity of cytosolic (peak A) TK activity is a necessary prerequisite and constitutes a biochemical marker for the development of overt colorectal carcinoma; it is likely that, otherwise, increased activity of the mitochondrial (peak B) isozyme alone, while sufficient to support slower growth of benign adenomas, is however insufficient to raise total TK levels high enough to support the demands of the rapidly replicating DNA for more nucleotide substrate in malignant lesions. Some FAP polyps also exhibit this pattern of increased peak A activity, in combination with increased total TK activity. These polyps may represent lesions that are still essentially benign but predisposed to malignant change or may be a precancerous condition that is already on its way to carcinogenesis. In any case, the synthesis of nucleic acids represents one final common pathway that must be activated for cell division to occur. It is our hope that further analysis of the events occurring at the molecular level that lead to the induction of cytosolic TK in FAP may shed light on the mechanisms underlying carcinogenesis in general and lead to novel therapeutic approaches aimed at the prevention of malignant transformation.

ACKNOWLEDGMENTS

We thank Professor Ryohei Okamoto and Professor Yoshio Mishima for their invaluable guidance, advice, and encouragement. This work was supported in part by a research grant no. 57570479, no. 59570565 and no. 62570599 from the Ministry of Education of Japan.

References

1. Kit S: Thymidine kinase, DNA synthesis and cancer. Mol Cell Biochem 11:161–182, 1978.
2. Bollum FJ, Potter VR: Nucleic acid metabolism in regenerating rat liver. VI. Soluble enzymes which convert thymidine to thymidine phosphates and DNA. Cancer Res 19:561–565, 1959.
3. Taylor AT, Stafford MA, Jones OW: Properties of thymidine kinase partially purified from human fetal and adult tissue. J Biol Chem 247:1930–1935, 1972.
4. Herzfeld A, Greengard O: Enzyme activities in human fetal and neoplastic tissues. Cancer 46:2047–2054, 1980.
5. Ferdinandus JA, Morris HP, Weber G: Behavior of opposing pathways on thymidine utilization in differentiating, regenerating, and neoplastic liver. Cancer Res 31:550–556, 1971.
6. Lai M-HT, Weber G: Increased concentration of thymidine kinase in rat hepatomas. Biochem Biophys Res Commun 111:280–287, 1983.
7. Greengard O, Herzfeld A: The undifferentiated enzy-

mic composition of human fetal lung and pulmonary tumors. Cancer Res 37:884–891, 1977.

8. Gronowitz JS, Steinholtz L, Kallander CFR, Hagberg H, Bergh J: Serum deoxythymidine kinase in small cell carcinoma of the lung. Cancer 58:111–118, 1986.

9. Ellims PH, Van der Weyden MB, Medley G: Thymidine kinase isoenzymes in human malignant lymphoma. Cancer Res 41:691–695, 1981.

10. Gronowitz JS, Hagberg H, Kallander CFR, Simonsson B: The use of serum deoxythymidine kinase as a prognostic marker, and in the monitoring of patients with non-Hodgkin's lymphoma. Br J Cancer 47:487–495, 1983.

11. Kallander CFR, Simonsson B, Hagberg H, Gronowitz JS: Serum deoxythymidine kinase gives prognostic information in chronic lymphocytic leukemia. Cancer 54:132–137, 1984.

12. Hagberg H, Gronowitz JS, Killander A, et al.: Serum deoxythymidine kinase in acute leukemia. Br J Cancer 49:537–540, 1984.

13. Bronzert DA, Monaco ME, Pinkus L, Aitken S, Lippman ME: Purification and properties of estrogen-responsive cytoplasmic thymidine kinase from human breast cancer. Cancer Res 41:604–610, 1981.

14. Sakamoto S, Kawasaki T, Yoshino H, Kudo H, Okamoto R: Effects of estrogen and prolactin on thymidine kinase isozyme activities in DMBA-induced rat mammary tumor. Toxicol Lett 21:91–96, 1984.

15. Sakamoto S, Iwama T, Ebuchi M, Tsukada K, Sagara T, Kawasaki T, Murakami S, Kasahara N, Kudo H, Okamoto R: Increased activities of thymidine kinase isozymes in human mammary tumors. Br J Surg 73:272–273, 1986.

16. Weber G, Lui MS, Takeda E, Denton JE: Enzymology of human colon tumor. Life Sci 27:793–799, 1980.

17. Weber G, Hager JC, Lui MS, Prajda N, Tzeng DY, Jackson RC, Takeda E, Eble JN: Biochemical programs of slowly and rapidly growing human colon carcinoma xenografts. Cancer Res 41:854–859, 1981.

18. Herzfeld A, Legg MA, Greengard O: Human colon tumors: Enzymic and histoogical characteristics. Cancer 42:1280–1283, 1978.

19. Sakamoto S, Iwama T, Tsukada K, Utsunomiya J, Kawasaki T, Okamoto R: Increased activity of thymidine kinase isozyme in human colon tumor. Carcinogenesis 5:183–185, 1984.

20. Sakamoto S, Sagara T, Iwama T, Kawasaki T, Okamoto R: Increased activities of thymidine kinase isozymes in human colon polyp and carcinoma. Carcinogenesis 6:917–919, 1985.

21. Sakamoto S, Kasahara N, Kawasaki T, Kudo H, Okamoto R, Kawachi Y, Murakami S, Iwama T, Yaegashi K, Mishima Y: Thymidylate synthetase and thymidine kinase activities in DMH-induced colon carcinomas in rats and effects of UFT. Bull Tokyo Med Dent Univ 33:137–144, 1986.

22. Sakamoto S, Kuwa K, Tsukada K, Sagara T, Kasahara N, Okamoto R: Relative activities of thymidylate synthetase and thymidine kinase in 1,2-dimethylhydrazine-induced colon carcinomas in rats. Carcinogenesis 8:405–408, 1987.

23. Thurnherr N, Deschner EE, Stonehill EH, Lipkin M: Induction of adenocarcinomas of the colon in mice by weekly injections of 1,2-dimethylhydrazine. Cancer Res 33:940–945, 1973.

24. Kowal EP, Markus G: Affinity chromatography of thymidine kinase from rat colon adenocarcinoma. Prep Biochem 6:369–385, 1976.

25. Weber G, Kizaki H, Tzeng D, Shiotani T, Olah E: Colon tumor: Enzymology of the neoplastic program. Life Sci 23:729–736, 1978.

26. Ferguson-Smith MA, Westerveld A: Report of the committee on the genetic constitution of chromosomes 13,14,15,16,17,18,19,20,21, and 22. Cytogenet Cell Genet 25:59–73, 1979.

27. Hashimoto T, Arima T, Okuda H, Fujii S: Purification and properties of deoxythymidine kinase from the Yoshida sarcoma. Cancer Res 32:67–73, 1972.

28. Masui H, Garren LD: On the mechanism of action of adrenocorticotropic hormone: The stimulation of thymidine kinase activity with altered properties and changed subcellular distribution. J Biol Chem 246:5407–5413, 1971.

29. Berk AJ, Clayton DA: A genetically distinct thymidine kinase in mammalian mitochondria. J Biol Chem 248:2722–2729, 1973.

30. Lee L-S, Cheng Y-C: Human deoxythymidine kinase: Purification and general properties of the cytoplasmic and mitochondrial isozymes derived from blast cells of acute myelocytic leukemia. J Biol Chem 251:2600–2604, 1976.

31. Deschner EE: Experimentally induced cancer of the colon. Cancer 34:824–828, 1974.

32. Balis ME, Higgins PJ, Salser JS: Enzymes of normal, premalignant, and malignant colonic cells. In Bruce WR, Correa P, Lipkin M, Tannenbaum SR, Wilkins TD (eds): Banbury Report 7: Gastrointestinal Cancer: Endogenous Factors. Cold Spring Harbor, NY: Cold Spring Harbor Laboratory, 1981, pp129–139.

33. Richards TC: Early changes in the dynamics of crypt cell populations in mouse colon following administration of 1,2-dimethylhydrazine. Cancer Res 37:1680–1685, 1977.

34. Maskens AP: Confirmation of the two-step nature of chemical carcinogenesis in the rat colon adenocarcinoma model. Cancer Res 41:1240–1245, 1981.

35. Bodmer WF, Bailey CJ, Bodmer J, Bussey HJR, Ellis A, Gorman P, Lucibello FC, Murday VA, Rider SH, Scambler P, Sheer D, Solomon E, Spurr NK: Localization of the gene for familial adenomatous polyposis on chromosome 5. Nature 328:614;–616, 1987.

36. Flemington E, Bradshaw HD, Traina-Dorge V, Slagel V, Deininger PL: Sequence, structure, and promoter characterization of the human thymidine kinase gene. Gene 52:267–277.

37. Barr FG, Rajagopalan S, MacArthur CA, Lieberman MW: Genomic hypomethylation and far-5′ sequence alterations are associated with carcinogen-induced activation of the hamster thymidine kinase gene. Mol Cell Biol 6:3023–3033, 1986.

38. Stewart CJ, Ito M, Conrad SE: Evidence for transcriptional and post-transcriptional control of the cellular thymidine kinase gene. Mol Cell Biol 7:1156–1163, 1987.

39. Knight GB, Gudas JM, Pardee AB: Cell-cycle-specific interaction of nuclear DNA-binding proteins with a CCAAT sequence from the human thymidine kinase gene. Proc Natl Acad Sci USA 84:8350–8354, 1987.

40. Dutrillaux B, Muleris M: Induction of increased salvage pathways of nucleotide synthesis by dosage effect due to chromosome imbalances may be fundamental in carcinogenesis: The example of colorectal carcinoma. Ann Genet 29:11–15, 1986.

39

The Role of Protein Kinase C in Colon Neoplasia

J.G. Guillem and I.B. Weinstein

Department of Surgery, Comprehensive Cancer Center (J.G.G.) and Institute of Cancer Research (I.B.W.), Columbia University, New York, New York

INTRODUCTION

Colon carcinogenesis in humans and in experimental animal models appears to proceed through multiple distinguishable stages of initiation, promotion, and progression. Advances in our understanding of the etiology, prevention, and treatment of this disease will come, in part, from the elucidation of the molecular mechanisms governing this multistage process.

During normal multicellular growth, the behavior of individual cells is coordinated with that of others via specific hormones, growth factors, and differentiating factors that act on distant tissues (endocrine system), neighboring cells (paracrine system), and the secretory cell itself (autocrine system). A variety of signal pathways exist by which extracellular messages received by the target cell are transmitted to the cytoplasm and nucleus, thereby altering gene expression. For example, certain growth factors (i.e., platelet-derived growth factor [PDGF], epidermal growth factor [EGF] mediate their effects by activation of a tyrosine kinase. The β-adrenergic pathway involves activation of an adenyl cyclase. A third pathway of signal transduction involves the activation of a phospholipid and Ca^{2+}-dependent protein kinase, designated *protein kinase C* (PKC) [1].

Since PKC is ubiquitous and is activated by a variety of growth factors, hormones, and neurotransmitters, it would seem that PKC plays a central role in signal transduction pathways [1]. In addition, since PKC has been shown to be a high-affinity receptor for the phorbol ester tumor promoters, and since it mediates the action of certain oncogenes [for review, see 2], it would appear that PKC also plays a central role in tumor promotion and disturbances in growth control in tumors. In this chapter, we review our data, as well as that of others, which implicate a role for PKC in colon carcinogenesis.

The etiology of colon cancer, like most human neoplasms is multifactorial in nature. Hereditary factors certainly play a predominant role in the development of familial adenomatous polyposis and familial nonpolyposis colon cancer. However, in the majority of the sporadic cases of colon cancer, dietary factors probably provide the overriding impetus for their development [4,7].

Evidence obtained from epidemiologic and experimental studies suggests that high-fat diets increase the risk of cancer of the colon [3,4,7]. The exact mechanism by which this occurs remains unclear, but several observations suggest both direct and indirect effects. An early theory that related diet and colon cancer suggested that dietary factors might act by altering the composition or metabolic activity of the gut flora and, thereby, the formation of putative mutagenic and carcinogenic factors by specific bacteria in the gut [28]. Mutagenic activity has indeed been demonstrated in fecal extracts of humans, and the level of this activity varies in different populations. In a recent summary of epidemiologic stud-

Familial Adenomatous Polyposis, pages 325–332

ies of fecal mutagens [28], Schiffman has concluded that several, but not all, of these studies show an apparent correlation between colon cancer risk and levels of fecal mutagens. On the other hand, he emphasized the need for further prospective studies to determine the possible causal significance of this correlation.

The mutagenic activity in human feces appears to be largely attributable to a group of compounds the fecapentaenes, which are potent direct acting mutagens in the Ames bacterial mutagenesis assay [28]. These compounds are produced by *Bateroides* species present in the human colon. At the present time, however, it is not clear whether fecapentaenes or other fecal mutagens play a causal role in human colon cancer, acting for example as an initiating agent.

Other types of evidence suggest that dietary lipid might increase colon cancer risk by enhancing cellular proliferation or acting through mechanisms analogous to those of certain known tumor promoters. In a mouse system, an orally administered fat bolus resulted in damage to the colonic epithelium and subsequent increased cell proliferation, suggestive of a promotion-like effect [5]. Several studies have documented an increased excretion of secondary bile acids in the feces of animals chronically fed a high-fat diet [6]. In addition, epidemiological studies have demonstrated a positive correlation between colon cancer incidence and elevated levels of secondary bile acids in the feces [7], suggesting that bile acids themselves may be directly involved in the carcinogenic process. In a bacterial test system, secondary bile acids are not mutagenic, although a comutagenic effect has been observed [8]. The bulk of experimental evidence, however, favors the concept that bile acids act as tumor promoters in colon carcinogenesis. Intrarectal injections or oral feeding of primary or secondary bile acids to rats that had been previously treated with MNNG or MNU enhanced the formation of colon tumors [9,10]. However, no tumor formation was seen in the rats treated with bile acids alone. This is in accordance with the definition of a tumor promoter as a compound that has weak or no carcinogenic activity when tested alone, but markedly enhances tumor yield when applied repeatedly following a low or suboptimal dose of an initiating carcinogen (Fig. 1).

The exact mechanism by which bile acids might function as tumor promoters is not known, but several observations suggest that they trigger a set of cellular responses somewhat similar to those seen with the intensively studied phorbol ester skin tumor promotor, designated TPA. Bile acids have been shown to increase ornithine decarboxylase (ODC) activity [11] and phospho-

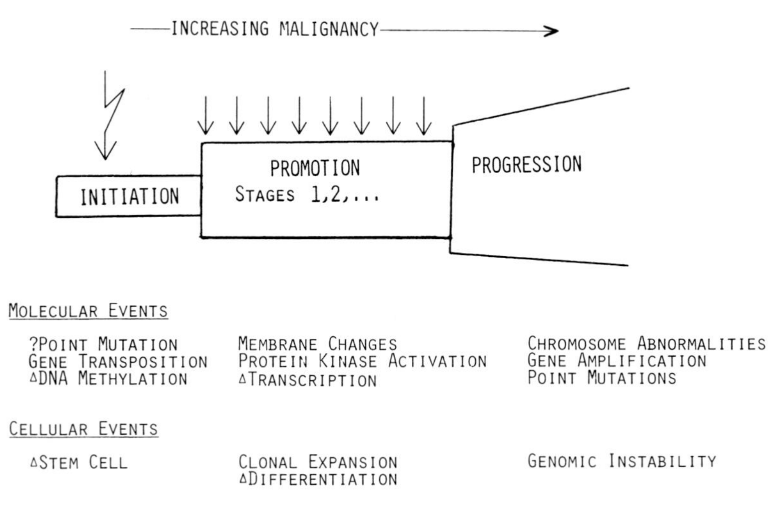

Fig. 1. Actions of tumor promoters.

lipid turnover in the rat colonic epithelium [12]. Since increased ODC activity, phospholipid turnover, and PKC activitation often occur as related events in cells undergoing a mitogenic stimulus [1], a PKC-mediated process for bile acid tumor promotion seems plausible.

In different cell types, a variety of agents, including TPA, EGF, PDGF, and serum elicit a pleiotypic mitogenic response that includes: increased transport of ions and hexoses; increased turnover of phospholipids; increased activity of rate-limiting enzymes such as ODC; increased mRNA production for several gene sequences, including *fos, myc,* actin, ODC and phorbin; and increased activity of several protein kinases, including PKC (Fig. 2).

The exact sequence of events in the mitogenic process have not been fully unraveled, but certain steps are now well described. After mitogenic growth factors interact with their respective membrane-associated receptors, phospholipase C is activated, which leads to the hydrolysis of phosphatidylinositol 4,5-diphosphate to yield diacylglycerol (DAG) and inositol 1,4,5-triphosphate (IP_3). DAG then activates PKC, and IP_3 triggers calcium release from storage sites in the endoplasmic reticulum, thus raising intracellular levels of Ca^{2+}. DAG activates PKC by binding to it and causing it to translocate to cell membranes, where in the presence of a phospholipid, such as phosphatidyl-serine, and calcium, the kinase becomes activated. Once activated, PKC phosphorylates several intracellular protein subtrates, including the EGF receptors, the insulin receptor, the cellular oncogene protein $pp60^{src}$, ion channels, and cytoskeletal proteins.

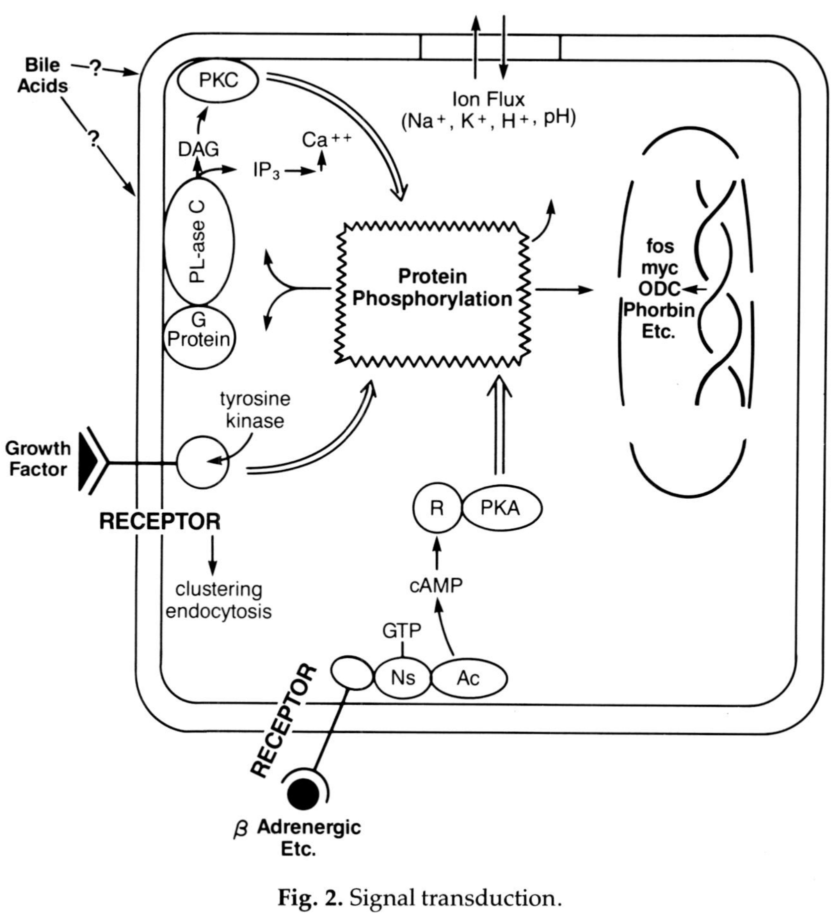

Fig. 2. Signal transduction.

Since several structurally diverse tumor promoters, in addition to the phorbol esters, can activate PKC, it appears plausible that endogenous tumor promoters such as bile acids could also mediate their biological effects through PKC. Our first set of experiments were aimed at addressing this question.

BILE ACID REGULATION OF PKC

Subcellular Studies

Using partially purified rat brain PKC, we tested nine different bile acids for their ability to activate or inhibit PKC in a cell-free system containing 1 mM Ca^{2+} and 30 μg/ml phosphatidylserine (PS). Under these conditions, deoxycholate and chenodeoxycholate acids inhibited PKC, whereas seven structurally related bile acids did not (Table 1). In addition, neither the glyco- nor tauro-conjugated derivatives of deoxy- and chenodeoxycholate acids inhibited PKC, suggesting specific structural requirements for PKC inactivation [13].

Since PKC activation is both Ca^{2+} and phospholipid dependent and since bile acids can form calcium soaps, it was conceivable that inhibition by bile acids of PKC was simply due to their Ca^{2+} chelating properties. This seemed unlikely, however, since the glyco-conjugated derivatives, which are stronger Ca^{2+} chelators than chenodeoxycholate and deoxycholate, did not inhibit PKC. To explore this aspect further, we increased the concentration of Ca^{2+} in our reaction mixture from 1 to 2 mM. We found that this doubling of Ca^{2+} concentration resulted not only in a relief of inhibition but an actual twofold enhancement of PKC activity. This effect was seen with nine different bile acids tested (Table 2). This finding is of particular biological significance since bile acids are normally present in the colon at mM concentrations, which is the concentration range at which we found bile acid activation of PKC.

Several studies have shown that low concentrations of deoxy- and chenodeoxycholate can perturb the membrane structure of rat colonic mucosal cells [14]. This would imply interaction with membrane phospholipids. We found a reduction in the cheno- and deoxycholate acid inhibition of PKC when we increased the phosphatidyl-serine (PS) concentration from 30 to 80 μg/ml in the subcellular reaction mixture. Our first set of studies in a subcellular system, suggested therefore, that the activation of PKC by chenodeoxycholate and deoxycholate acid resulted from a complex interaction between Ca^{2+}, PS, and specific bile acids. To extend our findings on isolated PKC to the *in vivo* situation, the following cellular studies were performed.

Cellular Translocation Studies

PKC is normally found in both the cytosolic and membrane compartments of cells at levels

TABLE 1.
Effects of Various Bile Acids on PKC Activity in the Presence of 1 mM Ca^{2+}

Bile acid	Concentration tested (mM)	Percent inhibition
Deoxycholate	1.4	50
Chenodeoxycholate	1.4	78
Cholate	2	<10
Glycholate	2	<10
Taurocholate	2	<10
Glycochenodeoxycholate	2	<10
Taurochenodeoxycholate	1.4	<10
Glycodeoxycholate	1.2	<10
Taurodeoxycholate	2	<10

TABLE 2.
Effects of Increased (2 mM) Calcium Concentration on Bile Acid Regulation of PKC

Bile acid	PKC fold stimulation
Deoxycholate	2.1
Chenodeoxycholate	1.4
Cholate	1.8
Glycocholate	1.7
Taurocholate	1.8
Glycochenodeoxycholate	1.6
Taurochenodeoxycholate	2.5
Glycodeoxycholate	2.6
Taurodeoxycholate	2.7

that vary from tissue to tissue and also with the physiological state of a tissue. Treatment of cells with TPA results in a translocation of PKC from the cytosol to the membrane fraction and subsequent down-regulation of enzyme activity, as well as down-regulation of phorbol ester receptor binding. The down-regulation results from proteolysis of the enzyme [for review, see 2]. Since bile-acid induced activation of isolated PKC mimicked that of TPA, it was of interest to compare the effects of bile acids with those of TPA on cellular levels and compartmentalization of PKC [15].

We found that treatment of mouse embryo fibroblasts (C3H 10T1/2 cells) with 200 μmol/Liter of deoxycholic acid (DOA) for 15 minutes caused a redistribution of PKC activity present in the cytosolic and particulate fractions (Fig. 3). This redistribution from the cytosol to the membrane fraction ranged from 24 to 43% of the cells' total PKC activity. Compared with

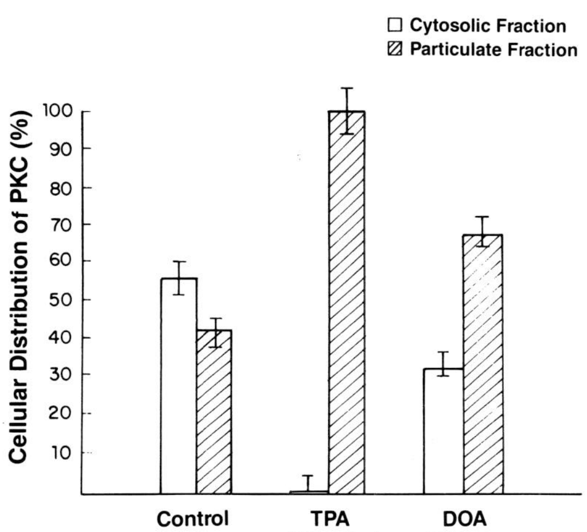

Fig. 3. Redistribution of protein kinase C (PKC) activity after C3H-10T1/2 cells were treated with either 12-O-tetradecanoyl-phorbol-13-acetate (TPA, 0.2 μmol/liter [100 μg/liter]) or deoxycholic acid (DOA, 200 μmol/liter) for 15 minutes. Control cells were treated with Dulbecco's phosphate-buffered saline (D-PBS) with or without dimethylsulfoxide for 15 minutes. Open bars indicate cytosolic fraction; hatched bars, particulate fraction.

TPA, DOA had a weaker, yet pronounced, effect on PKC translocation. Time course studies revealed that the effect of DOA on the translocation of PKC activity was rapid, and similar to the effect of TPA (Fig. 4). Maximal translocation occurred within 15 minutes of exposure of the cells to DOA.

Cellular Gene Expression Studies

ODC is the first and rate-limiting enzyme in the polyamine biosynthetic pathway [16]. Studies have shown increased ODC activity in human colon polyps and carcinomas [17,18]. In addition, ODC activity is increased in rat colonic mucosa exposed to colon carcinogens. It is also increased by the addition of bile acids or a high-fat diet [11], which as discussed above appear to act as tumor promoters. Because of the apparent role of ODC in colon carcinogenesis, knowledge of its regulation is important. Since, however, previous studies measured only ODC enzyme activity, it was not clear whether this bile-induced increase in ODC activity was mediated at a transcriptional or post-transcriptional level.

Previous studies have shown that the exposure of C3H 10T 1/2 cells to TPA causes an increase in ODC mRNA levels, that is maximal at about

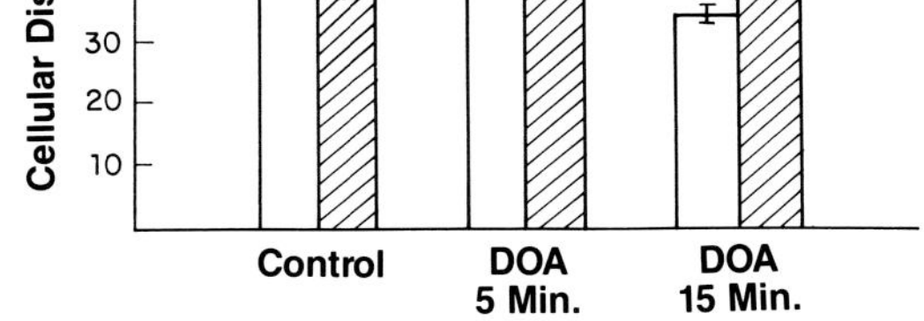

Fig. 4. Redistribution of protein kinase C (PKC) activity after C3H-10T1/2 cells were treated with deoxycholic acid (DOA, 200 μ mol/liter) for either 5 or 15 minutes. Control cells were treated with Dulbecco's phosphate-buffered saline (D-PBS) with or without dimethylsulfoxide for 15 minutes. Open bars indicate cytosolic fraction; hatched bars, particulate fraction.

4 hours [19]. We, examined therefore, the effects of DOA on ODC mRNA levels in the same cells after a 4 hour exposure time. In a manner analogous to TPA, DOA treatment of C3H-10T1/2 cells resulted in a dose-dependent increase in ODC mRNA levels. With increasing concentrations of DOA (10, 50, and 250 μM), the cells contained increasing levels of ODC mRNA (4, 15, and 18 times greater, respectively) when compared to control cells exposed to only to the solvent PBS (Fig. 5). These results suggest that the increased ODC enzyme activity induced by DOA may be due to an increase in expression of the ODC gene, either through increased transcription or mRNA stabilization. These results, along with those obtained on PKC activation and translocation, provide evidence that DOA can mimic TPA-like effects and thus it might also function as a tumor promoter through the activation of PKC.

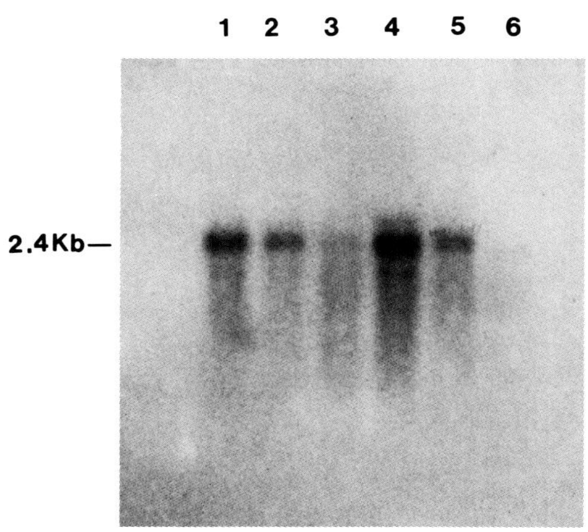

Fig. 5. Effects of 12-O-tetradecanoyl-phorbol-13-acetate and increasing concentrations of deoxycholic acid (DOA) on ornithine decarboxylase messenger RNA levels. Postconfluent C3H-10T1/2 cells were treated with one of the following solutions: lane 1,250 μmol/liter of DOA; lane 2, 50 μmol/liter of DOA; lane 3, 10 μmol/liter of DOA; lane 4, 0.2 μmol/liter (100 ng/mL) of 12-O-tetradecanoyl-phorbol-13-acetate in dimethylsulfoxide (DMSO) (final DMSO concentration, 0.1%); lane 5, 0.1% DMSO; and lane 6, phosphate-buffered saline. Total cellular RNA was isolated 4 hours after treatment, and 20 μg of each sample was fractionated by electrophoresis in a denaturing gel, transferred to Hybond-N membranes, hybridized to ^{32}P-labeled ornithine decarboxylase probe, and underwent autoradiography.

DOWN-REGULATION OF PKC

Time-course studies on a TPA-treated breast cancer cell line (MCF-7) have demonstrated an initial translocation of the enzyme from the cytosol to the membrane. Prolonged exposure to TPA resulted in decreased total PKC activity and apparent down-regulation of the PKC enzyme [20]. Since the colon cancer-promoting properties of bile acids can, in part, be explained through their interactions with PKC (see above), it was of interest to examine the phenomenom of PKC down-regulation in colon cancers. To do this, we compared the levels and compartmentalizations of PKC in the normal colon mucosa and colon tumors of patients with colon cancer.

Our initial results on nine human specimens demonstrated that PKC activity was uniformly reduced in all of the colon tumor samples examined, when each sample was compared with its normal adjacent colon mucosa [21]. The average specific PKC activity ratios were 5.1 (normal cytosolic/carcinoma cytosolic) and 3.7 (normal particulate/carcinoma particulate) [21]. Subsequent studies on a panel of 30 pairs of colon cancers and respective adjacent normal mucosa samples have corroborated our initial findings. All colonic tumors, irrespective of the Dukes' stage had reduced PKC activity. The average reduction was about threefold (unpublished data).

A POSSIBLE SYNERGISTIC INTERACTION BETWEEN ONCOGENES AND PKC DURING COLON CARCINOGENESIS

Other investigators have shown that rat kidney cells transformed by either the k-ras or sis oncogenes have elevated levels of diacylglycerol (DAG) [22], although the precise mechanism is not known. Since DAG is an endogenous activator of PKC [2], these results suggest that cells expressing an activated ras oncogene would experience persistent activation of PKC. This persistent exposure to increased levels of DAG might produce effects similar to those of chronic exposure to TPA, and thus result in down-regulation of PKC activity in transformed cells. A recent report demonstrated that transfection of C3H–10T1/2 fibroblasts with an activated human Ha-ras oncogene was associated with a significant decrease in the level of PKC [23]. These observations indicate that PKC is, indeed, down-regulated in ras-transformed cells. These findings might be directly relevant to our finding that colon tumors have decreased levels of PKC (21), since recent studies indicate that human colon tumors frequently have mutations in codon 12 of the c-k-ras oncogene [24,25]. Thus, the abnormal growth of colon tumors may be due, at least in part, to a synergistic interaction between the activated c-k-ras oncogene and PKC. Since only about 40% of human colon carcinomas display this c-k-ras mutation, and yet we found decreased levels of PKC in 100% of colon tumors, it is possible that the remaining 60% of colon tumors have mutations in another oncogene(s) that also leads to activation and down-regulation of PKC. It will be of interest, therefore, to search for these putative mutations in the latter set of colon tumors. We and others have found increased levels of c-myc RNA in both human [26] and rat [27] colon cancers. It is possible that this also reflects persistent activation of PKC, since the activation of PKC by treating cell with TPA or certain growth factors is known to activate c-myc expression [1]. Alternatively, the increased expression of c-myc in colon tumors may reflect additional disturbances in signal transduction that remain to be elucidated.

OVERVIEW AND FUTURE DIRECTIONS

The above results and speculations suggest how multiple factors might interact during the multistage process of colon carcinogenesis. Mutational changes in the c-k-ras oncogene, and possibly other oncogenes, resulting from the action of fecal mutagens or occurring spontaneously, could lead to persistent activation of PKC. In addition, increased levels of fecal bile acids associated with a lipid-rich diet could also activate PKC and thus enhance proliferation of the colonic epithelium. Since certain bacteria can produce high levels of specific phospholipases [28], we further speculate that this could lead to increased levels of DAG in the intestinal lumen, particularly in individuals on a lipid-rich diet. This could also stimulate PKC in the colonic epithelium and contribute to tumor formation. Studies are in progress to examine this possibility. Colon tumors in patients with familial polyposis, and also sporadic colon tumors, often display not only activation of the c-k-ras oncogene, but also deletions in specific cellular genes. The normal functions of these genes is not yet known, but it is possible that their loss also contributes to alterations in the PKC system, or other critical pathways of signal transductions that play a role in growth control. Obviously, much more research is required to understand the multiple environmental and genetic factors involved in human colon cancer causation. Nevertheless, rapid advances are being made through the application of methods and concepts of signal transduction and molecular genetics. Hopefully, this knowledge will lead to more effective approaches to the prevention and treatment of this major human cancer.

ACKNOWLEDGMENTS

This research was supported by National Cancer Institute grant CA26056 and an Award from the Aaron Diamond Foundation (to I.B.W.). J.G.G. is the recipient of a Phyllis Jacobs Rubenstein-Arthur Jacobs Fellowship in Surgical Oncology.

References

1. Weinstein IB: Growth factors, oncogenes and multistage carcinogenesis. J Cell Biochem 33:213–224, 1987.
2. Nishizuka Y: Studies and perspectives of protein kinase C. Science 233:305–312, 1986.
3. Bull AW, Soullier BK, Wilson PS, et al.: Promotion of azoxymethane-induced intestinal cancer by high-fat diets in rats. Cancer Res 39:4956–4959, 1979.
4. Doll R, Peto R: The causes of cancer: Quantitative estimates of avoidable risks of cancer in the United States today. J Natl Cancer Inst 66:1191–1308, 1981.
5. Bird RP, Medline A, Furrer R, Bruce WR: Toxicity of orally administered fat to the colonic epithelium of mice. Carcinogenesis (in press), 1988.
6. Reddy BS, Weisburger JH, Wynder EL: Effect of dietary fat level and dimethylhydrazine on fecal acid and neutral sterol excretion and colon carcinogenesis in rats. 52:507–511, 1974.

7. Reddy BS, Wynder EL: Large bowel carcinogenesis: Fecal constituents of populations with diverse incidence rates of colon cancer. J Natl Cancer Inst 50:1437–1442, 1973.

8. Silverman SJ, Andrews AW: Bile acids: Comutagenic activity in the salmonella-mammalian-microsome mutagenesis test. J Natl Cancer Inst 59:1557–1559, 1977.

9. Narisawa T, Magadia NE, Weisburger JH, Wynder EL: Promoting effects of bile acids on colon carcinogenesis after intrarectal instillation of N-methyl-N-nitrosoguanine in rats. J Natl Cancer Inst 53:1093–1095, 1974.

10. Sarwal AN, Cohen BI, Raicht RF, Takahashi M, Fazzini E: Effects of dietary administration of chenodeoxycholate on N-methyl-N-nitrosourea–induced colon cancer in rats. Biochim Biophys Acta 574:423–432, 1979.

11. Takano S, Akagi M, Bryan GT: Stimulation of ornithine decarboxylase activity and DNA synthesis by phorbol esters or bile acids in rat colon. Gann 75:29–35, 1984.

12. Craven PA, Pfanstiel J, Saito R, et al.: Relationship between loss of rat colonic surface epithelium induced by deoxycholate and initiation of the subsequent proliferative response. Cancer Res 46:5754–5759, 1986.

13. Fitzer CJ, O'Brian CA, Guillem JG, et al.: The regulation of protein kinase C by chenodeoxycholate, deoxycholate and several structurally related bile acids. Carcinogenesis 8:217–220, 1987.

14. Chadwick VS, Gagimella TS, Carlson JC, et al.: Effect of molecular structure on bile acid-induced alterations in absorptive function, permeability, and morphology in the perfused rabbit colon. J Lab Clin Med 94:661–674, 1979.

15. Guillem JG, O'Brian CA, Fitzer CJ, et al.: Studies on protein kinase C and colon carcinogenesis. Arch Surg 122:1475–1478, 1987.

16. Pegg AE, McCann PP: Polyamine metabolism and function. Am J Physiol 243:C212–221, 1982.

17. Luk GD, Baylin SB: Ornithine decarboxylase as a biologic marker in familial colonic polyposis. N Eng J Med 311:80–83, 1984.

18. Rozhin J, Wilson PS, Bull AW, Nigro ND: Ornithine decarboxylase activity in the rat and human colon. Cancer Res 44:3226–3230, 1984.

19. Verma AK, Pong RC, Erickson D: Involvement of protein kinase C in ornithine decarboxylase gene expression in primary culture of newborn mouse epidermal cells and in skin tumor promotion by 12-O-tetradecanoylphorbol-13-acetate. Cancer Res 46:6149–6155, 1986.

20. Darbon J, Issandou M, Delassus F, et al.: Phorbol esters induce both intracellular translocation and down-regulation of protein kinase C in MCF-7 cells. Biochem Biophys Res Commun 137:1159–1166, 1986.

21. Guillem JG, O'Brian CA, Fitzer CJ, et al.: Altered levels of protein kinase C and Ca^{2+}-dependent protein kinases in human colon carcinomas. Cancer Res 47:2036–2039, 1987.

22. Preiss J, Loomis CR, Bishop WR, et al.: Quantitative measurement of sn-1,2-diacylglycerols present in platelets, hepatocytes and ras- and sis-transformed normal rat kidney cells. J Biol Chem 261:8597–8600, 1986.

23. Weyman CM, Taparowsky EJ, Wolfson M, Ashendel CL: Partial down-regulation of protein kinase C in C3H-10T1/2 mouse fibroblasts transfected with the human Ha-ras oncogene. Cancer Res 48:6535–6541, 1988.

24. Forrester K, Almoguera C, Han K, et al.: Detection of high incidence of K-ras oncogenes during human colon tumorigenesis. Nature 327:293–297, 1987.

25. Bos JL, Fearon ER, Hamilton SR, et al.: Prevalence of ras gene mutations in human colorectal cancers. Nature 327:293–297, 1987.

26. Guillem JG, Levy MF, Hsieh LL, et al.: Overexpression of c-myc RNA may be a useful biomarker for studies on human colon cancer. Arch Surg (Submitted), 1988.

27. Guillem JG, Hsieh LL, O'Toole KM, et al.: Changes in expression of oncogenes and endogenous retroviral-like sequences during colon carcinogenesis. Cancer Res 48:3964–71, 1988.

28. Berk RS, Brown D, Coutinho I, and Meyers D: In vivo studies with two phospholipase C fractions from *Pseudomonas aeruginosa*. Infect Immun 1728–1730, 1987.

29. Schiffman MH: Epidemiology of fecal mutagenicity. Epidemiology Reviews. 8:92–105, 1986.

40

Monoclonal Antibodies and Carbohydrate Differentiation Antigens as Markers for Colonic Neoplasia

Andrea Quaroni, Lemuel Herrera, Milton M. Weiser, and Nicholas J. Petrelli

Section of Physiology, Cornell University, Ithaca, New York (A.Q.); Surgical Developmental Oncology, Roswell Park Memorial Institute, Buffalo, New York (L.H., N.J.P.); Division of Gastroenterology, Buffalo General Hospital, Buffalo, New York (M.M.W.)

INTRODUCTION

There is much evidence to suggest that alterations in the structure and/or distribution of cell surface glycoconjugates may be, at least in part, responsible for the abnormal behavior of tumor cells both in vivo and in vitro. These changes have been correlated with various properties of malignant cells such as loss of contact inhibition, a decrease in cell adhesion, increased growth rates, ability to form metastases in specific organs, escape from host immune surveillance, and expression of new antigens at the surface of the cells. Early studies of cell surface glycoproteins and glycolipids have focused mainly on virally or chemically transformed fibroblastic cells in culture, but similar alterations in cell surface glycoconjugates have been more recently demonstrated in tumor cells of epithelial origin in culture and in solid tumors in vivo. Of particular interest to colon cancer are changes in structure and histochemical staining properties of goblet cell mucins, which have been shown to represent early markers for intestinal dysplasia and/or neoplasia [1,2]. Lectins and antisera specific for human blood group antigens have been used extensively in these studies [3,4]. Tumors in the proximal colon have been shown to lack the blood group antigens present in the normal colonic mucosa, and the opposite situation has been described for the distal colon [5–9]. Differences in the structure of mucin, the major secreted glycoprotein in the colon, have been described using histochemical methods in normal colonic mucosa, cancerous tissues, and transitional mucosa located near colonic cancer [2,10,11]. The lectin from *Arachis hypogaea* (peanut agglutinin [PNA] was found to bind mucin in all the colonic cancers studied, but not to mucin in normal colon [10]. Similar changes in lectin binding patterns were observed in the transitional mucosa and in colonic polyps.

MONOCLONAL ANTIBODIES AND COLON CANCER

Application of the hybridoma technique to produce epitope-specific monoclonal antibodies to surface membrane antigens of tumor cells has increased enormously the panel of reagents that can be used to detect alterations in cell surface components associated with malignant transformation. As soon as this new methodology became established, a large number of studies were initiated with the hope of discovering unique cell surface antigens specific for different stages of oncogenesis, embryogenesis, and cellular differentiation. Although potentially interesting antibodies with the desired characteristics were readily obtained, detailed biochemical studies of the antigens for which they were specific have, in most cases, revealed that such antigens are

Familial Adenomatous Polyposis, pages 333–335

mainly carbohydrate structures of glycoproteins and glycolipids occurring in many different cell types. Many of them have been found to correspond to already known human blood group antigens, although the significance of this observation is still unclear [12].

Among the best known and extensively studied antigens of this type, detected using monoclonal antibodies prepared against tumor or embryonic cells, are the stage-specific embryonic antigen SSEA-1 (recognized by several monoclonal antibodies independently derived by different groups) [13–17], the gastrointestinal cancer-associated antigen (GICA) defined by antibody CA19.9 and identified as sialylated lacto-N-fucopentaose II [18,19], and various carbohydrate structures defined by monoclonal antibodies prepared against purified glycolipids, in many cases containing fucosylated type 1 or type 2 backbone groups and with di- or trimeric X determinants [20,21]. An antiserum against 3′-fucosyllactose has been used to stain human colonic adenocarcinomas by immunofluorescence [22]. In many cases, these "oncofetal" carbohydrate structures have been found to be associated with both glycolipids and glycoproteins produced by different normal and tumor cells [23].

A group of seven monoclonal antibodies prepared against brush border membranes purified from fetal rat intestine [24] and from the human colon tumor cell line Caco-2 [25] have revealed an intriguing relationship among fetal intestinal cells, normal small intestinal crypt cells, and colonic tumor cells. An attractive feature of the antigens they recognize is their occurrence in both rat and human colonic cancer, thus providing an important experimental model system for the study of their expression during tumor ontogeny. The antigen(s) recognized by these antibodies have been called *crypt cell antigens* (CCA), characterized as high molecular weight (glyco)proteins in both rat intestine and the human colon tumor cell line CaCo-2, and appear to be associated with unique carbohydrate structures and protein kinase activity [26]. In the fetal rat, the CCA were found to be first expressed at about day 15 of gestation, when intense staining of the epithelial–mesenchymal junction and of the entire epithelium was observed [27]. The antibodies to CCA were found to stain the rat large intestine only during a specific stage of development, comprising the last 3–4 days of fetal life and the first 7–10 days after birth [28]. No staining of any portion of both human and rat adult large intestine was observed. In contrast, the CCA were expressed in 13 of 14 human colon tumor cell lines examined [29]. In dimethylhydrazine-induced colonic and small intestinal rat neoplasms they were detected predominantly in poorly and moderately differentiated tumors [28]. Antigen expression was much less intense in well-differentiated tumors, and about one-half of them were negative. Essentially identical findings have been described in the case of human colonic tumors, providing valuable new markers for poorly differentiated human intestinal tumor cells, which have often been found not to react with other available antibodies or lectins.

To date, the basic cellular alteration(s) in cancer cells that are responsible for the expression of these and other monoclonal antibody-defined oncofetal surface antigens, and the biological function(s) of these altered cell products, have eluded the intense investigation to which they have been subjected. It is generally assumed that they may play a vital role in cellular interactions occurring at specific stages of embryogenesis and oncogenesis, but their mechanism(s) of action are essentially still unknown.

However, these newly characterized monoclonal antibodies have many potentially important applications as histological and clinical markers for colon cancer, including their use in serological assays, imaging of tumors and metastases in vivo, and histological classification of polyps and tumors.

References

1. Filipe MI: Mucous secretion in rat colonic mucosa during carcinogenesis induced by dimethylhydrazine. A morphological and histochemical study. Br J Cancer 32:60–77, 1975.
2. Filipe MI, Branfoot AC: Abnormal patterns of mucus secretion in apparently normal mucosa of large intestine with carcinoma. Cancer 34:282–290, 1974.
3. Jacobs LR, Huber PW: Regional distribution and alterations of lectin binding to colorectal mucin in mucosal

biopsies from controls and subjects with inflammatory bowel disease. J Clin Invest 75:112–118, 1985.

4. Yonezawa S, Nakamura T, Tanaka S, Sato E: Glycoconjugate with *Ulex euopaeus* agglutinin-I binding sites in normal mucosa, adenoma, and carcinoma of the human large bowel. JNCI 69:777–785, 1982.
5. Wiley EL, Mendelsohn G, Eggleston JC: Distribution of carcinoembryonic antigens and blood group substances in adenocarcinoma of the colon. Lab Invest 44:507–513, 1981.
6. Boland CR, Montgomery CK, Kim YS: A cancer-associated mucin alteration in benign colonic polyps. Gastroenterology 82:664–672, 1982.
7. Bresalier RS, Boland CR, Kim YS: Regional differences in normal and cancer-associated glycoconjugates of the human colon. JNCI 75:249–260, 1985.
8. Yuan M, Itzkowitz SH, Palekar A, Shamsuddin AM, Phelps PC, Trump BF, Kim YS: Distribution of blood group antigens A, B, H, Lewis[a], and Lewis[b] in human normal, fetal, and malignant colonic tissue. Cancer Res 45:4499–4511, 1985.
9. Kim YS, Yuan M, Itzkowitz SH, Sun QB, Kaizu T, Palekar A, Trump BF, Hakomori S: Expression of LeY and extended LeY blood-group related antigens in human malignant, premalignant, and nonmalignant colonic tissues. Cancer Res 46:5895–5992, 1986.
10. Boland CR, Montgomery CK, Kim YS: Alterations in human colonic mucin occurring with cellular differentiation and malignant transformation. Proc Natl Acad Sci USA 79:2051–2055, 1982.
11. Yamori T, Kimura H, Stewart K, Ota DM, Cleary KR, Irimura T: Differential production of high molecular weight sulfated glycoproteins in normal colonic mucosa, primary colon carcinoma, and metastases. Cancer Res 47:2741–2747, 1987.
12. Watanabe K, Hakomori SI: Status of blood group carbohydrate chains in ontogenesis and in oncogenesis. J Exp Med 144:644–653, 1976.
13. Solter D, Knowles BB: Monoclonal antibody defining a stage-specific mouse embryonic antigen. Proc Natl Acad Sci USA 75:5565–5569, 1978.
14. Knowles BB, Rappaport J, Solter D: Murine embryonic antigen (SSEA-1) is expressed on human cells and structurally related human blood group antigen I is expressed on mouse embryos. Dev Biol 93:54–58, 1982.
15. Shi ZR, McIntyre LJ, Knowles BB, Solter D, Kim YS: Expression of a carbohydrate differentiation antigen, stage-specific embryonic antigen 1, in human colonic adenocarcinoma. Cancer Res 44:1142–1147, 1984.
16. Hara A, Watanabe M, Kodaira S, Teramoto T: The expression of stage-specific embryonic antigen 1 in the noncancerous colorectal epithelia of familial polyposis coli. Dis Colon Rectum 30:440–443, 1987.
17. Fox N, Damjanov I, Knowles BB, Solter D: Immunohistochemical localization of the mouse stage-specific embryonic antigen 1 in human tissues and tumors. Cancer Res 43:669–678, 1983.
18. Magnani JL, Brockhaus M, Smith DF, Ginsburg V, Blaszczyk M, Mitchell KF, Steplewski Z, Koprowski H: A monosialoganglioside is a monoclonal antibody-defined antigen of colon carcinoma. Science 212:55–56, 1981.
19. Magnani JL, Nilsson B, Brockhaus M, Zopf D, Steplewski Z, Koprowski H, Ginsburg V: A monoclonal antibody-defined antigen associated with gastrointestinal cancer is a ganglioside containing sialylated lacto-N-fucopentaose II. J Biol Chem 257:14365–14369, 1982.
20. Fukushi Y, Hakomori S, Shepard T: Localization and alteration of mono-, di-, and trifucosyl alpha 1-3 type 2 chain structures during human embryogenesis and in human cancer. J Exp Med 160:506–520, 1984.
21. Feizi T: Mucin-type glycoproteins. Biochem Soc Trans 12:591–596, 1984.
22. Miyauchi T, Yonezawa S, Takamura T, Chiba T, Tejima S, Ozawa M, Sato E, Muramatzu T: A new fucosyl antigen expressed on colon adenocarcinoma and embryonal carcinoma cells. Nature 299:168–169, 1982.
23. Magnani JL, Steplewski Z, Koprowski H, Ginsburg V: Identification of the gastrointestinal and pancreatic cancer-associated antigen detected by monoclonal antibody 19-9 in the sera of patients as a mucin. Cancer Res 43:5489–5492, 1983.
24. Quaroni A: Crypt cell development in newborn rat small intestine. J Cell Biol 100:1601–1610, 1985.
25. Quaroni A: Crypt cell antigen expression in human tumor colonic cell lines. Analysis with a panel of monoclonal antibodies to CaCo-2 luminal membrane components. J Natl Cancer Inst 76:571–585, 1986.
26. Quaroni A, Weiser MM, Herrera L, Fay D: Crypt cell antigens (CCA): New carbohydrate markers for human colon cancer cells. Immunol Invest (in press), 1989.
27. Quaroni A: Fetal characteristics of small intestinal crypt cells. Proc Natl Acad Sci USA 83:1723–1727, 1986.
28. Quaroni A, Weiser MM, Lee S, Amodeo D: Expression of developmentally regulated crypt cell antigens in human and rat intestinal tumors. J Natl Cancer Inst 77:405–415, 1986.
29. Quaroni A: Expression of YBB3/10 antigen in human tumor colon cell lines and its induction by N,N-dimethylformamide. J Natl Cancer Inst 74:591–602, 1985.

41

Expression and Mutational Activation of the c-K-ras Oncogene in Human Colorectal Adenomas and Carcinomas

Kathleen Forrester, Concepcion Almoguera, Concepcion Lama, Jordan Dunitz, Hidenori Kawanishi, William E. Grizzle, and Manuel Perucho

Department of Biochemistry, State University of New York at Stony Brook, Stony Brook (K.F., C.A., C.L., J.D., M.P.) and Department of Pathology, Veterans Administration Medical Center, Northport (H.K.), New York; Department of Pathology, University of Alabama at Birmingham and the Birmingham Veterans Administration Medical Center, Birmingham, Alabama (W.E.G.); Research Program Director, California Institute of Biological Research, La Jolla, California (M.P.)

INTRODUCTION

It is becoming a paradigm in cancer research that combinations of genetic alterations leading to the activation of multiple cellular oncogenes, in conjunction with those resulting in the loss of suppressor functions of these activated oncogenes, are the underlying cause for neoplastic development [Bishop, 1987]. Oncogenes are a class of genes that have the potential to cause neoplastic growth and are the active forms of certain cellular genes (proto-oncogenes) involved in cell growth and differentiation. Diverse structural alterations in proto-oncogenes that lead to functional alterations in their encoded proteins are responsible for the activation of their oncogenic potential.

One of the most intense efforts in current cancer research is aimed at understanding the role that oncogenes play in the process of tumorigenesis. At the molecular genetic level, two main approaches are being used for this purpose. One is the use of carcinogen-induced animal tumor model systems in which, to some extent, the experimental parameters can be controlled. This allows a detailed dissection of the molecular events occurring during the carcinogenesis process. The other is the descriptive analysis of the association of particular oncogenes with defined types of spontaneous tumors, which therefore includes human cancer. An additional advantage of these studies is their potential for development of new approaches for cancer diagnosis and prognosis at the molecular genetic level.

It has become evident from these studies that the oncogenes more often associated with human cancer are the ras oncogenes, a group of closely related genes: c-H-ras, c-K-ras, and N-ras [for a recent review see Barbacid, 1987]. These highly conserved genes encode structurally similar proteins of 188–189 amino acids that are located in the inner surface of the cellular membrane, possess guanine nucleotide binding activity, and are able to hydrolize the bound guanosine triphosphate (GTP) to guanosine diphosphate (GDP) both in vitro and in vivo. These properties suggest that ras proteins belong to the group of G proteins involved in the process of signal transduction across the cell membrane. However, definitive characterization of ras proteins as G proteins in animal cells, as well as the metabolic pathway(s) through which they carry out their cellular function(s), remain to be determined.

The mechanism that activates the oncogenic potential of ras proto-oncogenes has been established as point mutations resulting in single amino

Familial Adenomatous Polyposis, pages 337–346

acid substitutions in the encoded proteins at several preferential positions. These mutations activate the transforming activity of ras genes in immortalized rodent fibroblasts [for review, see Varmus, 1984; Marshall, 1985]. This property was the reason for the rediscovery of ras genes by DNA transfection experiments in the early 1980s, because total genomic DNA from some tumor cell lines [Shih et al., 1979, 1981; Krontiris and Cooper, 1981; Perucho et al., 1981; Pulciani et al., 1982] and primary tumors [Pulciani et al., 1982] induced foci of morphologically transformed cells in NIH3T3 mouse fibroblasts. Alterations in the function of ras proteins resulting from those amino acid changes increase their oncogenic potential in vivo by at least two orders of magnitude. The mechanisms responsible for this drastic change in protein function are unknown. It is clear, however, that while mutant ras protein retain their ability to bind GTP, the GTPase activity of many of these oncogenic proteins is considerably decreased. It has been postulated that the inability of mutant ras proteins to hydrolyze the bound GTP might ''freeze'' them in their activated state, resulting in their oncogenic activation. In vitro, the decrease in GTPase activity is about 10-fold [McGrath et al., 1984; Sweet et al., 1984; Gibbs et al., 1984], while in vivo the activity is inhibited about 100-fold [Trahey and McCormick, 1987]. This difference is due to the specific association of ras proteins with a cellular protein factor termed GTPase activiting protein (GAP), which stimulates the GTPase activity of normal but not mutant p21 proteins [Trahey and McCormick, 1987; Adari et al., 1988; Cales et al., 1988].

Attempts to transform cultures of primary cells with ras oncogenes have been unsuccessful [Land et al., 1983; Ruley, 1983; Newbold and Overell, 1983], and human cells have been refractory to transformation by activated cellular ras oncogenes [Sager et al., 1983; Yoakum, et al, 1985]. Although activated ras oncogenes cannot transform primary rat embryo fibroblasts, they can readily do so if complemented with another class of oncogenes such as the members of the myc gene family, p53 and SV40 or polyoma large T [Land et al., 1983; Ruley, 1983]. These findings have been interpreted as supporting evidence for the multihit-multistep theory of carcinogenesis [Weinberg, 1983, 1985].

The initial studies using the NIH3T3 focus formation assay revealed the presence of activated ras oncogenes in about 10–15% of human tumors [Pulciani et al., 1982; Bishop, 1983; Varmus, 1984; Barbacid, 1986]. Activated ras oncogenes appeared randomly distributed without apparent association of the individual ras gene with the type of tumor [Varmus, 1984; Bishop 1983, 1987; Barbacid, 1986]. However, when more information became available by the use of other more sensitive diagnostic techniques for the detection of single point mutations in higher eukaryotic genes, it became apparent that the frequency of ras mutational activation in human cancer was underestimated in the original transfection experiments. In addition, associations between ras activation and some types of tumors are becoming apparent. Thus, N-ras is frequently associated with tumors of hematopoietic origin, while c-K-ras is found more often in carcinomas [Bos, 1988]. For instance, we recently found c-K-ras genes with mutations at codon 12 in 21 out of 22 primary human carcinomas of the exocrine pancreas [Almoguera et al., 1988] and in seven out of nine pancreatic carcinoma cell lines (unpublished results). The c-H-ras is the oncogene with lower incidence in human tumors [Barbacid, 1987; Bos, 1988]. We will describe here our recent studies on the frequency and timing of activation of c-K-ras oncogenes during human colorectal tumorigenesis.

RESULTS AND DISCUSSION

Frequency of Mutant c-K-ras Oncogenes in Primary Human Colorectal Tumors

We have used as a diagnostic assay a method previously developed in our group that is based on the ability of RNAse A to recognize and cleave a significant proportion of single base mismatches present in RNA:RNA heteroduplexes [Winter et al., 1985]. The RNAse A mismatch cleavage method is a powerful tool for the diagnostic detection and characterization of single point mutations in higher eukaryotic genes. The method allows the detection of not only the presence of a mutant gene but also the presence or absence of the normal allele in the cells, and it also allows the estimation of the relative expression levels of both normal and mutant alleles even when they differ by only a single nucleotide. In addition, the screening of primary tumors for the presence of mutant c-K-ras genes also provides information on the expression levels of this gene in tumor tissue relative to normal tissue from the same cancer patients, regardless of the presence or absence of mutant oncogenes in the tumors.

Total cellular RNA is prepared from frozen tumor specimens and hybridized with an antisense RNA probe corresponding to the first coding exon of the c-K-ras gene. The RNA hybrids are digested with RNAse A and the resistant products are analyzed by denaturing polyacrylamide gel electrophoresis. The presence of mutant c-K-ras genes is detected by the generation of mismatch-specific RNA subbands in the gels (Fig. 1).

In our initial studies we analyzed a panel of 66 primary tumors of the colon and rectum [Forrester et al., 1987]. Our results indicated that about 40% of human colorectal carcinomas contained c-K-ras genes with point mutations at codon 12. We have now analyzed a total of 104 colorectal adenocarcinomas of which 42 scored positive in the assay, confirming our original estimation of 40%. Similar frequency has been estimated by other groups using allelic-specific oligonucleotide (ASO) hybridization techniques [Bos et al., 1987; Vogelstein et al., 1988].

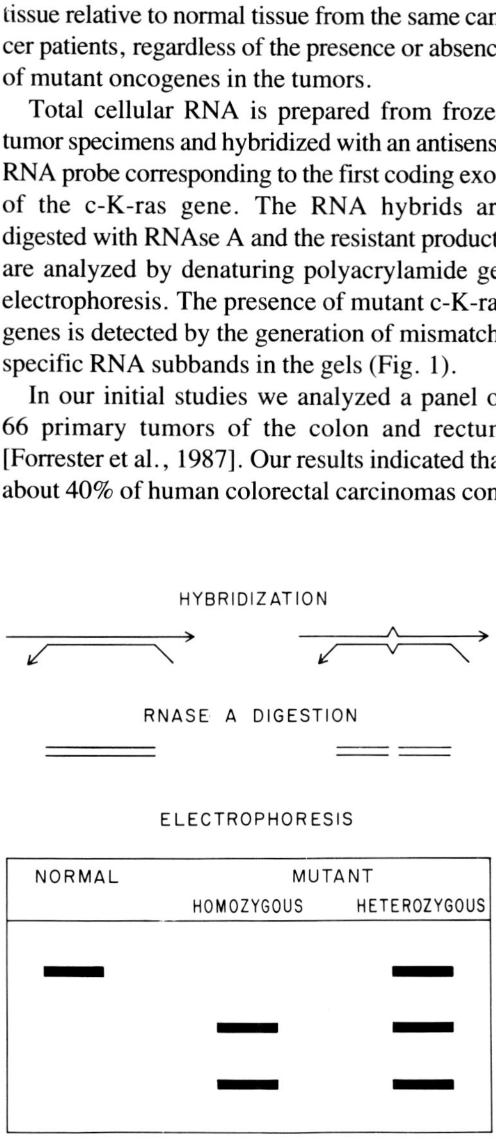

Fig. 1. Schematic representation of the RNAse A mismatch cleavage assay to detect single point mutations.

Because the RNAse A mismatch cleavage method does not depend on the position of the mutations, our results strongly suggest that point mutations in ras genes are not a secondary consequence of the high mutation rate of malignant cells [Duesberg, 1985]. If this were the case, we would expect to find other mutations randomly distributed in the region covered by the RNA probe used in our studies. It is reasonable to assume that some of these mismatches would have been cleaved by RNAse A. However, the mutations that we have detected were always located at codon 12, where point mutations activate the oncogenic potential of the encoded protein. Therefore, these results provide definitive evidence for a direct association of ras mutational activation with the tumorigenesis process in humans.

A typical result of this type of experiment is shown in Figure 2. The presence of RNA subbands of 67 and 46 nucleotides (indicated by arrows), diagnostic of a mismatch in the RNA hybrids, indicates that these colon tumors contain a c-K-ras gene with a single point mutation at the second position of codon 12 [Forrester et al., 1987]. In all cases analyzed, mutant c-K-ras oncogenes were found in tumor tissue (lanes T) but not in adjacent normal colonic tissues (lanes N) from the same individuals, demonstrating that ras mutations are somatic events that occur during tumor development.

Expression of c-K-ras in Human Colorectal Tumors

Figure 2 also shows that there are no major differences in the expression levels of the c-K-ras gene between tumor and normal tissue. The same result has been obtained in benign colorectal adenomas and regardless of the presence of a mutation in the c-K-ras gene. This result has been

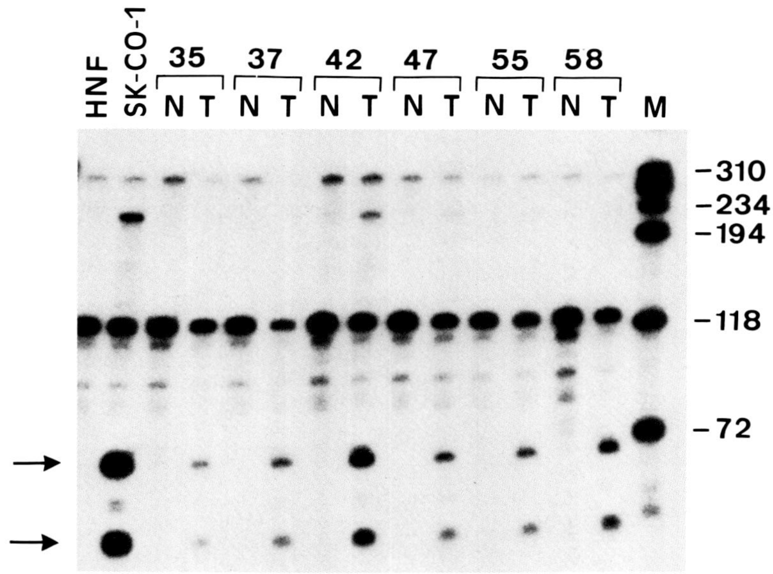

Fig. 2. RNAse A mismatch cleavage analysis of RNA from human colorectal carcinomas and normal tissue. Total cellular RNA was prepared from frozen tumor (T) or normal (N) tissue specimens from the cases indicated at the top, and 30 μg each were hybridized to an uniformely ^{32}P-labeled antisense RNA probe corresponding to the c-K-ras first coding exon. The probe contained a serine (G--A) mutation at the first position of codon 12. The samples were digested with RNAse A (20 μg/ml) for 30 minutes at 30°C, and the resistant products were analyzed by polyacrylamide gel electrophoresis as previously described [Forrester et al., 1987]. HNF, RNA from human normal fibroblasts; SK-CO-1, colon carcinoma cell line containing a c-K-ras gene with a valine (G--T) mutation at the second position of codon 12; M, molecular weight markers (0X 174 digested with HaeIII) with the size of the bands (in nucleotides) indicated at the right. Arrows indicate RNA subbands of 67 and 46 nucleotides.

confirmed in other experiments using a human γ-actin RNA probe as internal control to correct for variabilities in the amount of RNA used and/or recovered in the RNAse A mismatch experiments. Therefore, somatic mutational activation of the c-K-ras gene in human colorectal tumors is not preceded or accompanied by its transcriptional activation. In addition, an increase in the expression levels of the c-K-ras gene is not associated with the tumor phenotype in colorectal carcinomas. It is noteworthy that to date we have not found a single example of a human tissue, either tumor or normal, in which the c-K-ras gene is not expressed to detectable levels. In the case of colorectal carcinomas, no amplified c-K-ras genes have been found in over 100 cases. We interpret these results to indicate that activation of the oncogenic potential of ras genes in human cancer is mainly due to genetic alterations resulting in qualitative changes in their encoded proteins rather than a quantitative increase in their normal product. Therefore, in the absence of evidence for structural alterations (i.e., point mutations), the significance of studies implicating moderate fluctuations in the expression levels of the c-K-ras proto-oncogene with colon tumor development is not clear [Slamon et al, 1984; Spandidos and Kerr, 1984; Thor et al., 1984; Hand et al., 1984; Tanaka et al., 1986].

c-K-ras Oncogenes Are Dominant in Human Tumors

The result of the experiment shown in Figure 2 suggests that colon tumor cells are heterozygous for the mutant ras allele. However, because of the presence of contaminating nonneoplastic tissue (stromal, inflammatory, or muscular) in the tumor samples, these experiments do not give accurate information on the allelic ratio of the c-K-ras gene in the tumor cells. A more direct approach is provided by the analysis of tumor cell lines, because they are homogeneous populations of tumor cells without contaminating normal tissue. We and others have found that human tumor cells are frequently homozygous for the mutant ras allele (i.e., they have lost the normal allele) [Capon et al., 1983; Santos et al., 1984; Guerrero et al., 1985; Winter et al., 1985] or contain increased ratios of mutant versus normal alleles (i.e., the mutant allele has been amplified relative to the normal) [Capon et al., 1983; Winter et al., 1985; Forrester et al., 1987]. These results have been interpreted by some investigators as suggesting a recessive nature for activated ras oncogenes [Capon et al., 1983; Santos et al., 1984; Guerrero et al., 1985]. However, we have found several tumor cell lines derived from two lung and three pancreas carcinomas, and a colon carcinoma propagated in nude mice, in which both mutant and normal alleles are expressed to similar levels (manuscript in preparation). Therefore, human carcinoma cells can be heterozygous for the mutant c-K-ras allele, indicating that loss of the normal allele is not required for the expression of the malignant phenotype. Our results strongly support the concept that ras oncogenes act in a dominant but dose-dependent manner in human tumor cells.

c-K-ras and the Adenoma-Carcinoma Sequence

Our studies have revealed that mutational activation of the c-K-ras gene is independent of the age, sex, race, or anatomical localization of the tumors [Forrester et al., 1987]. This result supports the somatic nature of the activating mutations and suggests that they are induced by carcinogens in food.

In our initial experiments [Forrester et al., 1987] we found a strikingly high incidence of mutant c-K-ras genes in villous adenomas and in carcinomas originated in villous adenomas. These results indicated that somatic ras mutational activation can be a relatively early event during colon tumor development in humans.

To study in more detail the timing of activation of the c-K-ras gene during colon tumorigenesis, we analyzed several adenomatous polyps of the colon for the presence of mutant c-K-ras oncogenes (manuscript in preparation). We found mutant c-K-ras genes in three of four villous adenomas and in three of four villous adenomas with carcinoma in situ. On the other hand, we did not find activated c-K-ras oncogenes in ten tubular adenomas and in nine tubulovillous adenomas, indicating that mutant c-K-ras genes are not frequently involved in the development of these types of adenomas. Examples of a negative tubular adenoma and a positive villous adenoma are shown in Figures 3 and 4, respectively. In addition, mutant c-K-ras oncogenes were present in five of six carcinomas originated in villous adenomas and in one metastatic adenocarcinoma recurrent 3 years after surgical resection of a villous adenoma, in one of six carcinomas originated in tubulovillous adenomas, and in three of eight carcinomas originated in tubular adenomas. Therefore, the adenomas in which the activation of the ras gene had occurred appear to be those at higher risk to develop into overt carcinomas.

These results suggest two different possibilities. The first is that while development of tubular and tubulovillous adenomas does not require the previous activation of the ras gene, the development of villous adenomas might be initiated

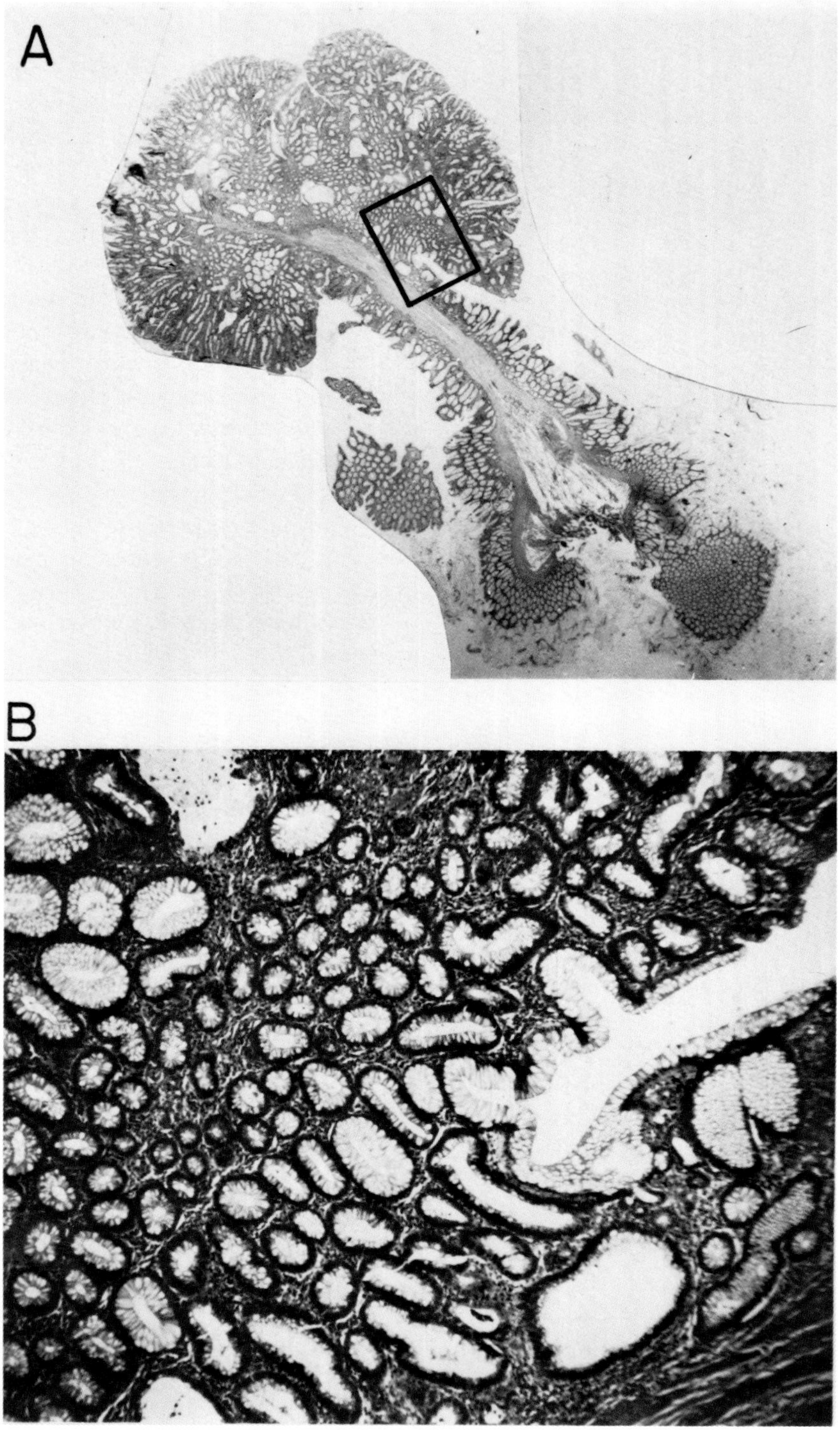

Fig. 3. **A:** Histology of a mutant c-K-ras–negative, tubular adenoma. **B:** Higher magnification of boxed area in A. Hematoxylin and eosin staining. A, ×10; B, ×200.

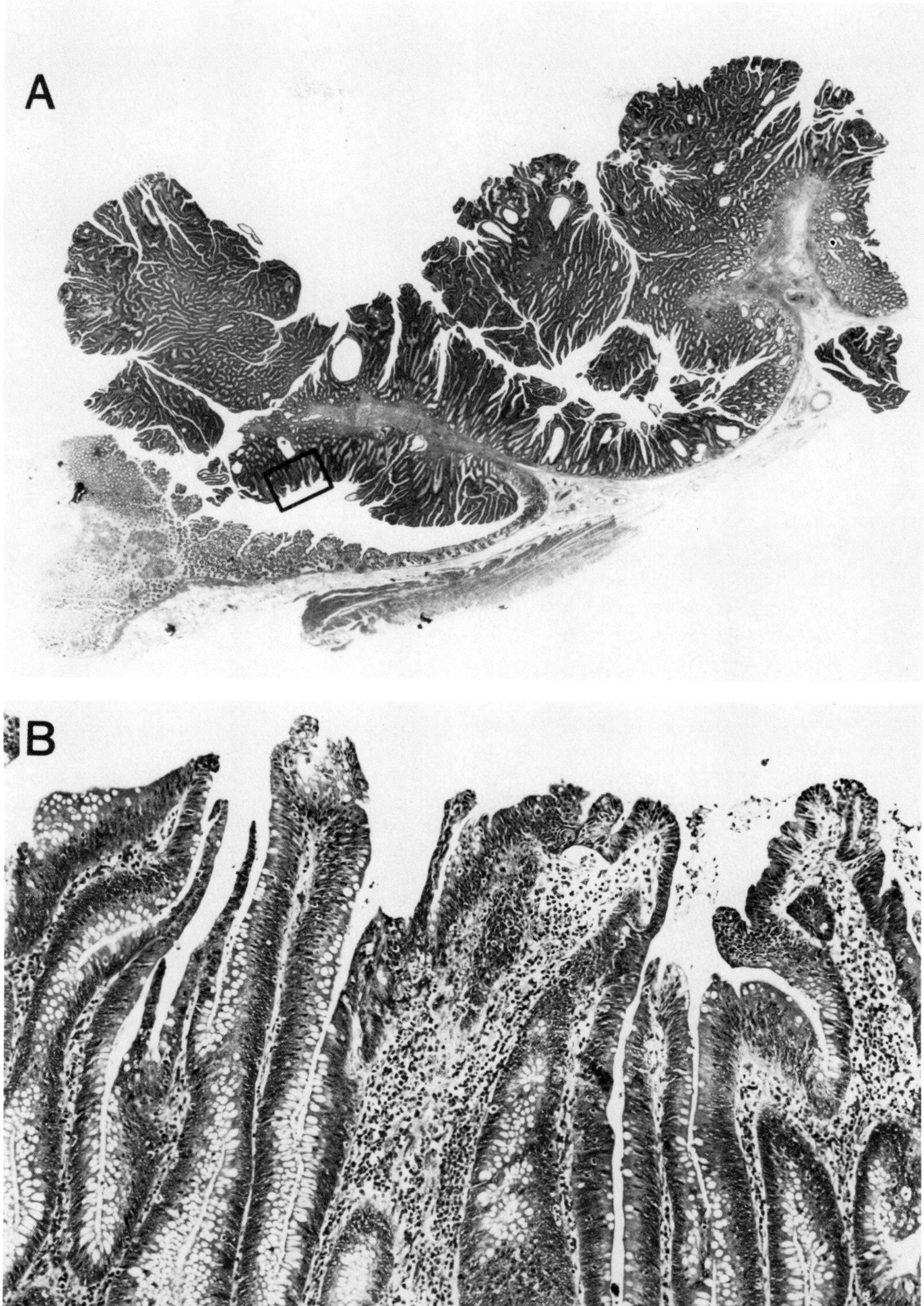

Fig. 4. **A:** Histology of a mutant c-K-ras positive, villous adenoma. Hematoxylin and eosin staining. There was no in situ carcinoma identified, and there was no invasion of the stalk. **B:** Higher magnification of boxed area in A. A, ×5; B, ×200.

by the mutational activation of the c-K-ras gene. The second is that the ras mutation occurs sometime after the development of the adenoma, its incidence increasing with the size of the tumor and/or its degree of dysplasia. Of the two possibilities, we favor the second for several reasons. First, the presence of the mutant c-K-ras oncogene correlates very well with the size of the adenoma (five of six adenomas larger than 3 cm in diameter, one of three between 2 and 3 cm, and none of the 16 smaller than 2 cm contained activated c-K-ras genes). Second, we have obtained evidence for the mutational activation of the c-K-ras gene at late stages of tumor development. For instance, while some primary tumors appear to contain only a minor proportion of cells carrying the mutant gene, their corresponding metastases contain a clearly higher proportion of tumor cells carrying the oncogene (unpublished results). In addition, the simultaneous activation of the c-K-ras and N-ras oncogenes was found in some colon tumors [Forrester et al., 1987], indicating that at least one of the activating mutations occurred after initiation of tumor development. Similar results have been found by other groups in other tumor systems [Janssen et al., 1987; Farr et al., 1988; Diamond et al., 1988]. Moreover, our results show that the incidence of c-K-ras oncogenes increases in tumors at more advanced stages of progression (Fig. 5). These results can be explained if mutations in the ras gene are accumulating along the tumorigenesis process, or if the tumors containing an activated oncogene possess more aggressive properties, or both. As mentioned above, we have evidence supporting the first interpretation. Further experiments, especially correlative follow-up studies comparing survival and recurrence rates, will be necessary to confirm or to rule out the second interpretation.

Based on these results, our current hypothesis postulates that somatic mutational activation of the c-K-ras gene can be both early (although probably not the initial event) and late during human colon carcinomatogenesis where it contributes in a dominant but dose-dependent manner to the manifestation of the tumor phenotype. The increased incidence of mutant c-K-ras genes

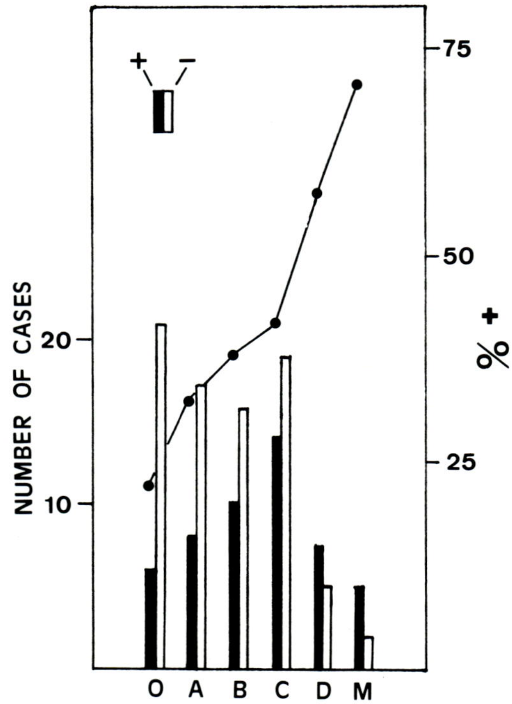

Fig. 5. c-K-ras incidence and colorectal tumor progression. The graph summarizes our current data on the screening of colorectal tumors positive (filled bars) or negative (open bars) for the presence of c-K-ras genes with mutations at codon 12. O, adenoma; A, carcinoma confined to muscularis propia; B, carcinoma extending through the colon wall; C, carcinoma metastatic to regional lymph nodes; D, carcinoma with distant, widespread metastatses; M, metastatic carcinoma. Eight cases have been included in D and M that were analyzed by RNAse A mismatch cleavage of PCR-amplified c-K-ras DNA sequences from formalin-fixed, paraffin-embedded tumor specimens obtained from autopsies, as previously described [Almoguera et al., 1988].

in colorectal metastases (both proximal and distal) also suggests that the oncogene is actively involved in tumor progression, including the metastatic process (Fig. 5 and unpublished results).

CONCLUSIONS

There are several questions that remain to be determined in relation to the role of ras activation in human colorectal cancer. We do not know if some villous adenomas containing a mutant c-K-ras gene will ever develop into malignant carcinomas. Further, we do not know what the other genetic alterations are that are undoubtedly required for the completion of the adenoma-carcinoma sequence or in which order they may occur. It is not clear either if there is a defined sequence of genetic alterations or if the sequence could be different as long as all the necessary steps are fulfilled. In a series of elegant experiments by Vogelstein and collaborators [1988], allelic deletions of chromosomes 17, 18, and to a lesser extent 5 have been characterized in a significant proportion of sporadic colorectal carcinomas. These genetic alterations accumulated during tumor progression, although the timing of the events was not invariant, supporting the second possibility mentioned above. We also do not know whether the subsequent amplification and overexpression of the mutant c-K-ras gene plays a role in conferring more aggressive growth properties to the colon tumor cells. The implication in that case will be that several important consecutive steps in the process of tumor progression are occurring in a single genetic locus, the c-K-ras. There is also the question of what other genetic alterations are playing the role of the ras oncogene in the negative tumors. Finally, it is not clear which is the nature of the event (or events) that induce the initial growth of the individual adenomas. These are some of the topics that will require further work.

In any case, the studies summarized here have significant implications in our understanding of the genetic alterations involved in development and progression of cancer of the large bowel. With about 140,000 new cases of colorectal cancer occurring every year in the United States, and with over 50,000 estimated deaths per year, it is clear that the most frequent, reproducible, and therefore predictable, well-characterized genetic aberration in human cancer of the colon and rectum is the somatic mutational activation at codon 12 of the c-K-ras gene. In addition, it is possible that the presence of activated ras oncogenes in human colorectal tumors may have useful applications not only for the diagnosis but also for the prognosis of this common type of human cancer.

ACKNOWLEDGMENTS

We thank Dr. Bert Vogelstein for his generous gift of a mouse xenograft of a human colon carcinoma and for sharing unpublished results. This work was supported by NIH grants ROI CA 38579 and CA 33021 and by a grant from Toyo Jozo Ltd. Co.

References

Adari H, Lowy DR, Willumsen BM, Der CJ, McCormick F (1988): Guanosine triphosphatase activating protein (GAP) interacts with the p21 ras effector binding domain. Science 240:518–521.

Almoguera C, Shibata D, Forrester K, Martin J, Arnheim N, Perucho M (1988): Most human carcinomas of the exocrine pancreas contain mutant c-K-ras genes. Cell 53:549–554.

Barbacid M (1986) Human oncogenes. In DeVita V, Hellman S, Rosenberg S (eds): Important Advances in Oncology. Philadelphia: J.B. Lippincot Company, pp3–22.

Barbacid M (1987): ras Genes. Annu Rev Biochem 56:779–827.

Bishop JM (1983): Cellular oncogenes and retroviruses. Annu Rev Biochem 52:301–354.

Bishop JM (1987): The molecular genetics of cancer. Science 235:305–311.

Bos JL (1988): The ras gene family and human carcinogenesis. Mutat Res 195:255–271.

Bos JL, Fearon ER, Hamilton SR, Verlaan-de Vries M, van Boom JH, van der Eb AJ, Vogelstein B (1987): Prevalence of ras gene mutations in human colorectal cancers. Nature 327:293–297.

Cales C, Hancock JF, Marshall CJ, Hall A (1988): The cytoplasmic protein GAP is implicated as the target for regulation by ras gene product. Nature 332:548–551.

Capon DJ, Seeburg PH, McGrath JP, Hayflick JS, Edman U, Levinson AD, Goeddel DV (1983): Activation of Ki-ras-2 gene in human colon and lung carcinomas by two different point mutations. Nature 304:507–512.

Diamond LE, Guerrero I, Pellicer A (1988): Concomitant K- and N-ras gene point mutations in clonal murine lymphomas. Mol Cell Biol 8:2233–2236.

Duesberg PH (1985): Activated proto-onc genes: Sufficient or necessary for cancer? Science 228:669–677.

Farr CJ, Saiki RK, Erlich HA, McCormick F, Marshall CJ (1988): Analysis of ras gene mutations in acute myeloid leukemia by polymerase chain reaction and oligonucleotide probes. Proc Natl Acad Sci USA 85:1629–1633.

Forrester K, Almoguera C, Han K, Grizzle WE, Perucho M, (1987): Detection of high incidence of K-ras oncogenes during human colon tumorigenesis. Nature 327: 298–303.

Gibbs JB, Sigal IS, Poe M, Scolnick EM (1984): Intrinsic GTPase activity distinguishes normal and oncogenic ras p21 molecules. Proc Natl Acad Sci USA 81:5704–5708.

Guerrero I, Villasante A, Corces V, Pellicer A (1985): Loss of normal N-ras allele in a mouse thymic lymphoma induced by a chemical carcinogen. Proc Natl Acad Sci USA 82:7810–7814.

Hand PH, Thor A, Wunderlich R, Muraro R, Caruso A, Schlom J (1984): Monoclonal antibodies of predefined specificity detect activated ras gene expression in human mammary and colon carcinomas. Proc Natl Acad Sci USA 81:5227–5231.

Janssen JG, Lyons J, Steenvoorden AM, Seliger H, Bartram CR (1987): Concurrent mutations in two different ras genes in acute myelocytic leukemias. Nucleic Acids Res 15:5669–5680.

Krontiris TG, Cooper GM(1981): Transforming activity of human tumor DNAs. Proc Natl Acad Sci USA 78:1181–1184.

Land H, Parada LF, Weinberg RA (1983): Tumorigenic conversion of primary embryo fibroblasts requires at least two cooperating oncogenes. Nature 304:596–602.

Marshall C (1985): Human oncogenes. In Weiss R, Teich N, Varmus H, Coffin J (eds): RNA Tumor Viruses, ed 2. Cold Spring Harbor, NY: Cold Spring Harbor Laboratory, pp 487–558.

McGrath JP, Capon DJ, Goeddel DV, Levinson AD (1984): Comparative biochemical properties of normal and activated human ras p21 protein. Nature 310:644–649.

Newbold RF, Overell RW (1983): Fibroblast immortality is a prerequisite for transformation by EJ c-Ha-ras oncogene. Nature 304:648–651.

Perucho M, Goldfarb M, Shimizu K, Lama C, Fogh J, Wigler M (1981): Human-tumor-derived cell lines contain common and different transforming genes. Cell 27:467–476.

Pulciani S, Santos E, Lauver AV, Long LK, Aaronson SA, Barbacid M (1982): Oncogenes in solid human tumors. Nature 300:539–541.

Ruley HE (1983): Adenovirus early region 1A enables viral and cellular transforming genes to transform primary cells in culture. Nature 304:602–606.

Sager R, Tanaka K, Lau CC, Ebina Y, Anisowicz A (1983): Resistance of human cells to tumorigenesis induced by cloned transforming genes. Proc Natl Acad Sci USA 80:7601–7605.

Santos E, Martin-Zanca D, Reddy E, Pierotti MA, Della Porta G, Barbacid M (1984): Malignant activation of a K-ras oncogene in lung carcinoma but not in normal tissue of the same patient. Science 223:661–664.

Shih C, Padhy LC, Murray M, Weinberg RA (1981): Tranforming genes of carcinomas and neuroblastomas introduced into mouse fibroblasts. Nature 290:261–264.

Shih C, Shilo BZ, Goldfarb MP, Dannenberg A, Weinberg RA (1979): Passage of phenotypes of chemically transformed cells via transfection of DNA and chromatin. Proc Natl Acad Sci USA 76:5714–5718.

Slamon DJ, de Kernion JB, Verma IM, Cline MJ (1984): Expression of cellular oncogenes in human malignancies. Science 224:256–262.

Spandidos DA, Kerr IB (1984): Elevated expression of the human ras oncogene family in premalignant and malignant tumours of the colorectum. Br J Cancer 49: 681–688.

Sweet RW, Yokoyama S, Kamata T, Feramisco JR, Rosenberg M, Gross M (1984): The product of ras is a GTPase and the T24 oncogenic mutant is deficient in this activity. Nature 311:273–275.

Tanaka T, Slamon DJ, Battifora H, Cline M (1986): Expression of p21 ras oncoproteins in human cancer. Cancer Res 46:1465–1470.

Thor RF, Hand HP, Wunderlich D, Caruso A, Muraro R, Schlom J (1984): Monoclonal antibodies define differential ras gene expression in malignant and benign colonic diseases. Nature 311:562–565.

Trahey M, McCormick F (1987): A cytoplasmic protein stimulates normal N-ras p21 GTPase, but does not affect oncogenic mutants. Science 238:542–545.

Varmus HE (1984): The molecular genetics of cellular oncogenes. Annu Rev Genet 18:553–612.

Vogelstein B, Fearon ER, Hamilton SR, Kern SE, Preisinger AC, Leppert M, Nakamura Y, White R, Smits AM, Bos JL (1988): Genetic alterations during colorectal tumor development. New Engl J Med 319:525–532.

Weinberg RA (1983): Cellular oncogenes and multistep carcinogenesis. Science 230:771–778.

Weinberg RA (1985): The action of oncogenes in the cytoplasm and nucleus. Science 230:770–776.

Winter E, Yamamoto F, Almoguera C, Perucho M (1985): A method to detect and characterize point mutations in transcribed genes: Amplification and overexpression of the mutant c-Ki-ras allele in human tumor cells. Proc Natl Acad Sci USA 82:7575–7579.

Yoakum GH, Lechner JF, Gabrielson EW, Korba BE, Malan-Shibley L, Willey JC, Valerio MG, Shamsuddin AM, Trump BF, Harris CC (1985): Transformation of human bronchial epithelial cells transfected by Harvey ras oncogene. Science 227:1174–1179.

Levels of ras Oncogene Protein Product in Familial Adenomatous Polyposis

Fabrizio Michelassi

Department of Surgery, University of Chicago Medical Center, Chicago, Illinois

INTRODUCTION

The occurrence of a colonic carcinoma in patients with familial adenomatous polyposis (FAP) follows a complex process involving malignant transformation of normal or preneoplastic epithelia. Much effort has been directed at understanding the transformation process, yet little is known about the mechanism involved. On the other hand, participation of a group of genes collectively known as oncogenes is believed to be required.

Of all the oncogenes known, the ras oncogene has been by far the most studied. By means of DNA transfection technology, the ras oncogene has been identified as capable of inducing malignant transformation of NIH 3T3 cell line [1–4] through production of a 21 kilodalton protein referred to as the p21 protein product [5]. Increased quantity of p21 protein product has been detected in human colon carcinomas via immunohistochemical techniques [6–8], spot hybridization [9], Western immunoblotting [10], and quantitative liquid competition radioimmunoassay [11], and it has been correlated with increased cell proliferation [12], histologic grade, nuclear anaplasia, and degree of undifferentiation [13].

There are no data about the relationship between ras oncogene protein product and premalignant lesions in FAP nor about the role p21 may play in malignant transformation. Therefore, we evaluated the levels of ras oncogene p21 product in histologic sections of tubular and villous adenomas from FAP patients and compared them with those in normal colonic epithelia.

MATERIALS AND METHODS

Archival formalin-fixed, paraffin-embedded specimens were retrieved from the files of the Department of Surgical Pathology of the University of Chicago Medical Center. The specimens included normal colonic mucosa (n = 15), tubular adenomas (n ± 12), and villous adenomas (n = 11). Specimens of normal colonic mucosa were obtained from patients who had undergone partial colectomy for trauma; specimens of tubular and villous adenomas were obtained from patients who had undergone proctocolectomy for FAP. Pathologic classification of the polyps was performed according to the method of Morson and Sobin [14].

The RAP-5 mouse IgG2a monclonal antibody to the ras p21 protein product was obtained from the National Institutes of Health (Bethesda, MD). A semiquantitative immunohistochemical assay was performed as previously reported. Briefly, 4 μm-thick paraffin sections were deparaffinized in xylene and rinsed in absolute alcohol. To block endogeneous peroxidase activity, tissue sections were placed for 10 minutes in methanol containing 0.3% hydrogen peroxidase. After rinsing in phosphate-buffered saline (PBS) adjusted to pH 7.4, nonspecific binding was blocked by preincubating tissue sections with 10% normal horse serum. The normal horse solution was then blotted off the slide, and the primary antibody was

Familial Adenomatous Polyposis, pages 347–350

applied. Primary incubation (30 minutes at 25°C) was carried out with serial dilutions of RAP-5 antibody from 1:5,000 to 1:160,000 in PBS, 0.1% bovine serum albumin, and 0.5% sodium azide in Tris buffer. Biotinylated antimouse IgG was used as the secondary antibody (30 minutes at 25°C). Following a PBS wash, the avidin–biotin complex was applied to the sections for 30 minutes. The peroxidase reaction was then initiated by the addition of 0.06% diaminobenzidine and 0.01% hydrogen peroxide for 5 minutes. Counterstaining was obtained with Gills' hematoxylin No. 3 for 15 seconds. One slide per case was used as a negative control by using leukocyte common antigen as the primary antibody. Human colon carcinoma with known increased levels of p21 protein product served as a positive control for ras p21 immunoreactivity.

A semiquantitative estimate of ras p21 expression was obtained by determining the highest dilution of antibody that elicited definitive cytoplasmic staining. Subtle, uniform, brown blushes were considered negative. Statistical comparison of data was based on Fisher's exact test [15].

RESULTS

The immunoperoxidase reaction for ras p21 protein appeared as a diffuse, brown cytoplasmic stain. At low dilutions, all epithelial and stromal elements within polyps and normal mucosa stained to some degree. At higher dilutions, normal stromal fibroblasts and smooth muscle cells did not stain, leaving the normal colonic epithelium and the benign colonic lesions exhibiting different degrees of stain. No mucosal reaction was obtained when RAP-5 was replaced by leukocyte common antigen.

Although there was a range of p21 titers observed for these categories of specimens, titers for normal colonic mucosa and tubular and villous adenomas in FAP clustered around low, intermediate, and high values of the spectrum, respectively.

Table 1 displays the p21 titer for all specimens and shows that titers of ras oncogene protein product in normal colonic epithelial cells were always less than 1:40,000. The tendency of individual groups to stain at titers higher or equal to 1:40,000 was compared using Fisher's exact test. The result of the analysis indicated that there was a significant increase in the titer of p21 found in tubular adenomas in FAP compared to normal colonic mucosa ($P < 0.05$) as well as in villous compared to tubular adenomas ($P < 0.05$).

DISCUSSION

This investigation has provided data on ras oncogene expression in lesions found in colons removed from patients with FAP and has established a statistically significant relationship between levels of expression of ras oncogene and different histological lesions. Using the aforementioned immunohistochemical assay, we found that ras p21 expression correlates significantly with the malignant potential of different human colonic premalignant conditions. For example, adenomatous polyps of the large bowel are thought to be premalignant, with a potential for malignant change from 5% for tubular adenoma to 40% for villous adenoma when patients are followed for up to 15 years [16]; our analysis demonstrated that there was a significant increase in the titer of ras p21 protein found in tubular adenomas and an even greater increase in the titer of villous adenomas compared with normal colonic epithelia.

Familial adenomatous polyposis is a hereditary disease characterized by multiple adenomas of the colon and a variety of extracolonic neoplasms. Adenocarcinoma of the colon or rectum occurs in virtually all untreated individuals. Studies of many family pedigrees have demonstrated inheritance by an autosomal dominant gene. The gross appearance consists typically of the entire mucosa of the colon and rectum replaced by hundreds or thousands of adenomas, which may vary in size from several millimeters to several centimeters in diameter and which may be sessile or pedunculated [17]. Histology of these adenomas may show tubular adenomas, villous adenomas, or tubulovillous adenomas, often all coexisting.

For many years, it was thought that the high incidence of colon adenocarcinoma in untreated FAP patients was just a direct consequence of the presence of hundreds of premalignant polyps, a mere quantitative relationship. On the other hand, a qualitative relationship has been sug-

TABLE 1.
Cellular ras Oncogene Protein Content in Specimens of Normal Colonic Mucosa and Polyps From FAP Patients

	<1: 5,000	1: 5,000	1: 10,000	1: 20,000	1: 40,000	1: 80,000	1: 160,000
Normal colonic mucosa (n = 15)	2	4	3	6	0	0	0
Tubular adenomas (n = 12)	0	0	1	3	8	0	0
Villous adenomas (n = 11)	0	0	0	0	4	4	3

gested recently by Bodner et al. [18], who have shown that the FAP gene is located on chromosome 5, and its heterozygosity may predispose to decreased FAP gene product, which, in turn, may allow deficient control of other factors responsible for initiation of neoplastic growth. The present study does not attempt to clarify whether the increased expression of ras oncogene is a necessary condition of the malignant transformation of benign colonic lesions in FAP, but, in view of previous studies showing that ras oncogene is capable of inducing malignant transformation in NIH 3T3 cells and in view of the recent suggestion that heterozygosity may predispose to a less effective control of factors responsible for neoplastic growth, it is tempting to postulate that increased levels of ras oncogene in a host characterized by thousands of premalignant lesions (quantitative change) and a decreased control on factors responsible for growth (qualitative change) will inevitably lead to malignancy.

SUMMARY

To investigate the role of ras oncogene in malignant transformation in FAP, we compared the levels of ras oncogene protein product p21 in specimens of normal human colonic mucosa (n = 15) to levels in specimens of tubular adenoma (n = 12) and villous adenoma (n = 11) in FAP. p21 Content was measured using the RAP-5 monoclonal antibody in a semiquantitative immunohistochemical assay. Titer was expressed as the highest dilution of antibody giving definitive staining using the avidin–biotin peroxidase method. Differences in p21 titer values among the three categories of specimens were statistically significant using Fisher's exact test (normal colonic mucosa < tubular adenomas in FAP < villous adenomas in FAP; $P < 0.05$). Since increased expression of cellular oncogene has been linked to malignant transformation, we conclude that different lesions in FAP have different potential for malignant transformation. This may be yet another important factor in the predisposition to cancer in FAP, together with the quantitative change represented by the multitude of polyps and the recently suggested qualitative change represented by the heterozygosity of the FAP gene.

ACKNOWLEDGMENTS

We thank Dr. J. Schlom, NIH, for the generous gift of monoclonal antibody RAP-5 and Mrs. Roberta Carden for her expert secretarial help. This work was supported by grant 87-100 from the American Cancer Society.

References

1. Cooper GM: Cellular transforming genes. Science 217:801–806, 1982.
2. Der CJ, Krontiris TG, Cooper GM: Transforming genes of human bladder and lung carcinoma cell lines are homologous to the ras genes of Harvey and Kirsten sarcoma viruses. Proc Natl Acad Sci USA 79:3637–3640, 1982.
3. Der CJ, Cooper GM: Altered gene products are associated with activation of cellular ras^{k} genes in human lung and colon carcinoma. Cell 32:201–208, 1983.
4. Murray MJ, Cunningham JM, Parada LF, et al.: The HL-60 transforming sequence: A ras oncogene consisting with altered myc genes in hematopoietic tumors. Cell 33:749–757, 1983.
5. Willingham MC, Pastan I, Shih TW, et al.: Localization of the srg gene product of the Harvey strain of MSV to plasma membrane of transformed cells by

electromicroscopic immunocytochemistry. Cell 19: 104, 1980.

6. Thor A, Hand PH, Wunderlich D, Caruso A, Moraro R, Schlom J: Monoclonal antibodies define differential ras gene expression in malignant and benign colonic diseases. Nature 311:562, 1984.

7. Hand PH, Thor A, Wunderlich D, Muraro R, Caruso A, Schlom J: Monoclonal antibodies of predefined specificity detected activated ras gene expression in human mammary and colon carcinomas. Proc Natl Acad Sci USA 81:5227, 1984.

8. Kerr IB, Lee FD, Quintanilla M, Balmain A: Immunocytochemical demonstration of p21 ras family oncogene product in normal mucosa and in premalignant and malignant tumours of the colorectum. Br J Cancer 52:695, 1985.

9. Spandidos DA, Kerr IB: Elevated expression of the human ras oncogene family in premalignant and malignant tumors of the colorectum. Br J Cancer 49:681, 1984.

10. Gallick GE, Kurzrock R, Kloetzer WAS, Arlinghaus RB, Gutterman JU: Expression of p21 ras in fresh primary and metastatic human colorectal tumors. Proc Natl Acad Sci USA 82:1795, 1985.

11. Hand PH, Vilasi V, THor A, Ohuchi N, Schlom J: Quantitation of Harvey ras p21 enhanced expression in human breast and colon carcinomas. JNCI 79:59, 1987.

12. Campisi J, Grah H, Pardee A, et al.: Cell cycle control in c-myc, but no c-ras expression is lost following classic chemical transformations. Cell 36:241–247, 1984.

13. Viola MV, Fromowitz F, Oravez S, et al.: Expression of ras oncogene p21 in prostate cancer. N Engl J Med 314:133–137, 1986.

14. Morson BC, Sobin LH: "Histologic Typing of Intestinal Tumors." Geneva: World Health Organization, 1976.

15. Thomas DG: Exact and asyntotic methods of the combination of two by two tables. Computer Biomed Res 8:423–426, 1975.

16. Moreson BD: Evolution of cancer of the colon and rectum. Cancer 34:845–851, 1974.

17. Bussey HJR: "Familial Polyposis Coli." Baltimore: Johns Hopkins University Press, 1975.

18. Bodner WF, Bailey CJ, Bodner AL, et al.: Localization of the gene for familial adenomatous polyposis in chromosome 5. Nature 328:614–616, 1987.

43

Oncogene Amplification in Colorectal Cancer

Manfred Schwab, Peter Schlag, Silke Brüderlein, and Kai van der Bosch

Institut für Experimentelle Pathologie, Deutsches Krebsforschungszentrum (M.S., S.B., K.V.D.B.) and Chirurgische Universitätsklinik, Sektion Chirurgische Onkologie (P.S.), Heidelberg, Federal Republic of Germany

INTRODUCTION

Colorectal cancer is among the most frequent solid malignant tumors in Western countries. The vast majority of colorectal cancers develops without well-known genetic background. But there is a small fraction of colorectal cancers for which susceptibility is inherited in an autosomal dominant manner. This form of cancer is familial adenomatous polyposis (FAP), also known as familial polyposis coli (FPC). The malignant change occurs in the colorectal mucosa, causing death in these patients at an average age of 41 years, with the youngest patient being only 12 years old [Watne, 1987]. FAP colon cancer develops at a much earlier age than the usual sixth to seventh decade for the general population. It seems clear that at least in the case of FAP/FPC cellular genes contribute to tumorigenesis. And cytogenetic studies of cells of nonhereditary forms of colorectal cancers have provided evidence for chromosomal abnormalities. The development of molecular probes for specific regions of the genome has facilitated a more refined analysis and has led to identification of nonrandom genetic alterations of cells of spontaneous colorectal cancers. It appears particularly significant that in spontaneous tumors deletion of genetic material is seen in chromosome 5q21-22, a region to which the gene responsible for FAP/FPC has been mapped by linkage analyses.

Among the chromosomal abnormalities indicating genetic changes in cells of colorectal tumors, "double minutes" (DMs) appear to be rather frequent. As we know, DMs indicate the presence of amplified cellular DNA. With the exception of metabolically specialized drug-resistant cells, DMs in cancer cells are indicators for amplified cellular oncogenes. This chapter will review major genetic changes that are found in cells of colorectal cancers, with primary reference to the role that amplification of cellular oncogenes might have in tumorigenesis.

AMPLIFICATION OF CELLULAR ONCOGENES—A HALLMARK OF MANY CANCER CELLS

The term *gene amplification* refers to the selective increase of the gene copy number and is better designated as *DNA amplification*. It should not be confused with elevated gene expression, although amplification generally does result in enhanced levels of the products encoded by the amplified gene. Amplification is one of the mechanisms by which cells can meet the demand for synthesis of specific gene products in amounts exceeding the transcriptional capacity of a single copy gene.

Cytogenetic studies of human and animal tumor cells have provided evidence for mysterious chromosomal abnormalities, including (DMs), C-bandless chromosomes (CMs), or homogeneously staining chromosomal regions (HSRs) diagnostic of amplified DNA [for details and photographs, see Schwab, 1985]. The first indications

Familial Adenomatous Polyposis, pages 351–360

for a causal relationship between the presence of DMs and CMs in tumor cells and the malignant phenotype emerged from work with murine SEWA cells (for review, see Levan et al., 1977]. The reproducibility with which SEWA cells generated CMs and DMs following transfer from tissue culture conditions into an animal host led to the suggestion that these chromosomal abnormalities contain genes that contribute to the malignant phenotype.

It is probably more than coincidence that proto-oncogenes are amplified consistently in animal and human tumor cells containing DMs, CMs, or HSRs. Historically the first case in which amplification of an oncogene has been discovered in DMs and in HSRs of a cancer cell is represented by the ras^K gene in the murine tumor cell line Y1 [Schwab et al., 1983b].

The list of amplified proto-oncogenes that have been identified so far includes myc, abl, ras^H, ras^K, N-myc, L-myc, erb, myb, and ras^N. However, they are not always present in DMs or HSRs [for review, see Alitalo and Schwab, 1986]. The copy number of amplified proto-oncogenes ranges form 5 to 700. (Data indicating amplification of less than fivefold should be viewed with caution.) Interestingly, myc genes account for over 90% of the amplifications that have been detected so far. The discovery of amplified oncogenes in direct preparations of human tumors not previously subjected to chemo- or to radiotherapy rules out the possibility that the amplified oncogenes they contain are artifacts generated by cell culture or therapeutical treament [Schwab et al., 1983a].

Cells derived from at least two different types of tumor have been found to carry two coexisting amplified proto-oncogenes. Both myc and ras^K were amplified in a human giant lung cell carcinoma [Taya et al., 1984], while amplified myc and ras^H genes have been detected in eight squamous cell carcinomas of the uterine cervix [Riou et al., 1984]. It is unclear, though, if the two oncogenes are coamplified in the same cell or if the tumor cell population is heterogeneous. Many copies of amplified ras^K were mutated at codon 12, which thus far appears to be one of the most common sites at which this gene becomes activated.

The topography of the amplified proto-oncogene is usually indistinguishable from that of the single-copy counterpart in the normal cell, in spite of the fact that the amplification is often associated with relocation of the DNA encompassing the proto-oncogene from its original chromosomal position to diverse locations on other chromosomes [Schwab et al., 1984a]. Enhanced levels of mRNA and, when tested, of protein have been found to be the general consequence of gene amplification. Only a few instances are known in which amplified proto-oncogenes have undergone structural rearrangements. These exceptional cases include abl in the myelogenous leukemia line K-562, myc in the APUDoma line COLO 320, and erb^B in the human epidermoid carcinoma cell line A431 and in several human brain tumors [for review, see Alitalo and Schwab, 1986]. The structural rearrangements are associated with the presence of an abnormal mRNA, but the data available at this point are insufficient to allow evaluation of the possible significance of such rearrangements in amplification or tumorigenesis.

Amplification gained particular significance as a genetic change associated with tumorigenesis when it was discovered that human neuroblastomas frequently contain an amplified oncogene N-myc localized in DMs or HSRs. N-myc is a member of a gene family referred to as *myc-box* genes [Schwab, 1988]. The discovery of myc-box genes was the outcome of the search for an oncogene that was assumed to be present in DMs or HSRs, which are a frequent feature of human neuroblastoma cells [Schwab et al., 1983a; for review, see Schwab, 1985]. N-myc was found using a viral myc probe and employing reduced stringency conditions for hybridization. Structural analyses revealed the presence of two highly conserved nucleotide boxes (designated *myc boxes*) in the 5′ end of v-myc, or myc, and N-myc. Amplification has been found in neuoblastoma cell lines and in tumors derived directly from patients not subjected to chemo- or to radiotherapy [for review, see Schwab, 1985]. DMs and HSRs, the presence of which originally stimulated the studies of neuroblastoma, are the sites of the amplified N-myc.

To determine the stage of tumor progression at which amplifications are first detectable, several groups have examined neuroblastomas that have been classified on the basis of various pathological and clinical criteria into Evans stages I–IV, with stage IV being the most advanced. In studies of more than 130 tumors, nearly all of the amplifications detected were present in the more advanced tumors (stages III and IV) [Brodeur et al., 1984; Seeger et al., 1985]. The estimated progression-free survival over a period of 18 months of standardized therapy was 70% for patients whose tumors lacked amplification and dropped to 30% in cases with 3–10 copies and to 5% in cases with more than 10 copies [Seeger et al., 1985]. It is conceivable that N-myc copy number may eventually turn out to be a useful marker for assessing prognosis of neuroblastoma and for devising specific therapeutical regimens. Taken together, neuroblastoma represents the first tumor in which amplification of one particular oncogene has been discovered to be related to tumor progression [Schwab et al., 1984a]. Neuroblastoma should provide an interesting system to study, because oncogene amplification is correlated with an advanced stage of disease and because the role of DNA amplification in tumor progression can be further investigated.

Similar principles of amplification of oncogenes have been found in other types of tumors, such as lung cancer and mammary cancer. Lung cancer is the most common fatal malignancy. Small cell lung cancer (SCLC) makes up approximately 25% of all lung cancers. Studies of cell lines established in culture have provided evidence for amplification of myc or, alternatively, of the myc-box genes N-myc or L-myc [for review, see Brooks et al., 1987]. Apparently in SCLC a growth advantage to the tumor cell is conferred by a more general myc function in contrast to neuroblastoma in which only N-myc has been found amplified.

In tissue culture two types of SCLC cell can be recognized, a classic form and a variant form. Although both types express neuroendocrine markers, the variant cell lines are characterized by their increased malignant potential. They have a shorter doubling time, higher cloning efficiency, increased tumorigenicity in nude mice, and are more resistant to radiation. While amplification of N-myc and L-myc has been found in both classic and variant forms of SCLC, amplification of myc seems to be associated exclusively with the variant forms.

Studies of direct preparations of tumors derived from patients have thus far failed to provide evidence for amplification. This does not mean that amplification seen in established cell lines is a tissue culture artifact. It is possible that progression in SCLC takes different routes of genetic changes and that the population of cells with amplification remains undetectable within the background of tumor cells that take other routes of progression. Nevertheless, the strong selection that apparently operates when cells are established in culture is a good indicator for a positive growth advantage that amplification of myc or the myc-box genes confers on the host cell.

In mammary cancers frequent amplification of the HER-2/neu oncogene has been encountered. The HER-2/neu oncogene is a member of the erb^B-like gene family and is related to the gene encoding the epidermal growth factor (EGF) receptor. The HER-2/neu gene has been found to be amplified between 2- and 20-fold in roughly 30% of cell mammary cancers [Slamon et al., 1987]. Like N-myc in neuroblastoma, the specificity at which HER-2/neu is amplified in mammary cancers suggests that this gene plays an important role in this disease.

A positive correlation of HER-2/neu amplification with involved lymph nodes was noted [Slamon et al., 1987], indicating a role of amplification in disease progression. In the same study a strong association between HER-2/neu amplification and relapse and survival was detected. This clearly makes HER-2/neu amplification a valuable parameter for assessment of prognosis. It would be interesting now to determine the status of amplification in primary tumors compared with metastases. Altogether, HER-2/neu amplification in mammary cancer provides a case in which amplification of an oncogene might contribute to the progression phase of tumorigenesis.

AMPLIFICATION IN COLORECTAL CANCERS

Colorectal cancers represent an interesting group of tumors in which cytogenetic evidence for amplification has been obtained but in which the identity of the amplified DNA is not known. Earlier studies on two cell lines had revealed amplification of myc in line COLO 320 [Alitalo et al., 1983] and of myb in line COLO 201/205 [Alitalo et al., 1984]. These two lines presumably represent nontypical cases, because COLO 320 cells possess neuroendocrine properties and are of unknown provenience, and COLO 201/205 cells lack cytogenetic evidence for amplification. In a recent study by Tal et al. [1988] amplification of the HER/neu gene was found in 2 of 45 tumors of the colon and in one of four tumors of the rectum. Cytogenetic analyses have not been performed, however.

In an effort to understand the role that gene amplification might have for development of colorectal cancers, we established a combined cytogenetic and molecular genetic program. At this point we have collected tumor material from more than 80 colorectal cancer patients and have established a series of cultures, some long-term, for cytogenetic and molecular analyses. We have identified at least eight cases in which cytogenetic evidence for gene amplification is evident. Usually DMs are easily detectable (Fig. 1a); in one case DMs were apparently replaced by an HSR during long-term culture (Fig.1b). While we could identify in one tumor (C77) as well as in cultured cells of this tumor roughly 20-fold amplification of the HER/neu oncogene (Fig. 2), most of the tumors that showed cytogenetic evidence for gene amplification were negative for amplification of HER/neu or of several other oncogenes like myc or ras that were tested as well (unpublished data). Additionally, we have been unable to identify amplification of a known oncogene in several cell lines obtained from the laboratory of Adi Gazdar [Park et al., 1988]. It is possible, therefore, that in many cases tumor cells that show cytogenetic evidence carry amplification of an as yet unidentified cellular oncogene.

In an attempt to define the identity of the genetic information in DMs, we are isolating amplified DNA. There are several strategies that can be used for isolation of amplified DNA in those cases in which molecular probes for identification are not yet available. One procedure originally developed by Roninson [1983], is based on the fact that the kinetics at which denatured DNA reassociates is proportional to the concentration of individual DNA sequences. Consequently amplified DNA isolated from one cell line carrying amplification is reasssociated earlier than the corresponding single copy sequences of a control cell line. When suitable conditions are chosen, amplified DNA is present in paired duplex form while the single copy DNA is still only partially or not at all paired. Subsequently nucleases specific for single strand DNA can be employed to digest the unpaired DNA, but leaving the paired DNA intact. The amplified DNA molecules can now be cloned into suitable plasmid or bacteriophage vector and are available for further studies of gene amplification. This strategy has been successfully employed in our laboratory for isolation of amplified DNA from melanoma (Kai van der Bosch, unpublished data). It is obvious, though, that this procedure works best when the degree of amplification is high (more than 35- to 50-fold).

In colorectal cancers, with few exceptions, the average degree of amplification appears to be moderate and may range up to 20-fold. After several as yet unsuccessful attempts with the Roninson procedure we have chosen to isolate DMs directly by micromanupulation procedures. Under microscopic inspection DMs were collected from metaphases by using a fine needle. The DNA was isolated again using micromanipulation and included into cloning vectors. Future studies should inform us about the chromosomal location of amplified DNA, the genetic complexity and nature, and should result in further understanding of the significance that gene amplification has for colorectal cancers.

ADDITIONAL GENETIC CHANGES IN COLORECTAL CANCERS

Early cytogenetic studies of cells of colorectal cancers have provided evidence for various chromosomal abnormalities that clearly point to

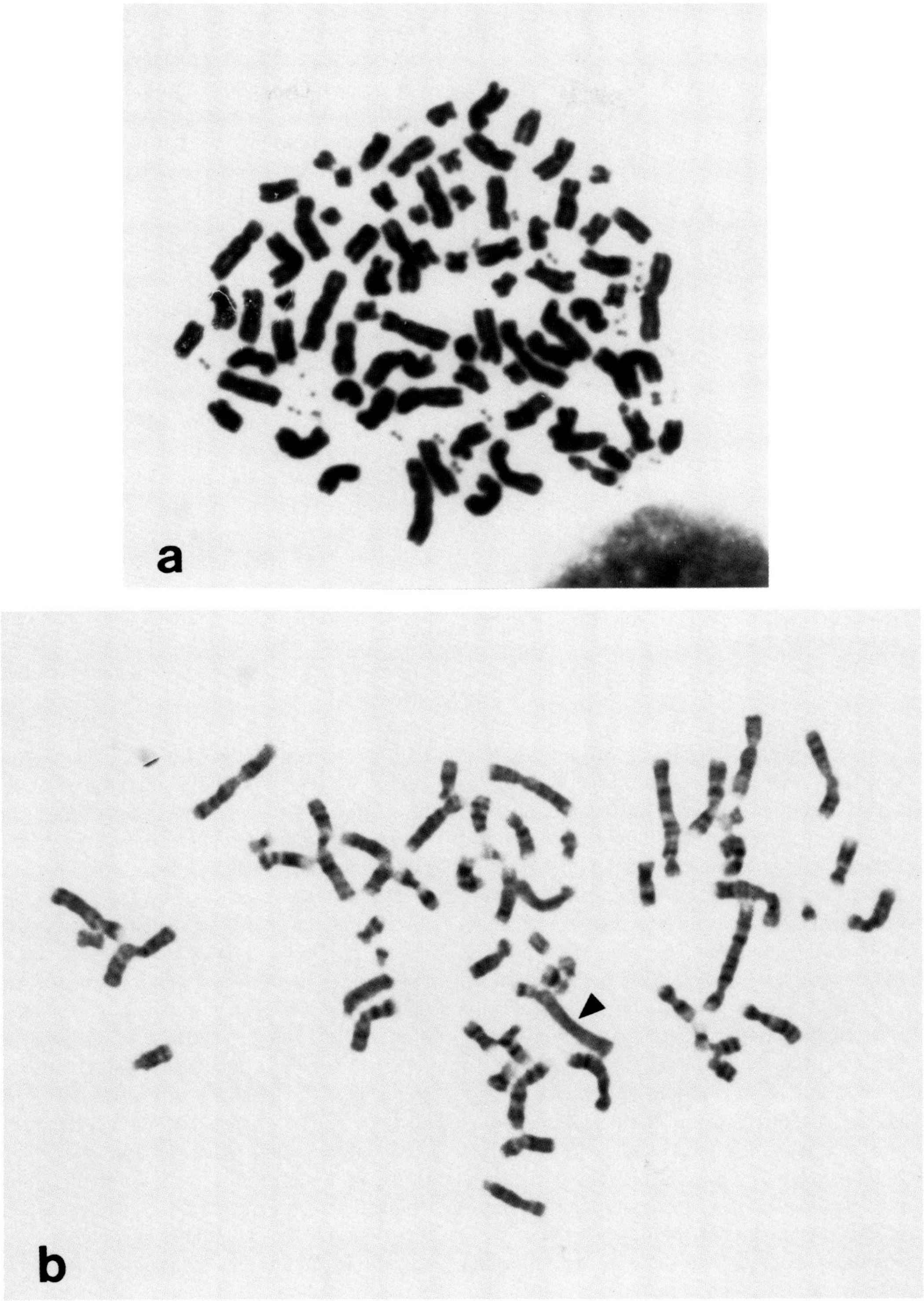

Fig. 1. Cytogenetic evidence for DNA amplification in colorectal cancers. **a:** Metaphase with numerous double minutes (DMs). **b:** Metaphase with a single homogeneously staining chromosomal origin (arrowhead).

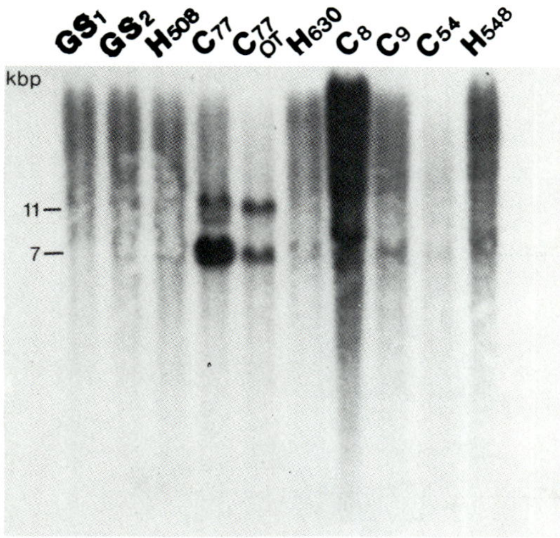

Fig. 2. Amplification of the HER-2/neu oncogene as a rare event in colorectal cancers. Tumor C77 carries approximately 20-fold amplification. DNA of other colon cancers is negative for HER-2/neu amplification, although evidence for DNA amplification is present as DMs. Tumor cell lines are indicated at the top.

genetic changes in the cancer cells. Because of the often bizarre complexity of chromosomal structures (Fig. 3), the significance of chromosomal abnormalities has long been enigmatic. Most of the chromosomal abnormalities found included complex translocations with generation of marker chromosomes of frequently unidentifiable genetic composition. A significant contribution is the observation of an intestitial deletion in chromosome 5 (5q13-22) in peripheral blood cells of a patient with Gardner's syndrome [Herrera et al., 1986]. This finding would indicate loss of genetic material.

By application of molecular biology techniques, genetic changes in cells of colorectal cancers are becoming more and more identified (Table 1). On the basis of the finding of interstitial deletion of 5q in a patient with Gardner's syndrome, a number of investigators have screened colorectal cancers with the aim of finding out whether loss of genetic material is a more frequent genetic change in colorectal cancers. Interestingly, by using a polymorphic minisatellite probe, at least 20% of a heterogeneous set of tumors analyzed had lost genetic material from the 5q region [Solomon et al., 1987]. Loss of genetic material in this region may be an important factor contributing to colorectal tumors and at the same time could point to a relationship between spontaneous colorectal tumors and FAP/FPC for which the gene has also been localized to the 5q region [Bodmer et al., 1987; Leppert et al., 1987]. The matter does become more complicated, though, considering the observation by Okamoto et al. [1988], who found loss of genetic material from colon carcinoma of patients with FAP/FPC not only in chromosome 5q but also in chromosome 22, with some additional losses in chromosomes 5,6,12q, and 15. For detection of loss of genetic material on chromosome 5 a molecular probe C11p11 was used that is closely linked to the FAP/FPC locus [Leppert et al., 1987; Bodmer et al., 1987] (Fig. 4). The relatively low frequency at which loss was detected could be explained by the assumption that the molecular probe C11p11 is, in molecular terms, still far away from the gene putatively deleted in colorectal cancers. Molecular probes from a region closer to the critical gene could in fact show loss at much higher frequency. Altogether, these results would suggest the possible involvement of more than one chromosomal locus in the development of familial and nonhereditary colon carcinomas.

That additional genetic changes are associated with colorectal cancers has been shown in studies by Bos et al. [1987] and Forrester et al. [1987]. A total of 93 colorectal tumors of various types was analyzed for mutational activation of ras genes. Roughly 40% of the tumors were found to contain a mutationally activated ras^K oncogene. No significant difference was found between mutation frequency and degree of differentiation or stage of progression. A high incidence of mutated ras^K was found in tumors originating in villous adenomas, which are common types of benign tumors. The mutations were specific for tumors and were not detected in normal surrounding colon tissue. Interestingly, in few cases both mutated ras^K and mutated ras^N coexisted in the same tumor [Forrester et al.,

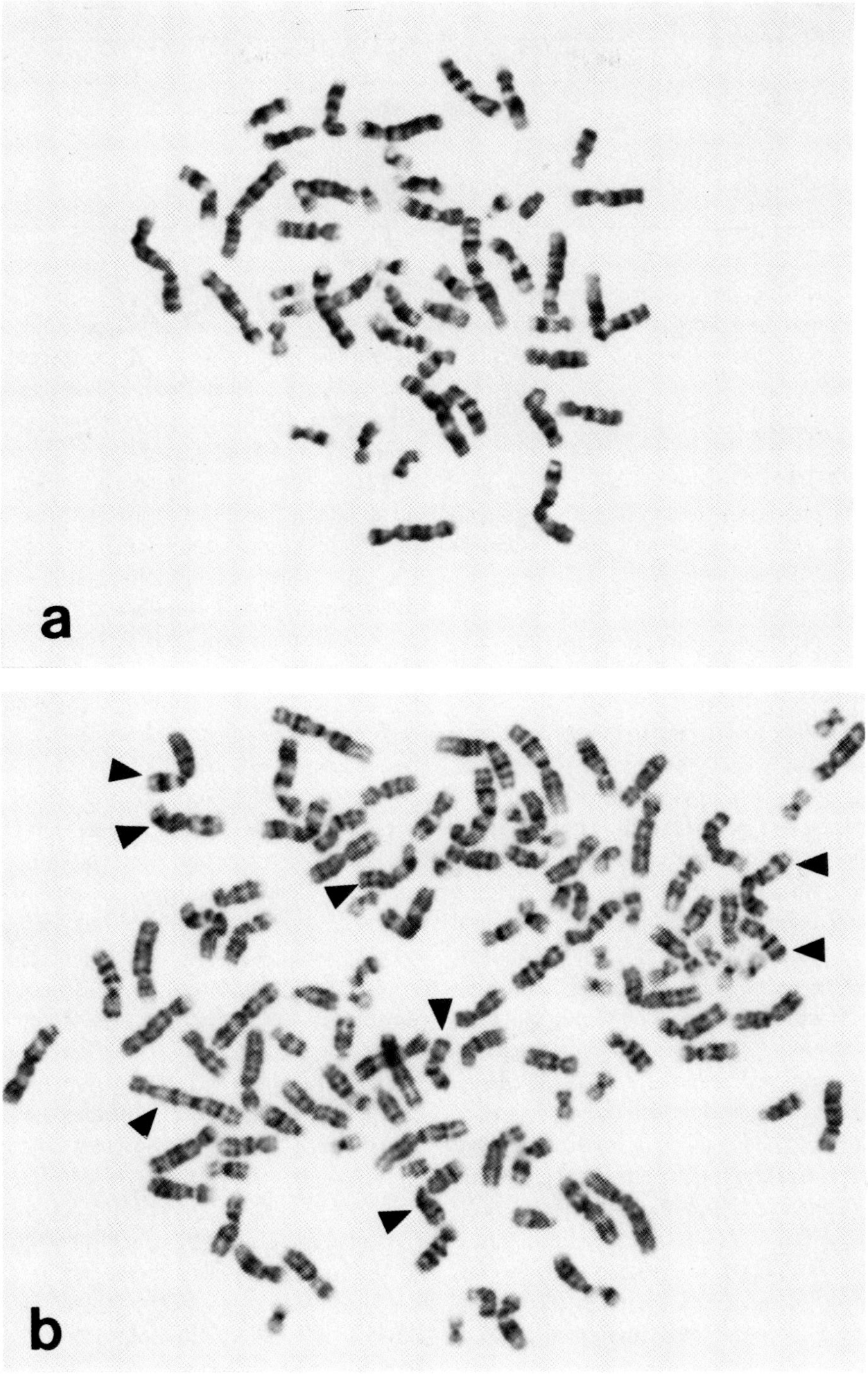

Fig. 3. Complex chromosomal rearrangements often found in cells of colorectal cancers. **a:** Normal constitutional karyotype. **b:** Tumor cell karyotype of the same patient showing complex marker chromosomes of unidentifiable composition (arrowheads).

TABLE 1.
Genetic Changes in Colorectal Cancers

Change	Chromosome	Reference
Deletion	5q	Herrera et al. [1986], Solomon et al. [1987], Okamoto et al. [1988]
	22, 6, 5, 12q, 15	Okamoto et al. [1988]
Mutation (ras^K)		Forrester et al. [1987], Bos et al. [1987]
Amplification	DMs	Reichmann et al. [1981], Tal et al. [1988], present study

1987], although the investigators failed to show that the two mutated ras genes were present in the same cell.

GENETIC CHANGES AND PROGRESSION OF COLORECTAL CANCERS

There is considerable evidence suggesting that at least most cancers arise from a single cell [Fialkow, 1979]. The progeny of this altered cell forms a neoplastic cell clone that is not necessarily malignant from the beginning. The acquisition of increasingly more malignant characteristics by the neoplastic cell, in particular the capacity to invade locally and to metastasize, represents what is generally referred to as *progression*. Progression describes the phenomenon that things that are bad get worse. It is conceptually important to note that the steps through which individual tumors progress may vary among tumors even when of the same type. A central issue in cancer research is to understand how tumors evolve and acquire a more aggressive phenotype. It is widely accepted that tumor cell populations progress by evolutionary change as a result of generation of a variant cell through genomic instability followed by selection of particular variant clones having a growth advantage within the particular tissue environment. Genetic instability appears to be characteristic of neoplastic cells and may be an important factor in tumor progression. As far as colorectal cancers are concerned, there are several stages that can be recognized during progression to malignancy. There is abundant evidence now that most colorectal cancers arise from pre-existing adenomas. Phenotypically progression can be observed from normal epithelium → adenoma → carcinoma. At this point there is little information about the stage of progression to which the different genetic changes may contribute. It appears though that loss of genetic material on chromosome 5 may be involved in development of carcinoma and not in the generation of benign adenomas. At least no adenomas have been found to have 5q material lost even not in the same patients that had lost 5q material in their colon carcinomas [Okamoto et al., 1988; Solomon et al., 1987]. In case of the ras mutations, with few exceptions, the same mutation was found in both the adenomatous (benign) and carcinomatous (malignant) regions of the tumor, suggesting that the mutation preceded the development of malignancy [Bos et al., 1987; Forrester et al., 1987]. There is good evidence that amplification in colorectal cancers, as in neuroblastoma and breast cancer, may be a genetic change associated with more aggressively growing tumors [Schwab, 1986]. In a cytogenetic study by Reichmann et al. [1981] on direct preparations of 31 cancers of the large bowel, six cases were detected with DMs. All three metastatic tumors contained DMs. Future studies employing sensitive methods of molecular biology should identify further the contribution of amplification to colorectal cancers.

CONCLUSIONS

A plethora of genetic changes has been found in various forms of colorectal cancer. As far as we know, there is no single genetic change that alone is associated with colorectal cancer. Progression to malignancy could be result of a combination of various types of genetic changes on different chromosomes. Of particular significance are what appear to be three types of genetic

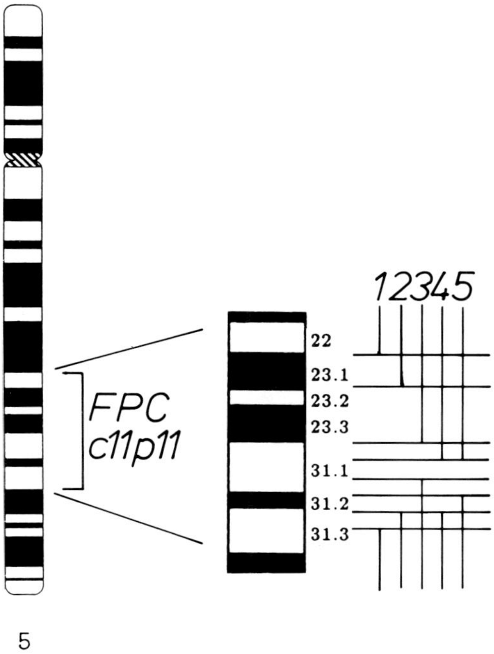

Fig. 4. Schematic illustration of the linkage of the FAP/FPC locus to molecular probe C11p11 on the short arm of chromosome 5. In spontaneous colorectal cancers the C11p11 sequence is deleted in roughly 20% of the cases. It is possible theoretically that the percentage of deletions is higher if molecular probes are employed that are localized closer to the critical gene. The size of the deletion presumably varies among different cancers (such as tumors 1–5). A high percentage of deletion is scored in case probes are used close to the critical gene hypothetically localized for illustrative purposes to chromosome 5q 31.1.

changes: 1) deletion of genetic material from chromosome 5q, a region to which the gene for FAP/FPC has been localized by linkage studies; 2) mutations in the ras^K gene; and 3) amplification of cellular oncogenes. Because amplification may be related to higher malignant phenotypes, application of amplified DNA probes could provide prognostic information. And further characterization of the genetic material deleted from 5q could result in molecular probes that in cases of FAP/FPC may be useful for identifying from the constitutional genotype susceptible individuals among members of families prone to FAP/FPC.

ACKNOWLEDGMENTS

Work referred to in this manuscript was supported by a grant through Heidelberg-Mannheim Comprehensive Cancer Center. We thank Ingrid Ulbrich for typing the manuscript.

References

Alitalo K, Schwab M (1986): Oncogene amplification in tumor cells. Adv Cancer Res 47:235–281.

Alitalo K, Schwab M, Lin CC, Varmus HE, Bishop JM (1983): Homogeneously staining chromosomal regions contain amplified copies of an abundantly expressed cellular oncogene MYC in malignant neuroendocrine cells from a human colon carcinoma. Proc Natl Acad Sci USA 80:1707–1711.

Alitalo K, Winqvist R, Lin CC, de la Chapelle A, Schwab M, Bishop JM (1984): Aberrant expression of an amplified c-myb oncogene in two cell lines from a colon carcinoma. Proc Natl Acad Sci USA 81:4534–4538.

Bodmer WF, Bailey CJ, Bodmer J, Bussey HJR, Ellis A, Gorman P, Lubicello FC, Murday VA, Rider SH, Scambler P, Sheer D, Solomon E, Spurr NK (1987): Localization of the gene for familial adenomatous polyposis on chromosome 5. Nature 328:614–616.

Bos J, Fearon E, Hamilton S, de Vries M, van Boom J, van der Eb A, Vogelstein B (1987): Prevalence of ras gene mutations in human colorectal cancers. Nature 327:293–297.

Brodeur J, Seeger RC, Schwab M, Varmus HE, Bishop JM (1984): Amplification of NMYC in untreated human neuroblastoma correlates with advanced disease stage. Science 224:1121–1124.

Brooks B, Battey J, Nau MM, Gazdar A, Minna J (1987): Amplification and expression of the myc gene in small cell lung cancer. Adv Viral Oncol 7:155–172.

Fialkow PJ (1979): Clonal origin of human tumors. Ann Rev Med 30:135–176.

Forrester K, Almoguere C, Han K, Grizzle W, Perucho M (1987): Detection of high incidence of K-ras oncogenes during human colon tumorigenesis. Nature 327:298–303.

Herrera L, Kakati S, Gibas L, Pietrzak E, Sandberg AA (1986): Brief clinical report: Gardner syndrome in a man with an interstital deletion of 5q. Am J Med Genet 25:473–476.

Levan A, Levan G, Mitelman F (1977): Double minutes and C-bandless chromosomes in a mouse tumor. In: Arrighi FE, Rao RN, Stubblefield E (eds): Genes, Chromosomes and Neoplasia. New York: Raven Press, pp223–251.

Leppert M, Dobbs M, Scambler P, O'Conell P, Makamura Y, Stauffer D, Woodward S, Burt R, Hughes J, Gardner E, Lathrop M, Wasmuth J, Lalouel J-M, White R (1987): The gene for familial polyposis coli maps to the long arm of chromosome 5. Science 328:1411–1413.

Okamoto M, Sasaki M, Sugio K, Sato C, Iwama T, Ikeuchi T, Tonomura A, Sasazuki T, Miyaki M (1988): Loss of constitutional heterozygosity in colon carcinoma from patients with familial polyposis coli. Nature 331:273–2177.

Park J-G, Oie HK, Sugarbaker PH, Henslee J, Chen T-R, Johnson BE, Gazdar AF (1987): Phenotypic variation of cell lines established from human colorectal carcinoma. Cancer Res 47:6710–6718.

Reichmann A, Martin P, Levin B (1981): Chromosomal banding pattern in human large bowel cancer. Int J Cancer 28:431–440.

Riou G, Barrois M, Tordjman I, Dutronquay V, Orth G (1984): Detection of papillomavirus genomes and evidence for amplification of the C-myc and C-Ha-ras invasive squamous cell carcinoma of the uterine cervix. C R Acad Sci Paris [Ser III] 14:575–580.

Roninson I (1983): Detection and mapping of homologous, repeated and amplified DNA sequences by DNA renaturation in agarose gels. Nucleic Acids Res 11:5413–5431.

Schwab M, Alitalo K, Varmus HE, Bishop JM, George D (1983b): A cellular oncogene (c-Ki-ras is amplified, overexpressed, and located within karyotypic abnormalities in mouse adrenocortical tumor cells. Nature 303:497–501.

Schwab M, Alitalo K, Klempnauer KH, Varmus HE, Bishop JM, Gilbert F, Brodeur G, Goldstein M, Trent J (1983a): Amplified DNA with limited homology to MYC cellular oncogene is shared by human neuroblastoma cell lines and a neuroblastoma tumor. Nature 305:245–248.

Schwab M, Varmus HE, Bishop JM, Grzeschik KH, Naylor S, Sakaguchi A, Brodeur G, Trent J (1984b): Chromosome localization in normal human cells and neuroblastomas of a gene related to c-myc. Natue 308:288–291.

Schwab M, Ellison J, Busch M, Rosenau W, Varmus HE, Bishop JM (1984a): Enhanced expression of the human gene N-myc consequent to amplification of DNA may contribute to malignant progression of neuroblastoma. Proc Natl Acad Sci USA 81:4940–4944.

Schwab M (1985): Amplification of N-myc in human neuroblastomas. Trends Genet 1:271–275.

Schwab M (1986): Amplification of proto-oncogenes and tumor progression. In Kahn P, Graf T (eds): Oncogenes and growth control. Berlin: Springer-Verlag, pp 332–339.

Schwab M (1988): The MYC-box oncogenes. In Reddy P, Skalka AM, Currah T (eds): The Oncogene Handbook. Amsterdam: Elsevier Science Publishers, pp. 381–391.

Seeger RC, Brodeur GM, Sather H, Dalton A, Siegel SE, Wong KY, Hammond D (1985): Association of multiple copies of the N-myc oncogene with rapid progression of neuroblastomas. N Engl J Med 313:1111–1116.

Slamon DJ, Clark GM, Wong GS, Levin WJ, Ullrich A, McGuire WL (1987): Human breast cancer: Correlation of relapse and survival with amplification of the HER-2/neu oncogene. Science 235:177–182.

Solomon E, Voss R, Hall V, Bodmer WF, Jass JR, Jeffreys AF, Lucibello FC, Patel I, Rider SH (1987): Chromosome 5 allele loss in human colorectal carcinomas.Nature 328:616–619.

Tal M, Wetzler M, Josefberg Z, Deutch A, Gutmann M, Assaf D, Kris R, Shiloh Y, Girol D, Schlessinger J (1988): Sporadic amplification of the HER2/neu protooncogene in adenocarcinomas of various tissues. Cancer Res 48:1517–1520.

Taya Y, Hosogai K, Hirohashi S, Shimosato Y, Tsuchiya R, Tsuchida N, Fushimi M, Sekiya T, Nishimura S (1984): A novel combination of K-ras and myc amplification accompanied by point mutational activation of K-ras in a human lung cancer. EMBO J 3:2943–2946.

Watne AL (1987): Patterns of inheritance of colon polyps. Semin Surg Oncol 3:71–76.

44

Amplification and Activation of the c-myc Oncogene in Adenocarcinoma of the Large Bowel

Kathleen M. Herold and Paul G. Rothberg

Department of Human Genetics, Roswell Park Memorial Institute, Buffalo, New York

INTRODUCTION

The human cellular myc gene (c-myc) was discovered because of its homology to the viral myc gene (v-myc) of the acutely oncogenic retrovirus MC29 [1]. The v-myc gene is responsible for the ability of MC29 to cause myelocytomatosis, sarcoma, carcinoma, and lymphoma in infected chickens [2,3]. In humans, the c-myc gene has been found altered in a variety of neoplasms [4], although a consistent association between myc gene mutations and neoplastic disease was found in only two cases. The myc gene is amplified (present in greater than one copy per haploid genome) in cell lines derived from an aggressive variant of small cell lung carcinoma [5]. Also, in Burkitt's lymphoma, a chromosomal translocation takes place that juxtaposes the myc gene with one of the immunoglobulin genes, and in many cases this results in a rearrangement in the immediate vicinity of the myc gene [6,7]. Both rearrangement and amplification of myc effect an increase in expression of the gene [8,9]. It is this overexpression, in which a normal cellular protein is produced in overabundance, or at an inappropriate time, that contributes to malignant growth. Elevated expression of the oncogene c-myc is often found in tranformed cells without concomitant rearrangement or amplification, but the molecular events that underlie this are unknown [10–12].

In previous work, we [12–14] and others [15–21] have shown that the oncogene c-myc is frequently expressed at an elevated level in adenocarcinoma of the colon. In a study of 29 primary human adenocarcinomas, we found that 21 (72%) had a level of mRNA fivefold or more of that in nonmalignant tissue from the same surgical specimen [12]. In each of the 21 colon tumors with elevated myc expression, the myc gene was neither amplified nor rearranged [12]. Subsequent studies of myc gene structure in colon cancer have confirmed our result on the absence of rearrangement, but have shown several instances of myc gene amplification [20–24]. In this paper we demonstrate that the colon carcinoma cell line WiDr has an amplified myc gene, and we explore the consequences of this alteration on the level of myc RNA. In addition, we examined methylation in the third exon of the c-myc gene and evaluated the effect of the differentiating agent sodium butyrate on the level of myc RNA in WiDr cells.

MATERIALS AND METHODS

Cells

WiDr, SW837, DLD-1, and SW1417 cell lines were obtained from the American Type Culture Collection (ATCC, Rockville, MD) and grown in RPMI 1640 medium (Gibco, Grand Island, NY) supplemented with 1 mM sodium pyruvate,

Familial Adenomatous Polyposis, pages 361–369

fetal bovine serum, and 5% Nu-Serum serum substitute (Collaborative Research, Bedford, MA). Cells were harvested when nearly confluent (>80%). Surgical specimens were received immediately after removal from the patient, flash frozen in liquid nitrogen, and stored at −70°C.

Preparation of RNA and DNA

RNA was prepared by lysis in guanidinium thiocyanate and centrifugation over a cesium chloride shelf as described by Rothberg et al. [11]. DNA from tissue culture cells was processed simultaneously from the same cells as described previously [11]. DNA from solid tissue was prepared by proteinase K digestion, phenol extraction, and ethanol precipitation as described by Davis et al. [25].

Southern and Northern Blots

Southern blots were prepared by incubating DNA with the appropriate restriction endonuclease according to the manufacturer's instructions (New England Biolabs, Beverly, MA), resolving the resulting fragments by gel electrophoresis, base denaturing in situ, transferring the size-separated DNA to a nylon hybridization membrane (Zetabind, AMF Cuno), and hybridizing with the appropriate radioactive DNA fragment [12]. Northern blots were done by denaturing 10 μg of total cellular RNA with glyoxal (50°C, 45 minutes), resolving by agarose gel electrophoresis, transferring the size-separated RNAs to a nylon hybridization membrane, and hybridizing at 65°C with the appropriate radioactive DNA fragment [26].

Hybridization and Probes

Hybridization and washing of nucleic acids immobilized on nylon membranes was carried out as described previously [26]. After removing unhybridized radioactive probe, the blots were exposed to XAR5 X-ray film (Kodak, Rochester, NY) at −70°C with a Cronex (Dupont, Wilmington, DE) intensifying screen. Densitometry of lightly exposed films was done with a Helena Laboratories Quick-scan Junior.

The c-myc probe was the third exon of the human myc gene contained in a 1.4 kbp (kilobase pair) ClaI–EcoRI fragment [11]. The N-myc probe was pNb-1, a 1.0 kbp EcoRI–BamHI fragment [27]. The mos probe was pHM2A, a 2.75 kbp EcoRI–EcoRI fragment [28]. ^{32}P-labeled probe was prepared by random primer labeling of DNA fragments purified by gel electrophoresis [26].

RESULTS

myc Gene Amplification

Amplification of cellular oncogenes is an important event that results in elevated expression of these cancer-inducing genes [9]. It has been demonstrated that the oncogene c-myc is occasionally amplified in adenocarcinoma of the colon [20–24]. To detect such a case, we chose to survey a group of colon carcinoma cell lines for changes in copy number of the c-myc gene. Figure 1 (upper panel) is a Southern blot analysis of the c-myc gene, and the related but distinct N-myc gene, in DNA fragments produced by the restriction endonuclease SacI. The equal intensities of the control N-myc bands confirms that equal quantities of DNA were loaded in each lane. However, the increased intensity of the c-myc gene signal from the WiDr adenocarcinoma cell line shows that extra gene copies were present, compared with normal colonic mucosa (SA), and colon carcinoma cell lines SW837, SW1417, and DLD-1. Two separate DNA preparations from WiDr are shown in Figure 1. After the initial discovery of myc gene amplification in WiDr (WiDr-2), we studied cells that were frozen ten generations earlier to determine if the amplification was present in cells that had gone through fewer passages since being received from the ATCC (WiDr-1). The intensity of the myc signal is about the same in both DNA preparations, indicating that the amplification was stable during the period of growth in tissue culture.

Polysomy of chromosome 8, which carries the c-myc gene [29], may possibly account for its amplification. This would also result in amplification of other genes on chromosome 8, including the c-mos oncogene [29]. The lower panel of Figure 1 is a Southern blot analysis of the mos gene that revealed no alteration in mos gene copy number. Thus, the myc amplification in WiDr was not due to multiple copies of chromosome 8.

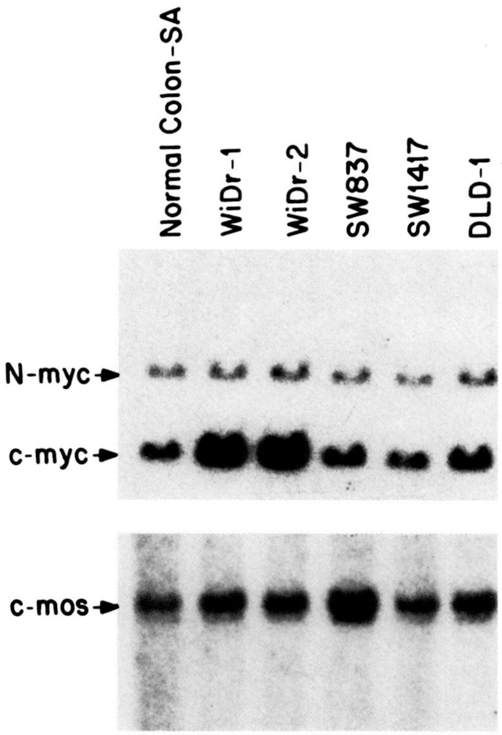

Fig. 1. Southern blot analysis reveals an amplification of the oncogene c-myc in colorectal adenocarcinoma cell line WiDr. **Upper panel:** Five micrograms of DNA from normal colonic mucosa (SA) and colon cancer cell lines WiDr, SW837, SW1417, and DLD-1 were cleaved with restriction endonuclease SacI, electrophoresed on a 0.8% agarose gel, and transferred to a solid support. The blot was hybridized with probes for c-myc and N-myc, washed to remove unhybridized radioactive probe, and exposed to X-ray film. The equal intensities of the N-myc signals confirms that equal quantities of DNA were loaded in each lane. The increased intensity of the c-myc band in WiDr indicates that the c-myc gene was amplified in both DNA preparations (WiDr-1 and WiDr-2). **Lower panel:** The same as above except using restriction endonuclease HindIII and a c-mos probe to show that the c-myc amplification was not due to polyploidy of chromosome 8.

To quantitate the degree of amplification, we prepared a Southern blot containing dilutions of WiDr DNA and several nonamplified samples. Figure 2 shows that the normal band intensity for myc, as exemplified by AN (normal lung), SA (normal colon), and SW1417 (colon cancer cell line), lies between the one-fourth and one-eighth dilution of WiDr. Therefore, we conclude that the WiDr adenocarcinoma cell line contains a four- to eightfold amplification of the myc gene, which corresponds to 8–16 copies per cell. Evaluation of the blot in Figure 1 with a scanning-integrating densitometer confirmed this result; normalizing for N-myc band intensities, the WiDr myc bands are 5.3-fold more intense than the

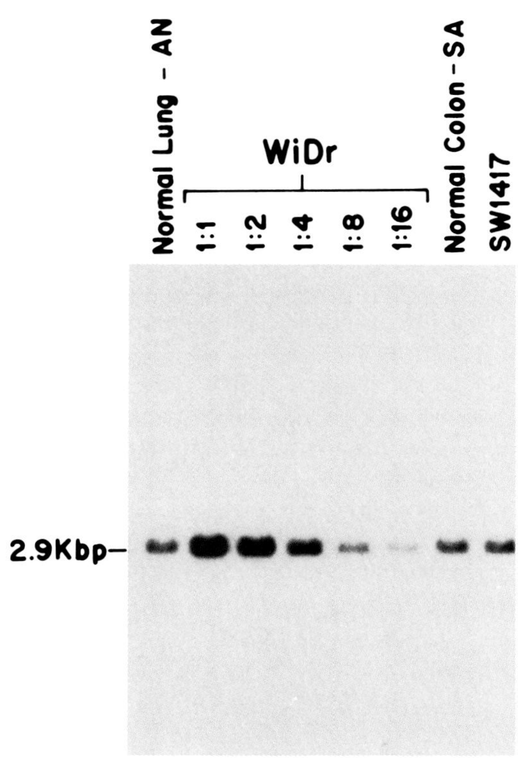

Fig. 2. Quantitation of c-myc gene amplification in WiDr. Five micrograms of DNA from normal human lung (AN), normal human colonic mucosa (SA), colon cancer cell lines SW1417 and WiDr, and the indicated dilutions of WiDr were cleaved with restriction endonuclease SacI, electrophoresed on a 0.9% agarose gel, and transferred to a solid support. The blot was hybridized with a c-myc probe. Successive WiDr lanes contained twofold serial dilutions of the 5 μg of DNA in the first (1:1) WiDr lane. The signal intensity of the normal DNAs fell between the 1:4 and 1:8 dilution of WiDr DNA.

average of the nonamplified samples. No rearrangements of myc or N-myc were detected using SacI (Fig. 1) or EcoRI (data not shown), which is in accord with previous work [12,16,18–24].

RNA Analysis

The expected consequence of gene amplification is increased expression. Figure 3 shows a Northern blot analysis of the level of myc mRNA in several patient samples and cell lines. In this experiment total RNA is denatured, separated by gel electrophoresis, transferred to a solid support, and hybridized with a radioactive myc probe. WiDr cells contained approximately a 10-fold greater abundance of myc RNA compared with the nonmalignant (N) portion of colectomy specimens from Fr and Se. Thus, the above raised expectation is fulfilled. The ~10-fold increase in RNA level and approximate fivefold DNA amplification may appear to indicate a slightly higher rate of transcription per myc gene copy in WiDr compared with normal colonic mucosa, but the low magnitude of the difference coupled with experimental error makes such an assumption hazardous. We conclude from this experiment that at least most of the increase in myc RNA level in WiDr can be attributed to its myc gene amplification.

We know from past work that myc RNA levels are often elevated in adenocarcinoma of the large bowel [12,21]. This is confirmed in Figure 3 by the carcinoma (CA) portion of colectomy specimens from Se and Pe. We wished to determine how WiDr, which has an amplification of the myc gene, compares with other colon cancer cell lines and patient samples with respect to myc RNA abundance. It can be seen in Figure 3 that WiDr gives a signal approximately equal to the other lines (SW837, SW1417, and DLD-1), which were shown (Fig. 1) to have a normal complement of myc genes. Thus, elevated expression of the myc gene occurs with and without concomitant amplification of the gene. The elevated level of myc RNA in WiDr cells was similar to that in one tumor (Pe) and below that in another (Se) of two randomly selected adenocarcinomas (Fig. 3).

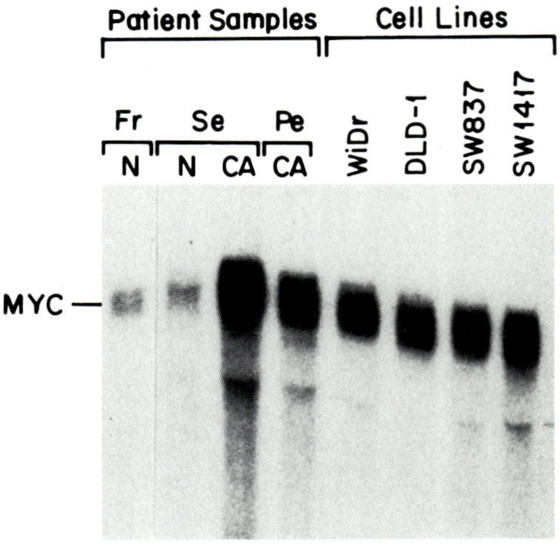

Fig. 3. Northern blot analysis of myc RNA in colectomy specimens and colon carcinoma cell lines. Ten micrograms of total RNA from nonmalignant mucosa (N) and adenocarcinoma of the large bowel (CA) derived from patients (Fr, Se, Pe) undergoing colectomy, as well as the cell lines WiDr, SW837, SW1417, and DLD-1 were denatured, resolved by electrophoresis on a 1.2% agarose gel, transferred to a solid support, and hybridized with a radioactive myc probe. The level of 2.4 kb (kilobase) myc RNA in the four colon cancer cell lines was approximately equal despite the fact that WiDr has four- to eightfold more myc DNA than the other lines (Fig. 1).

DNA Methylation

In vertebrate DNA the No. 5 carbon of C residues is often methylated in the sequence 5′-CG-3′. In many cases this methylation correlates with decreased gene expression, while demethylation is associated with a "turning on" of gene activity [30]. We analyzed the methylation state of a potential site in exon 3 of the myc gene, because previous work has shown that this site is subject to hypomethylation in several tumor types [31, 32]. In adenocarcinoma of the large bowel this site is hypomethylated in comparison with nonmalignant mucosa from the same surgical specimen (M.D. Erisman, P.G. Rothberg, and S.M. Astrin, data not shown). To be consistent with the hypothesis that myc expression per gene copy is essentially normal in WiDr cells, we predicted that this site would be methylated.

Our analysis was conducted by Southern blot hybridization after sequential digestion by EcoRI and HpaII. HpaII cuts the sequence CCGG but not C^{m}CGG. The potential HpaII sites (➧) in the 3′ half of the myc gene are illustrated in Figure 4A. A potential site in exon 2 is demethylated and is always cut by HpaII. If the variable site in exon 3 is also demethylated then 2.2 kpb and 1.0 kbp fragments will be generated as indicated in Figure 4A. If the exon 3 site is methylated, a 3.2 kbp fragment is generated (Fig. 4A). As seen in Figure 4B, WiDr cell DNA gave the 3.2 kbp fragment almost exclusively (lane H) and was therefore shown to be fully methylated in exon 3 as we predicted above. To demonstrate that this result was not due to incomplete cleavage by HpaII, the 3H lane reveals the same result with a threefold increase in the amount of restriction enzyme. This result is further supported by the complete cleavage of the exon 2 site. To prove that the lack of digestion at the CCGG site in exon 3 was due to methylation rather than to mutation, we substituted MspI for HpaII in the M lanes of Figure 4B. MspI cleaves the same CCGG sequence without regard to methylation at the internal C. The MspI digests gave the predicted 2.2 and 1.0 kbp fragments. Similar analysis of SW837 cell DNA demonstrated hypomethylation of the exon 3 site as compared with WiDr cell DNA (Fig. 4B).

Response to Butyrate

A variety of cell types have been shown to respond to agents that induce differentiation by reducing the level of c-myc RNA [33–37]. This phenomenon was also seen in colorectal carcinoma cells [26,38]. We reasoned that if the elevated level of myc RNA in WiDr cells is due to

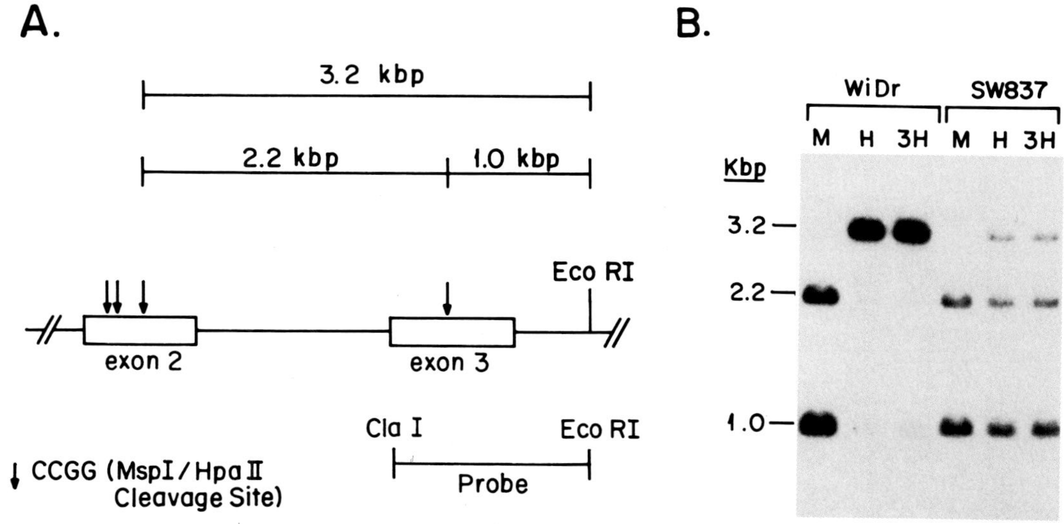

Fig. 4. Analysis of DNA methylation in exon 3 of the human myc gene. **A:** Diagram showing the location of potential HpaII sites in the 3′ half of the myc gene (➧) and the predicted fragments generated by endonuclease cleavage with EcoRI and HpaII. If the exon 3 site is fully methylated, a 3.2 kbp fragment will be detected. Molecules that lack methylation at the exon 3 site will give 2.2 and 1.0 kbp fragments. The 1.4 kbp ClaI–EcoRI fragment used to make radioactive probe is also indicated. **B:** DNA from WiDr or SW837, as indicated, was digested with EcoRI, purified by phenol extraction and ethanol precipitation, and then 5 μg aliquots were digested with 45 units of MspI (M), 35 units of HpaII (H), or 105 units of HpaII (3H). DNA was resolved by electrophoresis on a 1.2% agarose gel, then transferred and hybridized with a myc probe as described. WiDr cell DNA was fully methylated at the potential HpaII site in exon 3, while in SW837 cells this site lacked methylation on most molecules.

amplification of the encoding gene, then a short exposure to a differentiating agent should *not* result in reduced myc expression because the level of myc RNA in WiDr cells is already reduced to a normal level per gene copy. As shown in Figure 5, exposure of SW837 cells to 2 mM sodium butyrate for 24 hours resulted in a sharp reduction in the level of myc RNA. This contrasts with the lack of response of WiDr cells to the same conditions (Fig. 5). In further experiments (data not shown) we have demonstrated that the level of myc RNA in WiDr cells remains unchanged at butyrate levels up to 5 mM for 1 to 3 days. These results are in accord with our hypothesis that myc gene amplification is the cause of elevated myc expression in WiDr cells.

DISCUSSION

We have shown that WiDr, a cell line derived from a rectosigmoid adenocarcinoma [39], contains a four- to eightfold amplification of c-myc DNA (Figs. 1, 2), and an 8–16-fold elevated level of myc RNA (Fig. 3) compared with normal colonic mucosa. However, the elevated myc RNA level in WiDr was not exceptional when compared with other cell lines derived from colorectal carcinoma. The level of myc RNA in WiDr cells was similar to that in SW837, SW1417, and DLD-1 (Fig. 3), lines that contain the normal complement of one c-myc gene per haploid genome (Fig. 1). These results confirm that enhanced myc RNA levels can occur in the presence or absence of gene amplification in cancer of the large bowel [12]. Deregulation of myc expression without amplification or rearrangement of the gene has also been reported in leukemia [11], breast cancer [40], and hepatoma [41,42].

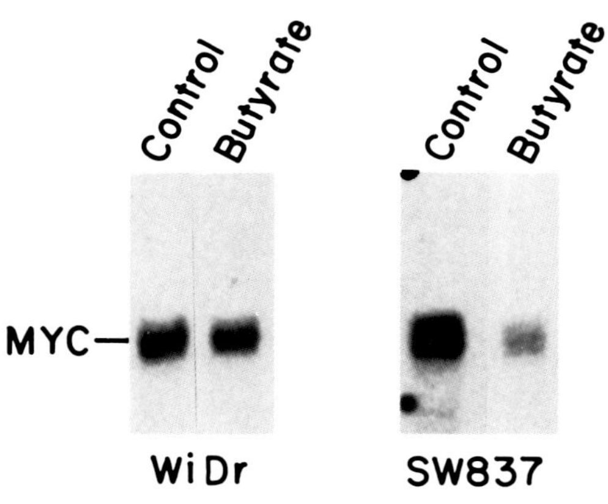

Fig. 5. Northern blot analysis of the effect of butyrate on the level of myc RNA in WiDr and SW837 cells. Cell cultures were exposed to 2 mM sodium butyrate (sodium salt of n-butyric acid) for 24 hours and then harvested for RNA preparation and Northern blot analysis with a myc probe. SW837 cells responded to butyrate with a marked decrease in expression of myc RNA. The level of myc RNA in WiDr cells remained unchanged.

WiDr has a normal, or near-normal, level of myc RNA per myc gene. The increased copy number of myc genes is apparently responsible for the increased level of myc RNA in WiDr. Two lines of evidence support this conclusion. One is the finding (Fig. 4) that a variable methylation site in exon 3 of the myc gene is fully methylated in WiDr cells. This fully methylated state is similar to the myc gene in normal colon, but different from the hypomethylated state of this site in colorectal carcinomas and the colorectal carcinoma cell line SW837 (Fig. 4). In addition, exposure to sodium butyrate caused a reduction of myc expression in SW837 but not in WiDr cells (Fig. 5). This is consistent with the hypothesis that the level of myc RNA in WiDr cells is already reduced to a normal level per gene copy. Despite these supportive data, we cannot exclude the possibility that a single mutated myc gene caused the increase in RNA while the other amplified myc genes are transcriptionally silent.

Another mechanism for activating myc expression is rearrangement, in which a promoter or other element capable of increasing gene expression in cis moves into the vicinity of the myc gene. The COLO 320DM cell line, which was derived from a neuroendocrine tumor of the large bowel, contains a rearrangement of the myc gene [43]. However, only one myc rearrangement has been found in a cell line [44] and none in a primary tumor of the 121 colorectal adenocarcinomas that have been reported on to date [12,16, 18,20–24,44].

How frequently is the myc gene amplified in

colorectal cancer? Table 1 is a summation of the literature regarding this question. Out of 14 cells lines and 107 patient samples, three and six respectively, had myc gene amplification (adjusting for the same cell line analyzed in more than one article and multiple lines developed from the same patient). Thus about 7% of the specimens analyzed contained excess myc genes. The lack of rearrangement and relative rarity of DNA amplification indicates that other molecular events must cause the increased myc RNA expression seen in the 70% or more of colorectal adenocarcinomas that have an elevated level of myc RNA.

What is the significance of elevated myc expression? Several lines of experimentation suggest that abnormal regulation of myc expression, with a consequent elevated RNA level, is a carcinogenic event. Keath et al. [45] used a mouse myc gene linked to a promoter derived from SV40 or Moloney murine leukemia virus to show that elevated expression of c-myc in two rodent fibroblast cell lines, NIH/3T3 and Rat2, made them capable of producing tumors in nude mice. The same SV40 construct was shown to block differentiation of mouse erythroleukemia cells [46]. In another type of experiment, transgenic mice, constructed using a c-myc gene linked to a strong promoter, suffered from increased rates of malignancy in several different tissues in which the fusion gene was expressed [47–49].

What is the significance of elevated myc expression in cancer of the large bowel? As described previously [13,14], the site distribution of unselected colorectal carcinomas with significantly elevated myc expression is similar to the site distribution of carcinomas in patients with familial adenomatous polyposis (FAP). This provides evidence that elevated myc expression plays a role in a genetically distinct form of sporadic colorectal cancer that involves the FAP gene. It is possible that the FAP gene, which is located on chromosome 5 [50], codes for a negative regulator of myc expression [51]. Alternatively, deregulated myc expression may be an independent event that is required for FAP tumorigenesis. In support of these possibilities, direct analysis of four independent adenocarcinomas of the large bowel from FAP patients has shown that all contain significantly elevated levels of myc RNA (M.D. Erisman and S.M. Astrin, personal communication; L. Herrera and P.G. Rothberg, unpublished data).

TABLE 1.
Frequency of c-myc Amplification in Adenocarcinoma of the Large Bowel

No. of samples	Type[a]	No. with amplification	Range[b]	References
21[c]	P	0	—	Erisman et al. [12]
6	L	0	—	Erisman et al. [12]
1	L	0	—	Yoshimoto et al. [16]
15	P	0	—	Sikora et al. [18]
14	P	1	26	Monnat et al. [20]
6	L	3	8–64	Untwale and Blick [21]
3	P	0	—	Untwale and Blick [21]
45	P	3	3–8	Yokota et al. [22], Meltzer et al. [24]
9	P	2	3–4	Alexander et al. [23]
7	L	2	3–5	Erisman et al. [44]
4	L	1	4–8	This study

[a]P, patient sample; L, cell line.
[b]Degree of amplification over normal.
[c]In Erisman et al. [12], only the 21 tumors that had an elevated level of myc RNA were analyzed for gene amplification.

CONCLUSIONS

Gene amplification (increased copy number) is an event that results in an increased quantity of the encoded protein. If the amplified gene is a cellular proto-oncogene, then its amplification and consequent overexpression are potentially carcinogenic events. We have found that the oncogene c-myc is amplified in the colon carcinoma cell line WiDr to a level of 8–16 copies per cell (four- to eightfold amplification). RNA transcribed from the myc gene was also elevated about 10-fold above that in normal colon, probably as a result of the DNA amplification. However, other colon carcinoma cell lines that did not contain c-myc amplification (SW837, SW1417, and DLD-1) also had an equally high level of myc RNA, confirming that enhanced myc RNA levels in cancer of the large bowel can occur in the presence or absence of gene amplification. Studies of DNA methylation in the myc gene and the response of myc RNA level to the differentiating agent sodium butyrate revealed differences between WiDr cells and SW837 cells that are consistent with gene amplification being responsible for the elevated level of myc RNA in WiDr cells.

ACKNOWLEDMENTS

We thank Dr. M. Schwab for plasmid pNb-1, Dr. G. Vande Woude for plasmid pHM2A, and G. Anderson, M.D. Erisman, and A. Mittelman for reviewing the manuscript, and N. Frame for its preparation. This work was supported by grants RR-05648-20 and P30CA16056-13 from the USPHS.

References

1. Roussel M, Saule S, Lagrou C, Rommens C, Beug H, Graf T, Stehelin D: Three new types of viral oncogene of cellular origin specific for haematopoietic cell transformation. Nature 281:452–455, 1979.

2. Graf T, Beug H: Avian leukemia viruses: Interaction with their target cells in vivo and in vitro. Biochim Biophys Acta 516:269–299, 1978.

3. Enrietto PJ, Payne LN, Hayman MJ: A recovered avian myelocytomatosis virus that induces lymphomas in chickens: Pathogenic properties and their molecular basis. Cell 35:369–379, 1983.

4. Nishimura S, Sekiya T: Human cancer and cellular oncogenes. Biochem J 243:313–327, 1987.

5. Little CD, Nau MM, Carney DN, Gazdar AF, Minna JD: Amplification and expression of the c-myc oncogene in human lung cancer cell lines. Nature 306:194–196, 1983.

6. Taub R, Kirsch I, Morton C, Lenoir G, Swan D, Tronick S, Aaronson S, Leder P: Translocation of the c-myc gene into the immunoglobulin heavy chain locus in human Burkitt lymphoma and murine plasmacytoma cells. Proc Natl Acad Sci USA 79:7837–7841, 1982.

7. Adams JM, Gerondakis S, Webb E, Corcoran LM, Cory S: Cellular myc oncogene is altered by chromosome translocation to an immunoglobulin locus in murine plasmacytomas and is rearrranged similarly in human Burkitt's lymphomas. Proc Natl Acad Sci USA 80:1982–1986, 1983.

8. Cory S: Activation of cellular oncogenes in hemopoietic cells by chromosome translocation. Adv Cancer Res 47:189–234, 1986.

9. Alitalo K, Schwab M: Oncogene amplification in tumor cells. Adv Cancer Res 47:235–281, 1986.

10. Campisi J, Gray HE, Pardee AB, Dean M, Sonenshein GE: Cell-cycle control of c-myc but not c-ras expression is lost following chemical transformation. Cell 36:241–247, 1984.

11. Rothberg PG, Erisman MD, Diehl RE, Rovigatti UG, Astrin SM: Structure and expression of the oncogene c-myc in fresh tumor material from patients with hematopoietic malignancies. Mol Cell Biol 4:1096–1103, 1984.

12. Erisman MD, Rothberg PG, Diehl RE, Morse CC, Spandorfer JM, Astrin SM: Deregulation of c-myc gene expression in human colon carcinoma is not accompanied by amplification or rearrangement of the gene. Mol Cell Biol 5:1969–1976, 1985.

13. Rothberg PG, Spandorfer JM, Erisman MD, Staroscik RN, Sears HF, Petersen RO, Astrin SM: Evidence that c-myc expression defines two genetically distinct forms of colorectal adenocarcinoma. Br J Can 52:629–632, 1985.

14. Rothberg PG: The role of the oncogene c-myc in sporadic large bowel cancer and familial polyposis coli. Semin Surg Oncol 3:152–158, 1987.

15. Slamon DJ, deKernion JB, Verma IM, Cline MJ: Expression of cellular oncogenes in human malignancies. Science 224:256–262, 1984.

16. Yoshimoto K, Hirohashi S, Sekiya T: Increased expression of the c-myc gene without gene amplification in human lung cancer and colon cancer cell lines. Jpn J Cancer Res (Gann) 77:540–545, 1986.

17. Stewart J, Evan G, Watson J, Sikora K: Detection of the c-myc oncogene product in colonic polyps and carcinomas. Br J Cancer 53:1–6, 1986.

18. Sikora K, Chan S, Evan G, Gabra H, Markham N, Stewart J, Watson J: c-myc oncogene expression in colorectal cancer. Cancer 59:1289–1295, 1987.

19. Tsuboi K, Hirayoshi K, Takeuchi K, Sabe H, Shimada Y, Ohshio G, Tobe T, Hatanaka M: Expression of the c-myc gene in human gastrointestinal malignancies. Biochem Biophys Res Commun 146:699–704, 1987.

20. Monnat M, Tardy S, Saraga P, Diggelmann H, Costa J: Prognostic implications of expression of the cellular genes myc, fos, Ha-ras and Ki-ras in colon carcinoma. Int J Cancer 40:293–299, 1987.

21. Untwale S, Blick M: Oncogene expression in adeno-

carcinomas of the colon and in colon tumor-derived cell lines. Anticancer Res 8:1–8, 1988.

22. Yokota J, Tsunetsugu-Yokota Y, Battifora H, Le Fevre C, Cline MJ: Alterations of myc, myb and ras^{HA} protooncogenes in cancers are frequent and show clinical correlation. Science 231:261–265, 1986.

23. Alexander RJ, Buxbaum JN, Raicht RF: Oncogene alterations in primary human colon tumors. Gastroenterology 91:1503–1510, 1986.

24. Meltzer SJ, Ahnen DJ, Battifora H, Yokota J, Cline MJ: Protooncogene abnormalities in colon cancers and adenomatous polyps. Gastroenterology 92:1174–1180, 1987.

25. Davis LG, Dibner MD, Battey JF: Basic Methods in Molecular Biology. New York: Elsevier Science Publishing Co., 1986.

26. Herold KM, Rothberg PG: Evidence for a labile intermediate in the butyrate induced reduction of the level of c-myc RNA in SW837 rectal carcinoma cells. Oncogene 3:423–428, 1988.

27. Schwab M, Alitalo K, Klempnauer K-H, Varmus HE, Bishop JM, Gilbert F, Brodeur G, Goldstein M, Trent J: Amplified DNA with limited homology to myc cellular oncogene is shared by human neuroblastoma cell lines and a neuroblastoma tumour. Nature 305:245–248, 1983.

28. Watson R, Oskarsson M, Vande Woude GF: Human DNA sequences homologous to the transforming gene (mos) of Moloney murine sarcoma virus. Proc Natl Acad Sci USA 79:4078–4082, 1982.

29. Neel BG, Jhanwar SC, Chaganti RSK, Hayward WS: Two human c-onc genes are located on the long arm of chromosome 8. Proc Natl Acad Sci USA 79:7842–7846, 1982.

30. Cedar H: DNA methylation and gene activity. Cell 53:3–4, 1988.

31. Cheah MSC, Wallace CD, Hoffman RM: Hypomethylation of DNA in human cancer cells: A site-specific change in the c-myc oncogene. JNCI 73:1057–1065, 1984.

32. Nambu S, Inoue K, Sasaki H: Site-specific hypomethylation of the c-myc oncogene in human hepatocellular carcinoma. Jpn J Cancer Res (Gann) 78:695–704, 1987.

33. Westin EH, Wong-Staal F, Gelman EP, Dalla-Favera R, Papas TS, Lautenberger JA, Eva A, Reddy EP, Tronik SR, Aaronson SA, Gallo RC: Expression of cellular homologous of retroviral onc genes in human hematopoietic cells. Proc Natl Acad Sci USA 79:2490–2494, 1982.

34. Reitsma PH, Rothberg PG, Astrin SM, Trial J, Bar-Shavit Z, Hall A, Teitelbaum SL, Kahn AJ: Regulation of myc gene expression in HL60 leukemia cells by a vitamin D metabolite. Nature 306:492–494, 1983.

35. Lachman HM, Skoultchi AI: Expression of c-myc changes during differentiation of mouse erythroleukemia cells. Nature 310:592–594, 1984.

36. deBustros A, Baylin SB, Berger CL, Roos BA, Leong SS, Nelkin BD: Phorbol esters increase calcitonin gene transcription and decrease c-myc mRNA levels in cultured human medullary thyroid carcinoma. J Biol Chem 260: 98–104, 1985.

37. Griep AE, DeLuca HF: Decreased c-myc expression is an early event in retinoic acid-induced differentiation of F9 teratocarcinoma cells. Proc Natl Acad Sci USA 83:5539–5543, 1986.

38. Mulder KM, Levine AE, Hernandez X, McKnight MK, Brattain DE, Brattain MG: Modulation of c-myc by transforming growth factor-β in human colon carcinoma cells. Biochem Biophys Res Commun 150:711–716, 1988.

39. Noguchi P, Wallace R, Johnson J, Earley EM, O'Brien S, Ferrone S, Pellegrino MA, Milstein J, Needy C, Browne W, Petricciani J: Characterization of WiDr: A human colon carcinoma cell line. In Vitro 15:401–408, 1979.

40. Escot C, Theillet C, Lidereau R, Spyratos F, Champeme M-H, Gest J, Callahan R: Genetic alteration of the c-myc protooncogene (myc) in human primary breast carcinomas. Proc Natl Acad Sci USA 83:4834–4838, 1986.

41. Hayashi K, Makino R, Sugimura T: Amplification and over-expression of the c-myc gene in Morris hepatomas. Jpn J Cancer Res (Gann) 75:475–478, 1984.

42. Huber BE, Thorgeirsson SS: Analysis of c-myc expression in a human hepatoma cell line. Cancer Res 47:3414–3420, 1987.

43. Schwab M, Klempnauer KH, Alitalo K, Varmus H, Bishop M: Rearrangement at the 5′ end of amplified c-myc in human COLO 320 cells is associated with abnormal transcription. Mol Cell Biol 6:2752–2755, 1986.

44. Erisman MD, Scott JK, Watt RA, Astrin SM: The c-myc protein is constitutively expressed at elevated levels in colorectal carcinoma cell lines. Oncogene 2:367–378, 1988.

45. Keath EJ, Caimi PG, Cole MD: Fibroblast lines expressing activated c-myc oncogenes are tumorigenic in nude mice and syngeneic animals. Cell 39:339–348, 1984.

46. Coppola JA, Cole MD: Constitutive c-myc oncogene expression blocks mouse erythroleukemia cell differentiation but not commitment. Nature 320:760–763, 1986.

47. Stewart TA, Pattengale PK, Leder P: Spontaneous mammary adenocarcinomas in transgenic mice that carry and express MTV/myc fusion genes. Cell 38:627–637, 1984.

48. Adams JM, Harris AW, Pinkert CA, Corcoran LM, Alexander WS, Cory S, Palmiter RD, Brinster RL: The c-myc oncogene driven by immunoglobulin enhancers induces lymphoid malignancy in transgenic mice. Nature 318:533–538, 1985.

49. Schoenenberger C, Andres A, Groner B, van der Valk M, LeMeur M, Gerlinger P: Targeted c-myc gene expression in mammary glands of transgenic mice induces mammary tumours with constitutive milk protein gene transcription. EMBO J 7:169–175, 1988.

50. Bodmer WF, Bailey CJ, Bodmer J, Bussey HJR, Ellis A, Gorman P, Lucibello FC, Murday VA, Rider SH, Scambler P, Sheer D, Solomon E, Spurr NK: Localization of the gene for familial adenomatous polyposis on chromosome 5. Nature 328:614–616, 1987.

51. Erisman MD, Scott JK, Astrin SM: Evidence that the FAP gene is involved in a subset of colon cancers with a complementable defect in c-myc regulation. Proc Natl Acad Sci USA (in press), 1989.

45

Genetic Markers in Colonic Neoplasia

Sandra R. Wolman, Patricia M. Camuto, and Andrew P. Feinberg

Program in Cancer Genetics, Michigan Cancer Foundation, Detroit, Michigan (S.R.W.); Department of Pathology, NYU School of Medicine, New York, New York (P.M.C.); Howard Hughes Medical Institute, Departments of Internal Medicine and Human Genetics, University of Michigan, Ann Arbor, Michigan (A.P.F.)

INTRODUCTION

In the development of tumors, the transformation from a normal to a malignant cell is thought to require several steps, at least some of which involve genetic alteration [for reviews, see 1,2]. Two important sources of information may help to define stages in the malignant progression of colonic neoplasia. They are 1) benign adenomatous polyps and 2) the inherited predisposition to colon cancer in certain families. If genetic markers can be identified that reliably define premalignant cells, either within the adenoma or within the predisposed individual, they may serve to illustrate the mechanism(s) of malignant progression and provide a basis for early intervention.

Acceptance that colonic polyps precede the development of frank malignancy is increasing. Evidence for the adenoma–carcinoma sequence comes from observations for the contiguity of benign polyps to malignant lesions, from the correlation of increasing adenoma size with relative risk of malignancy, and from statistical associations in prevalence of both diseases [3–5]. Multiplicity of bowel cancers is closely associated with adenomatous polyps [6]. Moreover, removal of polyps in a predisposed individual has been equated with prevention of further malignancy [5]. Studies of presumptively nonfamilial adenomatous polyps indicate that a familial component, probably with autosomal dominant inheritance, increases susceptibility to colon cancer [7]. The cosegregation and high incidence of both polyps and cancers of the colon within families lend support to the morphologic sequence of events and also reinforce the importance of marker identification in the antecedent lesion.

The association of benign and malignant lesions in individuals and the evidence for genetic determinants of common polyps both point to the value of the inherited polyposis syndromes, familial adenomatous polyposis (FAP) and Gardner's syndrome (GS), as models for cancer of the large bowel in general.[1] The gene responsible for inherited polyposis is present in all cells of an individual; to the degree that the gene is expressed or identifiable, it provides a genetic marker different from those of cells from nonafflicted persons. Gene expression may be limited to certain tissues, so that cells of the gastrointestinal mucosa may express markers not evident in skin or fibroblasts or other tissues. When expression is accompanied by formation of colonic adenomas, new markers may appear in those cells, and progression to frank malignancy could be expected to yield further signs of altered genotype as well as phenotype. Thus different tissues from the same individual may be representative of the steps in malignant transformation. Assuming that the markers of malignancy in the FAP cancers are similar to those in nonhereditary colon cancer, the events at earlier stages should be informative with respect to the cellular biology of precursor lesions and to possibilities for intervention.

[1]For this review, FPC is used to designate inherited polyposis syndromes except when the paper cited has specified otherwise.

Familial Adenomatous Polyposis, pages 371–382

The range of genetic markers extends from those that are genetic but not clearly relevant to the biologic processes in malignancy to those that are direct markers of tumor tissues. In the former class are those that by linkage may help to localize the gene(s) for susceptibility to FPC or other genetic determinants of colonic cancers. The latter include quantitative or qualitative alterations in the DNA of tumor cells that serve to identify them as such and may show specificity for tumors of the large bowel. For example, specific chromosome aberrations in the tumors could direct attention to potentially significant genetic sites in precursor states or lesions. In contrast, observations of genetic alterations that are more diffuse, such as increased cell proliferation, chromosome breakage, or altered methylation could serve to identify a precursor or premalignant condition and could also be part of the process of malignant transformation.

Cultured cells from patients with hereditary predisposition to colonic polyposis demonstrate differences in growth properties and in responses to tumorigenic agents, which indicates that the cells have acquired some of the characteristics of malignant transformation. Altered cellular organization, loss of contact inhibition, decreased dependence on serum, focus formation, and growth in soft agar are some of the differences from normal reported in cultured cells from polyposis syndrome patients [2]. These markers of transformation are indicators of abnormal gene expression in FAP cells and thus indirectly provide evidence of genetic alteration.

MARKERS

Linkage

Potentially, the most powerful tool for identification of a relevant cancer or susceptibility gene would be the demonstration of tight linkage between a specific fragment of DNA or altered chromosomal locus and segregation of the syndrome phenotype in a kindred with FAP. This type of approach was embodied in an examination of expression of heavy-chain allotypes of IgG [8]. Serum samples of FAP patients and normal blood donors were compared for Gm and Km allotypes. Allotypic differences may relate to disease susceptibility and have been found in association with specific, but nonhereditary, malignancies. The distribution of Gm phenotypes as a group differed in the FPC patients (all of whom were genetically unrelated) and the frequency of one phenotype was significantly increased with a more than twofold relative risk compared to controls. Such results could reflect statistical artifact or alternatively could provide the means for localization of susceptibility genes for FAP.

A similar approach was based on recognition that mutant alleles of oncogenes, particularly in the ras family, have been associated with several forms of human cancer, including sporadic colon cancer. It seemed plausible that such alleles might constitute a predisposing genetic factor in hereditary cancers. In early studies, two oncogene probes, for Ha-ras-1 or Ki-ras-2 coding sequences, were used to examine the polymorphisms in enzymic digests of DNA from members of the large GS kindred-109 [9]. Neither oncogene was linked to the GS locus, thus neither appeared likely to be the site of the causal mutation of the syndrome.

The power of linkage studies is obviously amplified when some degree of genomic localization is possible. Probes can then be selected with far greater specificity. Based on an informative case of FPC with a chromosome deletion [10], two laboratories independently demonstrated close association of heritability between FPC and a polymorphic variant of a genomic locus known as C11p11. LOD scores (measures of cosegregation; in this case the frequency of association of a genomic variant with disease expression within a family) of 3.26 in a study of six informative families [11] and of 3.37 from five kindreds [12] provided highly significant evidence of linkage and thus served to localize the FPC gene to the long arm of chromosome 5.

Chromosome Aberrations

Evidence that the FAP gene could be localized to chromosome 5 originated with a report of an individual with FAP as well as multiple developmental abnormalities who had an interstitial deletion of chromosome 5q [10].[2] This observation led to the studies of polymorphic genomic probes assigned to chromosome 5 in FAP families [11,12] described above. Because of close linkage with the C11p11 probe (developed for other studies by P. Scambler, unpublished), a gene for FAP could be localized to 5q21–q22, which is congruent with the chromosomal deletion originally described. Much of the work on chromosome aberrations in colorectal cancer has been summarized [1,13]. A large series of direct tumor analyses [13] did not show consistent abnormalities but emphasized the frequency of trisomies for chromosomes 7, 8, 13, 19, 20, and 21; loss of 17; and structural aberrations of 1 and 5. Others have observed trisomy for 7 [14], rearrangements of 12p [15], deletions of 12q [16], trisomy 12 [17], or inversion of 16—inv(16) (p13q22) [18]. Preferential involvement of 17 in chromosomal recombination was reported by Muleris et al. [19]. More recently, this group summarized their observations that monosomies 17p and 18 were the most frequent karyotypic changes in 18 near-diploid colorectal tumors [20,21]. In most tumors, additional monosomies, in order of decreasing frequency, involved chromosomes 1p, 4, 14, 5q, 6q, 2p, and 11q. Gains were observed in chromosomes 20, 8q, 13, 17q, and X, and a minority of cases showed combinations of aberrations.

Levin and Reichmann [13] also examined a number of adenomas in an attempt to correlate progression of chromosome aberrations with advancing malignancy. To some extent, their work demonstrated karyotypic progression. Of 18 lesions classified as adenomas, five were cytogenetically normal; five had only numerical aberrations, of which three were mosaic for normal cells; and seven showed both numerical and structural abnormalities. However, all these nonmalignant tumors were in the diploid range for chromosome number. In their larger series of adenocarcinomas, 9%, a much smaller proportion, were chromosomally normal, whereas another 12% of the malignancies showed only simple gains or losses of whole chromosomes [13]. Willson's group [22] have studied polyps and colonic cancers in primary culture and have developed a number of cell lines. Lines established from two tubular polyps had normal diploid karyotypes. Cell lines from six primary colorectal cancers and four metastases yielded karyotypic information that corroborates some of the observations from direct tumor study [23,24]. Several tumor lines showed trisomy 7, and rearrangements of chromosomes 1, 3, and 7 were also frequent.

Karyotypes of tumors from FAP patients have been reported rarely. The case report of an FAP carrier with 5q deletion is a notable exception that eventually led to localization of the FAP gene. Another, but less clearly relevant, case involving 5q was reported earlier [14]. Several polyps and an adenocarcinoma from a single FAP patient showed frequent abnormalities of chromosome 13 [25]. Lothe et al. [26] recently studied a duodenal adenocarcinoma from a patient with GS. The tumor had been established in nude mice and demonstrated loss of heterozygosity with respect to the p7 F12 allele, which is located on chromosome 13, as well as loss of one chromosome 13 by karyotypic analysis of a later passage. Cultured epithelial cell lines from an FAP-derived adenocarcinoma and three adenomas were examined for clonability, tumorigenicity and cytogenetics [27]. One line of adenoma-derived cells could not be passaged from single cells or grown as tumors in nude mice; the cells had a normal 46,XY karyotype. The carcinoma-derived line was clonogenic, tumorigenic in nude mice, and karyotypically abnormal. Findings included near-diploidy and isochromosomes for 1q, 14q and a translocation between chromosomes X and 17 in addition to some unidentified markers. Thus there are few data to show that colonic tumors in FAP patients display either the same spectrum of aberrations or ones that are significantly different from those of nonhereditary cancers. In the absence of such information, one must depend on the available observations on non-FAP large bowel malignancies, which are notable for their variety both within and between studies.

[2]Cytogenetic nomenclature is based on "An International System for Human Cytogenetic Nomenclature (Harnden DG, Klinger HP, eds) Basel: S. Karger, 1985.

In the absence of indicators from the malignant lesions, some investigators have followed a different approach based on the assumption that chromosome instability per se is an important aspect of predisposition to malignancy. Quantitative studies of chromosome aberrations on peripheral blood from FAP patients and derived epithelial, fibroblast, or tumor cells in culture have emerged from a number of laboratories, with focus on the incidence of tetraploidy in culture or elevated frequencies of numerical and structural aberrations [28,29]. Gardner and coworkers [29] reported numerical and structural chromosomal instability to be consistent markers for FAP gene carriers in certain kindreds. In contrast, examination of prometaphase chromosomes from cultured cells for structural aberrations, fragile sites, and sister chromatid exchanges revealed none of these parameters to be abnormal in five FAP patients examined [30].

Another aspect of potential susceptibility to chromosome damage in disorders predisposing to cancer was examined by evaluating the extent of damage after irradiation [31]. Patients with familial polyposis (or GS) showed a breakage incidence that was significantly higher than that for normal lines and significant incidence of chromatid gaps as well. No differences in postradiation repair time were observed. The authors' interpretation was that cell lines from cancer-prone individuals (including those with FAP) were deficient in excision repair of X-ray-induced DNA damage inflicted during the G2 phase of the cell cycle.

Loss of Heterozygosity

Use of restriction fragment length polymorphism (RFLP) analysis has extended our interpretation and understanding of specificity of chromosome markers. Recently, Monpezat and coworkers [32] reported specific loss of sequences on chromosomes 17 and 18 in 58% and 85%, respectively, of colon adenocarcinomas. RFLPs can detect variations in DNA sequence in the general population and can be used to distinguish the maternal and paternal copies of a given gene. Using this technique, if one observes a RFLP for a marker, such that the normal tissue shows two bands on Southern blot, representing the maternal and paternal alleles of a given gene, and the tumor shows only one of those bands, one can infer that one copy of the marker gene has been lost. Generally, it is assumed that this allelic loss represents loss of a large portion of a given chromosomal arm, or even an entire chromosome, and that a specific recessive tumor gene lies proximal to the given marker on that chromosome. By analogy with studies of retinoblastoma in which 13q markers show allelic loss in about 70% of tumors [33], over 10% of retinoblastomas were reported to show homozygous deletion of a specific cloned gene on the same chromosomal arm [34]. Similar apparently specific losses of alleles have been reported in bladder cancer [35], breast cancer [36], renal cell carcinoma [37], lung cancer [38], endocrine tumors [39], and neural tumors [40].

In a more detailed analysis, Thomas' group reported RFLP losses on chromosomes 17 and 18 in 75% and 86% of colon carcinomas, respectively [41]. Fearon et al. [42] showed somatic loss of chromosome 17p sequences in 75% of colorectal adenocarcinomas examined by means of RFLP. However, this was rarely observed in adenomas of either familial or spontaneous type. All tumors showed monoclonal patterns of X chromosome inactivation, which supports a monoclonal origin for these neoplasms whether malignant or benign, familial or sporadic. Some contradiction is apparent between recent RFLP reports and the cytogenetic literature, e.g., the work on chromosomes 17 and 12. The 17p loss by chromosome-specific RFLPs is far more common than can be accounted for by chromosome aberrations and mutations of Ki-ras more common than the frequency of chromosome 12 aberrations. Some of these may result from point or submicroscopic mutations; others may have evolved through loss of one pair member and reduplication of the remaining chromosome. Still others may reflect the very selective nature of karyotypic evaluation, which extends only to a small fraction of the tumor cell population. Although it is possible that karyotypic analysis may select for cells that are dividing and may not fully represent the native cells of a given tumor, the results from cytogenetic studies vary, and those of Muleris et al. [21] seem quite close to what would be expected from RFLP studies.

Solomon and coworkers [43] analyzed DNA preparations from paired samples of normal and tumor tissue from 45 individuals with sporadic colorectal carcinoma for RFLP losses with a variety of probes. Utilizing the locus-specific miniprobe λ MSS, which maps to 5q34-qter, they demonstrated that 20–40% of their patients showed partial or complete loss of an allele. The results were extended by analysis with another probe, L1.4, which maps to 5q31. Five of ten colonic cancer cell lines also showed loss of alleles on chromosome 5. Okamoto et al. [44] made a similar observation in 60% of their patients (albeit with a small sample size of five tumors). It was thus suggested that the FAP gene functions as a recessive tumor gene and that impaired function of one allele is transmitted vertically as a dominant trait and that inactivation of both alleles leads to cancer, akin to the mechanisms in retinoblastoma and Wilms' tumor.

However, in the study of colon cancer losses from chromosome 5, losses at lower frequency were also seen from chromosomes 6, 12, 15, and 22 [44]. The chromosome 17 and 18 allelic losses reported in some studies [41,42] were not seen in others [43,44]. Thus chromosomes 5, 17, and 18 have all been implicated in gene deletion or inactivation in colon carcinoma, but the studies reporting these losses are contradictory. The results from the studies of sporadic tumors provide additional support for a role of the 5q21–22 locus in the development of colonic cancers in general.

Analysis of DNA markers of human colorectal tumors is complicated by the fact that the tumors are largely contaminated by normal cellular elements. Often, when comparing tumor DNA to normal DNA, if a particular band representing an RFLP is reduced by more than 50% in intensity, it is assumed that the remaining band intensity is due to contaminating normal elements, although that assumption may be flawed. To overcome this assumption, Law and coworkers [45], in a recent study analyzed 35 colorectal cancers that were physically or biologically enriched by cryostat-sectioning or xenografting in nude mice. They found that only 19% of colorectal cancers showed loss of heterozygosity for chromosome 5 alleles; however, 56% showed allelic losses of chromosome 17, and 52% showed losses of chromosome 18. Interestingly, tumors with allelic loss on chromosome 5 also showed loss of heterozygosity on chromosomes 17 and 18, suggesting a complex model of carcinogenesis involving the cooperative action of tumor suppressor genes at multiple loci [45]. Efforts to identify other critical gene loci, using similar tools, will undoubtedly intensify. Large numbers of polymorphic variants distributed over the entire genome will be identified by restriction enzyme digestion in the near future.

Oncogene Alterations

There have been numerous attempts to identify altered, rearranged, or amplified oncogenes in sporadic and familial colonic neoplasms and in FAP families. Although mutated ras genes are activated oncogenes, transform primary cells in culture, and play a well documented role in tumorigenesis in animal models, their role in the development of human neoplasia is unclear. Fibroblast cultures from individuals with differing familial bases for colon cancer have been almost uniformly negative for transforming activity [46]. Gene activity, measured as the expression of mRNA for several oncogenes (c-fos and to a lesser extent c-myc, c-Ha-ras, and c-Ki-ras) was demonstrated in nine colonic cancers studied [47]. All these genes may subserve normal cellular functions, and expression per se does not imply causality. In contrast, direct examination of tumor DNA revealed oncogene alterations in a much smaller proportion of cases [48]. Southern blot analysis with probes for nine oncogenes and DNA from 32 colonic cancers showed amplification of c-myc in two tumors and evidence (by comparison with normal host tissues) of allelic deletion of c-ras or c-myb in two tumors. A recent abstract [49] reported structural DNA changes in 22% of 45 colon cancers probed with ten oncogenes.

Whereas transforming activity (usually ras) has been found in a few colonic cancer cell lines, the majority of fresh human tumors studied thus far have not demonstrated significant differences in oncogene activity by transfection assays. This method involves the transfer of tumor cell DNA into cultured mouse cells, which are then monitored for malignant transformation. It is limited by high rates of DNA degradation, by necrosis in vivo, by surgery and subsequent tissue handling, and by contamination of the specimen with nonneoplastic cells. The Ki-ras gene is 46 kb, so large that its size may preclude effective detection of changes by transfection methods.

More recently, oncogene-activating ras mutations have been reported in approximately 40% of human colorectal cancers in work from two independent laboratories [50,51]. Specifically, these were somatic mutations that occurred most frequently at codon 12 of the c-Ki-ras gene, an observation which had been noted earlier in 5 human colon tumor cell lines. The mutations were also present in early (Duke's A) as well as advanced stage (Duke's B and C) carcinomas and were frequent in histologically premalignant tissues, i.e., villous adenomas not associated with malignant tumors and the residual adenomatous regions of certain cancers. The question of whether Ki-ras mutation precedes carcinoma development is still unclear. Ki-ras mutations were not found in any of the normal tissues from all cases examined. With regard to the timing of the mutation, mutations were observed in adenomatous-appearing regions of cancers, and the authors concluded that these were the adenomas from which the tumor arose [51]. However, by the time a cancer is grossly visible, evidence of the original adenoma is often lost. Furthermore, isolated adenomas did not show c-Ki-ras mutations [51]. Many tumors show some degree of differentiation, and some tumors are capable of differentiating even into normal tissue [52], although this phenomenon has not been documented in colon cancer. Perucho's group [50] estimated that both mutant and normal alleles were expressed to the same degree in the cancer cell, which implies that the effects of the mutation are dominant and independent of regulation by the normal counterpart(s). The greater prevalence of altered activity in these tumors suggests that mutation of known oncogenes is more likely to play a common primary or causal role and to provide reliable genetic markers for stages of colon cancer than appeared true only a short time ago.

The limitations of the NIH 3T3 transfection assays used in the earlier studies are probably responsible for the differences in results. Both Bos' group [51] and Perucho's group [50] circumvented these problems by utilizing methods that permit direct detection of the specific ras mutation using the polymerase chain reaction, which allows selective amplifications in vitro of target sequences [53]. The mutated sequences are short; therefore, partial DNA degradation does not interfere with their analysis. Bos et al. [51] employed an oligomer hybridization assay in which mutation-specific oligonucleotide probes were hybridized with DNA extracted from frozen tissue tumor samples. Histologic examination of the tissue samples to be analyzed ensured that they contained a high proportion of neoplastic cells. Forrester et al. [50] utilized an RNAse A mismatch cleavage analysis in which total tumor cell RNA was hybridized to a serine RNA probe. The resulting hybrids were digested with RNAse A, which can recognize and cleave single base mismatches in RNA–RNA duplexes. The fragments were then analyzed by gel electrophoresis, and the mutation was localized in the gene transcript. Similar approaches could be used to study cases of colonic tumors associated with FAP in order to elucidate the functional significance of the Ki-ras mutations to neoplastic development and progression.

DNA Content and Cell Proliferation

Flow cytometric analysis of colon cancers shows nonuniformity of DNA content, which can contribute to prognostic evaluation [54]. Like other glandular and epithelial tumors, diploid tumors of colonic mucosa appear to be associated with a better outcome in terms of the development of progressive disease and overall survival [55–57]. Ploidy, as determined by flow cytometry, has been shown by some researchers to be a prognostic factor independent of histologic grade and pathologic stage. Although advanced-stage tumors (Duke's C) were found to be more often associated with aneuploidy, both diploid and aneuploid tumors were equally represented in the less advanced stages [57]. However, utilizing a cytophotometric technique, Cuvelier et al. [58] found that the nuclear DNA content of colonic adenocarcinomas in the setting of chronic ulcerative colitis did correlate with the degree of histologic differentiation and pathologic stage (Duke's classification). Several Scandinavian laboratories have reported that a high proportion of colon cancers are aneuploid, that metastases tend to show the same levels of ploidy as the primary tumors, and that aneuploidy could be predictive of cancer in dysplastic epithelium.

In general, the ploidy values of adenomas vary. In some studies aneuploidy is associated with increasing dysplasia, which supports a sequence of benign adenoma to dysplastic adenoma to cancer [59]. Other investigators have not found aneuploidy in adenomas [60]. McKinley et al. [61] demonstrated the presence of aneuploidy in a high-grade dysplastic lesion in a patient with Crohn's ileocolitis. Extensive sampling of the surgical specimen showed that it was not associated with carcinoma. Therefore, since diploid and aneuploid histograms from adenomas cannot be distinguished from those generated by carcinomas, the evidence suggests that DNA aneuploidy is not a reliable marker for either the neoplastic or the preneoplastic state.

Increased proliferation and cell turnover can be another indicator of quantitative DNA change. Loss of regulated DNA synthesis and increased size of the proliferating pool of cells is characteristic of tumor populations. The work of Deschner and Lipkin [62] showed expansion of the proliferative zone in mucosa from FPC patients. This was expanded to observations that DNA synthesis extends upward from the normal lower one-third toward the luminal surface of colonic crypts in other patients at risk for colonic cancer. Recent evidence that ornithine decarboxylase (ODC) may be a marker for premalignant colonic mucosa [63] also relates to cell turnover. The enzyme is necessary for polyamine synthesis, which, in turn, is required for DNA synthesis.

Methylation

A question posed with increasing frequency is whether a "genetic" change must involve a structural alteration in cellular DNA or whether (semi-)permanent, possibly regulatory modifications, such as methylation, could provide a basis for malignant or premalignant alterations in cell behavior. Decrease in methylation has been associated with gene activation, and increasing methylation appears to accompany tissue differentiation. Although studies of general hypomethylation in tumors have been inconclusive, investigation of specific genomic regions has shown hypomethylation in several human cancers [64]. The technique involves selective enzymic digestion of DNA; certain enzymes cannot cleave methylated bases and therefore yield smaller fragments on Southern blot when the DNA is less methylated. Probes for genes, which are unlikely to be expressed in colonic mucosa, such as crystallin or human chorionic gonadotrophin, were employed because they were expected to be highly methylated in normal colonic tissue. Comparison of normal bowel mucosa with benign polyps or malignant neoplasms of the colon from the same individuals generally revealed hypomethylation in both types of neoplasms, although with heterogeneity dependent on the gene and the specific neoplasm [65]. Since DNA from benign tumors was approximately as hypomethylated as that from malignant lesions, results were interpreted to indicate that altered methylation is an early change, preceding frank malignancy.

A paradox in the study of alterations in DNA methylation in colon cancer is an apparent discrepancy between the profound changes in DNA methylation when individual single copy sequences are analyzed using methylcytosine-sensitive restriction enzymes and the overall genomic 5-methylcytosine content of colon adenomas and carcinomas. Thus, whereas single-gene analysis shows apparently equal hypomethylation in adenomas and in carcinomas [65], studies of genomic 5-methylcytosine content do not [66]. Indeed, quantitative densitometric scanning of ethidium bromide-stained gels shows little or no change between normal and tumor, but, when the same gels are transferred to nitrocellulose and probed with specific genes, methylation at specific sites is decreased by 50–90% [64,65]. To address this dilemma, matched samples, from the same patients, of normal colonic mucosa and colon adenocarcinomas were digested to mononucleosides, and the 5-methylcytosine content was measured chromatographically [67]. In both adenomas and carcinomas, there was an 8–10% decrease in genomic methylcytosine content. This was apparent only when samples were matched from the same individuals, because there was a substantial variation in the normal mucosal 5-methylcytosine content among individuals. This variation did not correlate with age [67]. It appears that single copy genes preferentially have been hypomethylated, compared to repetitive sequences, which show little or no change. The difference between quantitative and qualitative studies is due partly to technical considerations and partly to biological differences. Thus repetitive sequences, which represent the majority of methylatable cytosines in the genome, do not appear to be as hypomethylated as single copy genes, which represent the minority of methylatable sites [65,67]. No difference was seen in 5-methylcytosine content between patients with adenomatous polyposis coli with patients with sporadic colon cancer. Most intriguing, however, was that three patients with nonpolypotic familial colon cancer (Lynch's syndrome) had the highest genomic 5-methylcytosine content among the 12 patients studied. It is not yet clear whether this preliminary observation will be borne out by study of additional patients, but, if it is seen consistently, it could be related to the increased activity of 5-methyltransferase in colon tumors, which has been hypothesized to serve a corrective role in disturbed DNA methylation [68].

TRANSFORMATION

The term "malignant transformation" in human disease generally refers to invasive cancer and includes both primary and metastatic malignancy. The definition of malignant transformation applied to cells growing in vitro is less clear, and the accuracy of its correlation with malignancy in vivo may be questioned. Cells in tissue culture that are characterized as transformed show features of growth and morphology that are, in many ways, analogous to cancer cells in vivo and, therefore, are often taken as models for the human disease. However, cells from human tumors often are unable to adapt to growth in culture, whereas transformed cells are expected to grow for indefinite periods. Clonability in soft agar is generally accepted as a marker for malignancy in vitro, whereas it is well known that cells from human tumors are clonable only in limited numbers. A third criterion for the definition of malignant transformation in vitro is the ability of cells to grow when transplanted into suitable host animals, such as the nude mouse. However, human tumors are not uniformly capable of growing by transplantation.

Studies of FAP (or GS) cells in culture have usually been based on fibroblasts. Although the mucosa of the large bowel is the tissue at greatest risk, it is evident that this genetic disorder is expressed in many cell types. The extracolonic lesions, first recognized as part of the syndrome by Gardner, include osteomas, epidermal cysts, adenomas of other parts of the gastrointestinal tract, and desmoid tumors. Since all cells from FAP patients may express the gene(s) to some extent, different tissues and cell types (as noted above) may also represent stages in the process of malignant transformation that are marked by different behavioral characteristics. One such marker is the biological response to tumor promoters by colonic mucosal cells from differing sources (normal individuals, FAP patients, patients with nonhereditary colon cancer). When mucosal epithelium is exposed to tumor promoters in short-term culture, there is enhancement of tritiated thymidine uptake in cells from FAP individuals [69]. This enhancement of a necessary precursor for cell proliferation is far greater in FAP mucosal cells than in cells from normal mucosa or cells derived from adenomas. The assumption is that the adenoma cells, derived from benign tumors, represent an early stage in tumor evolution and that FAP cells have bypassed one of the normal controls of proliferative response. The interpretation of these findings depends very much on the assumption that the sequence in tumor evolution is from the normal cell to a benign adenoma.

The difficulties in constructing such a sequence are illustrated by studies of intracellular actin cable formation [70,71]. One could define a sequence of progressive alteration from normal to morphologically normal but hyperproliferative mucosal cells of familial polyposis individuals to a benign adenomatous lesion to frank malignancy. However, studies of alterations in cytoskeleton indicate that actin is present in normal colonic mucosal cells, but there is considerable loss of cable formation in cells from familial polyposis. Cables are increased in benign adenomas and then lost in malignant cells [71]. The loss of actin cables in FAP epithelial cells is similar to that reported earlier for dermal fibroblasts from FAP [72].

A further distinction could also be made between cells from early- and late-stage benign adenomas. The cells differed in response to tumor promoters with respect to their ability to release plasminogen activator and acquire morphologic changes in vitro [70]. In response to a phorbol ester tumor promoter (TPA), cells from early adenomas retained their heavy and distinctive actin cables, whereas cells from later-stage adenomas in the presence of TPA were altered, and their cytoskeletons became disorganized. Morphologic distinctions in terms of size and tubular vs. villus histology are used in differentiating early- from late-stage adenomas. Although complex, the cytochemical studies of altered cellular skeleton, in general, support the idea that these modifications and consequent alterations in cell morphology are relevant expressions of the FAP gene.

Another recent study [73] examined several parameters of in vitro transformation in FAP fibroblasts using control cells from retinoblastoma patients and from normal sources. The different assays included evaluation of increased tetraploidy and chromosome aberrations, acquisition of anchorage independence in methocellulose or soft agar, growth within collagen gels, tumorigenicity in nude mice, and saturation density. Moreover, in recognition that tumor promoters may elicit features of transformation differently in normal cells than in cells genetically predisposed to cancer, many of these studies were performed with and without exposure of cells to TPA. The authors emphasized that the multiple markers of transformation were not necessarily expected to be acquired in a specific or orderly fashion. Several changes that are markers of transformation were fostered by TPA treatment (in cells from FAP). These included the formation of colonies in methocellulose, variable patterns of migration in collagen gels, and questionable increase in tetraploidy and chromosome aberrations. The latter were described as significantly different by t tests, but the number of mean breaks observed per cell did not appear to support induced differences in FPC that were greater than those in control material. The addition of tumor promoter in this study induced tetraploidy of comparable degrees in all cell types tested.

CONCLUSIONS

Major goals in identifying genetic markers to define precursor stages of large bowel cancer have already been achieved. Many markers have been described, both specific and nonspecific, direct and indirect, including undisputed markers of cell proliferation. They appear to be valid in both hereditary and nonhereditary conditions but, because of dependence on intestinal mucosal sampling and technical difficulties, have been of limited utility to the present time. Genetic markers such as chromosome aberrations are nonuniform and not always demonstrable even in malignant tumors. Nevertheless, they have served as critical signposts of localization of the FAP gene based on linkage with polymorphic DNA. The questions of interrelationship among the herditary bowel cancer syndromes appear to be resolved, and the relevance of FAP as a valid model for the sporadic presentation of colon cancer is established. This and other relevant gene(s) and gene products should provide tools for early diagnosis, and they suggest routes for intervention early in evolution of the disease.

At present, the most critical questions in the study of the molecular genetics of colon cancer are the identification and cloning of specific gene sequences and establishment of the exact order of alterations in multistep transformation. The most obvious model for colon carcinogenesis is that a series of molecular alterations takes place over many years in a given cell lineage and that these alterations include oncogene mutation, "antioncogene" or recessive tumor gene inactivation at multiple loci, and altered expression of other genes, possibly related to changes in DNA methylation. Of all of these changes, probably the earliest is a change in DNA methylation, since that is the only one consistently seen in adenomas. However, it has not been proved that changes in DNA methylation play a causal role in carcinogenesis. Alternative to this multistep molecular model, one or a very small number of genetic alterations could predispose to other changes. A prime candidate for such an alteration would cause genetic instability, hypothesized by many authors [74,75], including the patriarch of cancer genetics studies Teodor Boveri [76]. Genetic instability in cancer, however, despite its plausibility and some direct supporting evidence [77], has never been proved, and a number of experimental observations argue against a central role. Nevertheless, one should note that the hallmark of cancer is a change in chromosome number, because of reduplication of chromosomes, tetraploidy, and, possibly most important, considerable drift in chromosome number from cell to cell within a given tumor. Thus a critical event that we have not yet identified may set the stage for later genetic alterations that endow the cell with increasing proliferative and metastatic capacity. Let us hope that this so, because, if colon cancer indeed is extremely heterogeneous in its molecular cause, and in the combination of altered genes, then the hope for successful targeted gene therapy is unlikely to be fulfilled.

References

1. Wolman SR: Chromosomal markers in study of colon cancer. Digest Dis Sci 30:134S–140S, 1985.
2. Wolman SR: Determinants in malignant transformation: Studies in hereditary bowel cancer. In JRF Ingall, AJ Mastromarino (eds): "Prevention of Hereditary Large Bowel Cancer." NY: Alan R. Liss, Inc. 1983, pp 217–237.
3. Muto T, Bussey HJR, Morson BC: The evolution of cancer of the colon and rectum. Cancer 36:2251–2270, 1975.
4. Fenoglio CM, Lane N: The anatomical precursor of colorectal carcinoma. Cancer 34:819–823, 1974.
5. Morson BC: Genesis of colorectal caner. Clin Gastroenterol 5:505–525, 1976.
6. Cunliffe WJ, Hasleton PS, Tweedle DE, Schofield PF: Incidence of synchronous and metachronous colorectal carcinoma. Br J Surg 71:941–943, 1984.
7. Burt RW, Bishop DT, Cannon LA, Dowdle MA, Lee RG, Skolnick MH: Dominant inheritance of adenomatous colonic polyps and colorectal cancer. N Engl J Med 312:1540–1544, 1985.
8. Pandey JP, Ebbesen P, Bulow S, Svendsen JB, Fudenberg HH: IgG heavy-chain (Gm) allotypes in familial polyposis coli. Am J Hum Genet 38:133–136, 1986.
9. Barker D, McCoy M, Weinberg R, Goldfarb M, Wigler M, Burt R, Gardner E, White R: A test of the role of two oncogenes in inherited predisposition to colon cancer. Mol Biol Med 1:199–206, 1983.
10. Herrera L, Kakati S, Gibas L, Pietrzak E, Sandberg AA: Gardner syndrome in a man with an interstitial deletion of 5q, Am J Med Genet 25:473–476, 1986.
11. Bodmer WF, Bailey CJ, Bodmer J, Bussey HJR, Ellis A, Gorman P, Lucibello FC, Murday VA, Rider SH, Scambler P, Sheer D, Solomon E, Spurr NK: Localization of the gene for familial adenomatous polyposis on chromosome 5. Nature 328:614–616, 1987.
12. Leppert M, Dobbs M, Scambler P, O'Connell P, Nakamua D, Stauffer D, Woodward S, Burt R, Hughes J, Gardner E, Lathrop M, Wasmuth J, Lalouel JM, White R: The gene for familial polyposis coli maps to the long arm of chromosome 5, Science 238:1411–1413, 1987.
13. Levin B, Reichmann A: Chromosomes and large bowel tumors. Cancer Genet Cytogenet 19:159–162, 1986.
14. Ferti-Passantonopoulou A, Panani A, Avgerinos A, Raptis A: Cytogenetic findings in a large bowel adenocarcinoma. Cancer Genet Cytogenet 21:361–364, 1986.
15. Pathak S, Goodacre A: Specific chromosome anomalies and predisposition to human breast, renal cell, and colorectal carcinoma. Cancer Genet Cytogenet 19:29–36, 1986.
16. Becher R, Gibas Z, Sandberg AA: Involvement of chromosomes 7 and 12 in large bowel cancer: Trisomy 7 and 12q. Cancer Genet Cytogenet 9:329–332, 1983.
17. Ochi H, Takeuchi J, Douglass H, Sandberg AA: Possible specific chromosome changes in large bowel cancer, Cancer Genet Cytogenet 10:121–122, 1983.
18. Shabtai F, Sternberg A, Klar D, Riss R, Halbrecht I: Inversion(16) (p13q22) in tumor cells of sigmoid colon, Cancer Genet Cytogenet 27:171–175, 1987.
19. Muleris M, Salmon RJ, Zafrani B, Girodet J, Dutrillaux B: Consistent deficiencies of chromosome 18 and of the short arm of chromosome 17 in eleven cases of human large bowel cancer: A possible recessive determinism, Ann Genet 28:206–213, 1985.
20. Muleris M, Salmon RJ, Dutrillaux B: Existence of two distinct processes of chromosomal evolution in near-diploid colorectal tumors. Cancer Genet Cytogenet 32:43–50, 1988.
21. Muleris M, Salmon RJ, Dutrillaux A, Vielh P, Zafrani

B, Girodet J, Dutrillaux B: Characteristic chromosomal imbalances in 18 near-diploid colorectal tumors. Cancer Genet Cytogenet 29:289–301, 1987.

22. Willson JKV, Bittner GN, Oberley TD, Meisner LF, Weese JI: Cell culture of human colon adenomas and carcinomas. Cancer Res 47:2704–2713, 1987.

23. McBain JA, Weese JL, Meisner LF, Wolbert WH, Willson JKV: Establishment and characterization of human colorectal cancer cell lines. Cancer Res 44:5813–5821, 1984.

24. Willson JKV, Weese JL, Bittner GN, Meisner LF: The development of techniques that permit the selection and growth of malignant cells from human colonic carcinomas. In TG Pretlow, TP Pretlow (eds): "Cell Separation: Methods and Selected Applications." Orlando, FL: Academic Press, pp 277–293, 1987.

25. Reichmann A, Martin P, Levin B, Chromosomal banding patterns in familial polyposis associated with adenocarcinoma (abstract). Am J Hum Genet 34:139, 1982.

26. Lothe RA, Gedde-Dahl T, Lier ME, Aamdahl S, Bergan A, Stenwig AE, Broegger A: Loss of one chromosome #13 during development of a polyposis tumor. Cancer Genet Cytogenet 28:335–342, 1987.

27. Paraskeva C, Buckle BG, Sheer D, Wigley CB: The isolation and characterization of colorectal epithelial cell lines at different stages in malignant transformation from familial polyposis coli patients. Int J Cancer 34:49–56, 1984.

28. Delhanty JDA, David MB, Wood J: Chromosome instability in lymphocytes, fibroblasts, and colon epithelial-like cells from patients with familial polyposis coli. Cancer Genet Cytogenet 8:27–50, 1983.

29. Gardner EJ, Woodward SR, Hughes JP: Evaluation of chromosomal diagnosis for hereditary adenomatosis of the colorectum. Cancer Genet Cytogenet 15:321–334, 1985.

30. Nielsen KB, Bulow S, Tommerup N: Chromosomal studies in familial polyposis coli. Cancer Genet Cytogenet 17:355–357, 1985.

31. Parshad R, Sanford KK, Jones GM: Chromatid damage after G2 phase x-irradiation of cells from cancer-prone individuals implicates deficience in DNA repair, Proc Natl Acad Sci USA 80:5612–5616, 1983.

32. Monpezat J, Muleris M, Lefrancois D, Grunwald D, Salmon RJ, Frelat G, Dutrillaux B, Thomas G: Loss of heterozygosity in human colorectal adenocarcinoma indicates recessive mutations on chromosomes 17p and 18. Int Congress on Human Gene Mapping IX Paris, 1988, abstract #210.

33. Dryja TP, Cavenee W, White R, Rapaport JM, Petersen R, Albert DM, Bruns GA: Homozygosity of chromosome 13 in retinoblastoma. New Engl J Med 310:550–553, 1984.

34. Friend SH, Bernards R, Rogelj S, Weinberg RA, Rapaport JM, Albert DM, Dryja TP: A human DNA segment with properties of the gene that predisposes to retinoblastoma and osteosarcoma, Nature 323:643–646, 1986.

35. Fearon ER, Feinberg AP, Hamilton SH, Vogelstein B: Loss of genes on chromosome 11p in bladder cancer. Nature 318:377–380, 1985.

36. Lundberg C, Skoog L, Cavenee WK, Nordenskjold M: Loss of heterozygosity in human ductal breast tumors indicates a recessive mutation on chromosome 13. Proc Natl Acad Sci USA 84:2372, 1987.

37. Zbar B, Brach H, Talmadge C, Linehan M: Loss of alleles of loci on the short arm of chromosome 3 in renal cell carcinoma. Nature 327:721, 1987.

38. Yokota J, Tsunetsuga-Yokota Y, Battifora H, Le Fevre C, Cline MJ: Loss of heterozygosity on chromosomes 3, 13, and 17 in small-cell carcinoma and on chromosome 3 in adenocarcinoma of the lung. Proc Natl Acad Sci USA 84:9252, 1987.

39. Mathew CG, Smith BA, Thorpe K, Wong Z, Royle NJ, Jeffreys AJ, Ponder BA: Deletion of genes on chromosome 1 in endocrine neoplasia. Nature 328:524–526, 1987.

40. Seizinger BR, Matuza TI, Gusella JF: Loss of genes on chromosome 22 in tumorigenesis of human acoustic neuroma. Nature 322:644, 1987.

41. Monpezat J-P, Delattre O, Bernard A, Grunwald D, Remvikos Y, Muleris M, Salmon RJ, Frelat G, Dutrillaux B, Thomas G: Loss of alleles on chromosome 18 and on the short arm of chromosome 17 in polyploid colorectal carcinomas. Int J Cancer 41:404–408, 1988.

42. Fearon ER, Hamilton SR, Vogelstein B: Clonal analysis of human colorectal tumors. Science 238:193–197, 1987.

43. Solomon E, Voss R, Hall V, Bodmer WF, Jass JR, Jeffreys AJ, Lucibello FC, Patel I, Rider SH: Chromosome 5 allele loss in human colorectal carcinomas. Nature 328:616–619, 1987.

44. Okamoto M, Sasaki M, Sugio K, Sato C, Iwama T, Ikeuchi T, Tonumura A, Sasazuki T, Miyaki M: Loss of constitutional heterozygosity in colon carcinoma from patients with familial polyposis coli. Nature 331:273, 1988.

45. Law DJ, Olschwang S, Monpezat J-P, Lefrancois D, Jagelman D, Petrelli N, Thomas G, Feinberg AP: Concerted nonsyntenic allelic loss in human colorectal carcinoma. Science 241:961–965, 1988.

46. Needleman SW, Yuasa Y, Srivastava S, Aaronson SA: Normal cells of patients with high cancer risk syndromes lack transforming activity in the NIH3T3 transfection assay. Science 222:173–175, 1983.

47. Slamon DJ, DeKernion JB, Verma IM, Cline MJ: Expression of cellular oncogenes in human malignancies. Science 224:256–262, 1984.

48. Yokota J, Tsunetsugu-Yokota Y, Battifora H, LeFevre C, Cline MJ: Alterations of myc, myb and ras Ha protooncogenes in cancers are frequent and show clinical correlation. Science 231:261–265, 1986.

49. Meltzer SJ, Yokota J, Masuda H, Battifora H, Cline MJ: Oncogene alterations and the clinical behavior of colon cancer (abstract). Gastroenterology 90:1549, 1986.

50. Forrester K, Concepcion A, Kyuhyung H, Grizzle WE, Perucho M: Detection of high incidence of K-ras oncogenes during human colon tumorigenesis. Nature 8327:298–303, 1987.

51. Bos JL, Fearon ER, Hamilton SR, Verlaan-de Vries M, van Boom JH, van der Eb AJ, Vogelstein B: Prevalence of ras gene mutations in human colorectal cancers. Nature 327:293–297, 1987.

52. Pierce GB, Wallace C: Differentiation of malignant benign cells. Cancer Res 31:127, 1971.

53. Sailki R-K, Scharf S, Falcona F, Mullis K-B, Horn B-T, Erlich HA, Arnheim N: Enzymatic amplification of

beta-globin sequences and restriction site analysis for diagnosis of sickle cell anemia. Science 230:1350–1354, 1985.

54. Wolley RC, Schreiber K, Koss LG, Karas M, Sherman A: DNA distribution in human colon carcinomas and its relationship to clinical behavior. J Natl Cancer Inst 69:15–22, 1982.

55. Kokal W, Sheibani K, Terz J, Harada JR: Tumor DNA content in the prognosis of colorectal carcinoma. JAMA 255:3123–3127, 1986.

56. Banner BF, Tomas-De La Vega JE, Roseman DL, Coon JS: Should flow cytometric DNA analysis precede definitive surgery for colon carcinoma? Ann Surg 202:740–744, 1985.

57. Emdin SO, Stenling R, Roos G: Prognostic value of DNA content in colorectal carcinoma: A flow cytometric study with some methodologic aspects. Cancer 60:1282–1287, 1987.

58. Cuvelier CA, Morson BC, Roels HJ: The DNA content in cancer and dysplasia in chronic ulcerative colitis. Histopathology 11:927–939, 1987.

59. Goh HS, Jass JR; DNA content and the adenoma-carcinoma sequence in the colorectum. J Clin Pathol 39:387–92, 1986.

60. Whitehead F, Jarvis LR, Skinner JM, Whitehead R: Ploidy studies in adenomatous polyps of the colon. J Clin Pathol 38:1261–1264, 1985.

61. McKinley MJ, Budman DR, Kahn E: High grade dysplasia in Crohn's colitis characterized by flow cytometry, J Clin Gastroenterol 9:452–455, 1987.

62. Deschner EE, Lipkin M: Proliferative patterns in colonic mucosa in familial polyposis. Cancer 35:413–418, 1975.

63. Luk GD, Baylin SB: Ornithine decarboxylase as a biologic marker in familial colonic polyposis. N Engl J Med 311:80–83, 1984.

64. Feinberg AP, Vogelstein B: Hypomethylation distinguishes genes of some human cancers from their normal counterparts. Nature 301:89–92, 1983.

65. Goelz SE, Vogelstein B, Hamilton SR, Feinberg AP: Hypomethylation of DNA from benign and malignant human colon neoplasms. Science 228:187–196, 1985.

66. Gama-Sosa MA, Slagel VA, Trewyn RW, Ehrlich M: The 5-methylcytosine content of DNA from human tumors. Nucleic Acids Res 11:6883–6894, 1983.

67. Feinberg AP, Gehrke CW, Kuo KC, Ehrlich M: Reduced genomic 5-methylcytosine content in human colonic neoplasia. Cancer Res 48:1159–1161, 1988.

68. Kautiainen TL, Jones PA: DNA methylation in mammalian nuclei. Biochemistry 24:1193–1196, 1985.

69. Friedman E, Gillin S, Lipkin M: 12-0-Tetradecanoylphorbol-13-acetate stimulation of DNA synthesis in cultured preneoplastic familial polyposis colonic epithelial cells but not in normal colonic epithelial cells. Cancer Res 44:4078–4086, 1984.

70. Friedman E, Verderame M, Winawer S, Pollack R: Actin cytoskeletal organization loss in the benign-to-malignant tumor transition in cultured human colonic epithelial cells. Cancer Res 44:3040–3050, 1984.

71. Friedman E, Verderame M, Lipkin M, Pollack R: Altered actin cytoskeletal patterns in two premalignant stages in human colon carcinoma development. Cancer Res 45:3236–3242, 1985.

72. Kopelovich L, Conlon S, Pollack R: Defective organization of actin in cultured skin fibroblasts from patients with inherited adenocarcinoma. Proc Natl Acad Sci USA 74:3019–3022, 1977.

73. Gainer HStC, Schor S, Kinsella AR: Susceptibility of skin fibroblasts from individuals genetically predisposed to cancer, to transformation by the tumor promoter 12-0-tetradecanoylphorbol-13-acetate. Int J Cancer 34:349–357, 1984.

74. Nowell PC: The clonal evolution of tumor cell populations. Science 194:23–28, 1976.

75. Sandberg AA. "The Chromosomes in Human Cancer and Leukemia." New York: Elsevier, 1980.

76. Boveri T: "Zur Frage der Entstehung Maligner Tumoren." Jena: Fisher, 1914.

77. Cifone MA, Fidler IJ: Increasing metastatic potential is associated with increasing genetic instability of clones isolated from murine neoplasms. Proc Natl Acad Sci USA 78:6949–6952, 1981.

46

Loss of Alleles in Patients With Familial Adenomatous Polyposis and Colon Cancers

Mieko Okamoto, Chieko Sato, Takeo Iwama, and Michiko Miyaki

Department of Biochemistry, The Tokyo Metropolitan Institute of Medical Science, Honkomagome (M.O., C.S., M.M.) and Department of Surgery, Tokyo Medical and Dental University, Yushima (T.I.), Tokyo, Japan

INTRODUCTION

Recent studies have revealed a critical role of a specific gene loss in several embryonal tumors [1–6] and in certain adult cancers [7–17]. In retinoblastoma, hemizygosity or homozygosity of a recessive mutant allele results in the loss of normal gene product [18–20], and this seems to cause the manifestation of the disorder. Familial adenomatous polyposis (FAP) is an autosomal dominant trait characterized by numerous adenomatous polyps in the colon and rectum within the first few decades of life. The patients are at an extremely high risk of colorectal cancers if left untreated. The FAP gene has recently mapped to chromosome 5 [21,22]; however, little is known about the mechanisms of the tumorigenesis in FAP. Karyotype analyses have failed to detect specific deletion or translocation. Therefore, we chose a molecular genetic approach, using various polymorphic DNA markers, and have attempted to search for allele loss at a specific chromosomal region(s) in colorectal cancers from FAP patients. We also examined whether such loss is detectable in precancerous polyps. In this report, we demonstrate the loss of alleles on several different chromosomes in colon cancers and discuss the possible mechanisms of the carcinogenesis in FAP.

Familial Adenomatous Polyposis, pages 383–391

MATERIALS AND METHODS

Twenty-five FAP patients (ten with only polyps, five with colon cancers, and ten with both polyps and cancers) and 19 patients with sporadic colon cancers were examined to search for allele loss at a specific locus (loci). Table 1 represents the clinical features of several FAP patients. FAP can be subdivided into profuse and sparse types depending on the number of polyps. The majority of the patients we examined had the sparse type.

High-molecular-mass DNA was isolated by the method of sodium dodecyl sulfate (SDS)-proteinase K and phenol/chloroform treatment from surgical specimens of adenomatous polyps, colon cancers, and corresponding normal colon muscle, mucosa, or skin fibroblasts. In some cases, tumor specimens transplanted into nude mice were used as a source of tumor DNA. DNA was digested with appropriate restriction enzymes and fractionated by agarose gel electrophoresis, and Southern hybridization was performed with several polymorphic DNA markers as described previously [23]. In total, 30 probes for 13 human chromosomes, including four hypervariable locus-specific minisatellite probes, were used; 6929 (MYCL) [24] and pYNZ2 (D1S57) [25] for chromosome 1; p5G1 (CRYG) [26] for chromosome 2; pHF12-32 (D3S2) [27] for chromosome 3; L1.7 (D5S1) [26], pHF12-65 (D5S2) [27], C11p11 [21], L1.4 (D5S4) [21,28], PstI fragment of v-fms (FMS) [29], and λMS8

TABLE 1.
Clinical Features of Representative FAP Patients

Patient no.	Sex	Age (years)	Polyps	Colorectal Cancer
PLK 8	F	26	Sparse	+
PLK12	M	63		+
PLK15	F	20		−
PLK21	M	37	Sparse	+
PLK24	F	52	Sparse	+
PLK27	M	41	Sparse (~ 350)	+
PLK28	M	58	Sparse	+
PLK35	F	38		+
PLK36	F	52	Sparse (>1,000)	+
PLK41	M	44	Sparse	+
PLK43	F	34		+
PLK45	F	39	Sparse (>1,000)	+

(D5S43) [21,30] for chromosome 5; p23-0.6 (KRAS1P) [31] and 2.6 kb EcoRI fragment of c-myb (MYB) [32] for chromosome 6; NJ3.5 (COL1A2) [33] for chromosome 7; HindIII-BamHI fragment of v-bas [34] and VTR region of c-Ha-ras (HRAS1) [35] for chromosome 11; p23-0.6 and p640 (KRAS2) [31,36], pDL32B (D12S7) [26] and p7G11 (D12S8) [26] for chromosome 12; pAW101 (D14S10) [26] for chromosome 14; pMS1-14 (D15S1) [27] for chromosome 15; pHF12-2 (D17S1) [27], pYNZ-22 (D17S30) [26,37], and pTHH59 (D17S4) [38] for chromosome 17; pHF12-62 (D18S1) [27] for chromosome 18; and p22/34 (D22S9) [39], Hu-λ-C-RI-HindIII (IGLC) [26,40], a subclone pV3.3 from V4A (IGLV) [26], pMS3-18 (D22S1) [27], and Pst I fragment of v-sis (PDGFB) [26, 41] for chromosome 22.

RESULTS AND DISCUSSION

We have reported previously that loss of alleles in colon cancer seems to occur on several particular chromosomes [23]. Most frequent allele losses were observed in chromosome 22 (Table 2, Fig. 1). Fourteen FAP patients with colon cancer were informative for at least one of the five chromosome 22 markers (D22S9, IGLC, IGLV, D22S1, and PDGFB), and six of the 14 patients had lost the heterozygosity in their colon cancers (43%). Allele losses were observed only in malignant colon cancers, not in benign adenomas, even when the colon cancer had lost its heterozygosity. The same allele loss was observed also in sporadic colon cancers (four of 19 informative cases; 21%).

Fearon et al. [42] have reported that somatic loss of chromosome 17p sequences occurred in over 75% of the sporadic colon cancers. We also have detected similar loss of alleles for chromosome 17 markers, although our frequency was lower than theirs (data not shown). Eight FAP patients with colon cancers were informative for at least one of the two 17p markers (D17S1 and D17S30), and three of eight informative patients showed loss of the heterozygosity in their colon cancers (38%). Among these three, one colon cancer showed allele losses for the 17p markers, but it retained the heterozygosity for D17S4 mapped to 17q. This is consistent with the result of Fearon et al. [42]. The same allele losses were observed also in sporadic colon cancers (five of 15 informative cases; 33%)

Similar allele losses were observed for chromosome 12q markers (D12S7 and D12S8). Among 19 informative FAP patients, three colon cancers and one adenoma had lost the heterozygosity. Two of these four patients were also informative at the KRAS2 locus on 12p, and these two tumors retained heterozygosity at this locus. This suggests that the allele loss observed here is due to a partial deletion rather than to the entire loss of the chromosome. The same loss was also observed in two of 16 sporadic colon cancers.

Localization of the FAP gene on chromosome

TABLE 2.
Chromosome 22 Markers in Colon Cancers From FAP Patients*

Marker enzyme location	D22S9 TaqI q11	IGLC EcoRI q11	IGLV TaqI q11	D22S1 BglII q11–13	PDGFB HindIII q12–13
PLK 8 Ca	1/2	—		—	—
PLK12 Ca	—	2	—	—	—
PLK15 A	—	1/2	1/2	—	—
PLK21 Ca	—	—		1/2	—
PLK24 Ca	2	1	1	2	1
PLK25 A	—	1/2	—	1/2	—
PLK27 Ca	—	1/2	—	—	—
A		1/2	—		—
PLK28 Ca	1	1		—	—
A	1/2	1/2		—	—
PLK35 Ca	1/2	—		—	—
A	1/2	—		—	—
PLK36 Ca	1/2	—	—	1/2	—
A	1/2	—	—	1/2	—
PLK39 A	1/2	1/2	—	—	—
PLK41 Ca	—	1/2		1/2	—
A	—	1/2		1/2	—
PLK43 Ca	1/2	—	—	—	—
A1	1/2	—	—	—	—
A2	1/2	—	—	—	—
PLK45 Ca	—				
A1	—				
A2	—				
KuPL14 Ca	1	1	2	—	—
KuPL15 Ca	2	—	1	—	—
A	1/2	—	1/2	—	—
KuPL24 Ca1	—	—	1/2	—	1/2
Ca2	—	—	1	—	
A		—	1/2		—

*The phenotype observed in the tumor DNA is shown for every case when the normal DNA displayed heterozygosity. Heterozygosity is indicated by 1/2 (even though different pairs of alleles may be present for certain multiallele markers). 1 or 2 indicates tumor DNA that retained only the allele of higher or lower relative molecular mass, respectively. A dash indicates that the normal DNA was homozygous and therefore uninformative. Ca, carcinoma; A, adenomatous polyps. The numbers after these abbreviations (for example, Ca1) indicate tumors developed at different sites of the colon in a particular patient. For details refer to Figure 1 legend and Okamoto et al. [23].

5 [21,22] and allele losses on this chromosome in sporadic colon cancers [43] suggest the possible involvement of this gene locus in the tumorigenesis in FAP. Therefore, we examined, using the probe C11p11, which is closely linked to the FAP gene, whether such loss should occur in the tumorigenesis in FAP. Among 25 FAP patients, only one was informative for this probe, and this patient PLK45 had lost heterozygosity in the colon cancer but not in the two benign adenomas (Fig. 2). The same allele loss was observed in at least two sporadic colon cancers. Similarly, one patient with FAP showed allele loss at the c-fms locus in two independent colorectal cancers but, again, not in benign adenoma (data not shown).

To examine how frequently allele losses should occur in this chromosome region, we used another two highly polymorphic probes mapped to the distal to the FAP gene. An anonymous

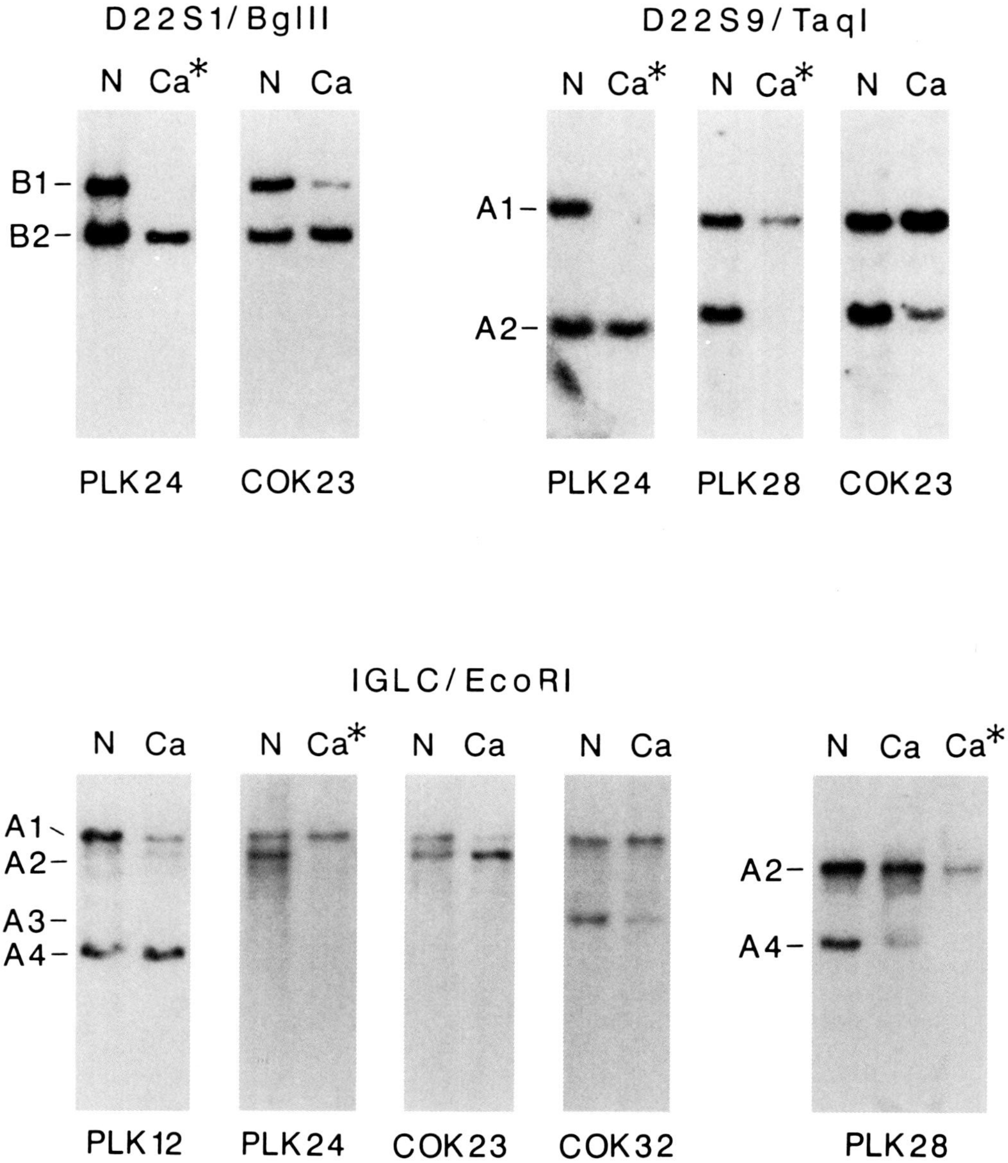

Fig. 1. Loss of alleles on chromosome 22 in familial and sporadic colon cancers. N, normal tissue; Ca, primary cancer obtained at surgery; Ca*, colon cancer grown in a nude mouse. PLK and KuPL indicate patients with FAP; COK and KuCO, patients with sporadic colon cancer. The letter and number on the left indicate a restriction fragment length polymorphism and polymorphic allele [for more details, see 23].

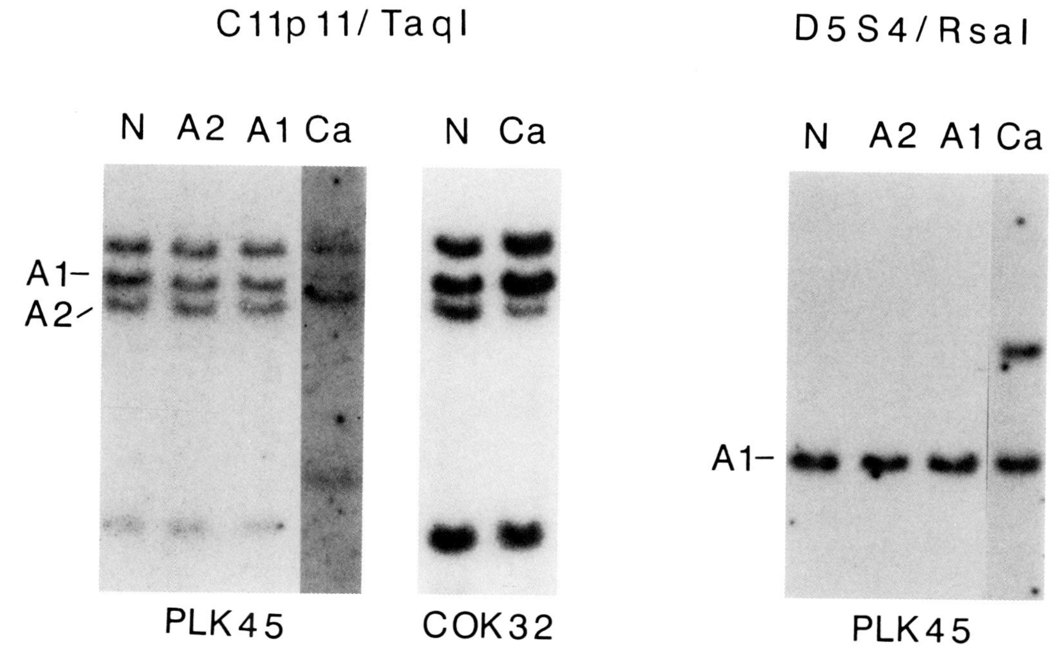

Fig. 2. Loss and alteration of alleles on chromosome 5 in familial and sporadic colon cancer (for details refer to Fig. 1 legend).

DNA segment D5S4, mapped to 5q31 [21], displayed multiple RFLPs with MspI, EcoRI, RsaI, or TaqI digests; D5S43, detected by a locus-specific minisatellite probe λMS8 [30] and mapped to 5q34-qter [21], displayed multiple alleles with a high degree of heterozygosity in HinfI-digested DNA. Among 15 patients examined, 12 were constitutively heterozygous for at least one of the two probes. PLK45 was constitutively homozygous for the marker D5S4, but, in the colon cancer that had lost one allele for the FAP gene-linked probe C11p11, D5S4 detected two fragments, one compatible with that in normal tissue and polyps and the other abnormally large (Fig. 2). This may suggest the rearrangment of one homologous chromosome 5, leading to the allele loss at the FAP gene. However, no allele loss or chromosomal alteration was observed in the other colon cancers, nor in the polyps from FAP patients.

Table 3 summarizes the allele losses for chromosome 5 markers in the colon cancer from FAP patients. Among 15 FAP patients with colon cancers, 11 were constitutively heterozygous for at least one of the chromosome 5 markers, and all were also informative for at least one of the markers near or distal to the FAP gene. Only two of the 11 patients showed loss of heterozygosity for these markers (18%). This apparently low frequency may be interpreted in three ways. 1) This may be the result of random drift from the limited number of the informative cases . 2) Chromosomal events leading to the hemizygosity or homozygosity of the FAP gene might occur as point mutation or very small deletion, so that most of these probes could not detect them. 3) Hemizygosity or homozygosity of the FAP gene may not be essential for the development of the colon cancer, although it is possible that loss of the normal gene homologue at this locus may favor the tumor progression. Further analyses are needed to exclude or substantiate either possibility.

The question of the frequency of allele loss

TABLE 3.
Chromosome 5 Markers in Colon Cancers From FAP Patients*

Marker enzyme location	D5S1 PstI 5	D5S2 MspI pter-q35	C11p11 TaqI q21-22	D5S4 MspI, RsaI q31	FMS EcoRI q34	D5S43 HinfI q34-qter
PLK 8 Ca	1/2	—	—	1/2	1/2	1/2
PLK12 Ca	1/2	—	—	—	—	1/2
PLK15 A	—	—	—	—	—	1/2
PLK21 Ca	—	—		1/2	—	1/2
PLK24 Ca	—	—	—	1/2	—	1/2
PLK25 A	—	—	—	—	1/2	—
PLK27 A	—	—	—	—	—	—
PLK28 Ca	—	—	—	1/2	—	1/2
PLK35 Ca	—	—	—	1/2	—	1/2
PLK36 Ca	1/2	—	—	1/2	—	1/2
A	1/2	—	—	1/2	—	1/2
PLK39 A	—	1/2	—	—	—	—
PLK41 Ca	—	—	—	1/2	1/2	1/2
A	—	—	—	1/2	1/2	1/2
PLK43 Ca	—	—	—	—	—	1/2
A1	—	—	—	—	—	1/2
A2	—	—	—	—	—	1/2
PLK45 Ca			2[a]	Re		—
A1	1/2		1/2	—		—
A2	1/2		1/2	—		—
KuPL24 Ca1		—	—	—	2	
Ca2		—	—	—	2	
A		—	—	—	1/2	

*Re indicates the allele of abnormal relative molecular mass. For details refer to Table 2 footnote.

was examined on other chromosomes. For each of chromosomes 1, 6, and 15, allele loss was observed in one colon cancer among three to eight informative FAP patients, whereas there was no such loss in chromosomes 2, 3, 7, 11, 14, and 18. Allele loss at the c-Ha-ras locus has been observed in several tumors [7,17,44], and its frequency has been reported to increase with tumor progression [45]. However, we did not observe any qualitative or quantitative changes at this locus, even in the DNAs extracted from tumors transplanted into nude mice [PLK8,21,24,28]. This suggests that the genome is remarkably stable and, therefore, that the allele losses observed here is not simply the result of chromosome instability in the colon cancers.

Most frequent allele loss was observed on chromosomes 17 and 22, whereas the FAP gene is on chromosome 5. An analogous case has been reported by Mathew et al. [46]; tumors from patients with MEN-2 had lost one allele at loci on chromosome 1, whereas the MEN-2 gene is on chromosome 10 [47,48]. These two cases showing unexpected allele losses suggest that the gene locus (loci) other than the primary mutation may be involved in the manifestation of the malignancy, and possibly these allele losses reflect the loss of a ''disease-specific tumor-suppressor gene(s).''

Loss of alleles on chromosome 22 has been reported in several tumors, such as meningioma [9,10], acoustic neuroma [8,9], Ewing's sarcoma [49], medullary thyroid carcinoma, and phaeochromocytoma of MEN-2 [12]. Most of these tumors are of neural crest origin. The incidence of brain tumors in FAP patients has been shown to be higher than that in non-FAP population [50]. Considering that there was no allele loss in colon cancers for chromosomes 3 and 11, for which several other cancers showed specific allele losses, we may speculate that the human genome contains a limited number of tumor-suppressor genes and that loss of the function of one or more of the genes may lead to particular cancers or, alternatively, that allele loss at a locus (loci) on chromosome 22 promotes tumor growth.

No allele loss in polyps, even when the colon cancer had lost its heterozygosity, strongly suggests that loss of heterozygosity is involved in carcinogenesis but not in polyp formation. Our observation of allele losses on more than one chromosome region may suggest that the carcinogenesis in FAP is not simple but multifactorial and complex. Evaluation of these chromosomal events, as well as the identification of the FAP gene on chromosome 5, will clarify the steps leading to the colon malignancy in FAP.

SUMMARY

With an aim to obtaining molecular clues about the tumorigenesis in FAP, we compared constitutional and tumor genotypes in colon cancers and polyps from 25 FAP patients using various polymorphic DNA markers on 13 human chromosomes. Frequent allele losses were observed in colon cancers at loci on chromosomes 12q, 17p, and 22, the frequencies being 23% (three of 13 informative cases), 38% (three of eight informative cases), and 43% (six of 14 informative cases), respectively. Molecular probes linked to or distal to the FAP gene on chromosome 5q also detected allele losses in two of 11 informative cases (18%). With a single exception, polyps retained their heterozygosity for these markers on 13 autosomes, even when allele loss was observed in the colon cancer. This suggests that allele losses on these chromosomes may be involved in carcinogenesis in FAP, but not in polyp formation. The same allele losses on these chromosomes were observed also in sporadic colon cancers, suggesting a common step(s) leading to the colon malignancy.

ACKNOWLEDGMENTS

We are grateful to the following for providing DNA probes: Y. Nakamura, R. White, J.D. Minna, L.-C. Tsui, P. O'Connell, P.L. Pearson, A.J. Jeffreys, C.J. Sherr, Y. Yuasa, P. Tuipouras, F. Ramirez, Y. Sakaki, R. Weinberg, N. Tsuchida, P. Leder, and J.D. Kaplan. The probes for D1S57, MYCL, D5S2, D14S1, D17S1, D17S30, D17S4, D18S1, and D22S1 were provided through the Japanese Cancer Research Resources Bank. This work was supported by a grant for cancer research from the Ministry of Education, Science and Culture of Japan.

References

1. Cavenee WK, Dryja TP, Phillips RA, Benedict WF, Godbout R, Gallie BL, Murphree AL, Strong LC, White RL: Expression of recessive alleles by chromosomal mechanisms in retinoblastoma. Nature 305:779–784, 1983.
2. Cavenee WK, Hansen MF, Nordenskjold M, Maumenee I, Squire JA, Phillips RA, Gallie BL: Genetic origin of mutations predisposing to retinoblastoma. Science 228:501–503, 1985.
3. Benedict WF, Srivatsan ES, Mark C, Banerjee A, Sparkes R, Murphree L: Complete or partial homozygosity of chromosome 13 in primary retinoblastoma. Cancer Res 47:4189–4191, 1987.
4. Solomon E: Recessive mutation in aetiology of Wilms' tumour. Nature 309:111–112, 1984.
5. Koufos A, Hansen MF, Copeland NG, Jenkins NA, Lampkin BC, Cavenee WK: Loss of heterozygosity in three embryonal tumours suggests a common pathogenetic mechanism. Nature 316: 330–334, 1985.
6. Scrable HJ, Witte DP, Lampkin BC, Cavenee WK: Chromosomal localization of the human rhabdomyosarcoma locus by mitotic recombination mapping. Nature 329:645–647, 1987.
7. Fearon ER, Feinberg AP, Hamilton SH, Vogelstein B: Loss of genes on the short arm of chromosome 11 in bladder cancer. Nature 318:377–380, 1985.
8. Seizinger BR, Martuza RL, Gusella JF: Loss of genes on chromosome 22 in tumorigenesis of human acoustic neuroma. Nature 322:644–647, 1986.
9. Seizinger BR, Rouleau G, Ozelius LJ, Lane AH, St. George-Hyslop P, Huson S, Gusella J, Martuza RL: Common pathogenetic mechanism for three tumor types in bilateral acoustic neurofibromatosis. Science 236:317–319, 1987.
10. Seizinger BR, de la Monte S, Atkins L, Gusella JF, Martuza RL: Molecular genetic approach to human meningioma: Loss of genes of chromosome 22. Proc Natl Acad Sci USA 84:5419–5423, 1987.

11. Zbar B, Brauch H, Talmadge C, Linehan M: Loss of alleles of loci on the short arm of chormosome 3 in renal cell carcinoma. Nature 327:721–724, 1987.

12. Takai S, Tateishi H, Nishisho I, Miki T, Motomura K, Miyauchi A, Kato M, Ikeuchi T, Yamamoto K, Okazaki M, Yamamoto M, Honjo T, Kumahara Y, Mori T: Loss of genes on chromosome 22 in medullary thyroid carcinoma and pheochromocytoma. Jpn J Cancer Res (Gann) 78:894–898, 1987.

13. Naylor SL, Johnson BE, Minna JD, Sakaguchi AY: Loss of heterozygosity of chromosome 3p markers in small-cell lung cancer. Nature 329:451–454, 1987.

14. Ali IU, Lidereau R, Theillet C, Callahan R: Reduction to homozygosity of genes on chromosome 11 in human breast neoplasia. Science 238:185–188, 1987.

15. Yokota J, Wada M, Shimosato Y, Terada M, Sugimura T: Loss of heterozygosity on chromosomes 3, 13, and 17 in small-cell carcinoma and on chromosome 3 in adenocarcinoma of the lung. Proc Natl Acad Sci USA 84:9252–9256, 1987.

16. Kok K, Osinga J, Carritt B, Davis MB, van der Hout AH, van der Veen AY, Landsvater RM, de Leij LFMH, Barendsen HH, Postmus PE, Poppema S, Buys CHCM: Deletion of a DNA sequence at the chromosomal region 3p21 in all major types of lung cancer. Nature 330:578–581, 1987.

17. Shiraishi M, Morinaga S, Noguchi M, Shimosato Y, Sekiya T: Loss of genes on the short arm of chromosome 11 in human lung carcinomas. Jpn J Cancer Res (Gann) 78:1302–1308, 1987.

18. Friend SH, Bernards R, Rogelj S, Weinberg RA, Rapaport JM, Albert DM Dryja TP: A human DNA segment with properties of the gene that predisposes to retinoblastoma and osteosarcoma. Nature 323:643–646, 1986.

19. Lee WH, Bookstein R, Hong F, Young LJ, Shew JY, Lee EY–HP: Human retinoblastoma susceptibility gene: Cloning, identification, and sequence. Science 235:1394–1399, 1987.

20. Fung Y–KT, Murphree AL, T'Ang A, Qian J, Hinrichs SH, Benedict WF: Structural evidence for the authenticity of the human retinoblastoma gene. Science 236:1657–1661, 1987.

21. Bodmer, WF, Bailey CJ, Bodmer J, Bussey HJR, Ellis A, Gorman P, Lucibello FC, Murday, VA, Rider SH, Scambler P, Sheer D, Solomon E, Spurr, NK: Localization of the gene for familial adenomatous polyposis on chromosome 5. Nature 328:614–616, 1987.

22. Leppert M, Dobbs, M, Scambler P, O'Connell P, Nakamura Y, Stauffer D, Woodward S, Burt R, Hughes J, Gardner E, Lathrop M, Wasmuth J, Lalouel J–M, White R: The gene for familial polyposis coli maps to the long arm of chromosome 5. Science 238:1411–1413, 1987.

23. Okamoto M, Sasaki M, Sugio K, Sato C, Iwama T, Ikeuchi T, Tonomura A, Sasazuki T, Miyaki M: Loss of constitutional heterozygosity in colon carcinoma from patients with familial polyposis coli. Nature 331:273–277, 1988.

24. Nau MM, Brooks BJ, Battey J, Sausville E, Gazdar AF, Kirsch IR, MacBride OW, Bertness V, Hollis GF, Minna JD: L-myc, a new myc-related gene amplified and expressed in human small cell lung cancer. Nature 318:69–73, 1985.

25. Nakamura Y, Culver M, Sergeant L, Leppert M, O'Connell P, Lathrop GM, Lalouel, J–M, White R: Isolation and mapping of a polymorphic DNA sequence (pYNZ2) on chromosome 1p (D1S57). Nucleic Acids Res, 16:4747, 1988.

26. Ninth International Workshop on Human Gene Mapping: Cytogenet, Cell Genet, 46:1–762, 1987.

27. Barker D, Schafer M, White R: Restriction sites containing CpG show a higher frequency of polymorphism in human DNA. Cell 36:131–138, 1984.

28. Bailey CJ, Rider SH, Bodmer WF: A new RFLP for L1.4 (D5S4) an anonymous genomic clone localised to chromosome 5. Nucleic Acids Res, 15:6762, 1987.

29. De Qi Xu, Guilhot S, Galibert F: Restriction fragment length polymorphism of the human c-fms gene. Proc Natl Acad Sci USA, 82:2862–2865, 1985.

30. Wong Z, Wilson V, Patel L, Povey S, Jeffreys AJ: Characterization of a panel of highly variable minisatellites cloned from human DNA. Ann Hum Genet 51:269–288, 1987.

31. Okamoto M, Sato C, Tsuchida N, Yoshida MC, Ezawa C, Miyaki M: Viral K-ras detects two TaqI polymorphisms, one for KRAS1 on chromosome 6 and the other for KRAS 2 on chromosome 12. Nucleic Acids Res, 16:2363, 1988.

32. Yuasa Y, Reddy ER, Rhim JS, Tronick SR, Aaronson SA: Activated N-ras in a human rectal carcinoma cell line associated with clonal homozygosity in myb locus-restriction fragment polymorphism. Jpn J Cancer Res (Gann) 77:639–647, 1986.

33. Tsipouras P, Myers JC, Ramirez F, Prockop DJ: Restriction fragment length polymorphism associated with the Proα2(1) gene of human type I procollagen. J Clin Invest, 72:1262–1267, 1983.

34. Andersen PR, Devare SG, Tronick, SR, Ellis RW, Aaronson SA, Scolnick EM: Generation of BALB-MuSV and Ha-MuSV by type C virus transduction of homologous transforming genes from different species. Cell 26:129–134, 1981.

35. Capon DJ, Chen EY, Levinson AD, Seeburg PH, Goeddel DV: Complete nucleotide sequences of the T24 human bladder carcinoma oncogene and its normal homologue. Nature 302:33–37, 1983.

36. Barker D, McCoy M, Weinberg R, Goldfarb M, Wigler M, Burt R, Gardner E, White R: A test of the role of two oncogenes in inherited predisposition to colon cancer. Mol Biol Med 1:199–206, 1983.

37. Nakamura Y, Leppert M, O'Connell P, Wolff R, Holm T, Culver M, Martin C, Fujimoto E, Hoff M, Kumlin E, White R: Variable number of tandem repeat (VNTR) markers for human gene mapping. Science 235:1616–1622, 1987.

38. Nakamura Y, Holm T, Gillilan S, Leppert M, O'Connell P, Lathrop GM, Lalouel J–M, White R: Isolation and mapping of a polymorphic DNA sequence (pTHH59) on chromosome 17q (D17S4). Nucleic Acids Res, 16:3598, 1988.

39. McDermid HE, Duncan AMV, Brasch KR, Holden JJA, Magenis E, Sheehy R, Burn J, Kardon N, Noel B, Schinzei A, Teshima I, White BN: Characterization of the supernumerary chromosome in cat eye syndrome. Science 232:646–648, 1986.

40. Hieter PA, Hollis GF, Korsmeyer SJ, Waldmann TA,

Leder P: Clustered arrangement of immunoglobulin λ constant region genes in man. Nature 294:536–540, 1981.

41. Gelmann EP, Wong-Staal F, Kramer RA, Gallo RC: Molecular cloning and comparative analyses of the genomes of simian sarcoma virus and its associated helper virus. Proc Natl Acad Sci USA, 78:3373–3377, 1981.

42. Fearon ER, Hamilton SR, Vogelstein B: Clonal analysis of human colorectal tumors. Science 238:193–197, 1987.

43. Solomon E, Voss R, Hall V, Bodmer, WF, Jass JR, Jeffreys AJ, Lucibello FC, Patel I, Rider SH: Chromosome 5 allele loss in human colorectal carcinomas. Nature 328:616–619, 1987.

44. Theillet C, Lidereau R, Escot C, Hutzell P, Brunet M, Gest J, Schlom J, Callahan R: Loss of c-H-ras-1 allele and aggressive human primary breast carcinomas. Cancer Res, 46:4776–4781, 1986.

45. Yokota J, Tsunetsugu-Yokota Y, Battifora H, LeFevre C, Cline MJ: Alterations of myc, myb, and Ha-ras proto-oncogenes in cancers are frequent and show clinical correlation. Science 231:261–265, 1986.

46. Mathew CGP, Smith BA, Thorpe K, Wong Z, Royle NJ, Jeffreys AJ, Ponder BAJ: Deletion of genes on chromosome 1 in endocrine neoplasia. Nature 328:524–526, 1987.

47. Mathew CGP, Chin KS, Easton DF, Thorpe K, Carter C, Liou GI, Fong SL, Bridges CDB, Haak H, Nieuwenhuijzen Kruseman AC, Schifter S, Hansen HH, Telenius H, Telenius-Berg M, Ponder BAJ: A linked genetic marker for multiple endocrine neoplasia type 2A on chromosome 10. Nature 328:527–528, 1987.

48. Simpson NE, Kidd KK, Goodfellow PJ, McDermid H, Myers S, Kidd JR, Jackson CE, Duncan AMV, Farrer LA, Brasch K, Castiglione C, Genel M, Gertner J, Greenberg CR, Gusella JF, Holden JJA, White BN: Assignment of multiple endocrine neoplasia type 2A to chromosome 10 by linkage. Nature 328:528–530, 1987.

49. Douglass EC, Valentine M, Green AA, Hayes FA, Thompson EI: t(11;22) and other chromosomal rearrangements in Ewing's sarcoma. JNCI 77:1211–1215, 1986.

50. Jagelman DG: Extracolonic manifestations of familial polyposis coli. Cancer Genet, Cytogenet, 27:319–325, 1987.

47

Closely Linked DNA Markers for Preclinical Prediction of Familial Adenomatous Polyposis

P. Meera Khan, C.M.J. Tops, C. Breukel, J.Th. Wijnen, H.M. vd Klift, I.S.J. van Leeuwen-Cornelisse, H.F.A. Vasen, G. Griffioen, F.C.A. den Hartog Jager, and C.B.H.W. Lamers

Human Genetics Institute, University of Leiden (P.M.K., C.M.J.T., C.B., J.Th.W., H.M.V.K., I.S.J.V.L.-C.), Clinical Genetics Center (I.S.J.V.L.-C.), National Familial Polyposis Registration Center (I.S.J.V.L.-C. H.F.A.V.), and, Department of Gastroenterology, University Medical Center (H.F.A.V., G.G., C.B.H.W.L.), Leiden, and Netherlands Cancer Institute, Amsterdam (F.C.A.D.H.J.), The Netherlands

Familial adenomatous polyposis (FAP), previously known as *familial polyposis coli,* is a dominantly inherited autosomal condition. The carriers of the gene have a tendency to develop hundreds of adenomatous polyps in the large bowel during their adolescence [Bussey, 1975]. On clinical diagnosis their large intestine is removed to prevent the otherwise inevitable development of colorectal adenocarcinoma and early death [for review, see Ingall and Mastromarino, 1983]. All of the first-degree relatives (especially the sibs and progeny) of the patients have a priori a 50% risk of developing the disease [Bussey, 1975]. The age at which the FAP carriers manifest characteristic symptoms leading to diagnosis is extremely variable. Therefore, markers for presymptomatic detection of the carriers with 100% reliability would relieve noncarrier relatives (who form one-half of the a priori at risk persons) from anxiety as well as the necessity of cumbersome and expensive periodic clinical investigations. Moreover, such markers would help clinicians to plan appropriate measures of treatment to prevent colon cancer in the remaining half. Single copy DNA markers with high polymorphism information content (PIC values) tightly linked to or situated within the disease locus would satisfy the above requirements [for a description of the rationale, see Gusella, 1986].

About 100,000 genes are dispersed on 22 autosomes and the sex chromosomes of humans. The gene determining FAP is one of them. If the chromosomal localization of the FAP gene were not known, its search by random linkage approach would have been like "looking for a needle in a haystack." Herrera et al. [1986] gave a detailed case report and suggested that a gene determining Gardner's syndrome (implicitly the FAP gene) is probably located either in the band region q13-q15 or q15-q22 on chromosome 5. Bodmer et al. [1987] obtained significant evidence for tight linkage between FAP and the polymorphic DNA marker c11p11 localized by in situ hybridization to the q21-q22 region on chromosome 5. Leppert et al. [1987] have independently investigated the FAP families in America and also obtained significant evidence for tight linkage between c11-p11 and FAP. These two groups observed no recombination between c11p11 and FAP in about 50 informative individuals. The investigators also included families with classical Gardner's syndrome and observed no indication for heterogeneity between families with respect to c11-p11-FAP linkage. Thus, these linkage studies did not contradict an earlier suggestion that the

Familial Adenomatous Polyposis, pages 393–396

classical familial polyposis coli and Gardner's syndrome represent different levels of molecular lesions in the same gene [For an interesting discussion, see McKusick, 1988, MIM No. 17510].

Because of its low PIC value, the TaqI polymorphism of C11p11 has been estimated to be informative for linkage only in about 20% of the random North European families. Moreover, the apparent absence of recombinants in 50 cases would not guarantee that recombination will not take place between the loci concerned. In fact, more recent studies revealed recombinants between C11p11 and FAP [Tops et al., 1989; Dr. M. Dunlop, Edinburgh, personal communication]. Therefore, there was an obvious need for new markers. Consequently, a further search for new markers has lead to the identification of additional markers mapping close to FAP. These markers are listed and relevant information on them is summarized in Table 1. Their allele frequencies are presented in Table 2.

TABLE 1.
Polymorphism Information Content (PIC) and Linkage Information on DNA Markers (=Probes) Thus Far Reported To Be Closely* Linked to the Gene Determining Familial Adenomatous Polyposis

Probe (locus)[a]	PIC (chrom.)[b]	Recombination fraction[c]	Peak LOD score[d]	References
C11p11 (D5S71)	0.14 (106)	0.00	3.26	Bodmer et al. [1987]
C11p11 (D5S71)	0.24 (?)	0.00	3.37	Leppert et al. [1987]
C11p11 (D5S71)	0.40 (96)[e]	0.06	4.39	Breukel et al. [1988] Tops et al. [1989]
Pi227 (D5S37)	0.75 (82)	0.04	12.29	Meera Khan et al. [1988], Tops et al. [1989]
YN5.48 (D5S81)	0.38 (?)	0.00	8.25	Nakamura et al. [1988]
YN5.64 (D5S82)	0.59 (?)	0.06	5.64	Nakamura et al. [1988]
MC5.61 (D5S84)	0.75 (?)	0.04	8.05	Nakamura et al. [1988]
KK5.33 (D5S85)	0.66 (?)	0.07	7.80	Nakamura et al. [1988]

*Linkage is described to be close (rather arbitrarily) when the recombination fraction ranges between 0.02 and 0.06. The one <0.02 is called *tight linkage.*

[a]The sites corresponding to the probe sequences in the chromosomes are conventionally designated by locus symbols. For example, D5S71 means the DNA sequence in chromosome 5 at site 71 that can be identified by the probe C11p11.

[b]Numbers in parentheses are number of chromosomes from random persons in a population screened by the probe to derive the corresponding PIC value. This number is necessary to evaluate the accuracy and reliability of allele frequencies from which the PIC value is estimated. In certain cases more than one site at a given locus might exhibit polymorphism, increasing its PIC value. The ones in this table are net PIC values. The PIC values of the markers indicate their relative usefulness in linkage studies. For example, C11p11 TaqI RFLP (see Table 2) with a PIC value of 0.14 in a given population will have a high probability of being informative for linkage with FAP in 14% of the FAP families in that population, while Pi227 with a net PIC value of 0.75 in another population will posses it in 75% of the FAP families in that population.

[c]Recombination fraction indicates the genetic distance between two loci (for example, a disease locus and a marker locus) considered for linkage analysis [see Ott, 1985]. Closest markers segregate together with the highest probability yielding a recombination fraction close to 0.00. Consequently, the inheritance of disease genes can be traced in the families through closely linked markers (see chapter 20, this volume) [Gusella, 1986].

[d]LOD represents log of odds in favor of linkage. A peak LOD of 3.00 means odds 1,000:1 in favor of linkage.

[e]The higher PIC value of C11p11 in this case is due to the net estimated value of both TaqI RFLP and the deletion polymorphism (DEL1) in C11p11 described in the Dutch population by Breukel et al. [1988, 1989]. Also it is important to note that PIC values may widely differ between divergent populations.

TABLE 2.
Allele Frequencies and Polymorphic Site-Specific Polymorphism Information (PIC) Values of DNA Markers Known To Map Close to FAP*

Probe	Site	Allele Size (kb)	Allele Symbol	Allele Freq.	No. of chromosomes	Population	PIC	References
C11p11	TaqI	4.4	A1	0.08	106	?		Bodmer et al. [1987]
		3.9	A2	0.92			0.14	
C11p11	TaqI	4.2	A1	0.17	?	?		Leppert et al. [1987]
		2.7	A2	0.83			0.24	
C11p11	TaqI	4.4	A1	0.11	142	Dutch		Breukel et al.
		3.9	A2	0.89			0.17	[1988, 1989]
	DEL1	0.070	B1	0.85	100	Dutch		Breukel et al.
		0.066	B2	0.15			0.22	[1988, 1989]
Pi227	BclI	8.6;1.2	A1	0.20	100	Dutch		Meera Khan et al.
		3.0	A2	0.37				[1988]
		1.8;1.2	A3	0.43			0.56	
	BstXI	2.7	B1	0.46	82	Dutch		Tops et al.
		2.3	B2	0.54			0.37	[1989]
	PstI	4.3	C1	0.16	92	Dutch		Meera Khan et al.
		3.0	C2	0.84			0.23	[1988]
	MboI	0.54	D1	0.44	18	Dutch		Meera Khan et al.
		0.46	D2	0.56			0.37	[1988]
YN5.48	TaqI	6.0	A1	0.50	?	?		Nakamura et al. [1988]
		3.6	A2	0.50			0.38	
YN5.64	PstI	5.2	A1	0.61	?	?		Nakamura et al. [1988]
		5.1	A2	0.39			0.36	
	TaqI	8.0	B1	0.15	?	?		Nakamura et al. [1988]
		6.0	B2	0.85			0.22	
MC5.61	MspI	5.5	A1	0.49	?	?		Nakamura et al. [1988]
		5.0	A2	0.51			0.38	
	TaqI	20.0	B1	0.54	?	?		Nakamura et al. [1988]
		18.0	B2	0.46			0.37	
KK5.33	TaqI	9.0	A1	0.43	?	?		Nakamura et al. [1988]
		8.0	A2	0.57			0.37	
	PstI	6.0	B1	0.23	?	?		
		8.0	B2	0.77			0.29	

*For locus symbols, see Table 1. Site, polymorphic site; note that the DEL1 site in C11p11 is not a conventional RFLP. It is a deletion polymorphism rapidly (in about 6 hours of laboratory time) detectable by a nonradioactive, directly visible staining procedure following polyacrylamide gel electrophoresis [Breukel et al., 1989]. Allele sizes are in kilobases (kbs). See the footnotes to Table 1 for further details.

The discovery of an additional polymorphic site within c11p11 [Breukel et al., 1988, 1989] (see Table 1, footnote e) has raised its PIC value to 0.40. Three of the four restriction fragment length polymorphism (RFLP) sites in the new probe pI227 (Stewart et al., 1987) gave a PIC value of 0.75 in a Dutch population [Meera Khan et al., 1988, Tops et al., 1989]. More recently, another set of four probes has been reported with PIC values ranging from 0.38 to 0.75 with recombination fractions estimated between 0.00 and 0.07 [Nakamura et al., 1988]. Available linkage information indicates that the listed loci c11p11, pI227, YN5.48, MC5.61, and KK5.33 are probably located on the same side of the FAP locus. Their respective 95% probability limits of recombination fractions are still fairly wide. Therefore the prediction of FAP gene carriers with 100% certainty is not yet possible. However, because of their high PIC values, with the help of the above probes it is possible to estimate the risk values with more than 90% of probability.

For the convenience of the groups and laboratories that might be interested in securing the probes for their use, we present the following addresses of the contact persons for the probes:

c11p11: Dr. Nigel K. Spurr
Clare Hall Laboratories
ICRF, Blanche Lane
South Mimms, Herts
EN6 3LD, United Kingdom

pI227: Dr. Gordon Stewart
Howard Hughes Medical Institute
University of Michigan
1150 Medical Center Dr. MSRBI, 3520
Ann Arbor, MI 48109-0650

YN5.48: Dr. Ysuke Nakamura
Howard Hughes Medical Institute
University of Utah Medical Center
603 Wintrobe
Salt Lake City, UT 84132

ACKNOWLEDGMENTS

Support by the Dutch Praeventie Fonds, The Hague (grant No. 28-1383), is gratefully acknowledged. We thank Mr. D. Scott Samuels for help with the preparation of the manuscript.

References

Bodmer WF, Bailey CJ, Bodmer J, Bussey HJR, Ellis A, Gorman P, Lucibello FC, Murday VA, Rider SH, Scambler P, Sheer D, Solomon E, Spurr NK (1987): Localization of the gene for familial adenomatous polyposis on chromosome 5. Nature 328:614–616.

Breukel C, Tops CMJ, Meera Khan P (1988): Search for novel DNA (C11p11) markers for presymptomatic prediction of familial adenomatous polyposis (FAP). Anticancer Res 8:1104–1105.

Breukel C, Tops CMJ, Meera Khan P (1989): Four base deletion polymorphism at D5S71 (probe C11p11) linked to familial adenomatous polyposis (FAP). Submitted for publication.

Bussey HJR (1975): Familial Polyposis Coli. Baltimore: Johns Hopkins University Press.

Gusella JF (1986): DNA polymorphism and human disease. Annu Rev Biochem 55:831–854.

Herrera L, Kakati S, Gibas L, Pietrzak E, Sandberg AA (1986): Gardner syndrome in a man with an interstitial deletion of 5q1. Am J Med Genet 25:473–476.

Ingall H. Mastromarino A (198e): Prevention of hereditary large bowl cancer. Progress in Clinical and Biological Research, Vol 115. New York: Alan R. Liss, Inc., pp 1–257.

Leppert M, Dobbs M, Scambler P, O'Connel P, Nakamura Y, Stauffer D, Woodward S, Burt R, Hughes J, Gardner E, Lathrop M, Wasmuth J, Lalouel M, White R (1987): The gene for familial polyposis coli maps to the long arm of chromosome 5. Science 238:1411–1413.

McKusick VA (1988): Mendelian Inheritance in Man, 8th ed. Baltimore: Johns Hopkins University Press.

Meera Khan P, Tops CMJ, vd Broek M, Breukel C, Wijnen JT, Oldenburg M, Box Jvd, van Leeuwen-Cornelisse ISJ, Vasen HFA, Griffioen, Verspaget HM, den Hertog Jagers FCA, Lamers CBHW (1988): Close linkage of a highly polymorphic marker (D5S37) to familial adenomatous polyposis (FAP) and confirmation of FAP localization on chromosome 5q21-q22. Hum Genet 79:183–185.

Nakamura Y, Lathrop M, Leppert M, Dobbs M, Wasmuth J, Wolff E, Carlson M, Fujimoto E, Krapcho K, Sears T, Woodward S, Hughes J, Burt R, Gardner E, Lalouel JM, White R (1988): Localization of the genetic defect in familial adenomatous polyposis within a small region of chromosome 5. Am J Hum Genet 43:638–644.

Ott J (1985): Analysis of Human Genetic Linkage. Baltimore: Johns Hopkins University Press.

Stewart GD, Bruns GAP, Wasmuth JJ, Kurnitt DM (1987): An anonymous DNA segment (Pi227) maps to the long arm of human chromosome 5 and identifies a BstXI polymorphism (D5S37). Nucleic Acids Res 15:3939.

Tops CMJ, Breukel C, vd Broek MH, Griffieon G, v Leewen ISJ, Vasen HFA, Wijnen JTh, Oldenburg M, vd Klift HM, Lamers CBHW, Meera Khan (1988): Preclinical prediction of familial adenomatous polyposis using the linked DNA marker Pi227. Anticancer Res 8:1103–1104.

Tops CMJ, Breukel C, Wijnen JTh, vd Klift HM, vd Broek MH, Oldenburg M, vd Bos J, v Leewen-Cornelisse ISJ, Vasen HFA, Griffieon G, Lamers CBHW, Meera Khan P (1989): Linkage relationships between APC, D5S37 (probe Pi227) and D5S71 (probe C11p11) in the Dutch polyposis families. Submitted to HGM10, New Haven, June 1989 (to be published in Cytogenet Cell Genet).

Index